MEDICINE FOR
EXAMINATIONS
A STREAMLINED APPROACH TO REVISION

KU-201-397

Gil

St 229 7383.

Chi 668 2413 D.D:

TFR 10 Hope Park Cres.
↑
wth no name !

R. J. Epstein graduated in medicine at the University of Sydney in 1978. In 1984 he was awarded the Sir Robert Menzies Memorial Scholarship to Cambridge University where he gained his PhD, and in 1987 was elected to Fellowship of the Royal Australasian College of Physicians. Currently he is a Lucille P. Markey Visiting Fellow at Harvard Medical School.

MEDICINE FOR
EXAMINATIONS
A STREAMLINED APPROACH TO REVISION

Second edition

R. J. Epstein MB PhD FRACP

CHURCHILL LIVINGSTONE
EDINBURGH LONDON MELBOURNE AND NEW YORK 1990

CHURCHILL LIVINGSTONE
Medical Division of Longman Group UK Limited

Distributed in the United States of America by
Churchill Livingstone Inc., 1560 Broadway, New York,
N.Y. 10036, and by associated companies, branches
and representatives throughout the world.

© Longman Group Limited 1985
© Longman Group UK Limited 1990

All rights reserved. No part of this publication may be
reproduced, stored in a retrieval system, or
transmitted in any form or by any means, electronic,
mechanical, photocopying, recording or otherwise,
without either the prior written permission of the
publishers (Churchill Livingstone, Robert Stevenson
House, 1–3 Baxter's Place, Leith Walk, Edinburgh EH1
3AF), or a licence permitting restricted copying in the
United Kingdom issued by the Copyright Licensing
Agency Ltd, 33–34 Alfred Place, London, WC1E 7DP.

First edition 1985
Second edition 1990

ISBN 0-443-04149-0

British Library Cataloguing in Publication Data
Epstein, R. J.
    Medicine for examinations. — 2nd ed.
    1. Medicine
    I. Title
    610

Produced by Longman Singapore Publishers (Pte) Ltd.
Printed in Singapore

Preface to the Second Edition

FIRST, PASS YOUR EXAM...

Many candidates approach medical examinations as gravely serious affairs. This is the wrong strategy. Medical exams are a sort of game and, as with all games, you make the most of them by ensuring you first know the rules. The catch is that the 'rules' of medical exams are largely unwritten. As a result, all too many candidates end up learning these rules only by going from one exam to the next — and that, plainly, isn't the most efficient approach. This second edition of *Medicine for Examinations* aims to transform the exam experience from one of academic 'musical chairs' to one which reflects the solid preparation undertaken by most candidates prior to the Big Day.

Since the last edition, it has remained sadly true that not even the most esoteric pearl of medical wisdom can be assumed 'unexaminable'. If you try flipping through any well-thumbed textbook in your medical library, however, you'll observe an interesting phenomenon: namely, that artistically-minded readers have taken the liberty of underlining discrete snippets of information. That so much is left unemphasized suggests that the important information is camouflaged within dense jungles of verbiage. How, then, can the prospective exam candidate overcome this handicap?

Certain subsets of information lend themselves to the exam format. You are more likely to be asked something which has a specific and topical answer, for instance, than something which is equivocal or passé. The second edition of *Medicine for Examinations* has been structured to take advantage of this bias, and several novel features have been created with this in mind. These include:

- A new chapter addressing common problems faced in the Short Case Viva
- A new chapter dealing with the approach to Long Cases
- A Long Case Format for organizing and streamlining case presentations
- Three new medical subject chapters (Pharmacology and toxicology, Psychiatry and Skin disease)
- Three new Physical Examination Protocols (Cranial nerves, Speech and higher centres, and Drug-addiction sequelae)

- Diagnostic Pathways: this feature has been added to demonstrate the mental strategies used in formulating a provisional diagnosis based on physical signs; the examples given are intended to be illustrative rather than definitive
- Fifteen Case Summaries (one for each chapter) outlining the commonest short cases to be encountered in each medical subspecialty
- Major new chapter subsections concerning topics such as ACE inhibitors, GnRH therapy, anti-idiotypic antibodies, liver transplantation, apolipoproteins, extracorporeal lithotripsy, non-tuberculous mycobacteria, genetic and nutritional disorders, HIV infection, magnetic resonance imaging, prostaglandins, Alzheimer's disease, blood gas analysis, fish oils, tumour staging, percutaneous angioplasty, atrial natriuretic factor, hormone replacement therapy, omeprazole, gut hormones, zoonoses, hypercoagulable states, urticaria, neurotransmitter abnormalities, amyloidosis, domiciliary oxygen therapy, megavoltage irradiation, passive smoking, thyroiditis, Barrett's oesophagus, antiphospholipid antibodies, chlamydial disease, acute mountain sickness, gut endocrine tumour syndromes, and many others
- A new Recommended Reading section suggesting techniques and sources for gleaning background information
- A thorough revision, expansion and updating of the entire text

Finally, a word on luck. It is true that luck plays a role in clinical examinations, and it is equally true that written examinations (particularly multiple-choice questions) can be ambiguously worded; in the overall scheme of things, however, the good candidate makes his/her own luck. Of course, there will be inevitable discrepancies between the results of comparable candidates in any single exam, but in the long run everything tends to even out. So don't be too down-hearted if events fail to go quite as ideally as you had hoped and, on the other hand, don't make the mistake of blaming Lady Luck when a little more preparation would have made the difference.

Instead, think positive — and pass.

Massachusetts, 1990   R. J. E.

Acknowledgements

Many of the improvements in this second edition of *Medicine for Examinations* have been contributed by readers and colleagues, and I would like to make special mention of the expert assistance rendered by Stewart Coltart, Sally Morgan, Graeme Howard and Neil McGill. Any inadvertent inaccuracies or oversimplifications, on the other hand, remain entirely my own doing, and I would be most grateful to any reader taking the trouble to bring such points of contention to my notice. Finally, I would like to thank Anne Epstein for her indispensable help throughout the five years spent revising this edition of *Medicine for Examinations*.

All efforts have been made to check the accuracy of drug dosages and scheduling in this book. It is recommended, however, that physicians consult the most recent manufacturer's guidelines prior to prescribing any medications mentioned herein.

Contents

The Short Cases

EVERYTHING YOU ALWAYS WANTED TO KNOW ABOUT THE SHORT CASE VIVA BUT WERE TOO SCARED TO ASK

Q: *Should I take beta-blockers before my viva?*

A: Inevitably, there will be some people who regard even the mention of beta-blockers as a tacit advocation of pill-popping, analogous to the illicit abuse of anabolic steroids by Olympic athletes. Let me make it clear from the outset, then, that *most* prospective clinical exam candidates will find the best preventative for disabling exam nerves to be plain hard work — practice, practice, and more practice.

Yet the fact remains that beta-blockers *are* used, and used by an increasing variety of people with the not-uncommon affliction of incapacitating stage fright. Understandably, many irrepressibly 'adrenergic' exam candidates have come to regard beta-blockers as a godsend. After all, if you find that every time you present a case you leave puddles of perspiration on the floor, your voice dries up, and your palpitations set the walls shaking, then you really can't be blamed for at least *thinking* about using a beta-blocker.

If the decision is made to try beta-blockers, several caveats apply. First, they should be prescribed in the ordinary way by your own physician (*not* yourself) in accordance with all the usual precautions and contraindications; don't simply filch them from the drug trolley on the ward. Second, you must *try* them (in precisely the same dosage that you plan to use) in a comparable situation *before* your exam — and preferably on several occasions. The horror stories you have heard about the candidate who became so hypotensive that she had to lie down on the floor during the viva, or about the one who had his first experience of acute asthma in the middle of the oral, are probably true. Do not, whatever you do, use benzodiazepines, alcohol or cannabis to calm your nerves; apart from anything else, remember that such drugs induce amnesia and obtundation.

Q: *What instruments do I need to carry into the exam?*

A: You should carry into the exam the same instruments that you've carried into all your previous practice cases; only in this way will you become familiar with your instruments and, more importantly, with your routines for using them. For if there's one situation where your well-practised routines are going to break down, it will be under the duress of an exam — and especially if your attention is distracted by the workings of an unfamiliar ophthalmoscope, causing you to forget to do something which would otherwise have won you lots of brownie points.

Most people will normally carry a watch (with a second hand) and a key (for plantar reflexes), while other items which could be secreted within your white coat include:

Stethoscope
Pen-light torch (with fresh batteries)
Tongue depressors
Red-topped hat pin
Cotton wool
Short ruler (6"/15 cm) or tape measure
Pocket visual acuity chart (read at 24"/60 cm)
Pen(s) and paper
Extra items which could be carried in a bag include:
Tendon reflex hammer
Ophthalmoscope
Tuning fork
Magnifying glass (for skin lesions)

There is no need to get carried away with your armamentarium, of course; no amount of instruments will compensate for lack of skill in using them. It is not necessary, for example, to invest in a massive (and expensive) stethoscope if you are happy you can hear the low-pitched rumbling diastolic murmur of mitral stenosis with your current model; proper positioning of the patient, and the experience to know what to listen for, are more important than the acoustics of your tubes. Nor is it mandatory to carry a white-topped pin for testing peripheral vision, or separate tuning forks for vibration and auditory testing (128 cps and 256/512 cps respectively). You won't be penalized if you can't afford your own ophthalmoscope, but it doesn't hurt if you have got one — the big advantage is that you are used to using it. Don't bother carrying your own auriscope, thermometer or blood pressure cuff; even in a long case, any diagnostic items not present can usually be requested from an attendant. Inevitably, some

1

long-case candidates will feel more secure in bringing along their own repertoire of diagnostic aids, including (in addition to the above):

Mydriatic drops

Urinalysis strips (plus MSU container)

Haemoccult tablets (glove, gauze, lubricant)

Schirmer's test papers

If you are expecting a neurological examination (speech or higher centres), it is also impressive to come prepared with the following:

Written orders, e.g. 'Stick out your tongue', 'Point to a chair'.

Card to read aloud, e.g. 'The war broke out last December'.

Illustrations, e.g. the Queen, Donald Duck, map of England.

Paper and pen for writing, drawing clockface, five-pointed star, etc.

But above all, irrespective of whether or not you carry your own instruments, do not neglect to mention that you would like to take the temperature and blood pressure, look at the fundi, test sensation, do a pelvic examination, urinalysis, etc.

Q: *How do I actually go about impressing the examiners on the day?*

A: Most of the books written about medical exams tell you to keep your fingernails clean, do not wear a low-cut dress (particularly if you are male), etc. More constructive advice, however, will depend on what sort of qualification you are in the market for. If you are sitting for medical school finals, the examiners will be (or at least should be) trying their hardest to pass you. They will expect only that your performance confirms:

Your knowledge is sound

Your demeanour is sensible

Your approach is safe

That is, they want to see that you have bothered to spend at least *some* time in the wards, and that you are not a Martian or some sort of lunatic.

If, on the other hand, you are sniffing around for a postgraduate qualification, then your examiners will predictably be more discerning — it's not only Martians and lunatics who find themselves poorly regarded in this setting. The successful candidate will certainly need to appear knowledgeable and sensible, but will also need to exude an aura of sufficient experience and maturity that their examiners would sleep happily at night if that candidate was looking after their patients. If you find this point difficult to grasp, try getting somebody to videotape you presenting a case; it may prove a constructive exercise in self-criticism.

Apart from these considerations, the best advice is still to be found in the old chestnuts which have been trotted out to prospective examinees for decades:

1 *More is missed by not looking than not knowing* (Riordan's corollary: if you don't put your finger in it, you put your foot in it.) The reassurance you can draw from this is that motivation and hard work are more important than talent, flair or genius — in medical exams, that is, though not necessarily in

other activities. Luck, as Pasteur once mumbled, favours the prepared mind. If you are given an ambiguous introduction to a short case (such as, 'Examine this man's chest'), err on the side of being too thorough — that is, go for the *systematic* approach wherever possible. At worst you'll get a growling reprimand (EXAMINER: 'I told you to examine his **chest**, didn't I, not his frigging hands!') which will make the instruction immediately clear.

Having said this, you should also try to get to the 'guts' of any one case in reasonable time, minimizing the time spent on parts of the examination which seem destined to be non-contributory. For example, if on examining a patient's legs you demonstrate fasciculations, wasting, brisk reflexes and extensor plantar responses, you are not automatically obliged to proceed to pin-sticking and cottonwool dabbing. Instead, don't be afraid to suggest to your examiners that you would now like to tap out the reflexes in the upper limbs and jaw, and to examine the bulbar musculature. After all, even if you *are* directed to persevere with the sensory examination, you will have at least given impressive evidence that you're capable of thinking on your feet.

2 *Common things are common* — even, it must be said, in medical exams. Don't speculate that the fundal haemorrhages might be due to hyperviscosity unless you have actively excluded diabetes, hypertension and suchlike first. Of course, the paradoxical (and somewhat ridiculous) aspect of short case vivas is that *certain* uncommon things appear relatively commonly, e.g. Argyll-Robertson pupils, motor neurone disease, pretibial myxoedema, Eisenmenger's syndrome, etc. Everyone is quick to admit that such conditions are rare in day-to-day clinical practice; but, oh boy, if there's one available at the time of the exam, you can be sure it will be included.

3 *Take your time,* especially at the beginning of each case. Show concern for the patient — this needs to be done as theatrically as any other aspect of the physical examination. Introduce yourself by name, shake hands, ask permission to examine them, help them get undressed and in position. Do not, whatever you do, treat the patient like a piece of meat. When exposing the area to be examined, for instance, at least pay lip service to their modesty by enquiring whether they are warm enough; while if you inadvertently happen to distress the patient during the performance (sorry, examination), be sure to display sufficient remorse to ensure that the examiners cannot accuse you of inhumane behaviour. Internalized anguish may win you a place in heaven, but it sure as hell won't help you through a short case viva.

When you have finished your examination and have been asked for your findings, *think before you speak*. A candidate who is seen to think before speaking will be regarded as thoughtful and safe, while one who speaks before thinking may come across as immature and foolhardy. If you are asked anything by the examiner, listen closely and answer the question — sounds simple, doesn't it? It is certainly a lot simpler if you get into the habit of making a conscious effort to think while you are examining. To do this well requires lots of practice; nonetheless, if you start describing your findings without *any* idea of how they fit together, you'll be unlikely to impress. Don't underestimate the value of information gleaned from the end of the bed — if you can see immediately that you are being asked to examine a patient with ascites, or exophthalmos, or hemiparesis, or a mastectomy, it makes life a lot easier. Indeed, the 'Diagnostic Pathways' in this book have been created specifically to illustrate how the recognition of an obvious physical sign such as this may serve as the focus around which a diagnostic pattern can be formed.

4 *Only state 'barn-door' clinical signs in the first instance* (i.e. avoid indecisive references to 'early clubbing', 'slight papilloedema', etc.). If the patient really does have cerebral metastases from a lung carcinoma, the examiners will generally re-direct your attention to the equivocal signs, e.g.:

EXAMINER: Did you ... ah ... think he was clubbed?

CANDIDATE: Sir, to be honest I *did* rather wonder whether he was clubbed — but the nailfold angle seemed relatively normal and there was less nailbed fluctuation than I would have expected ...

EXAMINER: I see. And, er, the fundi, you thought they were ... ah ...

CANDIDATE: Well, sir, I couldn't see any venous pulsations and the disc margins were somewhat indistinct, so I'd like to ... er ... examine for enlargement of the blind spot since this would ... ah ... be consistent with papilloedema.

EXAMINER (sighing): Mmmm, that won't be necessary. Perhaps you might like to take a look at this next patient's abdomen instead ...

If you can rationally justify your uncertainty, it is difficult for an examiner to penalize you too severely; whereas if you claim abnormalities which aren't there, you'll end up talking yourself into a corner from which there is no escape. In the event that you realize you have made an error, at least be decisive in admitting it — if you can rechannel the conversation quickly enough, the damage may be minimal.

Avoid mix-and-matching signs and 'cliché' jargon. If you think a patient with all the signs of pure aortic stenosis has a somewhat 'tapping' quality to his apex beat — irrespective of how beautifully the term may seem to describe this particular patient's sign — don't say so. Similarly, don't refer to the malar flush of a patient with a valvotomy scar as a 'butterfly rash', the high-stepping gait of a patient with footdrop as 'stamping', or the rusty sputum of a patient with pneumonia as 'anchovy sauce'. By the same token, of course, not all patients with hypopituitarism have 'alabaster' skin, just as not all acromegalics have bitemporal hemianopia — so don't get too tendentious.

You should also eschew the use of sloppy language, such as brand names (e.g. Lasix for frusemide, Tagamet for cimetidine) or abbreviations:

EXAMINER: All right then, how could your findings help explain this gentleman's symptoms?

CANDIDATE: Sir, I believe this man's neurological symptoms are due to MS, his lethargy to MF, his indigestion to his HSV, and his backache to PID.

The examiner may be less than impressed if he misinterprets your 'multiple sclerosis' acronym as 'mitral stenosis', your 'myelofibrosis' as 'mycosis fungoides', your 'highly selective vagotomy' as 'herpes simplex virus', and your 'prolapsed intervertebral disc' as 'pelvic inflammatory disease'!

5 *The greatest fool may ask questions which the wisest man can't answer* (it is best to avoid quoting this one during the interrogation). Don't get all defensive and uptight if you are completely ignorant about something; just say so, and get on to something else. You can be sure that there are plenty of things your examiners don't know either — some are notorious for saying things like, 'No, I don't know that either' after asking you something weird. Just don't waffle; instead, disarm them with candour. If the examiner persists in asking you 'difficult' questions, it could mean: (a) you are doing brilliantly, and they are simply trying to stretch your talents to the limit; (b) you have completely misunderstood the line of questioning and they are desperately trying to redirect you; or (c) you are stuck with a rotten examiner who wants to play the 'guess-what-I'm-thinking-of' game (they do exist) and who justifies such torture by alluding to the stresses of clinical practice. A reasonable ploy if you are in this fix is to ask for the question to be rephrased (rather than irritating them by demanding that it be 'repeated'), giving you a few more seconds to think and putting the onus on them to clarify what they are getting at. Alternatively, you can nod vigorously before temporizing with an equivocal response, such as:

CANDIDATE: Yes, that's a very difficult issue, isn't it, and I think there are a number of factors which need to be taken into consideration. On the one hand ...

Just don't cave in and moan, 'I don't understand', or they will be sure to take you for a ninny. On no account betray any sign of agitation throughout the ordeal; rather, concentrate on impressing the examiners with your professional imperturbability (as distinct, of course, from aloofness or overconfidence). Never give up, no matter how badly you feel things are going. Exams are too traumatic to be used simply as a tutorial for a repeat performance.

6 *It's all show biz.* The short case viva isn't a showcase for shrinking violets or wallflowers, it's a chance to be the centre of attention (if not quite famous) for 15 minutes. And that is a chance which you need to grasp with both hands. Exaggerate things a little bit, don't be shy. You are not there just to elicit physical signs, but also to be *seen* eliciting them — not unlike a magician is seen to pull a rabbit from a hat. If the liver is enlarged, or the jugular venous pulse elevated, don't just leave it at that: take out your ruler and (hey presto) measure the abnormality. If you are demonstrating a straightforward neurological deficit, do so with as much flair as you can muster, perhaps just short of declaring 'Voilà!'. If, after completing the examination requested, you are

asked if there is anything else you would like to look at, this is your cue to spring into action:

CANDIDATE: Sir, I would also like to examine the lungfields for basal crepitations, feel for sacral and peripheral oedema, check for ascites and hepatic distension, look for calf tenderness, take the temperature and blood pressure, examine the fundi, and perform a urinalysis.

When asked to present your findings, don't be coy if you are fairly sure you have twigged to the diagnosis: instead, try bowling them over at the outset with something solid like:

CANDIDATE: Sir, this patient has physical signs consistent with aortic stenosis of moderate severity. On general inspection . . .

On the other hand, if you are unsure of the diagnosis, limit yourself to describing the signs; volunteer a differential diagnosis (with all the attendant pros and cons of each one) only when asked. Use non-eponymous signs to describe your findings in the first instance, rather than insisting on baffling your examiners with biographical irrelevancies.

In summary:
BE CALM
BE PREPARED
BE THOROUGH
BE THEATRICAL
BE DECISIVE
THINK BEFORE SPEAKING

The Long Case

APPROACH TO THE LONG CASE

1 Your priority in the long case is to *keep the examiners entertained.* This requirement does not feature on the scorecard, of course, and may sound surprising to the paranoid candidate who instinctively feels that the examiners are hell-bent on finding an excuse to fail him/her. No, one of the better-kept secrets of the clinical examination system is that more often the *main* concern of the examiner is to resist nodding off during the case presentation. This is understandable when you realize that the examiner may be worried about his overdraft, behind schedule with his clinical research, due to deliver a lecture on an unrehearsed topic in three-quarters of an hour, and — most critically — partially mesmerized from having just sat through three soporific presentations of the same case that you are now about to describe.

How, then, does one go about entertaining one's examiners? The prerequisite is to make sure that the examiner does the minimal amount of *work.* In practice this means that you do the talking, that you ensure there are no embarrassing gaps in the monologue during which they have actively to compose a question for you, and that you refrain from exasperating them by talking stuff and nonsense.

Like nature itself, long case examiners abhor vacuums. The most ominous sign of a long case spiralling downward into oblivion is the protracted silence. Do not let things degenerate into a monosyllabic question-and-answer session. Show off your knowledge. Express concern for all possible aspects of your patient's plight — do not just mumble abstractly as if discussing a crossword puzzle. Explore every nuance of every problem. Prove to the examiners that you have experience, sensitivity, integrity, judgement; in short, sell yourself. By the time you have finished saying everything you have planned, the case should be all but over and the examiners too overwhelmed to fight back — and you may well be surprised to find that you have done your last-ever long case presentation. Just when it was (almost) getting to be fun, too.

2 *Success in the long case begins with a successful encounter with the patient.* People will give you all sorts of home-grown advice about how long to spend on the various sections of the case, but it clearly has to be *about* 20 minutes each for history, examination and writing up alike. Don't be concerned if you find yourself prompted to ask more historical details by the results of physical examination, or if when writing up you suddenly remember to examine something extra: real-life medicine is an organic process, not a stereotyped protocol. On the other hand, if you find yourself in the lion's den (i.e. being examined) and realized that you have irretrievably missed doing something which is critical to the case, then it may be best to make a clean breast of it rather than hoping to get off scot free — if you are lucky you may get to re-examine the patient.

Finally, don't forget to ask the patient the time-honoured 'long case' questions at the end (yes, the end) of the interview; after all, many of your less scrupulous colleagues will do exactly this, and it is obviously not in the public interest for you to concede any advantage to such degenerates. So, since you are morally obliged to do so, ask:

a) What do the doctors say is wrong with you?
b) What part of the body were the examiners most interested to examine when they visited you this morning?
c) What investigations or treatments are planned for you in the immediate future?
d) Is there anything else you think I should know?

In the event that the patient is under the misapprehension that they are not meant to give you such information, simply clarify for them that such precautions only apply to the candidates who come after you!

3 During the actual presentation of the long case, it is important to *show off* in the correct manner: one must, it seems, show off confidently but humbly. This means managing to communicate every iota of knowledge and clinical skill while at the same time avoiding any hint of smugness or complacency. If you have personally managed to see 23 cases similar to the one you are presenting, let your experience show. If you are familiar with the clinical research background relevant to the problem under discussion, use that knowledge to add authority and pizzazz to your conclusions; the 'Reviewing the Literature' sections in this book are designed for this purpose.

Keep in mind that what you are really seeking is approval, approval to be admitted into the exclusive club currently patronized by your examiners. Provided that you have got the case itself pretty well sorted out, don't be afraid to add a judicious pinch of charm and/or humour to your presentation, suitably peppered as it will need to be with deference and tact.

4 The eruption of an all-out, no-holds-barred argument with any examiner is obviously a dire prognostic indicator, but *a mature degree of self-assertion is a plus.* If challenged over some finding (or lack thereof) simply be honest: if you were a little dubious about it, say so, while if you were solidly convinced then stand your ground. Don't, in your paranoia, assume that the examiner will try to mislead you, but be prepared to have the strength of your conviction tested. If you have just claimed that a cardiac valve lesion is haemodynamically severe, be prepared to argue this from clinical facts rather than gut feeling. The biggest mistake is to assert something which you cannot substantiate — particularly if it is wrong.

5 *Don't be put off if the diagnosis doesn't appear clear-cut.* After all, even the consultant managing the case may not have worked things out, and the last thing he wants to hear is some young whippersnapper saying it's a cut-and-dried example of, say, mulibrey nanism or Gilles de la Tourette syndrome. If the definitive diagnosis is obscure, begin by giving a 'first-phase' diagnosis ('lower motor neurone lesion'), advancing then to the second phase ('involving lumbosacral nerve roots') and finally to a third-phase differential diagnosis ('polio', 'motor neurone disease', etc.) which may be clarified by relevant investigations. Rest assured that numerous clues (inadvertent or otherwise) can be given away by the examiners' subsequent questions. You should never be stuck for a differential diagnosis; have a mental list of generic causes ('tumour, trauma, infection, infarction . . .') which you can conjure up even when the cerebral computer has gone down in the heat of battle.

Never underestimate your ability to answer a question in the absence of specific knowledge. You may find yourself asked, for instance:

EXAMINER (smiling): Tell me then, what proportion of patients with this condition would you expect to have an elevated serum rhubarb?

to which you could answer,

CANDIDATE: I . . . I . . . (gulp) . . . don't know, sir.

[which would prompt the following reply:

EXAMINER (licking his lips): Ah. I see.]

or, alternatively, you could answer,

CANDIDATE: I believe it's around 10%, sir, if I recall correctly.

[which would prompt the reply:

EXAMINER (scowling): Hmm, I think you might find it's closer to 19% if you check on it. All right then, what about . . .]

Similarly, you could be asked about a drug you have never actually prescribed yourself, and your memory regarding its effects may need jogging:

EXAMINER: What do you know of the toxicity of amiodarone, then?

CANDIDATE: Ah yes, amiodarone. Well, sir, it can cause skin rashes in some individuals, nausea in others, at times vomiting, occasional diarrhoea . . .

EXAMINER: Yes, yes . . . what about . . . do you know of any . . . ah . . . *endocrinological* side-effects, by any chance?

Remember that even if one of the examiners insists in proving he knows more than you do about Binswanger's disease, say, or congenital hepatic fibrosis, there is at least one other examiner available to prevent undue emphasis being placed on such fringe knowledge. Don't let yourself be floored — by anything.

Have the justification(s) for any recommended investigation at the ready, including those that you know are often ordered 'routinely' (i.e. without thinking) in ordinary hospital practice. Furthermore, when presenting (say) a jaundiced patient, start by recommending the most conservative, non-invasive and inexpensive investigations (e.g. urinalysis, liver function tests) rather than the more definitive (ERCP, percutaneous cholangiogram). Simply imagine what you would do in real life, why you would do it, and the order in which you would do it; wisdom born of experience is undoubtedly the most impressive persona to create in a clinical viva.

In summary:
KEEP TALKING
SHOW OFF
SOUND AUTHORITATIVE
SELL YOURSELF
AVOID BEING OBNOXIOUS

PRESENTING THE LONG CASE: A FORMAT FOR EXAM CANDIDATES

One of the most time-honoured ways of frittering away precious minutes during preparation of a long case is to enter the patient's room armed only with blank sheets of paper. This means that you have automatically lost several minutes in having to write headings all the way through, such as 'allergies', 'pulse rate', 'main problems', 'prognosis', or whatever; moreover, you are constantly having to fret about whether you are doing everything in the conventional order, and whether you might not inadvertently be omitting a key finding.

This is not the way you would run things if you were trying to develop, say, an efficient private practice. It would make far more sense to have your own format for new case presentations already formulated and printed out, leaving you only with the task of information-gathering. This has the additional advantage of systematizing your approach to the case despite the pressures of the moment. Since there is no reason at all why such an approach shouldn't be used routinely in day-to-day clinical practice, there seems little theoretical objection to its use in a long case examination viva.

In the next few pages you will find an example of such a long case format. You may find that your own particular style is better suited to a custom-made version — in which case, write it up!

LONG CASE PROTOCOL: I HISTORY

EXAMINER: Hello there, I'm Professor Smith and this is Dr Jones— would you like to tell us about the patient you've just seen ?

CANDIDATE: Certainly, sir. I saw _____ who is a

NAME

_____ admitted to hospital _____

AGE   SEX   NATIONALITY   OCCUPATION   WHEN?

because of/for investigation of _____ . (S)he had been

PRESENTING SYMPTOM(S)

completely well until _____ when he developed

WHEN WERE THE VERY FIRST SYMPTOMS?

_____ He then/Since that time _____ (now go into

INITIAL SUSPICIOUS SYMPTOMS

(ENORMOUS DETAIL) _____

EXACT SEQUENCE OF EVENTS;   DURATION AND PERIODICITY OF SYMPTOMS;

_____

NATURE AND SEVERITY;   LOCATION AND RADIATION OF PAIN;   EXACERBATING AND RELIEVING FACTORS;

_____

RESPONSE TO PREVIOUS TREATMENT;   RESULTS OF PREVIOUS INVESTIGATIONS;

_____

HOW HAS THE DISEASE BEEN MONITORED?   ASSOCIATED FEATURES

_____

His main problem(s) in coping with this disease is/are _____

PAIN;

_____

DAY-TO-DAY INCAPACITY;   INABILITY TO WORK;   SOCIAL HANDICAP;

_____

SEXUAL PROBLEMS;   EFFECT ON FAMILY;   SUFFERING AND DEMORALIZATION

_____

His doctors have recently told him that he has _____

DIAGNOSIS IF KNOWN

and that the outlook is _____

PROGNOSIS IF KNOWN

Currently he remains in hospital because of _____

ONGOING MANAGEMENT;

_____

PLANNED INVESTIGATIONS   DISEASE COMPLICATIONS

Checklist:

short of breath
chest pain
palpitations
dizziness
orthopnoea
nocturnal dyspnoea
claudication
syncope
fatigue

wheeze
stridor
cough
sputum
haemoptysis
pleurisy
sweats

dysphagia
nausea
vomiting
diarrhoea
constipation
weight loss
heartburn
abdominal pain
jaundice
haematemesis
melaena
rectal bleeding

headache
photophobia
blurred vision
loss of vision
vertigo
deafness
funny turns
unconsciousness
paraesthesiae
numbness
weakness
paralysis
difficulty walking
dysarthria
dysphasia

haematuria
nocturia
dysuria
oliguria
polyuria
polydipsia
loin pain
pruritus
incontinence

skin rash
joint pain/
swelling

DIRECT QUESTIONS
RELATING TO
SYSTEM(S) INVOLVED
IN PRESENT ILLNESS
(positives and significant
negatives only)

DIRECT QUESTIONS
RELATING TO OTHER
SYSTEMS
(significant positives
and negatives only)

PAST MEDICAL
HISTORY

PREVIOUS OPERATIONS
AND BLOOD TRANSFUSIONS

DAILY LIFESTYLE
Past smoking
Current smoking
Past alcohol
Current alcohol
Analgesics
Laxatives
Oral contraceptives
Illicit drug use

OCCUPATIONAL
HISTORY

ACTIVITIES OF
DAILY LIVING
Functional capacity
Handicaps
Aids

MISCELLANEOUS
Allergies
Pets; animal contact
Recent travel
Diet
Menstrual/sexual
history (if relevant)

CURRENT MEDICATIONS
AND OTHER TREATMENT
Vitamins
Radiotherapy
Physiotherapy

FAMILY HISTORY

SOCIAL HISTORY

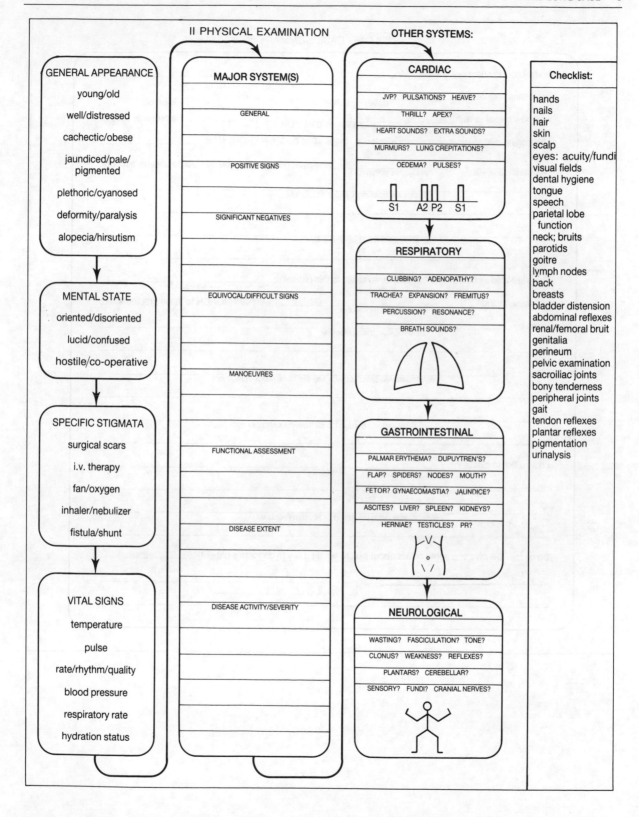

II PHYSICAL EXAMINATION

GENERAL APPEARANCE
young/old

well/distressed

cachectic/obese

jaundiced/pale/pigmented

plethoric/cyanosed

deformity/paralysis

alopecia/hirsutism

MENTAL STATE
oriented/disoriented

lucid/confused

hostile/co-operative

SPECIFIC STIGMATA
surgical scars

i.v. therapy

fan/oxygen

inhaler/nebulizer

fistula/shunt

VITAL SIGNS
temperature

pulse

rate/rhythm/quality

blood pressure

respiratory rate

hydration status

MAJOR SYSTEM(S)
GENERAL

POSITIVE SIGNS

SIGNIFICANT NEGATIVES

EQUIVOCAL/DIFFICULT SIGNS

MANOEUVRES

FUNCTIONAL ASSESSMENT

DISEASE EXTENT

DISEASE ACTIVITY/SEVERITY

OTHER SYSTEMS:

CARDIAC
JVP? PULSATIONS? HEAVE?

THRILL? APEX?

HEART SOUNDS? EXTRA SOUNDS?

MURMURS? LUNG CREPITATIONS?

OEDEMA? PULSES?

S1   A2 P2   S1

RESPIRATORY
CLUBBING? ADENOPATHY?

TRACHEA? EXPANSION? FREMITUS?

PERCUSSION? RESONANCE?

BREATH SOUNDS?

GASTROINTESTINAL
PALMAR ERYTHEMA? DUPUYTREN'S?

FLAP? SPIDERS? NODES? MOUTH?

FETOR? GYNAECOMASTIA? JAUNDICE?

ASCITES? LIVER? SPLEEN? KIDNEYS?

HERNIAE? TESTICLES? PR?

NEUROLOGICAL
WASTING? FASCICULATION? TONE?

CLONUS? WEAKNESS? REFLEXES?

PLANTARS? CEREBELLAR?

SENSORY? FUNDI? CRANIAL NERVES?

Checklist:
hands
nails
hair
skin
scalp
eyes: acuity/fundi
visual fields
dental hygiene
tongue
speech
parietal lobe
  function
neck; bruits
parotids
goitre
lymph nodes
back
breasts
bladder distension
abdominal reflexes
renal/femoral bruit
genitalia
perineum
pelvic examination
sacroiliac joints
bony tenderness
peripheral joints
gait
tendon reflexes
plantar reflexes
pigmentation
urinalysis

III LONG CASE SUMMARY

CANDIDATE: In summary, then, Mr/Mrs_____ is a very

NAME

interesting patient with a _____ history of _____

DURATION OF SYMPTOMS   SYMPTOMS

who now presents with_____ . He presents several

MAJOR SYMPTOMS AND SIGNS

challenging diagnostic/management problems. I believe that his MAIN PROBLEM is_____

SYMPTOM(S)?

_____. However, his case does present some unusual aspects:

PROVISIONAL DIAGNOSIS?   DIFFERENTIAL DIAGNOSIS?

_____

PROS AND CONS OF POSSIBLE DIAGNOSES

_____

_____

STRATEGIES FOR CLARIFYING DIAGNOSIS

_____

There are also a number of other problems related to this patient's_____,

MAIN PROBLEM

and these include _____ MY APPROACH to these problems is to

RELATED PROBLEMS

begin by _____

APPROACH TO MAIN PROBLEM;

_____

_____

INVESTIGATIONAL SEQUENCE (NON-INVASIVE FIRST) AND JUSTIFICATION;

_____

_____

MANAGEMENT STRATEGY (CONSERVATIVE MEASURES FIRST)

_____

I'd also like to discuss_____

APPROACH TO RELATED PROBLEMS

_____

_____

INVESTIGATION AND MANAGEMENT OF RELATED PROBLEMS

_____

So let me now give you some details about exactly what I'd like to do for this patient _____

_____

_____

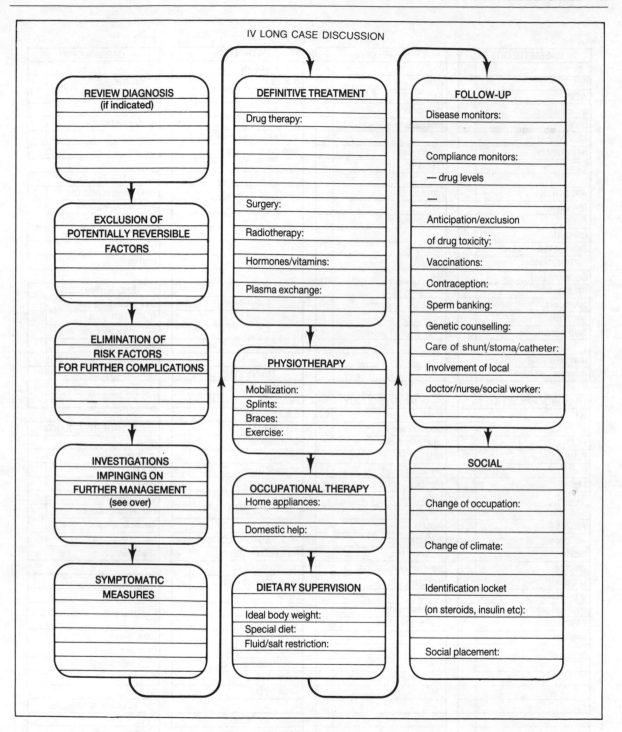

IV LONG CASE DISCUSSION

REVIEW DIAGNOSIS
(if indicated)

EXCLUSION OF POTENTIALLY REVERSIBLE FACTORS

ELIMINATION OF RISK FACTORS FOR FURTHER COMPLICATIONS

INVESTIGATIONS IMPINGING ON FURTHER MANAGEMENT
(see over)

SYMPTOMATIC MEASURES

DEFINITIVE TREATMENT

Drug therapy:

Surgery:

Radiotherapy:

Hormones/vitamins:

Plasma exchange:

PHYSIOTHERAPY

Mobilization:
Splints:
Braces:
Exercise:

OCCUPATIONAL THERAPY
Home appliances:

Domestic help:

DIETARY SUPERVISION

Ideal body weight:
Special diet:
Fluid/salt restriction:

FOLLOW-UP

Disease monitors:

Compliance monitors:
— drug levels
—

Anticipation/exclusion
of drug toxicity:

Vaccinations:

Contraception:

Sperm banking:

Genetic counselling:

Care of shunt/stoma/catheter:

Involvement of local
doctor/nurse/social worker:

SOCIAL

Change of occupation:

Change of climate:

Identification locket
(on steroids, insulin etc):

Social placement:

V LONG CASE INVESTIGATIONS

HAEMATOLOGY	
Hb	
film	
WCC	
differential	
platelets	
MCV/MCHC	
reticulocytes	
ESR	
PT	
APTT/PTTK	
fibrinogen	
FDPs	
folate/B_{12}	
Schilling test	
Fe/TIBC/ferritin	
Coombs' test	
haptoglobin	
NAP score	
lysozyme	
cold agglutinins	
marrow aspiration	
marrow trephine	

BIOCHEMISTRY	
Na^+	
K^+	
HCO_3^-	
BUN, S.Cr.	
Ca^{2+}	
Mg^{2+}	
albumin	
bilirubin	
AST/ALT	
alk. phos.	
GGT	
glucose	
uric acid	
cholesterol	
triglycerides	
CPK (-MB)	
amylase	
LDH	

RADIOLOGY	
CXR	
AXR	
SXR	
XR (specify)	
skeletal survey	
IVP	
myelogram	
CT scan:	
( )	
ultrasound:	
( )	
nuclear scan:	
( )	
angiogram:	
( )	
MRI	

MICROBIOLOGY	
MSU	
blood culture	
sputum culture	
AFB	
viral titres	
Mantoux	
VDRL, FTA	
HIV Ab	
HBsAg	
ASO titre	
thick/thin film	
darkfield examination	
Indian ink	
stool examination	
CSF examination	

PATHOLOGY	
review sections	
biopsy:	
( )	
cytology:	
( )	
immunofluorescence	
electron microscopy	

URINE STUDIES	
urinalysis	
microscopy	
culture sensitivity	
osmolality	
24-h calcium	
24-h urate	
serum iPTH	

IMMUNOLOGY	
ANA, dsDNA Ab	
rheumatoid factor	
lupus anticoagulant	
C_3 C_4	
EPG/IEPG	
Ig levels	
urinary BJP	
smooth muscle Ab	
antimitochondrial Ab	
cryoglobulins	
tissue typing	

EYE	
slit lamp examination	
fluorescein angiography	

CARDIOLOGY	
ECG	
echocardiography	
stress test	
ejection fraction	
cardiac catheter	
nuclear scan:	
( )	

NEUROLOGY	
EMG/nerve conduction	
muscle/nerve biopsy	
CSF studies	
EEG/evoked responses	
porphyrins	
lead level	

ENDOCRINOLOGY	
GTT	
fT_4/fT_3/TSH	
ACTH/urinary cortisol	
pituitary function tests:	
└TRH/GnRH/Arg/Synacthen	
hypothalamic function tests	

GASTROENTEROLOGY	
gastroscopy	
colonoscopy	
ERCP	
liver biopsy	
hepatitis serology	
oral cholecystogram	
i.v. cholangiogram	
fasting serum gastrin	
breath test(s)	

RESPIRATORY	
FEV_1/VC	
PEFR	
DL_{CO}	
blood gases	
bronchoscopy	
diagnostic lavage	
lung biopsy	

TUMOUR MARKERS	
AFP; βHCG	
paraprotein level	
CEA	
acid phosphatase	
thyroglobulin	
5HIAA, catecholamines	

VI SHORT CASE/LONG CASE SCORESHEET

SHORT CASES	unsatisfactory	borderline	good
APPROACH TO THE PATIENT			
WAS THE EXAMINATION TECHNICALLY SMOOTH ?			
WAS THE EXAMINATION SYSTEMATIC AND THOROUGH ?			
ACCURACY OF FINDINGS			
INTERPRETATION OF FINDINGS			

LONG CASE	unsatisfactory	borderline	good
HISTORY			
PHYSICAL FINDINGS			
INVESTIGATIONS			
MANAGEMENT			
CONCLUSIONS			

OVERALL ASSESSMENT: medical school finals (e.g. final MB) { This candidate is clinically safe to work under supervision } TRUE (pass) ☐ FALSE (fail) ☐

OVERALL ASSESSMENT: postgraduate internal medicine diploma (e.g.MRCP) { This candidate is clinically safe to work without supervision } TRUE (pass) ☐ FALSE (fail) ☐

Medicine for Examinations

CHAPTER 1

Cancer medicine

Physical examination protocol 1.1 You are asked to assess the current clinical status of a patient who has been receiving treatment for malignant disease

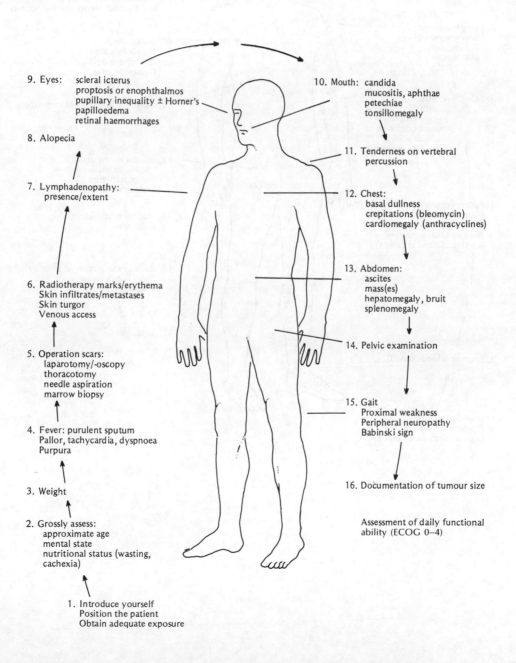

9. Eyes: scleral icterus
   proptosis or enophthalmos
   pupillary inequality ± Horner's
   papilloedema
   retinal haemorrhages

8. Alopecia

7. Lymphadenopathy:
   presence/extent

6. Radiotherapy marks/erythema
   Skin infiltrates/metastases
   Skin turgor
   Venous access

5. Operation scars:
   laparotomy/-oscopy
   thoracotomy
   needle aspiration
   marrow biopsy

4. Fever: purulent sputum
   Pallor, tachycardia, dyspnoea
   Purpura

3. Weight

2. Grossly assess:
   approximate age
   mental state
   nutritional status (wasting,
   cachexia)

1. Introduce yourself
   Position the patient
   Obtain adequate exposure

10. Mouth: candida
    mucositis, aphthae
    petechiae
    tonsillomegaly

11. Tenderness on vertebral
    percussion

12. Chest:
    basal dullness
    crepitations (bleomycin)
    cardiomegaly (anthracyclines)

13. Abdomen:
    ascites
    mass(es)
    hepatomegaly, bruit
    splenomegaly

14. Pelvic examination

15. Gait
    Proximal weakness
    Peripheral neuropathy
    Babinski sign

16. Documentation of tumour size

Assessment of daily functional
ability (ECOG 0–4)

Physical examination protocol 1.2 You are asked to examine a patient who has recently presented with metastatic disease of unknown primary aetiology

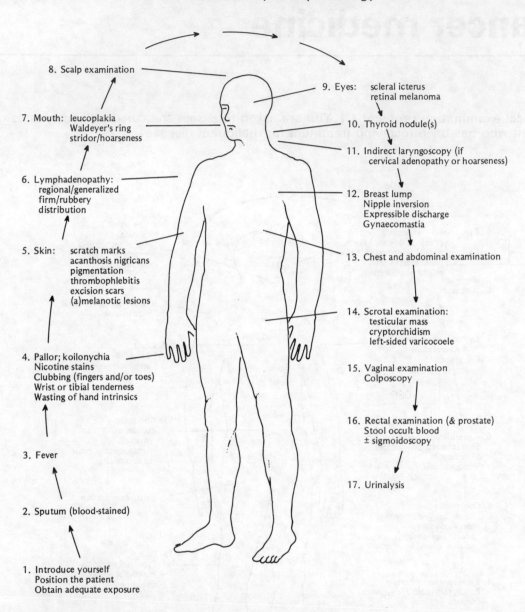

8. Scalp examination

7. Mouth: leucoplakia
   Waldeyer's ring
   stridor/hoarseness

6. Lymphadenopathy:
   regional/generalized
   firm/rubbery
   distribution

5. Skin: scratch marks
   acanthosis nigricans
   pigmentation
   thrombophlebitis
   excision scars
   (a)melanotic lesions

4. Pallor; koilonychia
   Nicotine stains
   Clubbing (fingers and/or toes)
   Wrist or tibial tenderness
   Wasting of hand intrinsics

3. Fever

2. Sputum (blood-stained)

1. Introduce yourself
   Position the patient
   Obtain adequate exposure

9. Eyes: scleral icterus
   retinal melanoma

10. Thyroid nodule(s)

11. Indirect laryngoscopy (if
    cervical adenopathy or hoarseness)

12. Breast lump
    Nipple inversion
    Expressible discharge
    Gynaecomastia

13. Chest and abdominal examination

14. Scrotal examination:
    testicular mass
    cryptorchidism
    left-sided varicocoele

15. Vaginal examination
    Colposcopy

16. Rectal examination (& prostate)
    Stool occult blood
    ± sigmoidoscopy

17. Urinalysis

Diagnostic pathway 1.1 This patient has ascites. What is the most likely cause?

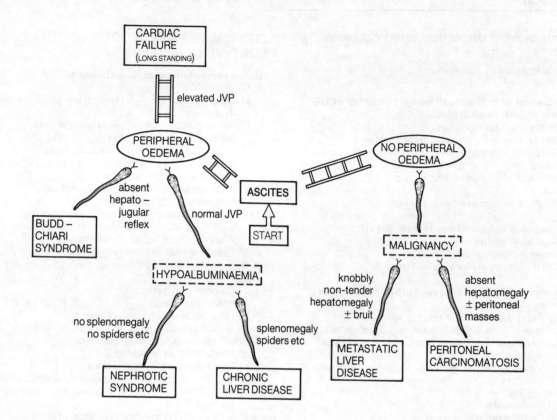

CLINICAL ASPECTS OF MALIGNANT DISEASE

COMMONEST ONCOLOGY SHORT CASES

1 Lung cancer
2 Metastatic liver disease

Assessment of patient well-being*: modified ECOG criteria (*'performance status')
1 Grade 0 — asymptomatic
2 Grade 1 — symptomatic, fully ambulant
3 Grade 2 — symptomatic, ambulant >50% waking hours
4 Grade 3 — symptomatic, in bed >50% waking hours
5 Grade 4 — symptomatic, bedfast

The palpable tumour: how to describe it
1 Site, size, shape
2 Fixation, fluctuation, firmness
3 Texture, temperature, tenderness

Differential diagnosis of fever in the cancer patient
1 Infection
  a) Septicaemia, esp.if neutropenic
  b) Intermittent bacteraemias, e.g. from central line
  c) Occult localized infections, e.g. cryptococcal meningitis
  d) Viraemia, esp. CMV (e.g. following marrow transplant)
2 Iatrogenic
  a) Bleomycin
  b) L-Asparaginase; interferon
  c) Transfusions
3 Primary disease manifestation (diagnosis of exclusion)
  a) Lymphoma
  b) Retroperitoneal tumours, e.g. renal cell carcinoma
  c) Metastatic liver disease; 'tumour necrosis'

Differential diagnosis of confusion in the cancer patient
1 Reversible metabolic derangements
  a) Hypercalcaemia
  b) Hyponatraemia (SIADH)
  c) Hyperviscosity
2 Reversible iatrogenic precipitants
  a) Opiates
  b) Steroids
  c) Procarbazine
  d) L-Asparaginase
3 Sepsis, esp.:
  a) Pneumonia
  b) Cryptococcal meningitis
  c) Progressive multifocal leucoencephalopathy
4 Tumour-related
  a) Paraneoplastic encephalopathy/dementia
  b) Cerebral metastases

Differential diagnosis of vomiting in the cancer patient
1 Iatrogenic

2 Gastrointestinal obstruction
3 Raised intracranial pressure
4 Hypercalcaemia and/or renal failure

CLINICAL PRESENTATIONS OF TUMOUR SUBTYPES

Clinical presentations of lung tumours
1 General
  a) Local symptoms — haemoptysis, stridor, dyspnoea
  b) Nerve palsy — recurrent laryngeal (esp. left-sided tumours); phrenic; T1 root plus Horner's syndrome (Pancoast tumour)
  c) Superior vena caval obstruction (esp. right-sided tumours)
  d) Metastatic presentations — jaundice, convulsions, tamponade
  e) Pleural effusion — uniform bloodstaining signifies pleural metastases, while chylous effusions may be non-metastatic
  f) Systemic manifestations — weight loss
2 Non-small-cell (i.e. chemoresistant) lung cancer (80%)
  a) Clubbing, hypertrophic osteoarthropathy ⎫
  b) Non-metastatic hypercalcaemia ⎬ esp. SCC
  c) Gynaecomastia (esp. adenocarcinoma)
3 Small-cell lung cancer (20%)
  a) Metastases at presentation
  b) Leucoerythroblastic anaemia
  c) Cerebral metastases, meningeal carcinomatosis
  d) SIADH (due to primary tumour or intracranial spread)
  e) Ectopic ACTH syndrome; Eaton-Lambert syndrome
  f) SVC obstruction (50% of cases)
4 Bronchioloalveolar cell carcinoma
  a) Copious clear sputum in a non-smoker
  b) Respiratory insufficiency ± pulmonary infiltrate
5 Bronchial adenoma (usually a carcinoid tumour)
  a) Haemoptysis with normal CXR (tumour usually central)
  b) Recurrent chest infections, e.g. abscess, pneumonia
  c) Incidental CXR finding in a non-smoker
  d) Brisk haemorrhage if biopsied (very vascular)

Clinical presentations of gastrointestinal tumours
1 Colorectal cancer
  a) Common — change of bowel habit, passage of blood per rectum
  b) Classical — iron-deficiency anaemia (esp. if right-sided)
  c) Rare — *Strep. bovis* endocarditis, *Clostridium septicum* myonecrosis
2 Pancreatic cancer
  'head' tumours:
  a) Common — progressive jaundice ± pain
  b) Classical — palpable non-tender gallbladder (Courvoisier's sign)
  'Tail' tumours:
  a) Common — weight loss

b) Classical — endogenous depression, *angor animi*
c) Rare — migratory thrombophlebitis (Trousseau's syndrome)
3 Gastric cancer
  a) Common — weight loss ± epigastric discomfort
  b) Classical
    — Troisier's sign (enlargement of Virchow's node)
    — Sister Mary Joseph nodule (umbilical mass)
    — Blumer's (prerectal) shelf on digital examination
    — Krukenberg tumours (ovarian metastases) at laparotomy
    — Acanthosis nigricans

Clinical presentations of liver tumours
1 Hepatoma
  a) Common
    — Onset of ascites in a previously stable cirrhotic
    — Unexplained weight loss in an alcoholic
    — Tender hepar with bruit (DDx: alcoholic hepatitis)
  b) Uncommon — polycythaemia, dysproteinaemia, porphyria
2 Hepatic adenoma (rare)
  Intraperitoneal rupture in a previously asymptomatic young woman taking combined (oestrogenic) oral contraceptives for at least five years
3 Hepatoblastoma (in infants only)
  Clubbing; precocious puberty

SYMPTOMS AND SIGNS OF SPECIFIC TUMOURS

Symptoms and signs of renal cell carcinoma
1 Common
  a) Haematuria, flank pain, flank mass
  b) Anaemia (25%)
2 Uncommon
  a) Polycythaemia (5%)
  b) Fever; thromboembolism
  c) Left-sided varicocoele
  d) Non-metastatic hypercalcaemia
  e) Non-metastatic liver dysfunction (Stauffer's syndrome)

Symptoms and signs of choriocarcinoma
1 Hyperemesis gravidarum
2 Bleeding metastases — haemoptysis, stroke
3 Painful gynaecomastia (in males)
4 Rare — mild hyperthyroidism (HCG shares TSH β-subunit)

Symptoms and signs of cervical carcinoma
1 Vaginal discharge
2 Pelvic pain (advanced disease)
3 Fistulas (e.g. rectovaginal: pneumaturia) — often iatrogenic
4 Obstructive uropathy (frequently terminal)

Symptoms and signs of ovarian tumours
1 Adenocarcinoma
  a) Ascites, bowel obstruction
  b) Peritoneal carcinomatosis at laparotomy
2 Stromal tumours (rare)
  a) Fibroma, thecoma — Meigs's syndrome
  b) *Struma ovarii* — thyrotoxicosis
  c) Granulosa cell tumour — vaginal bleeding
  d) Sertoli-Leydig tumour (arrhenoblastoma) — virilization

Symptoms and signs of melanoma
1 Common
  a) Cerebral metastases, meningeal carcinomatosis
  b) Pulmonary metastases
  c) Skin metastases (may be indolent)
2 Classical — hepatomegaly and unilateral scleral icterus (i.e. liver metastases from retinal primary; glass eye)

PATTERNS OF NEUROLOGICAL DEFICIT IN MALIGNANT DISEASE

Common presentations of intracranial neoplasms
1 Headaches (esp. morning; ± diplopia, projectile vomiting)
2 Convulsions (may be focal)
3 Cranial nerve deficit (may be mixed, or 'false localizing')
4 Personality change; dementia

Cerebrovascular manifestations of malignant disease
1 Intracranial haemorrhage — esp. in leukaemics
2 Bleeding metastases — melanoma, choriocarcinoma
3 Infarcts — non-bacterial endocarditis
4 Hyperviscosity — Waldenström's, myeloma
5 Sagittal sinus thrombosis — DIC (e.g. promyelocytic leukaemia)

Clinical features of meningeal carcinomatosis
1 Commonest causes
  a) Small-cell lung cancer
  b) Breast cancer
  c) Melanoma, lymphoma
2 Presentation
  a) Disseminated and/or mixed deficits (e.g. upper *and* lower motor neurone lesions)
  b) Bizarre sensory disturbances (e.g. unilateral jaw numbness)
3 Diagnosis
  a) CSF cytology; ↑ CSF protein ± ↓ CSF glucose
  b) Myelography may confirm nodules within spinal canal, but is only indicated to exclude a (treatable) compressive lesion

Clinical features of progressive multifocal leucoencephalopathy
1 Commonest cause — leukaemias, lymphomas
2 Pathology — deep cortical/cerebellar demyelination
3 Presentation — progressive cortical (visual, speech, higher centres) deficits, limb weakness, normal intracranial pressure
4 Diagnosis:
  a) CSF examination typically normal

b) Antibodies to JC virus (a papovavirus)
c) CT or NMR scanning may show lesions
d) Brain biopsy for viral studies (definitive)
5 Course — survival averages 3 months from diagnosis

Clinical features of Pancoast's syndrome
1 Commonest cause — lung cancer, esp. SCC
2 Symptoms — radicular arm pain (due to plexus invasion)
3 Signs — interossei wasting; T1 sensory loss; Horner's
4 Investigations — erosion of first and second ribs on CXR

Clinical features of myasthenic (Eaton-Lambert) syndrome
1 Commonest cause — small-cell lung cancer
2 Symptoms
   a) Weakness; myalgias, paraesthesiae
   b) Impotence; dry mouth
3 Signs
   a) Minimal wasting; hyporeflexia
   b) Augmenting pelvifemoral weakness
   c) Ocular/bulbar sparing
4 Diagnosis
   a) Negative edrophonium (Tensilon) test
   b) Post-tetanic facilitation on EMG
5 Treatment
   a) Ablation of underlying malignancy
   b) Corticosteroids, plasmapheresis
   c) Oral guanidine; diaminopyridine

Back pain: clinical features suggesting malignant aetiology
1 Insidious onset, progressive course, general ill health
2 Often worse at night
3 Thoracic or upper lumbar nerve root distribution
4 Disseminated sites of vertebral tenderness
5 Signs of multiple and/or bilateral nerve root lesions
6 Coexisting upper motor neurone signs
7 Associated sphincter dysfunction or perianal anaesthesia

INVESTIGATING MALIGNANT DISEASE

RADIOGRAPHIC ABNORMALITIES IN NEOPLASTIC DISEASE

Pulmonary infiltrates in the cancer patient
1 Infiltration (by tumour)
   a) Lymphangitis carcinomatosa (esp. in breast cancer)
   b) Lymphoma, bronchioloalveolar cell carcinoma
2 Infection (opportunistic)
   a) Neutropenic — Gram-negative or polymicrobial pneumonia
   b) Immunosuppressed — CMV, *Pneumocystis carinii*, fungi

3 Infarction (pulmonary) — thromboembolism
4 Collapse/consolidation (hypostatic) — obstructing primary tumour
5 Aspiration
   a) Intrinsic/extrinsic oesophageal obstruction by tumour
   b) Cytotoxic-induced emesis in a sedated patient
6 Iatrogenic
   a) Radiation pneumonitis
   b) Cytotoxic-induced lung disease (e.g. bleomycin)

Osteosclerotic lesions in the cancer patient
1 Metastatic prostate cancer
2 Metastatic breast cancer (esp. post-treatment) — typically mixed lytic/blastic
3 'Ivory vertebrae' or patchy sclerosis
   a) Hodgkin's disease
   b) Myelofibrosis
   c) Coincidental Paget's disease

Osteolytic lesions in the cancer patient
1 Metastatic carcinoma
2 Myeloma (focal lesions *or* generalized osteoporosis)
3 Primary bone tumours
4 *Generalized* osteopenia
   a) Old age
   b) Postmenopausal
   c) Immobilization
   d) Steroids

TUMOUR MARKERS

Diagnostic significance of tumour markers
1 AFP
   a) Non-seminomatous germ-cell tumours (80%)
   b) Hepatoma (50%) — specific but not sensitive
   c) Also elevated in normal pregnancy
2 β HCG
   a) Choriocarcinoma (100%)
   b) Non-seminomatous germ-cell tumours (50%)
   c) Seminoma (10% *only*)
3 CEA
   a) Colorectal cancer, *esp.* with liver metastases (poor sensitivity for early-stage disease)
   b) Often also elevated in advanced-stage gastric, breast and lung cancer
   c) *Occasionally* useful in postoperative follow-up of patients with preoperative elevations which normalize immediately following resection of primary, though no survival benefit of this strategy is recognized
   d) If elevated, may help distinguish undifferentiated carcinoma from lymphoma or amelanotic melanoma
4 Acid phosphatase (tartrate-resistant)
   a) Prostatic carcinoma, esp. bony secondaries (85% +ve)
   b) *Poor* sensitivity for early-stage disease
5 Prostate-specific antigen
   a) More sensitive but less specific than acid phosphatase

b) May be absent in poorly differentiated tumours

c) Levels reflect degree of extraprostatic extension

d) Elevation in asymptomatic elderly patients may indicate need for transrectal ultrasound ± needle biopsy

e) Better monitor of tumour activity than acid phosphatase

6 Alkaline phosphatase

a) Elevations may signify metastasis to bone or liver

b) In metastatic bone disease, the enzyme is heat-labile and there is no elevation of GGT or 5'-nucleotidase

c) Osteoblastic metastases (e.g. prostatic cancer) yield the greatest elevations, whereas lytic deposits (e.g. myeloma) tend to be associated with normal values

d) *Placental* isoenzyme is elevated in 50% of seminomas and also in dysgerminomas

7 Other

a) Calcitonin (medullary carcinoma of the thyroid) — invaluable in screening, diagnosis and follow-up

b) Thyroglobulin (papillary/follicular thyroid cancer) — useful in follow-up

c) Paraprotein (B-cell malignancy, esp. myeloma) — useful in initial diagnosis and follow up

d) ESR (Hodgkin's disease) — useful in follow-up

e) Urinary 5-HIAA (carcinoid syndrome) — useful in diagnosis and follow-up

f) Urinary/plasma catecholamines (phaeochromocytoma) — useful in initial diagnosis, less so in follow-up

g) Ca-125 (ovarian cancer)

h) Inhibin (granulosa-cell tumours)

i) S-100 (melanoma)

(NB: see also p. 119)

DETERMINING THE ORIGIN OF METASTATIC CANCER

Metastases from unknown primary*: investigative rationale

1 Diagnosis of treatable disease

a) Hormone-responsive disease

b) Chemosensitive disease

c) Radiosensitive disease

2 Avoidance of iatrogenic morbidity in resistant disease

3 Prevention of complications related to occult primary, e.g. bowel obstruction, pathological fracture

4 Prognostic clarification

Approach to evaluation of metastatic disease

1 Squamous cell carcinoma in cervical nodes

a) Meticulous inspection of scalp and skin

b) CXR (± barium swallow)

(* i.e no clue to organ of origin from symptoms, signs or CXR)

c) ENT examination: examination under anaesthesia with blind biopsies from nasopharynx and base of tongue

2 Anaplastic carcinoma in high cervical nodes

a) CXR; sputum cytology (most reliable in small-cell carcinoma)

b) Thyroid scan ± needle biopsy

c) Nasopharyngeal assessment

d) Consider missed diagnosis of poorly differentiated lymphoma, and exclude with monoclonal immunohistochemistry

3 Squamous cell carcinoma in inguinal nodes

a) Meticulous inspection of lower limbs and perineum

b) Proctoscopy and/or colposcopy

4 Metastatic adenocarcinoma

a) Oestrogen receptor (ER) status of biopsy tissue (in females)

b) Serum acid phosphatase (in males)

c) Serum AFP/HCG (if strongly positive, histology needs review)

d) Consider missed diagnosis of poorly differentiated lymphoma

5 ER-negative axillary node adenocarcinoma in a female — mammography

6 Retroperitoneal and/or mediastinal mass, or multiple pulmonary metastases, in a young male patient — AFP, β-HCG, testicular ultrasound

NB: presence of gynaecomastia in this context is virtually diagnostic of germ-cell tumour; if ultrasound negative, the patient should be treated with platinum-based therapy as a presumed extragonadal germ-cell tumour

Pathological characterization of metastatic tumour tissue

1 Light microscopy

a) Signet ring cells (favour gastric primary)

b) Keratin (favours SCC); melanin (melanoma)

c) Mucin — Common in gut/lung/ovarian/breast/endometrial Ca, rare in renal cell or thyroid cancer

d) Psammoma bodies
   — Ovarian cancer (mucin +)
   — Thyroid cancer (mucin −)

e) Amyloid — myeloma, medullary thyroid cancer

2 Immunoperoxidase

a) AFP, β HCG

b) Acid phosphatase, prostate-specific antigen

c) Neuron-specific enolase (neuroendocrine tumours)

3 Surface immunoglobulin
Antilight chain
   monoclonal antibodies } if lymphoma suspected
Phenotypic T-cell
   markers (e.g. CD_4)

4 Oestrogen receptor assay

5 Electron microscopy

a) Distinguishes
   — Adenocarcinoma and mesothelioma
   — Spindle-cell tumours (sarcomas, melanoma, SCC)

— Small round-cell tumours (see below)
b) *May* identify
— Amelanotic melanoma (melanosomes)
— Carcinoids (neurosecretory granules)
— Undifferentiated lymphomas, histiocytosis X

Differential diagnosis of small round-cell tumours
'LEMON':
1 Lymphoma
2 Ewing's tumour
3 Medulloblastoma
4 Oat-cell (small-cell) carcinoma
5 Neuroblastoma

SCREENING FOR MALIGNANT DISEASE

General principles of cancer screening
1 *Cost-effectiveness* of a screening test depends on
   a) the availability of effective treatment
   b) the ability to identify (and test) high-risk groups
2 The only test widely recognized as being *effective* in reducing morbidity is the Papanicolaou smear
3 Some authorities regard mammography of women aged 50–70 to be an effective public health screen, but the debate is complicated by unanswered questions of lead time and length time bias (see below and refs 1.5 and 1.6.)

Sources of bias in evaluating cancer screening tests
1 *Lead time bias* — i.e. by detecting disease at an earlier (presymptomatic) stage, subsequent survival is spuriously prolonged when compared with a cohort diagnosed at a later stage
2 *Length time bias* — i.e. by instituting mass screening programmes, a relative excess of patients with *indolent* disease will be detected initially (since at any one time the *prevalance* of detectable slowly-growing tumours will tend to be greater, even if the *incidence* of aggressive tumours is similar), leading to an illusory survival improvement in the screened cohort

Colorectal cancer: recommendations for 'high-risk' screening
1 Patients with ulcerative pancolitis of more than 10 years duration, or left-sided colitis of more than 20 years, should be monitored with 6-monthly sigmoidoscopy and annual colonoscopy with multiple biopsies. Proctocolectomy may be indicated if high-grade dysplasia is documented in any biopsy specimen, or if even low-grade dysplasia corresponds to an area of localized macroscopic abnormality
2 First-degree relatives of patients with multiple polyposis should be sigmoidoscoped annually after age 16. If polyps are noted, ileorectal anastomosis with rectal fulguration may be indicated
3 Patients with a past history of colorectal adenoma(s) or carcinoma may be monitored with 3-yearly colonoscopy. Occult blood testing has a purely supplementary role in follow-up of such patients
4 Patients presenting *de novo* with rectal bleeding should be investigated with sigmoidoscopy and

colonoscopy in the first instance unless contraindicated. Patients presenting with other colorectal symptoms should be evaluated with digital rectal examination and sigmoidoscopy, and the need for colonoscopy and/or barium studies assessed on the basis of these results

Current status of faecal occult blood testing
1 Not recommended for routine screening of standard-risk subjects (but see ref. 1.1b)
2 Two to five per cent of tests performed in standard-risk subjects will be positive, and of these 60% will be found to have no abnormality on full investigation, i.e. the false-positive rate for polyp/carcinoma detection is 60%; while the false-positive rate for carcinoma detection alone approaches 95%
3 The false-negative rate in *symptomatic* patients is 20% (i.e. this is an *inappropriate* investigation in such patients)
4 False-negatives may arise due to
   a) Sampling error
   b) Delay in test development
   c) Proximal site of bleeding
   d) Vitamin C ingestion
5 Less than 1% of screened standard-risk subjects will be found to have a carcinoma. Asymptomatic tumours detected in this way are twice as likely to be Duke's stage A or B than are *symptomatic* tumours; as yet, however, there is no evidence that screening (i.e. of asymptomatic patients) leads to improved survival

Further investigation of the abnormal cervical smear
1 Repeat smear (incl. endocervical curettage)
2 If abnormal, proceed to colposcopy and punch-directed biopsy
3 If doubt persists, proceed to cone biopsy

STAGING OF SOLID TUMOURS

Staging of testicular germ-cell tumours: MRC criteria
1 Stage I — involvement limited to testis
2 Stage II — abdominal nodal involvement
3 Stage III — mediastinal and/or supraclavicular nodes involved
4 Stage IV — extranodal disease (e.g. lung metastases)

Adverse prognostic features in testicular germ-cell tumours
1 Tumour bulk
   a) Infradiaphragmatic tumour mass > 10 cm diameter
   b) Supradiaphragmatic tumour mass > 5 cm diameter
2 AFP >1000 ng/l; β-HCG >50 000 mIU/ml
3 Non-pulmonary visceral spread (e.g. to liver, bone, CNS)
4 Extragonadal primary tumour

Staging of colorectal carcinoma
1 Duke's A — confined to (sub)mucosa

2 Duke's B — spread through muscularis layer
3 Duke's C — involvement of local nodes
4 Duke's D — distant metastases

Staging of cervix cancer
1 FIGO stage 0 — carcinoma in situ
2 FIGO stage 1 — confined to cervix
3 FIGO stage 2 — extends to upper vagina or parametrium
4 FIGO stage 3 — extends to lower vagina or pelvic sidewall
5 FIGO stage 4 — extends beyond true pelvis

Staging of small-cell lung cancer
1 Limited disease — confined to hemithorax (incl. ipsilateral supraclavicular nodes)
2 Extensive disease — spread beyond hemithorax (incl. ipsilateral pleural effusion)

Staging of breast cancer: the TNM classification
1 T—T1 = tumour < 2 cm diameter
    T2 = tumour 2–5 cm diameter
    T3 = tumour > 5 cm diameter
    T4 = tumour involving skin or chest wall
2 N—N0 = impalpable nodes
    N1 = mobile enlarged axillary nodes
    N2 = matted/fixed axillary nodes
    N3 = arm oedema (prior to radiotherapy or surgery) or involved supra/infraclavicular nodes
3 M—M0 = no evidence of metastases
    M1 = distant metastases
4 Stage 1 disease — T1N0
    Stage 2 disease — T1–2, N0–1
    Stage 3 disease — T3–4, N2–3
    Stage 4 disease — M1

Staging of malignant melanoma
1 Breslow thickness (depth of invasion) < 0.75 mm, i.e. confined to superficial dermis — good prognosis (95% cure)
2 Breslow thickness > 3.5 mm, i.e. invading subcutaneous fat — poor prognosis (20% cure only)

MANAGING MALIGNANT DISEASE

Therapeutic approaches in clinical oncology
1 Radical — maximal treatment, usually with curative intent*
2 Palliative — specific but submaximal antitumour treatment administered without anticipated survival prolongation
3 Symptomatic — non-specific measures
4 Adjuvant — prophylactic treatment of presumed micrometastases

---

*In some situations, e.g. advanced head and neck cancer, or locally recurrent breast cancer, radical (i.e. maximally tolerated) radiotherapy may be administered with palliative intent.

Malignancies curable with chemotherapy
1 70–90% cure rate
    a) Testicular teratoma or seminoma
    b) Choriocarcinoma (in women)
    c) Hodgkin's disease
    d) Wilms' tumour; embryonal rhabdomyosarcoma
2 40–60% cure rate
    a) Childhood acute lymphoblastic leukaemia
    b) Burkitt's lymphoma (endemic variety)
    c) Ewing's sarcoma; osteosarcoma
3 20–30% cure rate
    a) Non-Hodgkin's lymphoma (diffuse large-cell)
    b) Adult acute lymphoblastic leukaemia
4 5–15% cure rate — acute myeloblastic leukaemia

Malignancies responsive to palliative chemotherapy
1 Low-grade lymphomas; myeloma; chronic leukaemias
2 Breast cancer
3 Ovarian cancer
4 Small-cell lung cancer

Malignancies responsive to adjuvant chemotherapy
1 Wilms' tumour
2 Osteogenic sarcoma
3 Embryonal rhabdomyosarcoma
4 Premenopausal breast cancer with axillary nodal involvement (cf. postmenopausal breast cancer: adjuvant tamoxifen)

Malignancies curable with radical radiotherapy
1 Non-melanomatous skin cancer
2 Seminoma, dysgerminoma
3 Hodgkin's disease stages IA and IIA (unless bulky disease)
4 Non-Hodgkin's lymphoma stage I and II
5 Early-stage head and neck tumours (incl. laryngeal or lingual SCC, papillary/follicular thyroid cancer)
6 Early-stage carcinoma of the cervix or bladder

Malignant complications responsive to palliative radiotherapy
1 Painful bone metastases (local or hemibody irradiation)
2 Advanced refractory lymphomas (whole-body irradiation)
3 Neoplastic skin ulceration/fungation
4 Obstructed hollow viscus (esp. trachea, oesophagus, SVC)
5 Neural compression (cerebral, spinal cord, nerve)
6 Uncontrolled neoplastic bleeding (e.g. haemoptysis, haematuria)

Malignancies responsive to hormonal manipulation
1 Breast cancer
2 Prostate cancer
3 Endometrial cancer (progestogens)
4 Papillary/follicular thyroid cancer (T_4-suppression of TSH)

Malignancies resistant to treatment
1 Gastrointestinal adenocarcinomas, esp. pancreas
2 Renal cell carcinoma
3 Melanoma
4 Mesothelioma

5 Hepatoma
6 Soft-tissue sarcomas (in adults)

NB: 'radioresistance' of many of these tumours is technical rather than cellular in origin, i.e. the tumour may be 'sensitive', but toxicity to adjacent normal tissue precludes treatment

Malignancies which may undergo spontaneous regression
1 Neuroblastoma (esp. stage IV S)
2 Kaposi's sarcoma (endemic variety)
3 Rarely — melanoma, renal cell carcinoma

Fallacies in cancer management
1 A dire prognosis justifies toxic treatment even if therapeutic benefit unproven
2 Recognized tumour responsiveness (i.e. shrinkage) to a given therapy justifies treatment even if survival benefit unproven
3 Lack of therapeutic toxicity justifies presumptive treatment even if symptomatic benefit unproven

MECHANISMS OF CYTOTOXIC DRUG ACTIVITY

Classification of common chemotherapeutic agents
1 Alkylators
  a) Chlorambucil, cyclophosphamide
  b) Nitrogen mustard (mustine in MOPP)
  c) Melphalan (phenylalanine mustard), busulphan
2 Intercalators
  a) Anthracyclines (doxorubicin, daunorubicin)
  b) Anthraquinones (mitoxantrone); m-AMSA
3 Nitrosoureas (act by alkylating *and* crosslinking DNA) — BCNU, CCNU, streptozotocin
4 Antitumour antibiotics (variable mechanisms of action) — bleomycin, mithramycin, mitomycin C
5 Spindle toxins: vinca alkaloids — vincristine, vinblastine
6 Topoisomerase II inhibitors: podophyllotoxin derivatives — VP-16 (etoposide), VM-26
7 Inhibitors of protein synthesis — L-asparaginase
8 Antimetabolites
  a) Purine analogues — azathioprine, 6MP, 6TG
  b) Enzyme inhibitors
    — methotrexate (dihydrofolate reductase)
    — hydroxyurea (ribonucleotide reductase)
    — 5FU (thymidylate synthetase)
    — ara-C (DNA polymerase)
    — deoxycoformycin (cytosine deaminase)

Relationships of cytotoxic action to cell cycle kinetics
1 Non-cycle-specific (i.e. toxic to non-dividing cells in G_0) — radiotherapy
2 Cycle-specific but not phase-specific
  a) Alkylating agents (incl. cis-platinum)
  b) Tumour antibiotics (incl. anthracyclines)
3 Phase-specific
  a) S-phase (DNA synthesis) — antimetabolites
  b) G_1-phase (gap, or interphase) — L-asparaginase
  c) G_2, M (mitosis) — vinca alkaloids

Indications for corticosteroids in malignant disease
1 Oncolytic effect — B-cell malignancies, breast cancer
2 Intracranial neoplasm with raised intracranial pressure; nerve (incl. spinal cord) compression, esp. preradiotherapy
3 Hypercalcaemia (esp. in myeloma)
4 Dyspnoea due to lymphangitis carcinomatosa
5 Acute inflammation following radiotherapy, e.g. radiation proctitis (steroid enemas), non-candidal oesophagitis
6 Antiemetic; antipyretic (sometimes); appetite stimulation

Mechanisms of tumour resistance to anticancer drugs
1 General
  a) Tumour heterogeneity: genetic instability of primary tumour leads to clonal loss of sensitive drug targets
  b) Small growth fraction: many tumours replicate no faster than normal tissues, and are therefore no more sensitive to the non-specific cytotoxicity of many drugs
2 Specific
  a) Gene amplification (e.g. of the dihydrofolate reductase gene following methotrexate therapy)
  b) Reduced drug uptake (e.g. expression of P-glycoprotein, a membrane protein mediating drug efflux, in multidrug-resistant phenotype)
  c) Enhanced lesion repair (e.g. induction of alkyltransferase activity following alkylator therapy)
  d) Reduced requirement for metabolic product (e.g. acquired L-asparaginase resistance)
  e) Loss of specific receptors (e.g. some cases of tamoxifen resistance)

MORBIDITY OF CYTOTOXIC THERAPY

Common problems limiting use of cytotoxic therapy
1 Myelosuppression
  a) Alkylators, nitrosoureas
  b) Anthracyclines; ara-C; vinblastine
2 Severe nausea
  a) Cis-platinum (less with carboplatin)
  b) Anthracyclines; IV alkylating agents
3 Alopecia totalis
  a) Anthracyclines, cranial irradiation
  b) Cyclophosphamide; VP-16, ara-C
4 Mucositis, stomatitis
  a) Methotrexate
  b) Anthracyclines, bleomycin, 5FU
5 Pulmonary fibrosis
  a) Bleomycin, busulphan (dose-related)
  b) Methotrexate, etc. (idiosyncratic)
6 Radiation recall or potentiation
  a) Actinomycin D, anthracyclines
  b) Methotrexate
7 Extravasation necrosis
  a) Anthracyclines, actinomycin D
  b) Vincristine, vinblastine

8 Expense:
  a) New drugs, e.g. — carboplatin, vindesine, mitoxantrone
  b) Chronic therapy — hormones (e.g. megestrol, cyproterone)

Clinically significant interactions with cytotoxic therapy
1 Azathioprine ⎫ — four-fold potentiation by
  Oral 6MP   ⎭   allopurinol
2 Methotrexate
  a) Potentiated by aspirin, NSAIDs
  b) Potentiates radiation toxicity
3 Procarbazine — hypertension with tyramine-containing foods (MAO inhibition)
4 Cyclophosphamide — activated (potentiated) in liver by enzyme inducers, e.g. barbiturates

Genitourinary morbidity of cyclophosphamide/ifosfamide
1 Haemorrhagic cystitis (preventable by hydration or MESNA)
2 Bladder telangiectasia and/or fibrosis
3 Transitional cell carcinoma of the bladder
4 Azoöspermia, amenorrhoea
5 Inappropriate ADH secretion

Methotrexate toxicity: precipitants, potentiation and prevention
1 Precipitants (drugs competing for renal tubular secretion)
  a) Aspirin — also displaces drug from plasma protein binding
  b) Probenecid, phenylbutazone, cephalothin, trimethoprim
2 Potentiation — concurrent radiotherapy
3 Prevention (in high-dose regimens esp., e.g. for osteosarcoma)
  a) Forced diuresis (i.e. intravenous prehydration)
  b) Urinary alkalinization
  c) Oral folinic acid 'rescue' — 15 mg 6-hourly for six doses commencing 24 hours post-treatment (standard regimen)

Relative contraindications to anthracycline therapy
1 Frail and/or elderly patient
2 Obstructive jaundice
3 Left ventricular dysfunction
4 Severe hypertension
5 Past history of mediastinal irradiation and/or cyclophosphamide

Relatively non-myelosuppressive cytotoxics
1 Bleomycin
2 L-Asparaginase
3 Vincristine (cf. vinblastine)
4 Cis-platinum (cf. carboplatin)

TOXICITY OF RADIATION THERAPY

Modes of radiotherapy administration
1 External beam

  a) Superficial (25–150 kV)
    — Limited penetration
    — Used for skin cancers (BCC, SCC)
  b) Orthovoltage (250–350 kV)
    — Moderate penetration
    — Used to palliate painful bone metastases
    — Skin toxicity may be a problem
  c) Megavoltage (> 1 MV; usually 4–10 MV)
    — Produced by cobalt machines or linear accelerators
    — Excellent penetration ('skin-sparing' radiation)
2 Brachytherapy (interstitial)
  a) Unsealed sources
    — ^{32}P (polycythaemia vera)
    — ^{131}I (Graves' disease, thyroid cancer)
    — ^{137}Cs (Ca cervix)
  b) Sealed sources — ^{192}Ir (Ca breast, head and neck)

Determinants of radiation-induced toxicity
1 Volume irradiated
2 Tissue irradiated
3 Fraction size (i.e. dose per treatment session)
4 Total dose

Normal tissue tolerance: radiation dose thresholds
1 Brain — 50–60 Gy
2 Heart, small intestine — 40–50 Gy
3 Liver — 30 Gy
4 Lung, kidney — 20 Gy
5 Whole body — 3–5 Gy

(NB: These doses represent the 5% injury risk for an 'average' treatment volume and fractionation.)

Common problems following therapeutic irradiation
1 Acute local toxicity
  a) Erythema, desquamation, photosensitivity of overlying skin
  b) Hair loss (usually transient)
  c) Mucositis; inflammation of any organ
2 Acute systemic toxicity (radiation sickness)
  a) Fatigue and malaise
  b) Nausea, anorexia
3 Late toxicity caused by endarteritis obliterans, e.g.
  a) Radiation nephritis ⎫ acute syndromes
  b) Radiation pneumonitis ⎭ also occur
  c) Radiation myelopathy (cord ischaemia)
  d) ↓ Haemopoietic reserve (compromising future chemotherapy)
4 Mutagenicity — esp. leukaemogenesis (following megavoltage therapy or ^{32}P)

NB. **Late** toxicity is a major concern in **radical** treatment, but less so (or not at all) in **palliative** (short-term) treatment

Problems following abdominal or pelvic irradiation
1 Nausea, esp. in hepatic irradiation and whole-abdominal irradiation (e.g. for ovarian cancer, seminoma, lymphoma)
  Management — antiemetics (p. 28)

2 Diarrhoea, esp. in radical pelvic irradiation for gynaecological or genitourinary malignancies
Management — loperamide, codeine, low-residue diet
(NB: about 2% of patients receiving radical therapy for cervix cancer may require surgery for ischaemic rectosigmoid colitis.)
3 Tenesmus, rectal bleeding (radiation proctitis)
Management — prednisolone suppositories
4 Urinary frequency/dysuria
Management — exclude infection; anticholinergics; alkalinizers, analgesics; repeat cystoscopy if persistent
5 Vaginal discharge ± cervicitis
Management — actively exclude *Candida, Trichomonas* infections
Vaginal adhesions — treat with dilator
6 Nephrotoxicity (dose-related) — prevent by shielding

THERAPEUTIC USE OF CYTOTOXIC DRUGS

Points to discuss with patients prior to commencing treatment
1 Prognosis without treatment
2 Probability of therapeutic benefit (cure, complete or partial remission, disease-free interval, symptomatic improvement)
3 Risks of infertility/teratogenicity/premature menopause; availability of sperm banking
4 Probable severity of alopecia; availability of wig-making
5 Probable severity and duration of nausea; prophylaxis
6 Requirement for (and rationale of) maintenance allopurinol
7 Requirement for (and rationale of) regular blood tests
8 Urgent significance of fever or bruising/bleeding
9 Rationale of clinical trials and informed consent
10 Long-term risk of second malignancy, esp. in good-prognosis disease treated with alkylating agents (e.g. Hodgkin's)

Clinical assessment of the patient commencing treatment
1 Assessment and documentation of disease extent
  a) Measurement (and/or photography) of visible lesions
  b) Radiographic corroboration
  c) Measurement of tumour markers
  d) Invasive staging *if* stage-specific therapy exists (e.g. in Hodgkin's disease, breast cancer, or ovarian cancer)
2 Assessment of vital organ function
  a) Left ventricular function (pre-doxorubicin)
  b) Lung function (pre-bleomycin)
  c) Renal function (pre-platinum)
3 Assessment of immune status (in leukaemia or transplantation)
  a) CXR, Mantoux
  b) Viral (CMV, HSV, hepatitis B) and toxoplasma serology
4 Assessment of venous access; consideration of an implantable infusion port/catheter

5 Assessment of psychological adjustment to disease, and to disease- and treatment-related disability

Chemotherapeutic agents commonly used for solid tumours
1 Germ-cell tumours — cis-platinum, bleomycin, and VP-16 (or vinblastine)
2 Small-cell lung cancer
  a) VP-16
  b) Doxorubicin, cyclophosphamide
3 Breast cancer
  a) Doxorubicin
  b) Cyclophosphamide, methotrexate, 5FU
4 Ovarian cancer
  a) Cis-platinum or carboplatin
  b) Chlorambucil or cyclophosphamide
5 Choriocarcinoma — methotrexate and actinomycin D
6 Osteosarcoma — methotrexate, doxorubicin, platinum
7 Colorectal cancer — 5FU

Antiemetic regimens in cancer chemotherapy
1 Metoclopramide — incl. high-dose infusion (up to 2 mg/kg q2 h)
2 Dexamethasone — premedicate with 16 mg infusion over 10 min
3 Lorazepam — 2–3 mg orally pretreatment, then 2 mg i.v. q 4 h prn
4 Nabilone — 1–2 mg b.d. starting the night before treatment
5 Phenothiazines (etc.) e.g.
  a) Prochlorperazine, chlorpromazine, droperidol, haloperidol
  b) Fluphenazine 2.5 mg + nortriptyline 25 mg the night before

Infertility following cancer chemotherapy
1 MOPP chemotherapy for Hodgkin's disease
  a) Prepubertal children are less likely to be sterilized
  b) 80% of menstruating women will develop premature menopause
  c) 90% of men will become infertile without sperm banking
  d) Males may be rendered infertile by only 1–2 treatments
  e) Younger adults have better prospects for regaining fertility
2 Chemotherapy for germ-cell tumours
  a) Testicular tumour patients may be oligospermic pretreatment
  b) Virtually all are rendered infertile during PVB treatment
  c) 80% show partial recovery within 18 months of convalescence
  d) Gestational trophoblastic tumour therapy rarely sterilizes
3 Leukaemias and lymphomas
  a) High-dose *intermittent* treatment causes less sterility
  b) Long-duration maintenance therapy (incl. oral alkylating agents) is associated with a high incidence of sterility

SECOND PRIMARY MALIGNANCIES FOLLOWING CANCER THERAPY

Common antecedents of cytotoxic-induced malignancy
1 Treatment of haematological malignancy
   a) Hodgkin's disease, non-Hodgkin's lymphoma
   b) Multiple myeloma (melphalan)
   c) Polycythaemia vera (chlorambucil, ^{32}P)
2 Treatment of 'solid' tumours — ovarian cancer (chlorambucil)

Cytotoxic agents predisposing to second malignancies
1 Alkylating agents (e.g. chlorambucil, melphalan)
2 Nitrosoureas
3 Procarbazine
4 Azathioprine (via immunosuppression rather than mutagenicity; i.e. malignancies [skin SCCs, lymphomas] may be viral in origin)

Cytotoxic agents not implicated in genesis of second malignancies
1 Antimetabolites (except azathioprine)
2 Vinca alkaloids
3 Tumour antibiotics (but note that doxorubicin and actinomycin D may potentiate carcinogenicity of radiotherapy)

Cytotoxic-induced malignancies
1 Acute non-lymphocytic leukaemia* — esp. myelomonocytic
2 Non-Hodgkin's lymphoma — post-transplant/-Hodgkin's
3 SCC (skin, cervix) — post-transplant
4 TCC (bladder) — post-cyclophosphamide
5 Miscellaneous adenocarcinomas and soft-tissue sarcomas

Radiation-induced malignancies
1 Non-lymphocytic leukaemias (AML, CGL; *not* CLL)
2 Myeloma
3 Osteo- and soft tissue sarcoma
4 Thyroid carcinoma (after low-dose external radiation, *not* ^{131}I)
5 Breast cancer (e.g. following multiple fluoroscopies for TB)
6 Lung cancer, esp. small-cell (e.g. in Hiroshima survivors)
7 Hepatic angiosarcoma (Thorotrast)
8 Skin tumours (e.g. after scalp irradiation for ringworm)
9 CNS tumours (meningiomas and other neural tumours) following low-dose (1–2 Gy) scalp irradiation for tinea capitis

Hormone-induced neoplasms
1 Hepatocellular carcinoma — androgenic anabolic steroids
2 Hepatic adenoma — combined oral contraceptive
3 Endometrial carcinoma — exogenous oestrogens
4 Breast cancer — ?endogenous oestrogens
   Prostate cancer — endogenous androgens

*Up to 5% incidence within 10 years of treatment, especially if also treated with radiotherapy

5 Clear-cell vaginal carcinoma — maternal diethylstilboestrol
6 Testicular tumours — maternal obesity/?oestrogens

Familial syndromes predisposing to multiple malignancies
1 Medullary thyroid carcinoma, phaeochromocytoma (MEA II)
2 Pituitary/parathyroid/pancreatic islet cell tumours (MEA I)
3 Retinoblastoma, esp. bilateral (homozygous recessive gene) — associated also with osteosarcoma
4 Intestinal polyposis syndromes
   a) Hereditary (familial) polyposis — colorectal carcinomas
   b) Gardner's syndrome
      — small and large intestinal carcinomas
      — mesodermal tumours
   c) Turcot's syndrome
      — adenomatosis and brain tumours
5 Gorlin's (basal cell naevus) syndrome
   — multiple BCCs
   — medulloblastoma
6 High-incidence premenopausal breast cancer, esp. bilateral
7 'Cancer family syndrome'
   a) Colorectal carcinoma, esp. right-sided; no polyps
   b) Breast/ovary/endometrium/gliomas/sarcomas
8 Skin tumours (esp. melanoma) in dysplastic naevus syndrome

ONCOLOGICAL EMERGENCIES

Management of suspected spinal cord compression
1 Have a high index of suspicion *prior* to onset of paraparesis or urinary symptoms and confirm the diagnosis with urgent myelography. If lesions at multiple levels are demonstrated, surgical management is generally not appropriate
2 Refer the patient for immediate surgical decompression *if*
   a) Paraplegia and/or incontinence have not supervened, *and*
   b) The primary pathology is unknown, *or*
   c) The tumour is known to be radioresistant (e.g. melanoma) *or*
   d) The tumour has recurred following maximal cord irradiation
3 Refer the patient for immediate radiotherapy *if*
   a) The tumour is at least moderately radiosensitive, *and*
   b) Corticosteroids have been commenced
4 Refer the patient for cytotoxic therapy (rarely indicated) *if*
   a) The tumour is exquisitely chemosensitive, *and*
   b) The neurological deficit is neither serious nor fulminant, *or*
   c) Both surgery and radiotherapy are contraindicated

Management of superior vena caval obstruction
1 Confirm the diagnosis with CXR showing

mediastinal widening (or, if necessary, contrast venography or CT)

2 If the primary histological diagnosis is not known, this should be sought by either bronchoscopy with biopsy (shown to be safe in several studies) or, more traditionally, by mediastinotomy. Keep in mind that a small proportion (5%) of cases arise due to benign lesions (e.g. retrosternal goitre, aortic aneurysm)

3 If a tissue diagnosis cannot promptly be obtained, symptomatic relief can often be achieved using presumptive mediastinal irradiation ± steroid cover

4 Obstruction due to small-cell lung cancer or lymphoma may be best treated with systemic chemotherapy in the first instance

5 Although often described as an oncological emergency, the vast majority of SVC obstructions present subacutely and can be managed on a non-urgent (albeit prompt) basis

6 Intravenous lines (esp. if used for administration of vesicant cytotoxic therapy) should not be sited in the arms

Management of cancer-associated hypercalcaemia

1 Judiciously evaluate prospects for survival and quality of life before embarking upon definitive intervention

2 The mainstay of emergency management is intravenous *saline*, 1 litre every 3–4 hours; frusemide also promotes calcium excretion, and is particularly indicated if cardiac or renal failure supervene

3 This initial phase of management should also include
   a) Treatment of the underlying malignancy (e.g. with cytotoxics)
   b) Mobilization if feasible (ensuring adequate analgesia)
   c) Cessation of possible iatrogenic precipitants, e.g. tamoxifen, thiazides, vitamins A or D

4 *Corticosteroids* (prednisone 40 mg/day) may be adjunctive to therapy in myeloma. Myeloma patients with coexisting renal impairment are particularly suitable for treatment with calcitonin (100 U subcutaneously t.d.s.) and steroids; disadvantages of calcitonin include cost, need for parenteral administration, and short-lived effect

5 Intermittent *mithramycin* infusion (daily ×2, then weekly; 15–25 μg/kg) remains a highly effective method of controlling refractory hypercalcaemia in the short term. Potential side-effects include nausea, coagulopathy, and thrombocytopenia

6 *Biphosphonates* (e.g. disodium etidronate) may be given by intravenous infusion

Management of bleeding

1 Cytotoxic thrombocytopenia — platelet transfusion

2 Leucoerythroblastic thrombocytopenia — cytotoxic therapy

3 Hypersplenic thrombocytopenia (e.g. in hairy cell leukaemia) — splenectomy or splenic irradiation

4 Hyperviscosity — plasmapheresis

5 Obstructive jaundice — parenteral vitamin K

6 Uncontrolled neoplastic haemorrhage — radiotherapy

7 Disseminated intravascular coagulation
   a) Fresh frozen plasma (heparin contraindicated)
   b) Platelet transfusion if count $<80 \times 10^9$/l
   c) Cytotoxic therapy of underlying malignancy

Management of urological emergencies

1 Haemorrhagic cystitis — alum irrigation

2 Ureteric obstruction — stents or percutaneous nephrostomy (if prognosis warrants active intervention)

3 Priapism — control of underlying disease

4 Acute retention — catheterization

PAIN IN MALIGNANT DISEASE

Principles of treating malignant pain

1 Large doses

2 Regular rather than 'p.r.n.' administration

3 Oral route if possible

4 Single rather than multiple drugs

5 Hospital admission for severe pain control

6 Narcotic infusions for relief of refractory pain

Indications for parenteral/rectal analgesia

1 Inability to swallow (dysphagia, cachexia)

2 Persistent vomiting

3 Intractable pain despite optimal regular oral dosing

Suboptimal narcotic analgesics for malignant pain

1 Propoxyphene, pentazocine, oral pethidine — weak agonists which may precipitate dysphoria in opiate-dependent patients

2 Dextromoramide (Palfium)
   a) Short (2-hour) duration of action
   b) Rapid development of tolerance

3 Methadone (Physeptone) — prolonged (18–36 h) half-life → risk of cumulative toxicity

Clinical guidelines for use of narcotic analgesics

1 Approximate oral equivalents for 1 mg oral morphine
   a) 50 mg dextropropoxyphene
   b) 15 mg codeine phosphate
   c) 2 mg oxycodone
   d) 0.3 mg dextromoramide (peak effect)
   e) 1 mg methadone

2 Oxycodone suppositories — 30 mg every 8 hours is equipotent to 15 mg oral morphine every 4 hours

3 Morphine: oral-parenteral bioavailability ratio is about 1:3, though there is large variability in dosage requirements between individual patients. No advantage of using diamorphine (heroin) has been established

4 Nausea, if it occurs initially, usually settles after 72 hours of opiate use; constipation, on the other hand, is invariable and should be prevented by routine laxative administration

5 Addiction (cf. tolerance) is rarely a problem in malignant pain, nor is respiratory depression

Suggested oral analgesic regimens for cancer-associated pain

1 Mild — paracetamol 1 g q 4 h, and/or aspirin 600 mg q 4 h (for bone pain)
2 Moderate — dextropropoxyphene 50–100 mg q 4 h, or dihydrocodeine 30–60 mg q 4 h (constipating), or buprenorphine 0.2–0.4 mg q 6–8 h sublingually (emetic)
3 Severe — (dia)morphine 5–200 mg q 3–4 h

Specific indications for adjuvant non-narcotic drug therapy

1 Bone pain — NSAIDs, e.g. aspirin, diclofenac supps.
2 Nerve compression — corticosteroids (dexamethasone)
3 Neuralgias — carbamazepine, sodium valproate
4 Muscle spasm — baclofen, diazepam
5 Neoplastic ulcer — metronidazole (etc.)
6 Insomnia, depression — tricyclics
7 Opiate constipation — lactulose
8 Opiate augmentation ⎫ —phenothiazines,
  Opiate antiemesis ⎭ haloperidol

Neurosurgical approaches to intractable pain in cancer patients

1 Phenol nerve block — e.g. coeliac axis (pancreatic cancer)
2 Dorsal rhizotomy — for pain in trunk, neck or perineum
3 Percutaneous cordotomy — for unilateral pain below C5 dermatome
4 Thalamotomy — for 'central' pain
5 Epidural anaesthesia

Management of bony metastases

1 Bilateral cortical erosion on X-ray of long bone (esp. femur)
  a) Pin prophylactically
  b) Irradiate following surgical fixation
2 Bone pain without gross cortical erosion
  a) Systemic treatment, esp. if hormone-responsive disease
  b) Palliative irradiation
3 Intractable pain in resistant disease (widespread lesions, poor prognosis, adequate marrow reserve) — hemibody irradiation

SURGICAL ASPECTS OF MALIGNANT DISEASE

Potential indications for surgery in premalignant conditions

1 Orchiopexy in children with testicular maldescent Orchidectomy in adolescents or adults with cryptorchidism Bilateral orchidectomy in testicular feminization
2 Oöphorectomy in Turner's syndrome (incl. mosaics)

3 Colectomy in hereditary polyposis, or in long-standing ulcerative colitis with severe dysplasia on biopsy

Potential indications for cytoreductive (debulking) surgery

1 Prechemotherapy
  a) Ovarian cancer
  b) Burkitt's lymphoma
2 Post-chemotherapy
  a) Germ-cell tumours
  b) Osteosarcoma
3 Postradiotherapy
  a) Germ-cell tumours
  b) Head and neck tumours

Opportunities for surgical palliation in malignant disorders

1 Colostomy, gastrojejunostomy or feeding gastrostomy for neoplastic gastrointestinal obstruction
2 Placement of intraluminal silastic (e.g. Celestin) or infant feeding tube in oesophageal obstruction
3 Percutaneous insertion of biliary drainage catheter following transhepatic cholangiography for extrahepatic obstruction
4 Nephrostomy drainage, or passage of ureteric stent(s), for malignant ureteric obstruction
5 Creation of tracheostomy for obstructing laryngeal carcinoma
6 Insertion of Hickman's catheter or implantable infusion port
7 Le Veen shunt for intractable malignant ascites
8 Prophylactic pinning of impending pathological fracture
9 Ventriculoatrial or peritoneal shunt for hydrocephalus
10 Resection of (apparently) solitary metastasis, e.g. in germ-cell tumours, osteosarcoma, hepatic spread of bowel cancer

Approach to intestinal obstruction in the cancer patient

1 Commence nasogastric suction and intravenous fluids
2 If the obstruction does not rapidly resolve following such supportive measures, surgical palliation should be considered
3 Plain abdominal films may establish the obstructive site
4 Small bowel intubation may resolve incomplete obstructions
5 Right transverse colostomy is the treatment of choice for large bowel obstruction, and can be done under local anaesthesia without compromising prospects for subsequent tumour resection

Sexual morbidity of cancer treatment

1 Hysterectomy — infertility
2 Radical prostatectomy — infertility and impotence
3 Mastectomy ⎫ —disturbed sexual self-image,
  Intestinal stoma ⎭ impaired libido

4 Pelvic interstitial radiation — vaginal fibrosis
5 Abdominoperineal resection / Cystectomy } — impotence (exclude depression)
6 Para-aortic lymphadenectomy — retrograde ejaculation

MANAGEMENT ASPECTS OF LUNG CANCER

Contraindications to thoracotomy for lung cancer
1 Small-cell histology
2 Clinical evidence of local extrapulmonary invasion
   a) Hoarseness, bovine cough (recurrent laryngeal nerve palsy)
   b) Superior vena caval obstruction; dysphagia
   c) Pancoast's syndrome; Horner's syndrome
   d) Basal dullness due to pleural effusion (unless chylous) or phrenic nerve palsy
3 Investigational evidence of mediastinal involvement
   a) Carinal widening on chest X-ray
   b) Left main bronchus tumour within 2 cm of carina (bronchoscopy)
   c) Positive node biopsy on mediastinoscopy
4 Evidence of distant spread
   a) Positive liver/bone/brain scan
   b) Malignant cells in marrow or CSF
5 Inability to tolerate surgery
   a) Advanced age: >65 (for pneumonectomy), >70 (for lobectomy)
   b) FEV_1 <1.5 L (for pneumonectomy) or <1.0 L (for lobectomy)
   c) P_aCO_2 >45 mmHg *unless* due to distal collapse
   d) Pulmonary hypertension ± cor pulmonale
   e) General anaesthetic risk factors, e.g. ischaemic heart disease
6 Note that paraneoplastic syndromes *per se* are **not** a contraindication

NB: only 10% of patients are found to be suitable for surgery on initial assessment, and of those only a minority prove resectable

Favourable prognostic features in non-small-cell lung cancer
1 Age <60 years with no coexisting lung disease
2 Symptoms — minimal, no weight loss
3 Right-sided tumour with no demonstrable spread
4 Well-differentiated squamous cell histology
5 Small (<6 cm) primary removable by single lobectomy

Therapeutic modalities in non-small-cell lung cancer
1 Surgery if no contraindications
2 Observation only for minimally symptomatic patients with known extrapulmonary (metastatic or locally invasive) disease
3 *Palliative* irradiation for unresectable symptomatic disease
4 *Radical* irradiation for patients with small-volume localized disease and contraindications to thoracotomy

Adverse prognostic features in small-cell lung cancer
1 Symptoms, esp. weight loss (i.e. poor performance status)
2 Extensive disease, esp. CNS/liver/marrow metastases
3 Cytopenia, esp. thrombocytopenia
4 Mixed (small- and large-cell) histology
5 Failure to achieve complete remission with chemotherapy

Therapeutic modalities in small-cell lung cancer
1 Combination chemotherapy: radical in patients with limited-stage disease (q.v.), palliative if adverse prognostic features present
2 *Prophylactic* cranial irradiation for patients achieving complete remission following cytotoxic treatment
3 *Palliative* cranial irradiation for known cerebral metastases
4 Palliative intrathecal methotrexate ± neuraxis irradiation for meningeal carcinomatosis
5 Palliative irradiation for symptomatic chemoresistant disease

MANAGEMENT ASPECTS OF BREAST CANCER

Biological and prognostic considerations in breast cancer
1 Long-term follow-up of breast cancer patients suggests that there is no disease-free plateau; i.e. it is not strictly 'curable'
2 Axillary dissection is a valuable prognostic (but not therapeutic) measure, i.e. nodes do not 'limit' spread. Hence, breast cancer can be regarded as a systemic disease, the metastatic aggressiveness of which may be predicted by examining the regional nodes
3 The postmastectomy (lumpectomy, quadrantectomy) *disease-free survival* (relapse-free survival) is best predicted by:
   a) The **size** of the primary tumour
   b) The extent of **axillary node involvement**
4 The *postrelapse survival* is best predicted by the **response to hormonal manipulation**

Oestrogen receptor (ER) status and hormone-responsiveness
1 50% of primary breast tumours are ER+
2 50% of such tumours will respond to hormonal manipulation (cf. <5% for ER− tumours)
3 50% of ER+ tumours also have progesterone receptors (PR)
4 50% improvement in response rates is seen in tumours which are both ER+ and PR+ (i.e. 75% will respond)
5 50% of tumours responding to hormonal manipulation will respond to a second-line hormonal manipulation on relapse

Factors favouring response to hormonal manipulation
1 ER (PR)+

2 High absolute level of ER (>100 fmol/mg protein)
3 Response to previous hormonal manipulation
4 Long disease-free interval following resection of primary
5 Metastatic disease confined to bone/soft tissue/pleura
6 Postmenopausal status

Varieties of hormonal manipulation in breast cancer
1 Tamoxifen (an antioestrogen)
2 Progestogens (medroxyprogesterone, megestrol)
3 Aminoglutethimide (inhibits peripheral, but not ovarian, aromatization of androstenedione to oestrone) in *postmenopausal* patients only; esp. effective for painful bone metastases
4 Oöphorectomy (surgical or radiation) } in *premenopausal* patients only
  LHRH analogues (p. 96)
5 Androgens, oestrogens } rarely used now
  Hypophysectomy, adrenalectomy

Potential indications for cytotoxic therapy in breast cancer
1 Symptomatic ER-negative metastatic disease
2 Symptomatic ER-positive metastatic disease with no response to an adequate (six-week) trial of hormonal therapy
3 Metastatic liver disease and/or ascites
4 Lymphangitis carcinomatosa (lymphangitic pulmonary spread)
5 Mastitis carcinomatosa ('inflammatory' carcinoma)

Indications for adjuvant systemic therapy in breast cancer
1 Premenopausal (age <50) women with positive axillary nodes — adjuvant combination cytotoxic therapy (e.g. CMF)
2 Postmenopausal (age >50) women, esp. if ER-positive — adjuvant tamoxifen

(NB: see refs 1.7–1.9 for further discussion)

Surgical and radiotherapeutic aspects of primary breast cancer
1 Chest wall irradiation reduces the rate of local disease recurrence (25%–5%) but does not improve overall survival
2 Tumours less than 2 cm diameter may be treated with simple lumpectomy (± radiotherapy) in preference to mastectomy
3 Tumours more than 4 cm diameter may be treated with simple (rather than radical) mastectomy plus radiotherapy
4 The combination of axillary node dissection and postmastectomy axillary irradiation results in a high (and arguably unjustifiable) morbidity from ipsilateral arm lymphoedema
5 Routine postoperative irradiation is not of proven benefit in stage I (T1N0) disease

Breast cancer in pregnancy: management considerations
1 Prognosis (formerly thought to be grave) is probably little different from other premenopausal breast cancers
2 No role has been proven for therapeutic abortion in modifying the natural history of the disease; hence, it is not indicated
3 Surgery appears to be reasonably tolerated by mother and fetus alike at any stage of pregnancy
4 Chemotherapy is contraindicated in the first trimester; there is no definitive evidence of congenital anomalies due to later administration, but treatment is best postponed if possible
5 Ionizing radiation should be avoided throughout pregnancy
6 Subsequent pregnancies do not need to be discouraged (particularly if disease-free interval >3 years), though mothers should realize that their life expectancy remains reduced; further pregnancies, however, do not appear to affect the natural history of the disease

MANAGEMENT ASPECTS OF TESTICULAR GERM-CELL NEOPLASMS

Surgical considerations in testis tumours
1 Exploration of *any* undiagnosed testicular mass should be undertaken via a transinguinal (not scrotal) approach to prevent possible tumour spread to inguinal nodes; testicular ultrasound may be helpful in the preoperative workup
2 Tumour markers (AFP, β-HCG) should be sent prior to surgery for *any* undiagnosed testicular mass
3 Retrograde ejaculation and sterility may result from para-aortic lymphadenectomy for suspected stage II disease, esp. if bilateral lymphadenectomy is performed
4 Surgical debulking of residual (postchemotherapy) tumour may be of value therapeutically and diagnostically, since
  a) Further chemotherapy may be more effective after debulking
  b) Non-malignant masses may persist after successful therapy
5 Resection of pulmonary metastases may be of value in selected patients

Diagnostic considerations in testis tumours
1 Computed tomographic (CT) scanning of the abdomen and chest has become the staging procedure of choice in most institutions; >50% of teratoma patients will be found to have metastatic spread at presentation (cf. seminoma)
2 Residual abdominal lymph node enlargement on CT scanning following chemotherapy may signify benign differentiated teratoma rather than tumour persistence; nonetheless, provided that tumour markers have returned to normal, surgical exploration is indicated to exclude residual disease
3 Persistent elevation of markers (even in the absence of radiographic disease recurrence) is an indication for reintroduction of cytotoxic therapy
4 The plasma half-life of AFP is 5 days while that of HCG is 30 hours; the rate of decline of these

markers can therefore be used to predict the success or otherwise of therapy administered with curative intent

5 An elevated serum AFP is inconsistent with a diagnosis of pure seminoma. However, 5–10% of seminomas have an elevated β-HCG, indicating the presence of choriocarcinomatous elements

Therapeutic considerations in testis tumours

1 Frequent serial tumour markers should be assayed after *any* therapeutic intervention (if elevated pretreatment) to assess response and need for further treatment
2 Sperm banking should be offered prior to initiation ·of cytotoxic therapy (though the remaining testicle will frequently prove too azoöspermic for preservation of fertility)
3 There is an increased incidence of neoplasia in the remaining testicle; clinical and ultrasound monitoring may be of value
4 Radiotherapy may be curative in stage I and II seminomas
5 Platinum-based chemotherapy (cis-platinum or carboplatin) is the most effective therapeutic modality in teratoma (> stage I) and in seminoma (> bulky stage II); its efficacy may be enhanced by addition of vinblastine, bleomycin or VP-16
6 Grossly elevated tumour markers (AFP >500 ku/L, β-HCG >1000 IU/L, high LDH) indicate a lower probability of complete remission, especially in the context of bulky disease
7 Recent 'surveillance' studies of stage I teratoma suggest that deferral of further treatment ('adjuvant' para-aortic irradiation, or chemotherapy) may be appropriate

THERAPEUTIC MODALITIES IN MISCELLANEOUS MALIGNANCIES

Prostatic carcinoma

1 *Testicular* androgen ablation using either
   a) Bilateral orchidectomy, or
   b) Long-acting LHRH analogues
      — These include buserelin, goserelin, leuprolide
      — Induce continuous LH release, thus suppressing testosterone secretion which relies on cyclic LH pulsatility
      — Not thrombogenic (no decrease in AT-III; cf. oestrogens) but may cause disease 'flare'

   plus
   Adrenal androgen ablation using either
   a) Aminoglutethimide
      — Main action here is inhibition of pregnenolone synthesis from cholesterol, thus blocking adrenal androgen synthesis (cf. peripheral aromatase action in breast cancer)
      — Results in secondary ↑ LH with compensatory increase in testicular androgens; hence, best used in conjunction with orchidectomy or LHRH analogues
   b) Flutamide, nilutamide (non-steroidal

antiandrogens) — block peripheral androgen receptors and prevent disease 'flare'
   c) Ketoconazole
2 Progestational antiandrogens
   a) Cyproterone acetate
      — Reduces testicular *and* adrenal androgens
      — Also *reduces* LH levels
3 Oestrogens
   a) Stilboestrol (DES; 1 mg t.d.s.) — thrombogenic; losing popularity
4 Radical irradiation (for early-stage disease) Cytotoxic therapy (very limited efficacy)

(NB: endocrine therapy for prostate cancer, while relieving symptoms in about 60%, has not been shown to prolong survival)

Bladder carcinoma

1 Superficial tumours
   a) Cystoscopic fulguration
   b) Intravesical cytotoxics (thiotepa, doxorubicin, mitomycin C, BCG)
2 Invasive tumours — radical irradiation followed by salvage surgery (total cystectomy with creation of ileal conduit)
3 Extensive disease
   a) Palliative irradiation
   b) Cytotoxic therapy, e.g. cis-platinum (limited efficacy)

Ovarian cancer

1 Surgical staging and debulking
2 Systemic cytotoxic therapy
   a) Chlorambucil (for minor disease or frail patients)
   b) Cis-platinum/carboplatin (for major disease in fit patients)
3 Intraperitoneal cytotoxic therapy — remains an experimental approach
4 'Second-look' laparotomy
   a) Formerly undertaken if non-invasive staging was negative following 12 months cytotoxic therapy
   b) Has recently fallen into disfavour; no proven survival benefit

Papillary/follicular thyroid carcinoma

1 Subtotal thyroidectomy (if tumour <1 cm, otherwise total)
2 Ablation of metastases with high-dose (50–150 mCi) ^{131}I (i.e. *therapeutic* scan)
3 Long-term TSH suppression using oral thyroxine (200–300 μg/day)
4 Monitoring of disease with serum thyroglobulin estimations and/or whole-body iodine uptake scanning (i.e. *diagnostic* scan)

Medullary carcinoma of the thyroid

1 Total thyroidectomy (i.e. as for anaplastic carcinoma)
2 Exclusion of concomitant phaeochromocytoma/hyperparathyroidism
3 Family screening — plasma calcitonin levels following stimulation by pentagastrin, alcohol or calcium infusion

UNDERSTANDING MALIGNANT DISEASE

CLINICAL TRIALS IN ONCOLOGICAL PRACTICE

Types of clinical drug trials
1 Phase I study: *toxicological* study which ascertains maximum tolerated drug dose and side-effects; performed in heavily-pretreated poor-prognosis patients with informed consent
2 Phase 2 study: using doses found 'safe' in the phase 1 study, patients with various tumour types are treated to determine the new drug's *spectrum of anticancer activity* when used alone
3 Phase 3 study: 'sensitive' tumour types identified by the phase 2 study are treated with the new drug in a prospective randomized *comparison with standard treatment*

Factors confounding interpretation of clinical trials
1 Small numbers
2 Inadequate controls
3 Lack of endpoint definition
4 Insufficient long-term follow-up
5 Publication bias towards positive studies
6 Unstated criteria for patient exclusion/attrition

Strengths and weaknesses of epidemiological studies
1 Case-control studies
  a) Advantages
    — Cheap and quick
    — Relatively few participants required
    — Suitable for rare diseases
  b) Disadvantages — difficult to select control group with matching variables and without biased recall
2 Cohort studies
  a) Advantages
    — Minimal bias
    — Measures incidence as well as relative risk
  b) Disadvantages
    — Large number of participants needed
    — Long follow-up required
    — High attrition rate usual
    — Expensive and slow

AETIOLOGICAL FACTORS IN MALIGNANCY

Viruses implicated in tumorigenesis
1 Epstein-Barr virus
  a) Endemic Burkitt's lymphoma
  b) Nasopharyngeal carcinoma
  c) Primary cerebral lymphoma in immunosuppressed patients
2 Hepatitis B and hepatitis C — hepatoma
3 Papillomavirus (HPV), esp. serotypes 16 and 18
  a) Carcinoma of the cervix
  b) Penile, vulvar, anal carcinoma
  HPV serotype 5/8 — SCCs in renal transplant patients and epidermodysplasia verruciformis
4 HTLV-I and II — T-cell leukaemia/lymphoma
5 HIV — Kaposi's sarcoma in AIDS (indirect)

Premalignant syndromes of chromosomal instability
1 Xeroderma pigmentosum
  a) Ultraviolet light sensitivity
  b) Prone to skin SCCs
2 Ataxia telangiectasia
  a) X-radiation sensitivity
  b) Prone to leukaemias and lymphomas
3 Fanconi's anaemia
  a) DNA crosslinking drug sensitivity
  b) Prone to leukaemias
4 Bloom's syndrome
  a) Oncogenic virus sensitivity
  b) Prone to leukaemias

Cytogenetic aspects of tumour evolution
1 Certain tumours may be characterized by non-random chromosomal rearrangements. Examples include
  a) Hereditary retinoblastoma/osteosarcoma (13q deletion)
  b) Wilms' tumour (11p deletion; associated with aniridia and hemihypertrophy due to adjacent gene deletions)
2 Chromosomal translocations occurring in the vicinity of crucial regulatory genes (loosely called 'oncogenes'; see below) may underlie some malignancies; examples include
  a) Burkitt's lymphoma (8:14 translocation of c-*myc*)
  b) Chronic granulocytic leukaemia (9:22 translocation of c-*abl*)

So what exactly is an oncogene?
1 Cellular 'oncogenes' (c-*onc*), or proto-oncogenes, are normal regulatory genes which share some structural homology with transforming retroviral oncogenes (v-*onc*). Some of these genes can be identified by their ability to 'transfect' the malignant phenotype into partly-transformed cells *in vitro*
2 Putative mechanisms of oncogene action include:
  a) Cellular 'immortalization', e.g. *myc*
  b) Transformation of immortalized cells, e.g. *ras*
  c) Growth factor agonism (autocrine growth), e.g. *sis* (PDGF)
  d) Growth factor receptor production
    — *Erb*-B (EGF receptor)
    — *Erb*-A (oestrogen receptor)
3 Disease associations of oncogene activation include:
  a) *Abl/bcr* gene fusion in chronic granulocytic leukaemia
  b) *Sis* overexpression in myelofibrosis
  c) N-*myc* amplification in neuroblastoma, retinoblastoma
  d) L-*myc* amplification in small-cell lung cancer
4 Putative 'antioncogenes' (i.e. normal genes which, when functioning normally, prevent neoplastic transformation) have been implicated in the genesis of some malignancies, most notably in retinoblastoma (the Rb gene locus)

Tumour cell kinetics and their clinical relevance
1 Tumour too small to be detected by sensitive

screening tests:
a) 1 mm tumour diameter
b) 10^6 tumour cells
c) 20 tumour cell doublings
2 Tumour too small to be symptomatic; detectable by screening
a) 1 cm tumour diameter
b) 10^9 tumour cells
c) 30 tumour cell doublings
3 Tumour clinically evident; advanced disease, usually incurable
a) 1 kg tumour burden
b) 10^{12} tumour cells
c) 40 cell doublings

Malignancies associated with cigarette smoking

1 Lung cancer : SCC > small-cell > large-cell > adenocarcinoma*
2 Squamous cell carcinoma of mouth, larynx and oesophagus†
3 Transitional cell carcinoma of bladder and renal pelvis
4 Weaker associations
a) SCC cervix
b) Acute non-lymphocytic leukaemia
c) Pancreatic adenocarcinoma

OCCURRENCE AND PREVENTION OF CANCER

Incidence of malignant disease††

1 Western-world males
a) Lung cancer (25–30% cancer incidence, 35–40% mortality)
b) Colorectal cancer (10–15% cancer incidence and mortality)
c) Prostate cancer (10% cancer incidence and mortality)
2 Western-world females
a) Breast cancer (20–25% cancer incidence, 15–20% mortality)
b) Colorectal cancer (10–15% incidence and mortality)
c) Lung cancer (10% incidence, and rising; 15% mortality)
3 Commonest malignancies in third-world populations
a) Gastric cancer (commonest malignancy world-wide)
b) Oesophageal and oral cancer
c) Hepatoma
d) SCC cervix

Prognosis of treated malignancies (all stages)

1 Breast cancer ⎫
  Bladder cancer ⎬ 50–60% 5-year survival
  SCC cervix ⎭
2 Colorectal cancer ⎫ 30–40% 5-year survival
  Prostate cancer ⎭

---

*Neither bronchioloalveolar cell carcinoma nor mesothelioma is associated with smoking.
†Nasopharyngeal carcinoma is not associated with either smoking or alcohol ingestion.
††Excluding non-melanomatous skin cancer.

3 Ovarian cancer — 25% 5-year survival
4 Pancreatic cancer ⎫
  Gastric cancer ⎪ 0–10% 5-year survival
  Oesophageal cancer ⎬
  Lung cancer ⎭

Malignancies changing in incidence

1 Cancers increasing in frequency
a) Lung cancer (in third world)
b) Melanoma
c) Early-onset (<35-years-old) SCC cervix
d) Kaposi's sarcoma
e) Testicular tumours
2 Cancers declining in frequency
a) Gastric cancer
b) Lung cancer (in Western middle classes, esp. males)

Geographical clustering of various cancers

1 Hepatoma — Mozambique, South-east Asia
2 Gastric cancer — Japan, Chile, China, USSR
3 Oral cancer — India, South-east Asia
4 Oesophageal cancer — Iran, Turkey, Afghanistan, China
5 Nasopharyngeal cancer — South China; Eskimos
6 Skin cancer — Australia
7 SCC cervix — Chile; Latin America, Asia
8 Penile cancer — Uganda

Preventable cancers

1 Lung cancer and other cigarette-induced neoplasms
2 Skin cancer, esp. non-melanomatous (reduction of uv exposure)
3 Hepatoma (hepatitis B vaccination)
4 SCC cervix (cytological screening, barrier contraception)
5 Oral cancer (vitamin A supplements, cessation of betel-nut)
6 Penile cancer (circumcision)

Dietary factors implicated in carcinogenesis

1 Betel-nut/tobacco chewing ⎫ — oral cancer
  Alcohol, incl. mouthwashes ⎭
2 Alcohol and tobacco ⎫
  Opium; dietary deficiencies ⎬ — oesophageal cancer
  Bracken fern (in Japanese) ⎭
3 Salted fish — nasopharyngeal carcinoma
4 Aflatoxin — hepatoma
5 Over-nutrition (obesity) — endometrial and gallbladder cancer

Major risk factors for various cancers

1 Breast
a) Affected first-degree relative(s)
b) Late age of first full-term pregnancy
2 Endometrial
a) Unopposed exogenous oestrogen administration
b) Long-term adjuvant tamoxifen therapy (ref. 1.9)
c) Obesity, nulliparity, high social class
3 Cervix
a) Early and/or promiscuous sexual activity
b) Low social class

4 Hepatoma
   a) Macronodular cirrhosis (hepatitis B and C, haemochromatosis, α-1-antitrypsin deficiency
   b) Alcohol, aflatoxin, anabolic steroids
   Hepatic adenoma — oestrogens
   Angiosarcoma — Thorotrast, arsenic, vinyl chloride monomer
5 Gallbladder
   a) Gallstones (chronic cholecystitis); obesity
   b) 'Porcelain' (calcified) gallbladder
6 Bile ducts
   a) Inflammatory bowel disease
   b) *Clonorchis sinensis* infestation
7 Colorectal
   a) Affected first-degree relative(s)
   b) Ulcerative colitis, hereditary polyposis
   c) Villous adenoma; Gardner's syndrome
8 Oesophageal
   a) Cigarettes, alcohol; corrosive ingestion
   b) Achalasia, coeliac disease, Plummer-Vinson
   c) Tylosis (rare); Barrett's oesophagus (SCC)
9 Lung
   a) Cigarettes; nickel, chromium, radiation
   b) Asbestos* (synergy with cigarettes)
   c) Scars (predispose to adenocarcinoma)
   d) Scleroderma (predisposes to alveolar-cell)
10 Mesothelioma — asbestos*, esp. 'blue' (crocidolite)
11 Bladder (TCC)
   a) Male sex; past history of bladder cancer
   b) Aromatic dye/naphthalene exposure
   c) Cigarettes, analgesics, cyclophosphamide
   Bladder (SCC) — *Schistosoma haematobium* infestation
12 Thyroid
   a) Low-dose (<2000 rad) irradiation
   b) Multinodular goitre
   c) Gardner's/Cowden's/Werner's syndromes
13 Lymphoma
   a) Radiotherapy, chemotherapy
   b) Sjögren's syndrome
14 Osteosarcoma — Paget's disease; osteogenesis imperfecta
15 Testicular tumours — cryptorchidism, testicular feminization
16 Melanoma — dysplastic naevus syndrome; repeated sunburn in childhood

*Incidence of asbestos-related neoplasms does **not** appear to be dose-related

BACKGROUND FEATURES OF SPECIFIC MALIGNANCIES

The solitary thyroid nodule: factors favouring malignancy
1 Positive family history of medullary thyroid cancer
2 Past history of *low-dose* neck irradiation, esp. in childhood
3 Clinical features — stony hard, non-tender nodule, fixed firm regional lymphadenopathy
4 Elevated serum thyroglobulin (papillary/follicular cancer); calcitonin (medullary carcinoma)
5 'Cold' nodule on scintigraphy
6 Solid lesion on ultrasound

Medullary carcinoma of the thyroid (MTC): clinical considerations
1 80% arise sporadically (i.e. no family history of multiple endocrine adenomatosis: MEA)
2 *Familial* MTC may be either
   a) Isolated familial MTC (least aggressive type)
   b) MTC associated with type IIa MEA
   c) MTC associated with type IIb MEA (rarest and most aggressive)
3 Familial transmission is autosomal dominant — 90% get MTC by age 60; up to 50% have hyperparathyroidism
4 Serum calcium remains normal despite gross elevation of serum calcitonin ± diarrhoea
5 Screen family members (i.e. of *all* index cases) using
   a) Pentagastrin-stimulated calcitonin
   b) Calcium-stimulated calcitonin
   c) Alcohol-stimulated calcitonin
6 Prognosis
   a) Calcitonin <1000 pg/ml: 95% cure
   b) Calcitonin <5000 pg/ml: 90% cure
   c) Calcitonin >10 000 pg/ml: 5% cure

Factors distinguishing osteosarcoma from Ewing's sarcoma
1 Osteosarcoma — usually affects metaphysis (Ewing's: diaphysis)
2 Osteosarcoma — usually affects long bones (Ewing's: flat bones)
3 Osteosarcoma X-ray — Codman's triangle (Ewing's: onionskinning)
4 Osteosarcoma — usually radioresistant (Ewing's: radiosensitive)
5 Osteosarcoma associated with other tumours (e.g. retinoblastoma)

Reviewing the Literature: Cancer Medicine

1.1 Aldridge M C, Sim A J W 1986 Colonoscopy findings in symptomatic patients without X-ray evidence of colonic neoplasms. Lancet 2: 833–834

Study of 97 patients confirming that colonscopy should be the first-line investigation in patients with colonic symptoms, particularly PR bleeding
Hardcastle J D et al 1989 Randomised, controlled trial of faecal occult blood screening for colorectal cancer. Lancet i: 1182–1184
Study of 107 349 asymptomatic subjects showing >10% pick-up rate for cancers and >50% for adenomas in subjects with positive tests. Screening effectively 'down-staged' the detected cancers compared with non-screened controls, but survival benefit is not yet proven

1.2 Caygill C P J, Hill M J, Kirkham J S, Northfield T C 1986 Mortality from gastric cancer following gastric surgery for peptic ulcer. Lancet 1: 929–931

Viste A et al 1986 Risk of carcinoma following gastric operations for benign disease. Lancet 2: 502–504

These studies suggest that patients operated upon for chronic benign gastric ulcer have an increased incidence of adenocarcinoma development subsequently. In the first study, 4466 patients were followed for 20 years postsurgery and found to have a 4.5-fold increased relative risk of gastric cancer; in the second, 3470 patients were reviewed 45 years postoperatively and found to have a 7-fold increased risk

1.3 Giardiello F M et al 1987 Increased risk of cancer in the Peutz-Jeghers syndrome. New England Journal of Medicine 36: 1511–1514

Manchul L A, Jin A, Pritchard K I et al 1985 The frequency of malignant neoplasms in patients with polymyositis-dermatomyositis: a controlled trial. Archives of Internal Medicine 145: 1835–1839

The first of these two studies showed a 20-fold increased risk of gastrointestinal and non-gastrointestinal cancer alike in a cohort of 31 patients with Peutz-Jeghers syndrome. In the second study (71 patients), an excess of many tumour subtypes was confirmed prior to or simultaneous with the diagnosis of polymyositis or dermatomyositis, but no subsequent excess in patients who appeared cancer-free at diagnosis. There was no particular tumour type(s) associated with the development of myositis, no predilection for either sex, and no significant difference in the proportion of dermatomyositis and polymyositis

1.4 Sarrazin D et al 1984 Conservative treatment versus mastectomy in breast cancer. Cancer 53: 1209–1213

Preliminary evidence that small (<2 cm diameter) tumours may best be treated by local excision and chest wall irradiation (many therapists now also treat T2 primary tumours in this way). The evidence for routine nodal irradiation is also questioned, particularly in patients who have undergone axillary dissection

1.5 Tabar L, Fagerberg C J G, Gad A et al 1985 Reduction in mortality from breast cancer screening with mammography: randomized trial from the Breast Cancer Screening Working Group of the Swedish National Board of Health. Lancet 1: 829–832

This trial reported an observed 31% reduction in mortality from breast cancer, and a higher proportion of early-stage tumours, in women offered screening every 2–3 years. Other studies have suggested a 40% reduction in mortality following 3-yearly screening of women aged over 50

1.6 UK Trial of Early Detection of Breast Cancer Group 1988 First results on mortality reduction in the UK trial of early detection of breast cancer. Lancet ii: 411–416

Andersson I et al 1988 Mammographic screening and mortality from breast cancer: the Mälmo mammographic screening trial. British Medical Journal 297: 943–948

Neither the British nor the Swedish trial confirmed a significant effect of mammography on reducing overall mortality from breast cancer, though the Swedish trial suggested a possible benefit in a subset of patients >55 years old

1.7 Nolvadex Adjuvant Trial Organization (NATO) 1985 Controlled trial of tamoxifen as single adjuvant agent in management of early breast cancer. Lancet 1: 836–840

Randomized trial of 1312 patients treated for 5 years with adjuvant tamoxifen; there was a highly significant delay in relapse seen in the adjuvant arm of the study. This general conclusion was later supported by Danish and Scottish studies

Early Breast Cancer Trialists' Collaborative Group 1988 Effects of adjuvant tamoxifen and of cytotoxic therapy on mortality in early breast cancer. New England Journal of Medicine 319: 1681–1692

Overview of 68 clinical trials (involving approximately 30 000 women and 8000 deaths) of adjuvant hormonal or cytotoxic therapy demonstrating the value of this approach. Combination chemotherapy reduced the annual risk of death for women under 50 by about 25% during the first 5 years, while adjuvant tamoxifen reduced this risk by about 20%

1.8 Padmanabhan N, Howell A, Rubens R D 1986 Mechanism of action of adjuvant chemotherapy in early breast cancer. Lancet 2: 411–414

Study of 411 patients showed prolongation of time to recurrence and survival only in ER/PR+ve premenopausal patients, suggesting that adjuvant chemotherapy acts via ovarian suppression rather than via a direct cytolytic effect

1.9 Fornander T et al 1989 Adjuvant tamoxifen in early breast cancer: occurrence of new primary cancers. Lancet i: 117–120

Of 931 patients treated with tamoxifen for an average of 4.5 years, 13 developed endometrial cancer, whereas only 2 out of 915 untreated controls did so in this Swedish study
Bergkvist L et al 1989 The risk of breast cancer after oestrogen and oestrogen-progestin replacement. New England Journal of Medicine 321: 293–297

Apparent two-fold increased risk of breast cancer in women taking oestradiol (but not conjugated oestrogens) for six years, increasing to four-fold if combined with progestins. The debate continues

1.10 Rosenberg S A, Lotze M T, Muul L M et al 1985 Observations on the systemic administration of autologous lymphokine-activated killer cells and recombinant interleukin-2 to patients with metastatic cancer. New England Journal of Medicine 313: 1485–1492

Preliminary report of 25 patients transfused with autologous killer cells activated by recombinant-derived IL-2; there were 10 partial responses and 1 complete response. Fluid retention was the major toxicity. Subsequent studies have been less euphoric

CHAPTER 2
Cardiology

Physical examination protocol 2.1 You are asked to examine the patient's cardiovascular system

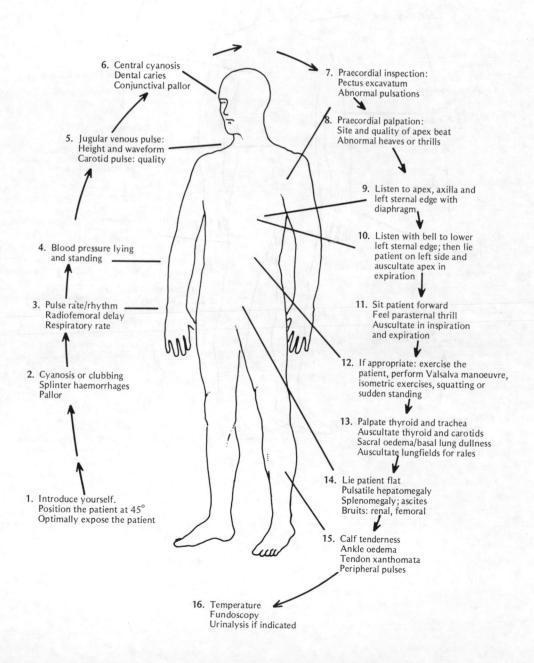

6. Central cyanosis
   Dental caries
   Conjunctival pallor

7. Praecordial inspection:
   Pectus excavatum
   Abnormal pulsations

8. Praecordial palpation:
   Site and quality of apex beat
   Abnormal heaves or thrills

5. Jugular venous pulse:
   Height and waveform
   Carotid pulse: quality

9. Listen to apex, axilla and
   left sternal edge with
   diaphragm

10. Listen with bell to lower
    left sternal edge; then lie
    patient on left side and
    auscultate apex in
    expiration

4. Blood pressure lying
   and standing

11. Sit patient forward
    Feel parasternal thrill
    Auscultate in inspiration
    and expiration

3. Pulse rate/rhythm
   Radiofemoral delay
   Respiratory rate

12. If appropriate: exercise the
    patient, perform Valsalva manoeuvre,
    isometric exercises, squatting or
    sudden standing

2. Cyanosis or clubbing
   Splinter haemorrhages
   Pallor

13. Palpate thyroid and trachea
    Auscultate thyroid and carotids
    Sacral oedema/basal lung dullness
    Auscultate lungfields for rales

14. Lie patient flat
    Pulsatile hepatomegaly
    Splenomegaly; ascites
    Bruits: renal, femoral

1. Introduce yourself.
   Position the patient at 45°
   Optimally expose the patient

15. Calf tenderness
    Ankle oedema
    Tendon xanthomata
    Peripheral pulses

16. Temperature
    Fundoscopy
    Urinalysis if indicated

Physical examination protocol 2.2 You are asked to examine a patient with refractory hypertension

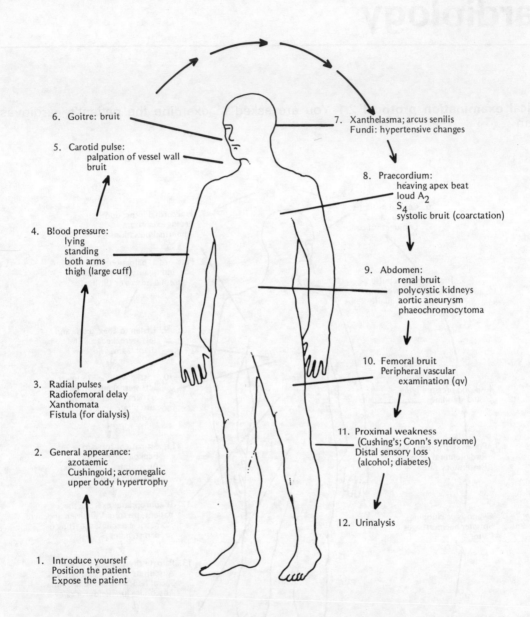

6. Goitre: bruit

5. Carotid pulse:
    palpation of vessel wall
    bruit

4. Blood pressure:
    lying
    standing
    both arms
    thigh (large cuff)

3. Radial pulses
    Radiofemoral delay
    Xanthomata
    Fistula (for dialysis)

2. General appearance:
    azotaemic
    Cushingoid; acromegalic
    upper body hypertrophy

1. Introduce yourself
    Position the patient
    Expose the patient

7. Xanthelasma; arcus senilis
    Fundi: hypertensive changes

8. Praecordium:
    heaving apex beat
    loud A_2
    S_4
    systolic bruit (coarctation)

9. Abdomen:
    renal bruit
    polycystic kidneys
    aortic aneurysm
    phaeochromocytoma

10. Femoral bruit
    Peripheral vascular
    examination (qv)

11. Proximal weakness
    (Cushing's; Conn's syndrome)
    Distal sensory loss
    (alcohol; diabetes)

12. Urinalysis

Physical examination protocol 2.3 You are told that the patient is known to have aortic incompetence, and asked to examine him from that point of view

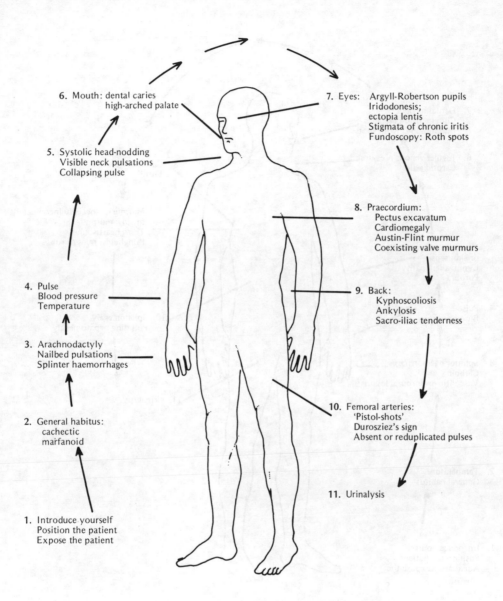

6. Mouth: dental caries
   high-arched palate

7. Eyes: Argyll-Robertson pupils
   Iridodonesis;
   ectopia lentis
   Stigmata of chronic iritis
   Fundoscopy: Roth spots

5. Systolic head-nodding
   Visible neck pulsations
   Collapsing pulse

8. Praecordium:
   Pectus excavatum
   Cardiomegaly
   Austin-Flint murmur
   Coexisting valve murmurs

4. Pulse
   Blood pressure
   Temperature

9. Back:
   Kyphoscoliosis
   Ankylosis
   Sacro-iliac tenderness

3. Arachnodactyly
   Nailbed pulsations
   Splinter haemorrhages

10. Femoral arteries:
   'Pistol-shots'
   Durosziez's sign
   Absent or reduplicated pulses

2. General habitus:
   cachectic
   marfanoid

11. Urinalysis

1. Introduce yourself
   Position the patient
   Expose the patient

Physical examination protocol 2.4 You are asked to examine the patient looking specifically for signs of bacterial endocarditis

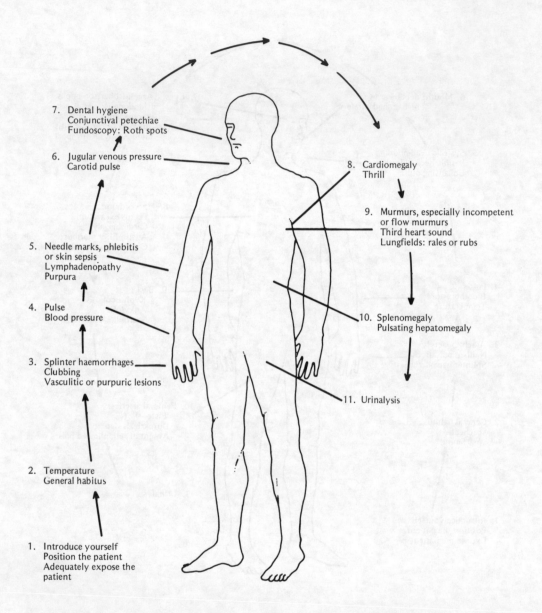

7. Dental hygiene
    Conjunctival petechiae
    Fundoscopy: Roth spots

6. Jugular venous pressure
    Carotid pulse

5. Needle marks, phlebitis
    or skin sepsis
    Lymphadenopathy
    Purpura

4. Pulse
    Blood pressure

3. Splinter haemorrhages
    Clubbing
    Vasculitic or purpuric lesions

2. Temperature
    General habitus

1. Introduce yourself
    Position the patient
    Adequately expose the
    patient

8. Cardiomegaly
    Thrill

9. Murmurs, especially incompetent
    or flow murmurs
    Third heart sound
    Lungfields: rales or rubs

10. Splenomegaly
    Pulsating hepatomegaly

11. Urinalysis

Physical examination protocol 2.5 You are asked to examine the patient's peripheral vascular system

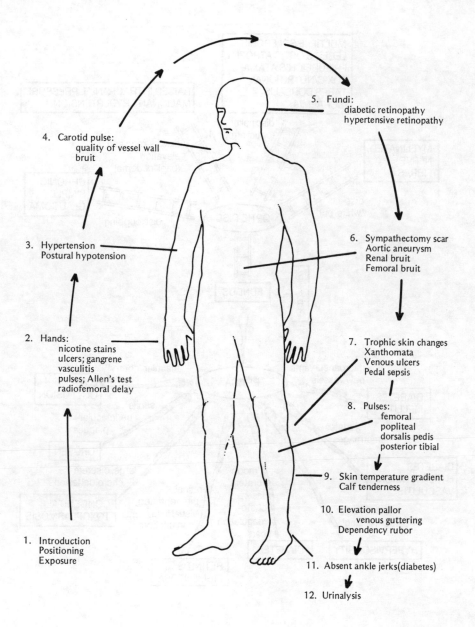

4. Carotid pulse:
   quality of vessel wall
   bruit

5. Fundi:
   diabetic retinopathy
   hypertensive retinopathy

3. Hypertension
   Postural hypotension

6. Sympathectomy scar
   Aortic aneurysm
   Renal bruit
   Femoral bruit

2. Hands:
   nicotine stains
   ulcers; gangrene
   vasculitis
   pulses; Allen's test
   radiofemoral delay

7. Trophic skin changes
   Xanthomata
   Venous ulcers
   Pedal sepsis

8. Pulses:
   femoral
   popliteal
   dorsalis pedis
   posterior tibial

9. Skin temperature gradient
   Calf tenderness

10. Elevation pallor
    venous guttering
    Dependency rubor

1. Introduction
   Positioning
   Exposure

11. Absent ankle jerks(diabetes)

12. Urinalysis

Diagnostic pathway 2.1 This patient has a fundoscopic abnormality. How would you characterize this?

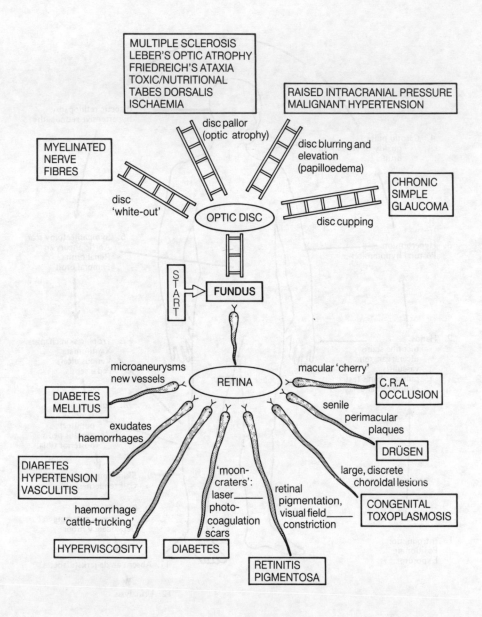

CLINICAL ASPECTS OF CARDIOVASCULAR DISEASE

> **COMMONEST CARDIAC SHORT CASES**
> 1 Mitral and/or aortic valve disease
> 2 Cardiac failure/cardiomyopathy

THE HISTORY

Assessment of cardiorespiratory capacity
(New York Heart Association — NYHA — criteria)
1 NYHA I — dyspnoeic only on severe exertion
2 NYHA II — dyspnoeic walking up hills, stairs
3 NYHA III — dyspnoeic walking on the flat
4 NYHA IV — dyspnoeic at rest

Assessment of chest pain
(modified Canadian Cardiovascular Society criteria)
1 Grade I—angina only on strenuous or prolonged exertion
2 Grade II—angina climbing two flights of stairs
3 Grade III—angina walking one block on the level
4 Grade IV—angina at rest

Pain: how to describe it
1 When?
  a) First onset?
  b) Duration of individual episodes?
  c) Periodicity?
2 Where?
  a) Site of origin?
  b) Radiation?
  c) Effect of different postures?
3 How?
  a) Severity?
  b) Nature?
  c) Exacerbating and relieving factors?

THE PULSE

Clinical abnormalities of pulse character
1 Paradoxical—tamponade/constrictive pericarditis; asthma
2 Collapsing—aortic incompetence, patent ductus arteriosus
3 Plateau—aortic valvular stenosis
4 Bisferiens—mixed aortic valve disease
5 Jerky—hypertrophic cardiomyopathy (HOCM)
6 Alternans—severe left ventricular failure

Differential diagnosis of unequal radial pulses
1 Cervical rib
2 Proximal coarctation
3 Takayasu's arteritis
4 Dissecting aneurysm

The irregularly irregular pulse: differential diagnosis
1 Atrial fibrillation
2 Sinus arrhythmia

3 Multiple atrial or ventricular premature beats
4 Atrial tachycardia or atrial flutter with varying block

Clinical signs of atrial fibrillation
1 Irregularly irregular pulse in time and amplitude
2 Absent 'a' waves in jugular venous pulse
3 Variation in intensity of first heart sound
4 Associated signs of mitral valve disease, cardiomyopathy, thyrotoxicosis

Analysing the jugular venous pulse
1 Normal
  a) 'a' wave — (right) **a**trial systole
  b) 'v' wave — **v**enous filling
  c) 'x' descent — systolic collapse (atrial relaxation)
  d) 'y' descent — diastolic collapse (tricuspid opening)
2 Abnormal 'a' wave
  a) Absent — atrial fibrillation
  b) Giant* — tricuspid stenosis, pulmonary stenosis/hypertension
  c) Solitary — complete heart block
3 Cannon waves
  a) Regular — nodal rhythm
  b) Irregular — complete heart block, ventricular ectopic beats
4 Systolic (ventricular) waves — tricuspid incompetence
5 Rapid 'y' descent — tricuspid incompetence, constrictive pericarditis
6 Slow/absent 'y' descent — tricuspid stenosis, cardiac tamponade
7 Rapid 'x' descent — constrictive pericarditis, cardiac tamponade
8 Fixed elevation — superior vena caval obstruction
9 Absent hepatojugular reflux — inferior vena caval obstruction, Budd-Chiari

THE PRAECORDIUM

Cardiac significance of a left thoracotomy (cf. sternotomy) scar
1 Previous mitral valvotomy
2 Previous repair of aortic coarctation
3 Previous repair of patent ductus arteriosus

Reasons for failure to palpate the apex beat
1 Poor technique
2 Dextrocardia — any cause, incl. right pneumonectomy
3 Pericardial disease — effusion, constrictive pericarditis
4 Other — emphysema, obesity

Palpable heart sounds
1 Palpable S_1 — 'tapping' apex beat (mitral stenosis)
2 Palpable S_4 — 'double' apex beat (HOCM/severe aortic stenosis)
3 Palpable P_2 — pulmonary diastolic 'shock' (pul. hypertension)

---

*Associated with right atrial S_4.
†**Not** 'v' waves; associated with pulsatile liver.

Miscellaneous abnormalities of the apex beat
1 Heaving (sustained): LV pressure load — aortic stenosis, long-standing hypertension
2 Hyperdynamic, displaced: LV volume load — mitral/aortic incompetence, patent ductus arteriosus
3 Dyskinetic — left ventricular aneurysm
4 Displaced to right — dextrocardia, right pneumonectomy
5 Impalpable — pulmonary emphysema, pericardial effusion, constrictive pericarditis

THE HEART SOUNDS

Conditions causing a soft first heart sound
1 Mitral regurgitation
2 Mitral stenosis with rigid valve
3 Cardiomyopathy, left ventricular failure
4 First degree heart block
5 Large pericardial effusion

Conditions causing a loud first heart sound
1 Mitral stenosis with mobile valve
2 Sinus tachycardia (e.g. thyrotoxicosis)
3 Wolff-Parkinson-White syndrome

Splitting of the second heart sound
1 Physiological (i.e. A_2 pre-P_2) — widens on inspiration
2 Paradoxical (P_2 pre-A_2, narrows on inspiration) — LBBB
3 Widely split — RBBB
4 Wide fixed split — ASD
5 Narrow split with loud P_2— pulmonary hypertension
6 Wide split with soft P_2— pulmonary stenosis
7 Loud A_2— systemic hypertension
8 Single S_2 (inaudible A_2) — calcific aortic stenosis

Differential diagnosis of the fixed split second heart sound
1 Atrial septal defect (secundum or primum)
2 Partial anomalous pulmonary venous drainage (rare)
3 Misdiagnosis
   a) Opening snap (mitral stenosis) simulating P_2
   b) Midsystolic click (mitral valve prolapse) simulating A_2

Differential diagnosis of a third heart sound
1 Opening snap in mitral stenosis
2 Fixed split second sound in atrial septal defect
3 Mitral valve prolapse with systolic click simulating S_2

MURMURS OF THE HEART

Features of an 'innocent' murmur
1 Systolic ejection murmur
2 Short (duration <50% systole)
3 Soft, low-pitched and well-transmitted
4 Supine position best for auscultation
5 Single S_2 during expiration while standing
6 Satisfactory ECG and CXR

Characteristics of a venous hum
1 Best heard when sitting up
2 More common on right side
3 Increases during inspiration
4 Louder in diastole
5 Maximal with head turned away
6 Abolished by finger pressure over internal jugular vein

Causes of a late systolic murmur
1 Mitral valve prolapse
2 Aortic coarctation
3 Pulmonary arterial stenosis
4 Hypertrophic cardiomyopathy
5 Papillary muscle dysfunction

Systolic murmur following myocardial infarction?
1 Papillary muscle dysfunction or partial rupture (common) — soft apical murmur, no thrill; clinically stable
   Rupture of chorda tendineae (uncommon) — loud apical murmur, ± thrill; clinically variable
   Complete rupture of papillary muscle (uncommon) — loud apical murmur, prominent thrill; usually fatal
2 Ruptured interventricular septum (common) — loud medial murmur, prominent thrill; may be operable
3 Functional mitral incompetence due to cardiac dilatation
4 Pulmonary systolic murmur due to pulmonary embolism
5 Misdiagnosis: pericardial rub — transmural infarction; Dressler's syndrome

MITRAL STENOSIS

Signs of valve mobility in mitral stenosis
1 Loud S_1
2 Opening snap

Radiographic features of mitral stenosis
1 P-A film
   a) Straight (or convex) left heart border (unless auricle removed at valvotomy)
   b) Double shadow of left atrium behind right atrium
   c) Splaying of subcarinal angle greater than 90°
   d) Dilated upper lobe veins
   e) Prominent pulmonary conus
   f) Pulmonary haemosiderosis
2 Lateral
   a) Left atrial/right ventricular enlargement
   b) Valvular calcification
   c) McCallum's patch (left atrial calcification)
   d) Oesophageal indentation on barium swallow

Echocardiography in mitral stenosis
1 Thickened leaflets; calcification
2 Left atrial enlargement
3 Loss of 'A' point, if in atrial fibrillation
4 Excursion of anterior leaflet less than 20 mm
5 Sustained anterior position of posterior leaflet during diastole (most specific sign)
6 Reduced EF slope (semiquantitative for severity)

Indicators of severity in mitral stenosis
1 Symptoms
2 Signs
  a) Length of diastolic murmur
  b) Proximity of opening snap to S_2
  c) Signs of pulmonary hypertension/congestion
  d) Functional pulmonary incompetence
    (Graham-Steell murmur) or tricuspid
    incompetence
3 CXR
  a) Left atrial/right ventricular enlargement
  b) Pulmonary hypertension and congestion
4 ECG
  a) Atrial enlargement
  b) Right ventricular strain pattern
5 Echo: M-mode
  a) Flattening of EF slope: more than 30 mm/s is
    mild, less than 10 mm/s is severe
6 Catheter
  a) Mitral valve gradient
  b) Elevated right heart pressures
  c) Decreased cardiac output during exercise

Severity of mitral stenosis assessed by 2–D echocardiography
1 Cross-sectional valve area > 2.5 cm^2 —
  asymptomatic
2 Cross-sectional valve area 1.5–2.5 cm^2 —
  symptoms on exercise only
3 Cross-sectional valve area 0.5–1.5 cm^2 —
  symptoms at rest
4 Cross-sectional valve area < 0.5 cm^2 — severe
  stenosis

Contraindications to valvotomy in mitral stenosis
1 Lack of symptoms
2 Significant mitral incompetence
3 Rigid valve
4 Heavily calcified leaflets on
  fluoroscopy/echocardiography
5 Suspicion of left atrial thrombus

Indications for surgery in mitral stenosis
1 Progressive symptomatic deterioration due to
  pulmonary congestion in the absence of
  identifiable reversible factors
2 Recurrent embolic episodes

Mitral stenotic diastolic murmur: differential diagnosis
1 Austin-Flint murmur — non-stenotic mitral flow
  murmur in severe aortic incompetence
2 Graham-Steell murmur — pulmonary incompetent
  murmur in severe mitral stenosis with pulmonary
  hypertension; maximal on inspiration
3 Carey-Coombs murmur — non-stenotic mitral flow
  murmur in acute rheumatic valvulitis
4 Flow murmur in cardiac volume overload (i.e. like
  Austin-Flint)
  a) Severe mitral incompetence
  b) VSD, PDA
  c) Renal failure with fluid overload
5 Tricuspid flow murmur with secundum ASD
6 Left atrial myxoma

Signs favouring an Austin-Flint murmur
1 Cardiomegaly; apex not tapping
2 Soft S_1
3 S_3, no opening snap
4 Murmur reduced by nitrates
5 ECG — left ventricular dominance
6 Echo — flutter on anterior mitral valve leaflet,
  posterior diastolic motion of posterior valve leaflet

MITRAL INCOMPETENCE

Signs of dominance in mixed mitral valve disease
1 Soft S_1; S_3
2 Left ventricular enlargement with thrusting apex
3 ECG showing left ventricular hypertrophy and left
  axis deviation

Clinical assessment of severity in mitral incompetence
1 Degree of left ventricular enlargement
2 Presence of S_3
3 Mid-diastolic flow murmur
4 Thrill; loudness of murmur; pulmonary
  congestion/hypertension

Causes of mitral incompetence
1 Rheumatic
2 Infective endocarditis
3 Mitral valve prolapse
4 Functional (left ventricular dilatation)
5 Ischaemic
  a) Papillary muscle dysfunction
  b) Ruptured chorda tendineae
6 Rheumatoid arthritis; ankylosing spondylitis
7 Associations — Marfan's; 1° ASD; hypertrophic
  cardiomyopathy

Signs favouring acute rather than chronic mitral incompetence
1 Sinus tachycardia
2 Large 'a' wave
3 Minimally displaced apex beat
4 Right ventricular heave with apical systolic thrill
5 Normal intensity S_1; S_4; loud P_2
6 Short (non-pansystolic) murmur radiating well to
  base

LEFT ATRIAL MYXOMA

Diagnostic clues to left atrial myxoma
1 Symptoms
  a) Constitutional
  b) Sudden onset; episodic
  c) Postural
2 Signs
  a) Pansystolic murmur; may be postural
  b) Loud or soft S_1; 'tumour plop'
  c) Sinus rhythm
3 Investigations
  a) Normal CXR
  b) Left atrial mass on 2–D echocardiogram
  c) Positive embolus histology

Echocardiographic differential diagnosis of left atrial myxoma

1 Left atrial thrombus
2 Large mitral valve vegetation (e.g. staphylococcal, fungal)
3 Ruptured chorda tendineae; thick or redundant valve leaflets

MITRAL VALVE PROLAPSE

Clinical associations of mitral valve prolapse

1 Marfan's syndrome; Ehlers-Danlos syndrome
2 Ostium secundum atrial septal defect
3 Wolff-Parkinson-White syndrome
4 Hypertrophic cardiomyopathy
5 Polyarteritis nodosa
6 Adult polycystic disease
7 Postvalvotomy
8 Ischaemic or rheumatic heart disease

Manoeuvres intensifying the murmur

1 Sudden standing
2 Valsalva (phases 2 and 3)

Manoeuvres intensifying the click

1 Squatting
2 Isometric handgrip

ECG abnormalities in mitral valve prolapse

1 Non-specific ST-T wave changes, esp. in inferior leads
2 Frequent atrial or ventricular ectopic beats
3 Prolonged $Q\text{-}T_c$; episodic ventricular tachycardia
4 Wolff-Parkinson-White syndrome (type A)
5 False-positive stress test

Approach to management of mitral valve prolapse

1 Incidental finding / Asymptomatic patient } — reassure and follow up
2 Atypical (non-anginal) chest pain / Normal ECG } — propranolol
3 Exertional chest pain / Exertional dyspnoea } — stress test
4 'Funny turns' / ECG: ST-T wave changes, prolonged $Q\text{-}T_c$ } — Holter monitor
  'Funny turns' with neurological signs / Normal ECG and Holter } — antiplatelet therapy
5 Systolic murmur present — antibiotic prophylaxis
6 Severe mitral incompetence — valve repair/prosthesis

AORTIC INCOMPETENCE

Eponymous signs associated with aortic incompetence

1 Quincke's — capillary pulsation visible on nail compression
2 Corrigan's (pulse) — collapsing pulse
3 Corrigan's (sign) — visible carotid systolic pulsation
4 De Musset's — systolic head nodding
5 Austin-Flint (murmur) — functional mitral diastolic murmur

6 Duroziez's — to-and-fro bruit audible on lightly compressing femoral arteries with diaphragm
7 Traube's — systolic 'pistol-shots' heard over femoral arteries
8 Marfan's (syndrome), Argyll-Robertson (pupils) — aetiologic associations

Clinical indicators of severity in chronic aortic incompetence

1 Presence of symptoms
2 Pulse character, pulse pressure
  Absolute value of diastolic blood pressure
3 Degree of cardiomegaly
4 S_3; Austin-Flint murmur
  Length of diastolic murmur

Indicators of severity in acute aortic incompetence

(e.g. due to infective endocarditis, ruptured chorda)
1 Symptoms and signs of pulmonary venous congestion
2 Secondary mitral valve dysfunction
  a) Soft S_1
  b) Austin-Flint murmur
  c) Premature closure of mitral valve on echocardiography

NB: pulse pressure may *not* be wide despite severe (acute) aortic incompetence

Indications for valve replacement in aortic incompetence

1 Symptoms
2 Increasing heart size on CXR
3 Development of left ventricular strain pattern on ECG
4 Declining exercise tolerance on stress testing
5 Echocardiogram showing left ventricular end-systolic diameter greater than 55 mm in an asymptomatic patient
6 Fall in ejection fraction on exercise gated blood pool scan

Causes of aortic incompetence

1 Valvulitis
  a) Rheumatic
  b) Infective endocarditis
  c) Rheumatoid arthritis
2 Aortitis
  a) Syphilis
  b) Ankylosing spondylitis
3 Annuloaortic ectasia: Marfan's syndrome
4 Hypertension
5 Bicuspid aortic valve
6 Aortic dissection; trauma

Predictors of heart failure following aortic valve surgery

1 Symptoms preoperatively
2 Echo
  a) Fractional shortening less than 25%
  b) Left ventricular end-systolic diameter greater than 55 mm
3 Gated blood pool scan
  a) Left ventricular dysfunction
  b) Fall in ejection fraction on exercise

AORTIC STENOSIS

Indicators of severity in aortic stenosis
1 Pulse character (slowly rising, 'plateau')
  Pulse pressure (narrow)
  Absolute value of systolic blood pressure (reduced)
2 Signs of left ventricular failure
3 S_2: soft, single, or paradoxically split
4 Presence of S_4; thrill; long late-peaking murmur
5 Cardiac catheter — systolic transvalvular gradient
  > 60 mmHg

NB: accurate assessment may be *impossible* without catheterization. Pulse pressure width is unreliable in elderly patients; murmurs may become inaudible in patients with valve calcification, tight stenosis, or cardiac failure; while even the transvalvular gradient measured at catheterization may decline if left ventricular dysfunction supervenes

Prognosis: symptom-related actuarial outcome of aortic stenosis
1 Angina: death within three years (if untreated)
2 Syncope: death within two years
3 Dyspnoea: death within one year
4 Overt cardiac failure: death within six months

Signs of dominance in mixed aortic valve disease
1 Minimal cardiomegaly
2 Anacrotic pulse and narrow pulse pressure
3 S_4; no S_3

Causes and differential diagnosis of aortic stenosis
1 Valvular
  a) Rheumatic
  b) Calcific (degenerative)
  c) Congenital bicuspid valve
  d) Congenital aortic stenosis (with ejection click)
2 Subvalvar
  a) Hypertrophic cardiomyopathy
  b) Congenital subaortic membranous stenosis
3 Supravalvar
  a) Congenital aortic coarctation
  b) Congenital supravalvar aortic stenosis with or without elfin facies and hypercalcaemia

TRICUSPID VALVE DISEASE

Diagnostic clues to tricuspid stenosis
1 History — unexplained symptomatic improvement in context of known mitral stenosis
2 Examination
  a) Giant 'a' waves but no parasternal heave or loud P_2
  b) Diastolic murmur increases on inspiration
  c) Hepatomegaly with presystolic pulsation
3 Investigations
  a) Clear CXR despite marked clinical venous engorgement
  b) Isolated right atrial enlargement on CXR and ECG

Tricuspid incompetence: distinction from mitral incompetence
1 Murmur increases on inspiration

2 Murmur does not radiate well to axilla
3 Systolic waves and steep 'y' descents in jugular venous pulse
4 Pulsatile liver
5 No left ventricular enlargement (i.e. in isolated lesions*
6 Aetiological stigmata
  a) Cyanosis and fixed split S_2— Ebstein's anomaly
  b) Nodular hepatomegaly, telangiectasia — carcinoid syndrome
  c) Needle marks — intravenous drug abuse

INVESTIGATING CARDIOVASCULAR DISEASE

CHEST X-RAYS

Differential diagnosis of pulmonary plethora
1 Atrial septal defect
2 Ventricular septal defect
3 Patent ductus arteriosus (i.e. any left-to-right shunt)

Differential diagnosis of pulmonary oligaemia
1 Pulmonic valvular stenosis
2 Pulmonary atresia
3 Primary pulmonary hypertension (peripheral oligaemia)
4 Massive pulmonary embolism
5 Eisenmenger syndrome; Fallot's tetralogy; transposition (i.e. any right-to-left shunt)

Differential diagnosis of globular cardiomegaly
1 Congestive cardiac failure
2 Congestive cardiomyopathy
3 Pericardial effusion
4 Multiple valvular defects

The 'normal' chest X-ray: checklist
1 Patient's name; film date; correct siding
2 Adequate inspiration; optimal exposure; clavicles centred
3 Relative transradiancy of lungfields (?mastectomy, Swyer-James)
4 *Actively* look for
  a) Retrocardiac mass
  b) Valvular calcification
  c) Rib resection/notching/erosions/fractures
  d) Small pneumothorax, effusion
  e) Gastric air bubble on right (situs inversus)
  f) Nipple shadow (absent on lateral)
5 Ask to see lateral/decubitus/expiratory/erect/apical lordotic views if clinically indicated

ECHOCARDIOGRAPHY

Diagnostic uses of echocardiography
1 Pericardial effusion
2 Mitral valve disease (esp. prolapse or stenosis)
3 Hypertrophic cardiomyopathy

---

*Tricuspid valve lesions most commonly occur in conjunction with other valvular lesions.

4 Infective endocarditis (40% false-negative rate)
5 Cardiac tumours
6 Other
   a) LV aneurysm/clot; aortic dissection
   b) Cardiomyopathies
   c) Bubble contrast study to confirm shunts

Echocardiographic features of left ventricular dysfunction
1 Left ventricular enlargement
2 Reduced fractional shortening
3 Paradoxical septal motion
4 'B' notch; reduced EF slope
5 Premature aortic valve closure

Differential diagnosis of paradoxical septal motion
1 Congestive cardiomyopathy
2 Septal infarction
3 Right ventricular volume overload (e.g. ASD)
4 Conduction disturbance
   a) LBBB
   b) WPW
   c) Right ventricular pacing

Conditions better assessed with M-mode echocardiography
1 Left ventricular hypertrophy
2 Hypertrophic cardiomyopathy

Conditions better assessed with 2–D echocardiography
1 Tricuspid and pulmonary valve disease
2 Measurement of mitral/aortic valve *area*
3 Aortic root lesions (e.g. dissection, ectasia)
4 Regional left ventricular dysfunction

Asymmetric septal hypertrophy: differential diagnosis
1 Hypertrophic cardiomyopathy
2 Infarction of left ventricular free wall
3 Asymptomatic relatives of patients with hypertrophic cardiomyopathy
4 Rarely: left ventricular hypertrophy due to systemic hypertension or valvular aortic stenosis

Valve surgery indicated by echo alone: prerequisites
1 Young patient (<30 years)
2 Single valve involvement (esp. mitral)
3 Consistent clinical picture
4 Technically good echocardiogram

NUCLEAR CARDIOLOGY

Clinical utility of 'hot-spot' ($^{99}Tc^m$ pyrophosphate) scanning
1 Suspected infarct with negative enzymes (e.g. late presentation)
2 Suspected infarct with equivocal enzymes (e.g. postsurgery, intramuscular injection)
3 Suspected infarct with non-diagnostic ECG
   a) Previous infarction
   b) Pacemaker in situ
   c) Left bundle branch block, Wolff-Parkinson-White syndrome
4 Suspected right ventricular or true posterior infarct

NB: Usefulness of hotspot scanning in acute phase of myocardial infarction is limited, since it may take 48 hours to become positive.

Indications for 'cold-spot' (thallium) scanning
1 Preangiographic evaluation of chest pain
   a) Non-diagnostic stress ECG
   b) Male with typical angina and negative stress ECG
   c) Male with atypical chest pain and positive stress ECG
   d) Female with chest pains and positive stress ECG
2 Postangiography
   a) To ascertain exact site of ischaemia in patient with multivessel disease, some of which are ungraftable
   b) To assess functional significance of stenoses seen at angiography and adequacy of collateral circulation
   c) To assess the viability of myocardium apparently jeopardized by stenosis at angiography
3 Postbypass assessment of chest pain
   a) Graft occlusion vs post(peri)cardiotomy syndrome
   b) Graft occlusion vs chest wall pain
   c) Graft occlusion vs ungrafted stenosis
4 Prior to thrombolytic therapy — to assess extent of jeopardized myocardium (may become positive within 4 hours of infarction; cf. hotspot scanning)

Value of gated cardiac blood pool scanning ('equilibrium technique')
1 Assessment of left ventricular function prior to valve replacement or coronary artery surgery
2 Detection of ventricular aneurysms in patients with recurrent ventricular arrhythmias or refractory cardiac failure
3 Distinguishing global cardiomyopathy from segmental ventricular dysfunction (arguably academic)
4 Diagnosis of right ventricular infarction

CARDIAC CATHETERIZATION

Rationale in valvular heart disease
1 To define the nature and severity of the suspected lesion
2 To detect coexisting valvular lesions
3 To assess left ventricular function
4 To determine the state of the coronary arteries
5 To assess pulmonary vascular resistance and/or pulmonary capillary wedge pressure

Other indications for cardiac catheterization
1 Detection and quantification of shunts
2 Electrophysiologic studies
3 Endomyocardial biopsy
   a) Cardiomyopathy/myocarditis
   b) Intracardiac tumour
   c) Post-transplant

Specific indications for coronary angiography
1 Typical angina refractory to medical therapy

2 Typical angina and/or myocardial infarction in a patient younger than 40 years
3 Angina following myocardial infarction
4 Strongly positive exercise test
5 Atypical chest pain
   a) In a male with a positive stress test
   b) In a female with a positive exercise thallium scan

Morbidity of cardiac catheterization
1 Brachial or femoral arterial occlusion; median nerve palsy
2 Coronary dissection; aortic dissection; tamponade
3 Left ventricular perforation
4 Cerebral embolism
5 Ventricular dysrhythmias; death, especially in the setting of left main disease (mortality rate: 2–5/1000)

EXERCISE STRESS (ECG) TESTING

Indications for exercise testing
1 Diagnosis of ischaemic heart disease in patients in whom the diagnosis cannot be made on clinical grounds (e.g. atypical chest pain)
2 Investigation of symptoms suggesting exercise-induced arrhythmias
3 Objective evaluation of symptoms (and/or degree of incapacity) in patients with known coronary artery disease
4 Assessment and rehabilitation of patients following myocardial infarction
   a) Submaximal (symptom-limited) test prior to hospital discharge
   b) Maximal test 6 weeks later (prior to return to work)
5 Assessment of 'at-risk' individuals prior to commencement of an exercise programme

Exclusion criteria
1 Recent prolonged ischaemic chest pain
2 Known severe left main coronary artery disease
3 Severe hypertension, cardiac failure or aortic stenosis
4 Documented recurrent ventricular tachyarrhythmias
5 Left bundle branch block
6 Digoxin administration in the previous seven days

Indicators of test positivity
1 Development of angina
2 Inability to achieve reasonable workload
3 >1 mm downward-sloping ST segment depression
4 Failure of blood pressure to rise

Indications for premature cessation
1 Dizziness, leg pains, severe dyspnoea and/or angina
2 Fall in systolic blood pressure of more than 10 mmHg
3 Ventricular tachyarrhythmias

Causes of false-positive tests
1 Female
2 Anaemia; myxoedema; hypokalaemia; hyperventilation

3 Mitral valve prolapse, valvular stenosis, hypertension or cardiomyopathy
4 Left bundle branch block; WPW; LV 'strain' pattern on resting ECG
5 Recent treatment with digoxin or beta-blockers

Variations on the exercise test theme
1 Combined test — exercise ECG + radionuclide angiography + ^{201}Tl(thallium)scintigraphy
2 ^{201}Tl scintigraphy + dipyridamole — coronary vasodilatation → ↑ ^{201}Tl myocardial uptake *if* coronary arteries normal
3 'Dobutamine test' (= pharmacological exercise test) — may precipitate ischaemia in coronary disease

ELECTROCARDIOGRAPHY (ECG)

Common cardiac rhythm anomalies in athletes
1 Sinus arrhythmia
2 Sinus bradycardia
3 First-degree heart block
4 Wenckebach phenomenon
5 Junctional rhythm

ECG effects of carotid sinus massage
1 Sinus tachycardia — transient slowing
2 Paroxysmal atrial (junctional re-entrant) tachycardia (PAT) — termination (sinus rhythm)
3 Atrial tachycardia/flutter/fibrillation — A-V block
4 Wenckebach phenomenon — A-V nodal block (intra-His block)
5 Tachycardia-dependent bundle branch block — disappearance of block
6 Bradycardia-dependent bundle branch block — appearance of block
7 Demand pacemaker — reinitiation of pacemaker rhythm
8 Ventricular tachycardia — no effect

Causes of a low-voltage ECG
1 Pulmonary emphysema; pericardial effusion
2 Cardiomyopathy; global ischaemia; amyloid heart disease
3 Myxoedema
4 Incorrect calibration

Voltage criteria for left ventricular hypertrophy
1 None is absolute
2 $S(V_1) + R(V_6) > 35$ mm
3 Any R >25 mm; any R + any S >45 mm
4 R(lead I) >20 mm
   R(aVl) >13 mm if cardiac axis normal
   R(aVl) >16 mm if there is left axis deviation

Diagnostic criteria for right ventricular hypertrophy
1 Dominant R wave in V_1; $R(V_1)$ amplitude >7 mm
2 Diagnosis supported by T-wave inversion in V_{1-4} ('strain')
3 Exclusion of other causes of tall $R(V_1)$
   a) RBBB
   b) WPW type A
   c) Dextrocardia

d) Posterior infarction
e) Hypertrophic cardiomyopathy

Left anterior hemiblock: diagnosis and significance
1 Left axis deviation without other cause (LBBB, LVH)
2 Small 'q' in lead I, small 'r' in III
3 May mask inferior infarct

Left posterior hemiblock: diagnosis and significance
1 Axis to the right of +100° without other cause
2 Small 'r' in I, small 'q' in III
3 May mask anterior infarct

Complete heart block: important causes
1 Lenegre's disease: sclerodegeneration of the conduction system
2 Lev's disease: fibrocalcareous encroachment onto the conduction system; often associated with calcific aortic stenosis and preceded by first-degree heart block
3 Ischaemic heart disease; inferior infarct
4 Digoxin toxicity, esp. when associated with ischaemia
5 Congenital (proximal block, narrow QRS, usually asymptomatic)

Criteria for pathological 'Q' wave in standard lead III
1 Duration of 'Q' greater than 0.04 s
2 Presence of 'Q' (aVf) >0.02 s in duration
3 Presence of 'Q' in lead II
4 'Q' (III) >2.5 mm amplitude (unless R(III) >5 mm and P(III) upright)

Some causes of pathological 'Q' waves
1 Transmural myocardial infarction of indeterminate age
2 Left bundle branch block
3 Hypertrophic cardiomyopathy; WPW
4 Hyperkalaemia
5 Amyloid heart disease
6 Cardiac contusion; myocarditis
7 Dextrocardia; reversed limb leads; high lead placement

Causes of an elevated ST-segment
1 Acute myocardial infarction
2 Pericarditis
3 Ventricular aneurysm
4 Coronary spasm
5 Early repolarization

Non-specific ST-T wave changes: some causes
1 Ischaemic heart disease
2 Post-tachycardia
3 Hyperventilation; anxiety
4 Postprandial; cold drinks
5 Mitral valve prolapse
6 Subarachnoid haemorrhage
7 Smoking
8 Phaeochromocytoma
9 Digoxin therapy; hypokalaemia

Causes of a prolonged Q-T$_c$
(in general, Q-T interval <50% R-R interval)
1 Ischaemic heart disease

2 Hypocalcaemia; hypothyroidism; hypothermia
3 Rheumatic carditis
4 Mitral valve prolapse
5 Pulmonary embolism
6 Increased intracranial pressure
7 Heredofamilial
8 Quinidine; tricyclics, phenothiazines, amiodarone

Absent 'p' waves
1 Atrial fibrillation
2 Nodal rhythm; sinoatrial block
3 Severe hyperkalaemia

Inverted 'p' waves in standard lead I
1 Nodal rhythm
2 Dextrocardia
3 Reversed limb leads

ECG manifestations of digoxin therapy
1 Prolonged P-R interval
2 Shortened Q-T$_c$
3 S-T depression ('reverse-tick'); T-wave flattening

ECG manifestations of quinidine therapy
1 Increased QRS width (25% increase may denote toxicity)
2 Prolonged Q-T$_c$; prolonged P-R interval; low wide T-wave
3 Torsade de pointes (polymorphous VT with prolonged Q-T$_c$)

ECG manifestations of hyperkalaemia
1 Peaked ('tent-shaped') T waves
2 P wave flattening
3 Broad QRS
4 Non-specific ST-T wave abnormalities
5 Asystole

ECG localization of acute myocardial infarction
1 Anterior — Q waves/ST elevation V$_{2-4}$
2 Extensive anterior — Q waves/ST elevation I, aVL, V$_{1-6}$
3 Anteroseptal — Q waves/ST elevation V$_{1-3}$
4 Anterolateral — Q waves/ST elevation V$_{4-6}$
5 Inferior — Q waves/ST elevation II, III, aVF
6 True posterior — abnormalities in V$_{1-2}$ (see below)
7 Right ventricular — ST elevation in V$_{4R}$

ECG in true posterior infarction
1 Dominant widened 'R' (V$_{1-2}$)
   — no RBBB/RVH/WPW
2 Tall widened 'T' (V$_{1-2}$)
3 Concave-up ST depression (V$_{1-2}$)
4 Usually associated with signs of inferior infarction

ECG in cor pulmonale
1 Right axis deviation
2 Clockwise rotation
3 P pulmonale (in 20% only)
4 R:S >1 in V$_1$ and aVR
   R:S <1 in V$_6$
5 Right bundle branch block

ECG in rheumatic fever
1 Tachycardia: sinus or idionodal

2 Heart block: first degree or Wenckebach
3 Prolonged Q-T$_c$

ECG with reversed limb leads
1 Lead I appears to have reversed polarity
2 Leads II and III appear interchanged
3 aVr and aVl appear interchanged; aVf is normal

ECG in myotonic dystrophy
1 Sinus bradycardia
2 First degree heart block
3 Left axis deviation

MANAGING CARDIOVASCULAR DISEASE

SURGERY AND THE HEART

Cardiovascular risk factors in general surgery
1 Major
  a) Age >70 years
  b) Myocardial infarction within previous 6 months
  c) Clinical
    — Third heart sound
    — Elevated jugular venous pressure
  d) Catheterization data
    — Ejection fraction <30%
    — Triple vessel/left main disease
2 Minor
  a) Duration of anaesthesia >3 hours
  b) Thoracic or upper abdominal surgery
  c) Aortic stenosis
  d) Hypertension

Potential morbidity of open-heart surgery
1 Left ventricular dysfunction ± perioperative myocardial infarction
2 Cerebral sequelae
  a) Embolism with infarction
  b) Personality change, confusion
3 Bleeding tendency ('post-pump'; syndrome; see below)
4 Delayed complications
  a) Postcardiotomy syndrome
  b) Endocarditis (after valve surgery)
  c) CMV viraemia
  d) Hepatitis

Coronary artery bypass grafting: survival benefit
1 Definite
  a) Left main coronary artery disease
  b) Symptomatic triple-vessel disease
2 Probable
  a) Symptomatic double-vessel disease *plus* impaired left ventricular function
  b) Double-vessel disease *plus* high-grade proximal stenosis of left anterior descending branch of left coronary artery
  c) *Reversible* segmental wall motion abnormalities demonstrable on left ventriculography
(NB: There is **no** hard evidence that coronary artery bypass grafting improves left ventricular function in **any** patient subset)

Factors influencing surgical approach to coronary disease
1 Presence of symptoms uncontrollable by optimal medical therapy (i.e. unstable angina)
2 Size of left anterior descending branch of left coronary artery
3 Amount of myocardium jeopardized by coronary stenoses

Contraindications to coronary artery grafting
1 Lack of symptoms (left main disease is the exception)
2 Inadequate trial of medical therapy
3 Severe left ventricular dysfunction
4 Myocardial infarction within previous month
5 Technically ungraftable vessels

Operability criteria in coronary artery grafting
1 Satisfactory general medical condition
2 Adequate left ventricular function
3 Presence of discrete proximal stenoses with good distal run-off

The 'post-pump' (cardiopulmonary bypass) syndrome: pathogenesis
1 Coagulopathy (may respond to dextran or dDAVP)
  a) Heparin effect
  b) Thrombocytopenia
  c) Massive transfusion (see p. 141)
  d) Coagulation factor depletion
2 Anaemia, leucopenia — mechanical intravascular haemolysis
3 Systemic inflammatory reactions — e.g. 'shock lung' (due to complement activation)

Postcardiotomy (Dressler's) syndrome: clinical features
1 Acute febrile illness within 6 months of heart surgery/infarct
2 Chest pain: pleuritic or pericarditic
3 CXR may show pleural effusion(s), cardiomegaly; ECG often normal
4 Antiheart antibodies may be measurable in plasma
5 Self-limiting; may need NSAIDs, aspirin, steroids, aspiration
6 Diagnosis made by exclusion (DDx: acute myocardial infarction)

PACEMAKING

Indications for permanent pacing
1 Symptomatic bradyarrhythmia (e.g. sick sinus)
2 Acquired (distal) complete heart block — if symptomatic
3 Intermittent Möbitz type II A-V block (wide QRS) documented on Holter monitor
4 Symptomatic patient with bi- or trifascicular block and prolonged H-V interval on electrophysiologic study
5 Alternating RBBB and LBBB
6 Drug-resistant tachyarrhythmias

Indications for transvenous pacing in anterior infarcts
1 Second- or third-degree A-V block

2 New RBBB with pre-existing first-degree heart block/LAHB/LPHB
3 New LBBB with pre-existing first-degree heart block
4 Alternating RBBB and LBBB

Sources of interference
1 Intraoperative unipolar diathermy
2 Arc welding
3 Metal detectors at (some) airports
4 Pectoralis overactivity (rare)
5 Microwave ovens (rare)
6 NMR scanners

Reasons for apparent failure
1 Failure of stimulus artefact
2 Failure of ventricular capture
3 Failure of demand function
   a) Undersensing
   b) Oversensing
4 Symptoms not due to cardiac arrhythmia

Features of the 'pacemaker syndrome'
1 Symptoms include dizziness, syncope, and episodic dyspnoea
2 Caused by ventricular pacemaker inducing *atrial* contraction leading to increased atrial pressure and reduced cardiac output
3 Such retrograde ventriculoatrial conduction may occur despite blockage of anterograde conduction

PROSTHETIC VALVES

Factors influencing valve selection
1 Topographic considerations
   a) Problems in mitral/tricuspid position — thrombosis ± obstruction/embolism
   b) Problems in aortic position — intravascular haemolysis (more so if combined with mitral prosthesis)
2 Ball-in-cage (Starr-Edwards), cloth-covered
   a) Disadvantages — thromboembolism, haemolysis (Silastic > steel)
   b) Advantage — durability
3 Ball-in-cage, non-cloth covered
   a) Disadvantages — audibility, flow impediment (esp. with exercise)
   b) Advantage — less thromboembolism
4 Tilting disc (e.g. Björk-Shiley, St Jude)
   a) Disadvantages — prone to massive thrombosis; audibility
   b) Advantage — excellent haemodynamics
5 Tissue valves (e.g. Hancock, Carpentier-Edwards, Ionnescu)
   a) Disadvantages — lack of durability; prone to calcification, esp. in young patients
   b) Advantage — may obviate necessity for anticoagulation

Features of valvar haemolysis
1 Diagnosis
   a) Signs of gross (para)valvular regurgitation
   b) Normochromic (rarely, hypochromic) anaemia
   c) Blood film: schistocytes, no spherocytes

   d) ↓ Haptoglobin with negative Coombs'/Ham's tests
   e) Haemosiderinuria (implies long-standing haemolysis)
2 Management
   a) Transfusion to normal Hb
   b) Long-term iron (±folate) supplementation
   c) Limitation of activity and/or beta-blockade
   d) Systemic corticosteroids
   e) Valve repair or replacement

Tissue valves: indications for use
1 Elderly patient requiring aortic valve replacement
2 Elderly patient in sinus rhythm with normal size left atrium requiring mitral valve prosthesis
3 Young woman in sinus rhythm desiring pregnancy
4 Any patient with absolute contraindication to anticoagulation

Anticoagulant management of the pregnant patient
1 Use subcutaneous heparin prophylaxis (10 000 U b.d.) throughout first trimester in order to avoid warfarin embryopathy
2 Switch to warfarin at start of second trimester, and maintain until halfway through third trimester (prolonged use of heparin prophylaxis may result in severe osteoporosis)
3 Change back to heparin (subcutaneous at home, infusion in hospital) and monitor closely using protamine sulphate neutralization test and platelet count, esp. prior to delivery (neonatal intraventricular haemorrhage is a major risk)
4 Avoid use of epidural anaesthesia throughout confinement. At delivery, reverse heparin promptly with protamine sulphate.
5 Recommence subcutaneous heparin immediately following delivery
6 Recommence warfarin one week following delivery (not contraindicated in lactation; cf. phenindione)

HEART TRANSPLANTS

Relative contraindications to transplantation
1 Currently acceptable quality of life
2 Age greater than 50
3 Severe pulmonary hypertension
4 Past history of thromboembolism
5 Insulin-dependent diabetes
6 Renal or hepatic insufficiency
7 Major systemic or psychiatric illness
8 Positive cytotoxic crossmatch with donor organ

Signs of rejection
1 Fever (early sign)
2 CXR: cardiomegaly
3 ECG: conduction disturbances, reduced QRS voltage
4 Cardiac failure (late sign)

Indications for heart-lung transplantation
1 Pulmonary hypertension — primary (advanced)
2 Pulmonary hypertension — congenital heart disease (Eisenmenger's)
3 Pulmonary hypertension — secondary to cystic fibrosis

INTERVENTIONAL CARDIOLOGY

Percutaneous transmural coronary angioplasty (PTCA): state of the art
1 80% of angiographic lesions are suitable for attempted PTCA
2 80% of such lesions can be successfully dilated
3 30% of dilated lesions will reocclude within 3 months
4 3–5% of patients will require urgent thoracotomy post-PTCA

Potential indications for PTCA
1 Unstable angina in a patient with single-vessel disease
2 Unstable angina in a patient with multivessel disease and relative (but not absolute) contraindications to thoracotomy
3 Following thrombolytic therapy for acute myocardial infarction

DRUG THERAPY

Elimination pathways of cardioactive drugs
1 Initial hepatic metabolism
  a) Digitoxin
  b) Quinidine
  c) Lignocaine
  d) Anti-anginals
   — Nitrates
   — Propranolol
   — Verapamil
2 Initial renal excretion
  a) Digoxin
  b) Disopyramide
  c) Procainamide

Popular drug combinations in cardiological practice
1 Nifedipine + β-blocker
2 ACE inhibitor + thiazide
3 Sodium nitroprusside + dopamine/dobutamine

Cardiovascular effects of tricyclic antidepressants
1 Tachycardia (anticholinergic effect)
2 Hypotension (esp. postural)
3 Prolonged Q-T$_c$ (quinidine-like effect)
4 Prolonged P-R interval
5 Antagonism of guanethidine and methyldopa
6 Precipitation of ventricular arrhythmias (esp. in overdose)

CALCIUM ANTAGONISTS

Verapamil: absolute contraindications
1 High-degree A-V block
2 Sick sinus syndrome
3 Wolff-Parkinson-White syndrome with anterograde conduction manifesting as recurrent atrial fibrillation/flutter
4 Digoxin toxicity
5 Hypotension, heart failure (some reports indicate that prophylactic i.v. calcium may eliminate negative inotropy)
6 Simultaneous i.v. use with β-blockers

Calcium antagonists: which one?
1 Verapamil
  a) Supraventricular tachycardia
  b) Hypertrophic cardiomyopathy
  c) Angina with tachycardia
2 Nifedipine
  a) Left ventricular dysfunction/cardiac failure
  b) Hypertension — systemic or pulmonary
  c) Sinus bradycardia; impaired AV conduction
  d) Coronary artery spasm
  e) Peripheral vasospasm (Raynaud's)
  f) Peripheral vascular disease
  g) With β-blockers

ANTIARRHYTHMIC THERAPY

Practical classification of antiarrhythmic drugs
1 'AV node' drugs
  a) Digoxin
  b) Verapamil
  c) β-blockers
2 'Ventricle' drugs
  a) Lignocaine
  b) Mexiletine, tocainide
  c) Phenytoin
3 'Whole-heart' (incl. bundle of Kent) drugs
  a) Amiodarone
  b) Disopyramide
  c) Quinidine, procainamide

Electrophysiological classification of antiarrhythmic drugs
1 # I
  a) Block membrane Na$^+$ transport
  b) Reduce rate of action potential rise (phase O depolarization)
  c) E.g. quinidine, procainamide, disopyramide; lignocaine
2 # II
  a) Sympathetic nervous system blockers
  b) Reduce phase 4 depolarization
  c) E.g. β-blockers
3 # III
  a) Prolong duration of action potential and refractory period
  b) No effect on phase O depolarization
  c) E.g. amiodarone
4 # IV
  a) Calcium blockers
  b) E.g. verapamil (*not* nifedipine — no antiarrhythmic action)

Drugs reducing ventricular rate in atrial fibrillation
1 Digoxin
2 Verapamil
3 Amiodarone
4 β-blockers (contraindicated if heart failure likely)

Quinidine: contraindications to use
1 Single agent use in atrial flutter/fibrillation
2 Prolonged Q-T$_c$
3 Hypotension
4 Sick sinus syndrome
5 Intravenous use
6 Myasthenia gravis

Quinidine: toxicity

1 Diarrhoea
2 Nausea, vomiting, abdominal pain; fever
3 Thrombocytopenia, agranulocytosis
4 Cinchonism: tinnitus, deafness, vertigo; toxic amblyopia; sweats, flushing, urticaria
5 Potentiation of digoxin and warfarin toxicity

Disopyramide: toxicity

1 Anticholinergic, esp. urinary retention in males
2 Negative inotropy, esp. when given as an i.v. bolus
3 Ventricular tachyarrhythmias (usually preceded by Q-T_c prolongation)

DIGOXIN THERAPY

Side-effects of digoxin

1 Gastrointestinal: diarrhoea, abdominal pain, intestinal ulceration
2 Central: nausea, anorexia; confusion, convulsions, depression
3 Visual: xanthopsia, haloes, blurring
·4 Headache; facial pain
5 Metabolic: gynaecomastia; hyperkalaemia (rare)

Contraindications to digoxin therapy

1 Wolff-Parkinson-White syndrome
2 A-V block
3 Hypertrophic cardiomyopathy in sinus rhythm (similarly, severe valvular aortic stenosis)
4 Constrictive pericarditis; acute myocarditis
5 Prior to elective cardioversion

Indications for serum digoxin estimation

1 Suspected toxicity
2 Refractory atrial fibrillation
3 Appearance of new arrhythmia(s)
4 Change in renal function
5 Initiation of new treatment, esp. quinidine; amiodarone; verapamil, spironolactone

Metabolic predispositions to digoxin toxicity

1 General
  a) Old age
  b) Pre-existing myocardial disease
  c) Hypoxia, acidosis
2 Renal impairment
3 Hypokalaemia, hypomagnesaemia, hypercalcaemia
4 Hypothyroidism
5 Cardiac amyloidosis

Arrhythmias in digoxin toxicity

1 'Classical'
  a) Atrial fibrillation with slow ventricular response
  b) Non-paroxysmal AV junctional tachycardia
2 Common in elderly patients: increased automaticity
  a) Frequent ventricular ectopic beats (seen in 50%)
  b) Ventricular bigeminy
  c) Ventricular tachycardia (seen in 5%)
3 Common in young patients, esp. overdoses: increased AV block
  a) Junctional rhythm (seen in 20%)
  b) Wenckebach phenomenon

c) Atrial tachycardia with varying block ('SVT with block')
d) Sinus bradycardia

Management of digoxin toxicity

1 Cease digoxin administration
2 Correct electrolyte imbalance. Aim to maintain serum potassium between 4.5 and 5.5 mmol/l. Do not administer potassium in presence of A-V block. Infuse potassium in saline (not in dextrose)
3 A-V block
  a) Atropine, phenytoin
  b) Temporary pacing
4 Supraventricular tachycardia: propranolol
5 Ventricular arrhythmias
  a) Lignocaine, phenytoin
  b) Temporary pacing
  c) (Emergency) cardioversion
6 Antibody (Fab) fragments in refractory cases

SYMPATHOLYTIC AND SYMPATHOMIMETIC THERAPY

Physiological manifestations of adrenergic stimulation

1 α-1 (postsynaptic) stimulation
  a) Peripheral vasoconstriction, pressor effects
  b) Prazosin is a peripheral α-1 antagonist
2 α-2 (presynaptic) stimulation
  a) Sympathetic inhibition
  b) Clonidine is a central α-2 agonist
3 β-1 (predominantly cardiac) stimulation
  a) Tachycardia, positive inotropy
  b) Increased AV conduction
  c) 'Cardioselective' blockers — metoprolol, atenolol, acebutolol
4 β-2 (predominantly peripheral) stimulation
  a) Peripheral vasodilatation
  b) Bronchodilatation
5 Dopaminergic
  a) Low-dose — mesenteric/coronary/cerebral/renal vasodilatation
  b) Moderate-dose — predominantly β-1 effects
  c) High-dose — predominantly α-1-mediated vasoconstriction

Hazards of combining β-blockers with other therapy

1 Verapamil* — depression of myocardial contractility and conduction
2 Ergotamine, dopamine — non-selective blockade of β-1-mediated vasodilatation →severe vasoconstriction and necrosis
3 Prazosin — accentuation of 'first-dose' hypotension
4 Clonidine — exacerbation of withdrawal hypertension
5 Adrenaline — immediate severe hypertension
6 Indomethacin — antagonism of therapeutic hypotensive effect
7 Cimetidine — potentiation of therapeutic hypotensive effect
8 Antianginal therapy of coronary artery spasm — putative antagonism by β-blockade.

---

*Especially parenteral administration.

Rationale of β-blockade in myocardial infarction
1 Within 4 hours of commencement
 (± streptokinase/angioplasty)
 a) May reduce chest pain
 b) May reduce infarct size (and ?cardiogenic shock)
 c) May prevent some arrhythmias (incl. SVT, VF)
2 Subacute phase
 a) Appears to reduce incidence of arrhythmias
 b) No effect on infarct size
3 Postinfarct (maintenance) — reduced mortality and reinfarction rate, esp. in patients with
 a) Modest LV dysfunction
 b) Positive exercise test prior to discharge (this may also indicate need for catheterization and consideration of coronary bypass)
 c) Old age

ANGIOTENSIN-CONVERTING ENZYME (ACE) INHIBITORS

Currently available ACE inhibitors
1 Captopril
 a) Rapid onset of action, short half-life
 b) Requires b.d./t.d.s. dosage regimen (on empty stomach)
2 Enalapril
 a) Hepatically bioactivated to enalaprilat
 b) Slower onset of action; once-daily dosage
3 Lisinopril
 a) Substitution of lysine for proline in enalaprilat
 b) 24-hour duration of action; once-daily dosage
4 Others
 a) Alecapril (prodrug for captopril)
 b) Pentopril, ramipril (long duration of action)

Proposed mechanisms of action of ACE inhibitors
1 Reduction of angiotensin II levels
 a) Vasodilatation
 b) ↓ renin release
 c) ↓ aldosterone secretion
2 Increase in bradykinin levels — vasodilatation
3 Increase in prostacyclin and prostaglandin E2 levels — vasodilatation

Indications for ACE inhibition
1 'Classical' indications
 a) Severe refractory heart failure
 b) Severe refractory hypertension
 c) Renovascular hypertension
 d) Hypertension in scleroderma
 e) Unacceptable toxicity using multidrug regimens
2 Additional (current) indications
 a) First-line therapy of mild-to-moderate hypertension
 b) First-line therapy of congestive cardiomyopathy
 c) ?cardioprotection in acute myocardial infarction

Advantages of ACE inhibitors over conventional antihypertensives
1 Peripheral vascular resistance is reduced
2 Renal, cardiac, and cerebral perfusion is maintained or increased due to selective vasodilating activity
3 No effect on myocardial conductivity or contractility
4 No effect on metabolism of glucose, urate, lipids or electrolytes; safe to use in diabetes and gout
5 Reduce proteinuria and retard nephropathy in hypertensive diabetics
6 Safe to use in asthma and depression
7 Do not cause drowsiness, fatigue or impotence; hence, patient compliance is high

Proven benefits of ACE inhibitors in refractory heart failure
1 Improved haemodynamics — no reflex tachycardia (vasodilating action includes ↓ preload)
2 Improved exercise tolerance and angina threshold — ↓ myocardial oxygen utilization despite ↑ cardiac output
3 Improved renal function and electrolyte balance — no secondary hyperaldosteronism
4 Improved survival

Side-effects of ACE inhibitors
1 Sulfhydryl moiety-related (i.e. seen with captopril/alecapril)
 a) Rash (dose-related; commoner in renal failure)
 b) Taste disturbance
 c) Mouth ulcers
 d) Neutropaenia/agranulocytosis ⎫ Unusual at
 e) Proteinuria/nephrosis ⎬ doses now used
 f) Euphoria ⎭
2 'Class' effects (more common with longer-acting ACE inhibitors)
 a) Hypotension (see below)
 b) Hyperkalaemia (esp. in renal failure)
 c) Cough (may necessitate changing therapy)
 d) Angio-oedema (may be fatal)
 e) Renal insufficiency (esp. in bilateral renal artery stenosis or concurrent loop diuretic therapy)

High-risk scenarios for 'first-dose' hypotension with ACE inhibitors
1 Current diuretic therapy
2 Low-salt diet
3 High-renin hypertension
4 Haemodialysis

VASODILATOR THERAPY

Indications for vasodilator therapy
1 Cardiac failure*
 a) Cardiogenic shock, cardiomyopathy
 b) Acute valvular incompetence; septal rupture
 c) Hypertensive heart failure
2 Hypertension
 a) Crisis (incl. encephalopathy)
 b) Refractory hypertension
3 Angina

Predominant preload reducers
1 Nitrates
2 Frusemide
3 Morphine (in pulmonary oedema)

NB: Frusemide causes initial rapid venodilatation, followed by slower offloading effect due to diuresis

*Hypotension and/or reflex tachycardia do *not* usually occur when vasodilators are used appropriately for CCF

Predominant afterload reducers
1 Hydralazine
2 Minoxidil
3 Nifedipine
4 Prostacyclin (PGI_2)

Pre- and afterload reducers
1 Prazosin
2 ACE inhibitors, e.g. captopril
3 Sodium nitroprusside ('SNIP')
4 Atrial natriuretic factor (ANF)
NB: Nitroprusside best for 'forward failure', e.g. in septal/chordal rupture, acute mitral/aortic incompetence due to endocarditis

Toxicity of prolonged (>48 hour) nitroprusside infusions
1 Cyanide intoxication
2 Lactic acidosis
3 Hypothyroidism

THROMBOLYTIC THERAPY

Potential indications for thrombolytic therapy
1 Massive pulmonary embolism: more than 40% of the vascular bed obliterated
2 Pulmonary embolism with life-threatening haemodynamic deterioration
3 Massive iliofemoral thrombosis (treatment reduces incidence of postphlebitic syndrome)
4 Hyperacute phase of myocardial infarction

Contraindications to thrombolytic therapy
1 Surgery within the last 10 days
2 Cerebrovascular accident within the last 2 months
3 Recent gastrointestinal bleeding, peptic ulcer or arterial puncture
4 Probable intracardiac thrombus (e.g. mitral stenosis with AF)
5 Severe hypertension
6 Proliferative diabetic retinopathy
7 Pregnancy and puerperium
8 Severe chronic liver disease

Monitors of thrombolytic therapy
1 PTTK/APTT, (pro)thrombin time, euglobulin lysis time
2 Resolution of condition requiring treatment (i.e. as determined by lung scan, blood gases, etc.)
3 Overdosage may be corrected by administration of fresh frozen plasma or epsilonaminocaproic acid (EACA)

Indications for pulmonary angiography
1 Suspected massive pulmonary embolus in a patient considered suitable for thoracotomy and thrombectomy
2 Suspected pulmonary emboli in a patient with a relative contraindication to anticoagulation
3 Symptomatic pulmonary hypertension of obscure cause

CORONARY THROMBOLYSIS

Postinfarct thrombolytic therapy: the GISSI criteria
1 No known contraindication to thrombolysis
2 Symptom duration less than 3 hours
3 Patient younger than 65
4 No previous infarcts
5 Anterior infarct

Coronary recanalization efficiency
1 Intravenous streptokinase — 50%
2 Intracoronary streptokinase — 70%
3 Intravenous TPA (tissue plasminogen activator) — 70%

TPA or streptokinase? Points to consider
1 TPA is a recombinantly-produced, naturally-occurring substance which binds to fibrin in clots then activates (cleaves) plasminogen to plasmin, causing localized thrombolysis. Streptokinase (or urokinase) similarly binds to fibrin in clots, but also degrades fibrinogen, leading to **generalized** fibrinolysis
2 Despite the apparently greater specificity of TPA, neither its efficacy nor its safety record have been proven superior to that of streptokinase; both are complicated by cerebral haemorrhage in 0.5–1.0% of cases
3 Clinical trials of TPA have shown 50% (the TIMI-1 study) and 26% (the ASSET study) reductions in death from myocardial infarction
4 Clinical trials of streptokinase have shown 25% (the ISIS-2 study) and 18% (the GISSI study) reductions in death from myocardial infarction, the latter increasing to 50% if given in the first hour of symptoms
5 TPA is far more expensive than streptokinase

UNDERSTANDING CARDIOVASCULAR DISEASE

TACHYARRHYTHMIAS

Management of atrial flutter
1 Slow ventricular rate with digoxin (or intravenous ouabain)
2 If tachycardia persists despite full digitalization, beta-blocker or verapamil may be added provided there is no contraindication.
3 If reversion to sinus rhythm does not occur despite digitalization, quinidine or disopyramide may be added. If quinidine is commenced, the maintenance dose of digoxin should be reduced by 50% pending the attainment of a new steady state
4 If above measures fail, prepare the patient for elective synchronized cardioversion. Commence heparin infusion 48 hours beforehand, and cease digoxin 24 hours prior to cardioversion. Following cardioversion, commence quinidine and maintain for three months.

Cardioversion: indications and contraindications

1 Indications
   a) Coarse ventricular fibrillation
   b) Ventricular tachycardia or rapid atrial fibrillation of recent onset with haemodynamic deterioration
   c) Atrial flutter or paroxysmal atrial tachycardia resistant to medical therapy
2 Contraindications
   a) Suspected intracardiac thrombus
   b) Atrial fibrillation if
      — Long-standing
      — Asymptomatic
      — Associated with thyrotoxicosis
   c) Digoxin toxicity

Rapid atrial fibrillation resistant to digoxin: causes to exclude

1 Inadequately treated cardiac failure ± myocardial infarction
2 Thyrotoxicosis
3 Wolff-Parkinson-White syndrome
4 Mitral stenosis with pulmonary congestion
5 Pulmonary embolism
6 Myocarditis, congestive cardiomyopathy
7 Intracardiac (or pericardial) metastases
8 Digoxin toxicity (**very** rare)

Palpitations in young patients

1 Anxiety; idiopathic
2 Thyrotoxicosis; phaeochromocytoma
3 Pre-excitation
   a) Intranodal bypass tract (commonest)
   b) Wolff-Parkinson-White syndrome
   c) Atrio-His bypass (Lown-Ganong-Levine syndrome)
   d) Intra-atrial/sinus node re-entry

Indications for electrophysiologic study in tachyarrhythmias

1 Wide-complex tachycardias unable to be distinguished from ventricular tachycardia
2 Recurrent ventricular tachycardia
3 Recurrent supraventricular tachycardia with
   a) Haemodynamic compromise
   b) Syncopal episodes
   c) Wolff-Parkinson-White syndrome on resting ECG

Differential diagnosis of wide-complex tachycardia

1 Ventricular tachycardia
2 Wolff-Parkinson-White syndrome with anterograde conduction
3 Supraventricular tachycardia with aberrant conduction

Ventricular tachycardia or SVT with aberrancy? Factors favouring ventricular tachycardia

1 Past history of ventricular disease (e.g. aneurysm)
2 Heart rate <170/min; no effect of carotid sinus massage
3 Clinical evidence of A-V dissociation
   a) Cannon waves in JVP; 'a' waves slower than apex
   b) Beat-to-beat variation in systolic blood pressure
   c) Varying intensity of S_1
4 ECG evidence of A-V dissociation
   a) Dissociated 'P' waves
   b) Fusion beats, capture beats
      — Left axis deviation
      — QRS duration >140 ms
      — QRS morphology different to previous tracings

NB: If unsure, do **not** give verapamil (dangerous in VT); try procainamide instead or, if urgent, cardiovert

WOLFF-PARKINSON-WHITE SYNDROME (WPW)

Associations of WPW

1 Mitral valve prolapse
2 Hypertrophic cardiomyopathy (uncommonly)
3 Ebstein's anomaly; secundum ASD
4 Thyrotoxicosis
5 Male sex; familial

Arrhythmias encountered in WPW

1 Paroxysmal atrial tachycardia — 70%
2 Atrial fibrillation — 10–15%
3 Atrial flutter — 5% (development of one-to-one conduction is considered highly suggestive of the diagnosis)
4 Sinus bradycardia — 1%

Subtypes of WPW

1 Type A
   a) QRS above the isoelectric line in V_1
   b) Simulates posterior or inferior infarction
   c) Accessory pathway connects left atrium and ventricle
2 Type B
   a) QRS below isoelectric line in V_1
   b) Simulates anterior or inferior infarction
   c) Pathway connects right atrium and ventricle (e.g. Ebstein's anomaly)

Management of WPW

1 Observe if minimally symptomatic
2 Medical therapy
   a) Amiodarone
   b) Disopyramide
   c) β-blockers
3 Avoidance of digoxin and carotid sinus massage
4 Surgical division of bundle of Kent (following His-bundle studies) if refractory to medical measures

BRADYARRHYTHMIAS

Causes of bradyarrhythmias

1 Sinoatrial dysfunction ('sick sinus')
   Nodal rhythm
   Complete heart block
2 β-blockade
3 Increased intracranial pressure
4 Metabolic

a) Hypothyroidism
b) Hypothermia
c) Hyperbilirubinaemia (severe)

Indications for electrophysiological study in bradyarrhythmias

1 Normal Holter monitor study in symptomatic patient
2 Cardiac arrest in the absence of myocardial infarction
3 Syncopal episodes associated with
a) Sinus bradycardia
b) Möbitz type I A-V block
c) Bifascicular block with prolonged P-R interval
4 Asymptomatic patient with
a) Möbitz type I and bundle branch block
b) Mobitz type II A-V block
c) 2:1 or 3:1 block with wide QRS

NB: Significant false-positive and -negative rate

ECG manifestations of sick sinus syndrome

1 Prolonged episodes of sinus bradycardia
a) Absolute (<40/min)
b) Relative (e.g. <50/min going up stairs)
2 Profound sinus arrhythmia with symptoms of tissue hypoperfusion
3 Periods of sinus arrest (>2 s)
4 Junctional escape rhythms
5 'Brady-tachy' syndrome: background bradycardia punctuated by paroxysmal bursts of rapid atrial flutter/fibrillation
6 Chronic atrial fibrillation (end-stage sinus node dysfunction)

Diagnosis and management of sick sinus syndrome

1 Holter study (see above)
2 Stress test: excessive tachycardia at submaximal load
3 β-blockade/digoxin: may lead to atropine-resistant bradycardia
4 Electrophysiological study: rapid atrial pacing followed by sinus arrest (2–3 s)
5 Management
a) Repeated emboli — warfarinization
b) Repeated syncope — ventricular demand pacing

AORTIC DISSECTION

Predispositions to aortic dissection

1 Hypertension
2 Congenital bicuspid aortic valve
3 Coarctation
4 Marfan's syndrome
5 Pregnancy

Acute severe chest pain: features suggesting aortic dissection

1 Ascending aorta dissection
a) Marfanoid habitus
b) New aortic incompetent murmur
c) Signs of cardiac tamponade
d) ECG — inferior infarction (right coronary occlusion)[†]

2 Aortic arch dissection
a) Reduced pulse in left arm
b) Asymmetric blood pressure readings
c) Carotid occlusion, esp. left
3 Descending aortic dissection
a) Reduced femoral pulse, esp. on left
b) Microhaematuria (renal infarction)
c) Left basal dullness (haemothorax)

Management priorities in aortic dissection

1 General measures
a) Confirm diagnosis with echo or aortography
b) Transfer to specialist cardiac surgery unit
2 Ascending (de Bakey type I) dissection
a) Reduce aortic filling pressure
— IV propranolol ± nitroprusside infusion
— Nifedipine ± nitroprusside infusion
— Labetalol infusion
b) Urgent thoracotomy to prevent intrapericardial rupture
c) Vascular graft ± aortic valve replacement
3 Descending (de Bakey type III) dissection
a) Urgent treatment of hypertension ± negative inotrope
b) Consider non-operative management
c) Long-term propranolol prophylaxis

AORTIC COARCTATION

Congenital associations of coarctation

1 Bicuspid aortic valve (~90%)
2 Congenital aortic valvular stenosis
3 Ventricular septal defect
4 Patent ductus arteriosus (→ differential cyanosis)
5 Male sex (M:F = 2:1); Turner's syndrome

Radiological features of aortic coarctation

1 Rib notching affecting inferior aspects of posterior ribs (nos 3–8) due to collateralizing anastomoses between internal mammary and inferior epigastric arteries (Dock's sign); not usually present until adolescence.
2 Rib notching confined to right hemithorax indicates coarctation proximal to left subclavian
3 Dilatation of ascending aorta and left subclavian artery visible at the left mediastinal border
4 Poststenotic aortic dilatation (→ 'reverse-3' sign)

Complications of coarctation

1 Intracranial haemorrhage (subarachnoid or intracerebral)
2 Refractory hypertension (normoreninaemic)
3 Aortic dissection/rupture (esp. during pregnancy)
4 Accelerated coronary artery disease
5 Infective endarteritis
6 Perioperative catastrophes
a) Mesenteric infarction
b) Renal ischaemia
c) Paraplegia (due to anterior spinal artery occlusion) — more likely if absent collaterals on angiography

---

[†] Classically the ECG is normal in aortic dissection.

ATRIAL SEPTAL DEFECT (ASD)

Murmurs encountered in ASD
1 Pulmonary flow murmur
2 Tricuspid flow murmur (usually implies large shunt)
3 Pulmonary incompetent (Graham-Steell) murmur of pulmonary hypertension
4 Associated lesions
   a) Late systolic murmur (mitral valve prolapse associated with secundum ASD)
   b) Mitral incompetence (primum lesion)
   c) Mitral stenosis (Lutembacher's syndrome)
   d) Tricuspid incompetence
     — Pulmonary hypertension
     — Primum defect
     — Ebstein's anomaly (with secundum defect)

NB: auscultatory hallmark of ASD is fixed splitting of the second sound

Diagnostic work-up of suspected ASD
1 CXR
   a) Pulmonary plethora
   b) Right ventricular/pulmonary artery enlargement
2 Fluoroscopy: 'hilar dance'
3 ECG
   a) Right axis deviation and incomplete RBBB (secundum)
   b) Left axis deviation and complete RBBB (primum)
   c) First degree heart block (sinus venosus type)
4 Echo
   a) Paradoxical septal motion
   b) Right ventricular enlargement
   c) Visualization of shunt using bubble contrast/indocyanin green
5 First-pass nuclear scan: shunt quantification
6 Cardiac catheterization
   a) Shunt size (oximetry, dye dilution curve)
   b) Pulmonary hypertension
   c) Associated lesions

Indications for surgery in ASD
1 Pulmonary : systemic blood flow >1.5 : 1.0
2 Pulmonary : systemic vascular resistance <0.7 : 1.0

Determinants of shunt magnitude in ASD
1 Relative ventricular compliance
2 Relative resistance of pulmonary and systemic vasculature

OTHER ASPECTS OF CONGENITAL HEART DISEASE

Common congenital heart diseases
1 VSD (30%)
2 ASD (10%)
3 PDA (10%)

Indications for surgery in ventricular septal defect
1 Pulmonary: systemic blood flow >1.5:1.0
2 Pulmonary: systemic vascular resistance <0.5:1.0

Determinants of shunt magnitude in ventricular septal defect
1 Defect size
2 Relative resistance of pulmonary and systemic vasculature

Signs of a developing Eisenmenger complex
1 Decreasing intensity of pulmonary/tricuspid flow murmurs
2 Increasing intensity of P_2; development of single S_2
3 Appearance of Graham-Steell murmur
4 Development of central cyanosis; clubbing (late)

Eisenmenger's syndrome: causes of death
1 Right ventricular failure
2 Massive haemoptysis
3 Cerebral embolism/abscess
4 Pregnancy
5 Anaesthesia

NB: Infective endocarditis rarely occurs in patients with established Eisenmenger's syndrome

Congenital causes of left axis deviation on ECG
1 Ostium primum atrial septal defect
2 Tricuspid atresia
3 A-V communis (endocardial cushion defect)
4 Myotonic dystrophy
5 VSD, PDA

Congenital lesions particularly prone to endocarditis
1 Bicuspid aortic valve
2 Patent ductus arteriosus
3 **Small** ventricular septal defect (*maladie de Roger*)
4 Ostium primum atrial septal defect

INFECTIVE ENDOCARDITIS

Occurrence of infective endocarditis
1 Primary — 40%
2 Previous rheumatic valve damage — 30%
3 Congenital heart disease — 10%
4 Prosthetic valve — 10%
5 Intravenous narcotic abuse — 10%

Features of endocarditis in i.v. drug abusers
1 Predominant valve involvement
   a) Tricuspid
   b) Valve damaged initially by starch/lactose drug contaminants
   c) Subsequently colonized by bacteraemias/fungaemias from unhygienic injection technique
2 Predominant micro-organisms
   a) *Staph aureus*
   b) Enterococci (group D streptococci, e.g. *St. faecalis*)
   c) *Pseudomonas* spp. (e.g. *Ps cepacia, Ps aeruginosa*)
   d) *Candida parapsilosis*
   e) *Bacillus cereus*
   f) *Serratia marcescens*

Predispositions to various organisms
1 Normal valve (± bedsores, i.v. drug abuse) — *Staph. aureus*
2 Rheumatic heart disease (± dental surgery) — *Strep. viridans* (alpha-haemolytic)
3 Sigmoidoscopy/cystoscopy/intrauterine device — *Strep. faecalis*
4 Cardiac surgery, valve prosthesis
   a) *Staph. albus*
   b) Fungi, esp. *Candida* spp.
   c) *Pseudomonas* spp.
   d) JK organism
5 Colonic carcinoma — *Strep. bovis* (classically)

Streptococcal endocarditis: organisms implicated
1 Viridans streptococci, esp.
   St. mitior
   St. sanguis } account for 50% of strep. endocarditis
2 *St. mutans*
   St. bovis } account for 30%
3 *St. milleri*
   Enterococci } account for 15%
4 Group B
   Group A
   Pneumococci } account for <1% each

Factors worsening prognosis of infective endocarditis
1 Prosthetic valve as nidus
2 Cultures negative (40% mortality)
3 *Staph. aureus* isolated from blood cultures
4 Hypocomplementaemia

Negative blood cultures? Some considerations
1 Prior antibiotic therapy
2 Fastidious organism or inappropriate culture medium:
   a) L-forms
   b) Fungi
   c) Rickettsiae, esp. Q fever
   d) Anaerobes
   e) Pyridoxine-dependent streptococci
3 Right-sided endocarditis
4 Sampling error (cultures taken in abacteraemic phase)
5 Misdiagnosis: atrial myxoma, marantic endocarditis
6 Presumptive therapy (? as for *St. faecalis*)

Reasons for fever recrudescence in treated endocarditis
1 Antibiotic inappropriate
   Antibiotic levels subtherapeutic
   Antibiotic resistance
   Antibiotic allergy
   Antibiotic use complicated by superinfection (e.g. fungal)
2 Extensive valve ring infection
3 Metastatic abscesses — splenic, cerebral, myocardial
4 Pulmonary emboli — septic or bland
5 Phlebitis, esp. infected central line

Indications for surgery in infective endocarditis
1 Suspected extensive valve ring infection
2 Refractory heart failure, esp. with aortic incompetence
3 Repeated septic emboli, e.g. due to *H. parainfluenzae*
4 Persistent bacteraemias/fevers despite optimal therapy
5 Massive vegetations demonstrated on echocardiogram
6 Prosthetic valve involvement (esp. fungal or early post-op)

Monitors of established endocarditis
1 Symptoms
2 Temperature
3 Daily physical examination
4 Urinalysis
5 White cell count, haemoglobin, ESR
6 Blood cultures as indicated during antibiotic therapy and following cessation thereof
7 Weekly estimations of minimum bactericidal concentration (MBC) of antibiotic (see below)
8 Neutrophil alkaline phosphatase if abscess formation suspected

Determination of antibiotic dosage in infective endocarditis
1 Streptococcal endocarditis — maintain peak antibiotic level >8x MBC
2 Neutropaenic patients — maintain peak antibiotic level >16x MBC
3 Staphylococcal or pseudomonal endocarditis
   a) Maintain trough antibiotic level >16x MBC
   b) Maintain peak antibiotic level > 32 × MBC

Recommended initial antibiotic therapy if organism unknown
(i.e. if presumptive treatment considered essential)
1 'Community-acquired' endocarditis { — Ampicillin + gentamicin
2 Prosthetic valve
   Drug addict { —Ampicillin + gentamicin + flucloxacillin
3 Elderly patient
   Renal failure { —Ampicillin + netilmicin
4 Major penicillin allergy — vancomycin

Patients requiring procedural antibiotic prophylaxis
1 Past medical history of infective endocarditis
2 Prosthetic heart valves
3 Rheumatic heart disease
4 Most congenital heart disease (exception: secundum ASD)
5 Mitral valve prolapse with incompetence (i.e. with murmur)
6 Hypertrophic cardiomyopathy

Procedures for which prophylaxis recommended
1 Dental surgery with expected gingival bleeding
2 Tonsillectomy, adenoidectomy
3 Rigid bronchoscopy or oesophagoscopy; variceal sclerotherapy
4 Cystoscopy, and most genitourinary surgery
5 Colonoscopy, and most lower gastrointestinal surgery
6 Any surgery involving incision of septic tissue

CARDIAC FAILURE

Concepts and definitions
1 Cardiac failure: a condition in which an adequate cardiac output can only be maintained at the cost of an abnormal elevation of the venous filling pressure
2 Preload: left ventricular end-diastolic pressure
3 Afterload: left ventricular systolic wall tension

Components of afterload
1 Peripheral resistance
2 Arterial compliance
3 Blood viscosity and volume

Radiological signs of cardiac failure
1 Dilated upper lobe veins
2 Kerley 'B' lines
3 Perihilar alveolar opacities
4 Cardiomegaly
5 Effusion(s), esp. on right

Right ventricular failure with a normal chest X-ray
1 Constrictive pericarditis
2 Tricuspid stenosis
3 Pulmonary embolism
4 Restrictive cardiomyopathy
5 Right ventricular infarction

Pulmonary oedema with normal cardiac size on chest X-ray
1 Myocardial infarction
2 Mitral stenosis
3 Constrictive pericarditis
4 Toxic
   a) Chlorine inhalation
   b) Heroin use
   c) Oxygen toxicity
5 Intracranial catastrophe
6 Pneumonia; aspiration; septicaemia; fat emboli

Precipitants of cardiac failure in valvular disease
1 Onset of atrial fibrillation
2 Infective endocarditis
3 Recrudescence of rheumatic fever
4 Lower respiratory tract infection
5 Pregnancy; anaemia; lack of compliance with medication

Diagnostic considerations in refractory heart failure
1 Silent myocardial infarction
2 Pulmonary emboli
3 High-output failure in elderly: thyrotoxicosis, Paget's disease
4 Left ventricular aneurysm
5 Silent valvular stenosis
6 Thiamine deficiency
7 Anaemia
8 Myocarditis
9 Cardiac tamponade; constrictive pericarditis
10 Iatrogenic
   a) Overvigorous diuresis
   b) Tachyarrhythmia due to digoxin toxicity

CXR correlation with pulmonary capillary wedge pressure (PCWP)
1 Dilated upper lobe veins — PCWP = 15 mmHg
2 Kerley B lines — PCWP = 20 mmHg
3 Pulmonary oedema — PCWP = 25 mmHg

NB: Therapeutic normalization of PCWP may precede CXR normalization by up to 48 hours

Therapy according to PCWP
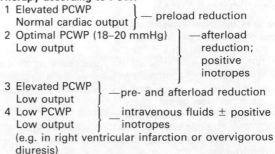
1 Elevated PCWP / Normal cardiac output } — preload reduction
2 Optimal PCWP (18–20 mmHg) / Low output } —afterload reduction; positive inotropes
3 Elevated PCWP / Low output } —pre- and afterload reduction
4 Low PCWP / Low output } —intravenous fluids ± positive inotropes
(e.g. in right ventricular infarction or overvigorous diuresis)

Differential diagnosis of a low central venous pressure (<-3 cm)
1 Warm extremities
   a) Drug overdose
   b) Brainstem lesion
   c) Septic shock
2 Cool extremities, low haemoglobin — haemorrhage
3 Cool extremities, normal/high haemoglobin
   a) Gastrointestinal fluid losses (diarrhoea, vomiting)
   b) Renal fluid loss (e.g. diabetic ketoacidosis)
   c) Third spacing (e.g. rapid accumulation of ascites)

Differential diagnosis of nocturnal dyspnoea
1 Cardiac
   a) Left ventricular failure
   b) Hypertrophic cardiomyopathy; coronary spasm
2 Pulmonary: asthma; extrinsic allergic alveolitis; emboli
3 CNS/pharyngeal: sleep apnoea

ATRIAL NATRIURETIC FACTOR

Atrial natriuretic factor (ANF): its significance in cardiac failure
1 Increased ANF levels are seen in cardiac failure and other oedematous states; this is thought to be *compensatory* rather than pathogenetic
2 Increased atrial filling pressure (esp. right atrium) leads to increased ANF secretion
3 ANF levels are inversely proportional to left ventricular function; deterioration is associated with further ANF elevation
4 Reduction in ANF is seen following successful treatment of cardiac failure

Functions of atrial natriuretic factor
1 Diuretic
   a) Inhibits distal tubular reabsorption of sodium
   b) Promotes excretion of sodium and water (but *not* potassium)

c) May also increase GFR (see below)
2 Vasodilator
  a) Inhibits vasoconstriction mediated by angiotensin II and noradrenaline, suppressing renin-aldosterone axis; also → ↓ ADH
  b) Does not *lead* to reflex tachycardia despite lowering BP

CARDIOMYOPATHY

Features distinguishing restrictive cardiomyopathy from constrictive pericarditis
1 Pulse — no paradox
2 JVP — normal 'y' descent, no Kussmaul's sign
3 Apical impulse — prominent
4 Auscultation — associated A-V valvular incompetence (often)
5 Extra sounds — S_3 (low-pitched)
6 CXR — no pericardial calcification; cardiomegaly
7 ECG — LVH, 'Q' waves, intraventricular conduction disturbances
8 Echo — no pericardial thickening/effusion; LV thickening
9 Catheter
  a) LV end-diastolic pressure >RV end-diastolic pressure
  b) RV systolic pressure >60 mmHg
10 Endomyocardial biopsy — abnormal
11 Therapeutic response — reduction in height of JVP with diuretics

NB: May be *impossible* to distinguish without cardiac catheterization or even thoracotomy

Features distinguishing hypertrophic cardiomyopathy from aortic valvular stenosis
1 Family history — premature sudden death
2 Pulse — jerky (steeply rising)
3 Blood pressure — normal
4 Apex beat — double impulse
5 S_2 — normal quality and splitting
6 Murmur — late systolic (not ejection), maximal at sternal edge
7 Radiation — murmur inaudible in carotids
8 Manoeuvres
  a) Murmur increased by Valsalva/standing/nitrates
  b) Murmur reduced by squatting/isometric exercise
9 Associated sounds — mitral incompetent murmur (often); no click
10 CXR — no valvular calcification or post-stenotic dilatation
11 ECG — septal 'Q' waves; WPW (rarely)

Clinical features favouring myocarditis over cardiomyopathy
1 Young patient
2 Recent history of fevers and myalgias prior to cardiac symptoms
3 Minor cardiomegaly only
4 Episodes of ventricular tachycardia
5 Elevated viral titres (e.g. Coxsackie B, mumps, ECHO, CMV)

HYPERTROPHIC CARDIOMYOPATHY (HOCM)

Causes and associations of HOCM
1 Familial (increased penetrance in males)
2 Friedreich's ataxia
3 Hypertension; aortic stenosis
4 Phaeochromocytoma; thyrotoxicosis
5 Pompe's disease; familial lentiginosis

Echocardiography of HOCM
1 Asymmetric septal hypertrophy (septum more than 12 mm thick, and more than 130% of posterior wall thickness)
2 Systolic anterior motion of anterior leaflet of mitral valve
3 Premature closure of the aortic valve
4 Reduced EF slope due to reduced ventricular compliance

Features of catheterization for HOCM
1 Distorted left ventricular cavity with systolic obliteration
2 Elevated left ventricular end-diastolic pressure
3 Thickened papillary muscles
4 Ejection fraction greater than 85%
5 Postectopic reduction in intra-aortic pressure

Drugs contraindicated in HOCM
1 Digoxin (unless in atrial fibrillation)
2 Other positive inotropes
3 Atropine; other positive chronotropes
4 Nitrates; other vasodilators
5 Diuretics (unless in cardiac failure)
6 Verapamil, if left atrial pressure (or PCWP) is elevated

Principles of management in HOCM
1 Echocardiographic screening of all family members
2 Detection (Holter) and treatment (amiodarone) of ventricular arrhythmias
3 Minimization of strenuous activity *if* obstruction documented
4 Prophylaxis against infective endocarditis
5 Symptoms: β-blockers (do *not* reduce risk of sudden death)
6 Symptoms refractory to medical therapy: septal myomectomy

ISCHAEMIC HEART DISEASE

Reversible independent risk factors for premature heart disease
1 LDL-hypercholesterolaemia
2 Hypertension
3 Smoking

Irreversible risk factors for ischaemic heart disease
1 Increasing age
2 Male sex
3 Positive family history

Unstable angina: definition(s)
1 Recent symptomatic progression
   a) Increasing frequency and/or duration of angina
   b) Development of pain at rest/nocturnally/postprandially
   c) Development of nitrate-resistant angina
2 Recurrent angina despite maximal medical therapy
3 Clinically suspected infarct with negative ECG and enzymes

Clinical features of coronary artery spasm (variant angina)
1 Symptoms (including dizziness) often occur at rest or at night
2 ECG (classically) shows ST-elevation before and during pain
3 Stress ECG typically negative if no associated coronary disease
4 Angiography — absent collateralization, varying stenotic sites
5 Ergometrine test — usually positive, but risky and non-specific
6 Pain relieved by sublingual nitrates, or by prophylaxis with calcium antagonists; may be exacerbated by β-blockers due to unopposed α-adrenergic coronary vasoconstriction

SMOKING

Plasma and urinary markers of cigarette smoke exposure
1 Cotinine (and/or nicotine)
2 Carbon monoxide
3 Thiocyanate
4 Urinary mutagenesis assays

Physiological sequelae of cigarette smoking
1 Increased platelet adhesion/aggregation/whole blood viscosity
2 Increased heart rate; increased catecholamine sensitivity/release
3 Increased carboxyhaemoglobin level, increased haematocrit
4 Decreased level of HDL-cholesterol/vascular compliance
5 Decreased threshold to ventricular fibrillation

Cardiovascular sequelae of cigarette smoking
1 Increased incidence of
   a) Sudden death
   b) Coronary artery disease
   c) Malignant hypertension
   d) Subarachnoid haemorrhage
   e) Ischaemic stroke
2 Increased mortality due to aortic aneurysm
3 Increased morbidity from peripheral vascular disease
4 Increased thromboembolism in patients taking oral contraceptives

Drugs antagonized by cigarette smoking
(due to induction of hepatic microsomal enzymes by smoking)
1 Propranolol
2 Theophylline
3 Lignocaine
4 Imipramine

PASSIVE SMOKING

Passive smoking: characteristics of sidestream smoke
1 Contributes 85% of cigarette smoke in an average 'smoking' room (cf. 15% from exhaled 'mainstream' smoke)
2 Exposure of non-smoking individual living or working with smokers averages 1–2 cigarettes/day
3 Sidestream smoke is of higher pH and contains smaller particles than does mainstream smoke
4 Sidestream smoke contains higher carbon monoxide concentrations than does mainstream smoke

Consequences of passive smoking
1 Increased incidence of lung cancer
2 Worsening of angina and coronary artery disease
3 Exacerbation of asthma
4 Impairment of lung function ($\downarrow$ FEV_1 and forced midexpiratory flow rate) in adults and children
5 $\uparrow$ Bronchitis
   $\uparrow$ Chronic otitis media   } in children of smoking mothers
   $\uparrow$ Tonsillectomy/adenoidectomy

ACUTE MYOCARDIAL INFARCTION

Cardiac arrest: principles of management
1 Praecordial 'thump' — reverts asystole but not VF
   'Blind' defibrillation — reverts VF but not asystole
2 Asystole is treated with intravenous adrenaline
   Fine VF can be 'coarsened' with intravenous adrenaline
   Coarse VF is treated with cardioversion ± i.v. lignocaine
3 Acidosis may often be managed with hyperventilation alone
   Hazards of intravenous sodium bicarbonate administration include pulmonary oedema and hyperosmolality

Cardiac arrest in sinus rhythm (electromechanical dissociation): differential diagnosis
1 Cardiac rupture
2 Cardiac tamponade
3 Massive pulmonary embolism

Bad prognostic indicators in acute myocardial infarction
1 Advanced age
2 Previous infarct
3 CPK — >2000 i.u./ml
4 ECG — development of new intraventricular conduction defects or complex arrhythmias
5 Angiogram — absent collaterals to jeopardized myocardium
6 Cardiogenic shock

'Cardiogenic shock': could it be anything else?

1 Hypovolaemia
  a) Overvigorous diuresis
  b) Third-spacing
  c) Haemorrhage
2 Cardiac tamponade
3 Ruptured interventricular septum or papillary muscle
4 Pulmonary embolism
5 High output failure; adrenal failure; septic shock
6 Anaphylaxis

Common mechanisms of death following myocardial infarction

1 First few hours — VF
2 First few days — pump failure
3 First few months — reinfarction

Myocardial infarction: complications by site

1 Anterior infarction (10% have another infarct)
  a) Ventricular arrhythmias (incl. late-onset VF)
  b) Left ventricular aneurysm or thrombus formation
  c) Cardiac rupture
2 Inferior infarction (20% have another infarct)
  a) Bradycardia; complete heart block
  b) Papillary muscle dysfunction (common)
  c) Papillary muscle/chorda tendineae rupture (rare)
  d) Associated right ventricular infarction
3 Non-transmural infarction (50% have another infarct); i.e. 'subendocardial' infarction
  a) Fewer acute complications than in transmural infarcts
  b) Higher incidence of subsequent infarcts
  c) Similar long-term prognosis

Myocardial infarction without demonstrable coronary artery disease?

1 Coronary microvascular disease
  Coronary artery spasm
  Coronary angiography
2 Aortic stenosis
  Aortic dissection (ascending)
3 Severe hypertension
4 Thyrotoxicosis
5 Arteritis: Takayasu's, PAN

Drugs reducing mortality in acute myocardial infarction

1 Proven benefit
  a) β-blockers
  b) Thrombolytic therapy (strepto-/urokinase, tPA)
2 Suspected benefit
  a) Aspirin
  b) Nitrates

Prevention of reinfarction

1 Stop smoking
2 β-blockade (timolol, metoprolol, propranolol)
3 Aspirin for patients with unstable angina
4 Coronary artery bypass grafting for patients found to have left main disease following positive convalescent stress ECG

HYPERLIPIDAEMIA

Macroscopic appearance of hyperlipidaemic serum

1 Chylomicronaemia — lipaemic supernatant
2 Increased VLDL/IDL — diffusely lipaemic
3 Increased LDL — clear

Incidence and genetics of primary hyperlipidaemias

1 Common hyperlipidaemias
  a) Autosomal dominant transmission (familial)
  b) WHO types IIa, IIb, IV
  c) Major excesses of *cholesterol* and *triglycerides*
    — IIa: — cholesterol (↑ LDL)
    — IIb: — cholesterol (↑ LDL) + triglyceride (↑ VLDL)
    — IV: — triglycerides (↑ VLDL) + cholesterol
2 Uncommon hyperlipidaemias
  a) Autosomal recessive transmission
  b) WHO types I, III, V
  c) Major (primary) excesses of *lipoproteins*:
    — I: — chylomicrons (→ ↑ ↑ triglycerides, ↑ cholesterol)
    — III: — IDL 'remnants' (→ ↑ ↑ cholesterol, ↑ ↑ triglycerides)
    — V: — VLDL (→ ↑ triglycerides), chylomicrons, cholesterol

Clinical characterization of hyperlipidaemias

1 Fasting hypertriglyceridaemia
  a) With chylomicronaemia (I, V) due to lipoprotein lipase (or apo C-II) deficiency
  b) With excess VLDL (IIb, IV, V)
  c) **Not** associated with accelerated atherosclerosis
  d) Symptoms and signs of hypertriglyceridaemia:
    — Eruptive xanthomata (usually regress with therapy)
    — Abdominal pain ± pancreatitis
    — Hepatosplenomegaly
    — Lipaemia retinalis (whitish arteriolar discolouration)
2 Hypercholesterolaemia with excess LDL (IIa, IIb)
  a) Due to primary LDL receptor defect and/or LDL overproduction
  b) Strongly associated with accelerated atherosclerosis
  c) Symptoms and signs of hypercholesterolaemia:
    — Tendinitis, polyarthritis
    — Tendon xanthomata (usually *persist* despite therapy)
    — Planar xanthomata (in homozygotes only)
    — Arcus senilis: pathological if younger than 40
    — Xanthelasma
3 Broad-beta 'remnant' hyperlipidaemia with excess IDL (III)
  a) Strongly associated with accelerated atherosclerosis
  b) Responds well to clofibrate (xanthomata regress)
  c) Symptoms and signs:
    — Tuberous xanthomata (esp. elbows, knees)
    — Linear palmar-crease (planar) xanthomata
    — Peripheral vascular disease

Secondary hyperlipidaemias

1 Predominantly increased cholesterol
  a) Hypothyroidism
  b) Cholestasis (esp. PBC)
  c) Anorexia nervosa
2 Predominantly increased triglycerides
  a) Alcohol abuse
  b) Diabetes mellitus
  c) Chronic renal failure
3 Increased cholesterol and triglycerides
  a) Nephrotic syndrome
  b) Paraproteinaemic states (rarely)
  c) High-dose steroid therapy

Drugs adversely affecting blood lipids

1 Thiazides
2 Non-selective beta-blockers
3 Isotretinoin (for acne)
4 Norgestrel-containing oral contraceptives

} ↑ triglycerides, and/or ↓ HDL-cholesterol

Factors affecting HDL-cholesterol levels

1 Factors associated with low levels
  a) Obesity, dietary sugar
  b) Progestogens, androgens, male sex
  c) Cigarette smoking
  d) Drugs (see above), incl. probucol
  e) Tangier disease, familial LCAT deficiency
2 Factors associated with high levels
  a) Regular exercise (↑ HDL-2)
  b) Oestrogens, female sex
  c) Moderate alcohol intake (↑ HDL-3)
  d) Increasing age/education status
  e) Phenytoin use
  f) Fish oil (e.g. cod liver oil; see below)

Hypolipidaemic states in clinical medicine

1 Bassen-Kornzweig syndrome
  a) ↓ Apolipoprotein B and all lipid fractions except HDL
  b) Characterized by red cell acanthocytosis, ataxia, retinopathy, steatorrhoea and death before middle life
  c) Treatable with vitamin E (± A, D, K) and medium-chain triglycerides
2 Tangier disease
  a) ↓ HDL but no cardiovascular complications; no treatment
  b) Manifests with orange tonsils, neuropathy, splenomegaly, and corneal opacities
3 LCAT deficiency
  a) ↓ HDL, ↑ VLDL
  b) Manifests with atheroma, uraemia, haemolysis

APOLIPOPROTEINS

Apolipoproteins in cardiovascular disease

1 *Apolipoproteins* are the polypeptide components which make up lipoproteins; the 11 apolipoproteins are A-I, A-II, A-IV; B48, B100; C-I, C-II, C-III; D, E, F

2 *Lipoproteins* are water-soluble protein complexes which envelop and transport lipids (cholesterol and triglycerides) in plasma; they comprise LDL, VLDL, HDL, IDL and chylomicrons;
  Lipoprotein (a) antigen [Lp(a)] is a variant LDL which is associated with coronary artery disease
3 *Apolipoprotein B* is the main lipid transport protein:
  a) *Apo B100* is the sole protein constituent of LDL and the major protein constituent of VLDL
  b) *Apo B48* is the major protein of chylomicrons
  c) ↑ Apo B → coronary artery disease
  d) ↓ Apo B → Bassen-Kornzweig syndrome
4 *Apo A-I* is the major protein constituent of HDL
  a) ↓ Apo A-I → hypertriglyceridaemia (#IV, V)
  b) ↓ Apo A-I : apo B → coronary artery disease
5 *Apo C-II* is an activator of lipoprotein lipase
  a) ↓ Apo C-II → fasting chylomicronaemia (#I, V)
6 *Apo E* consists of three isoforms: E3, E4, E2
  a) *Apo E3* is the commonest allele; an abnormal form is found in IDL 'remnants' (#III)
  b) ↑ *Apo E4* → high LDL and cholesterol
  c) ↑ *Apo E2* (uncommon) → low LDL and cholesterol

HYPOLIPIDAEMIC DRUGS

Mechanisms underlying hypolipidaemic therapy

1 Cholestyramine, colestipol
  a) Non-absorbable anion-exchange resins binding bile acids
  b) Reduce LDL (but increase VLDL/triglycerides if used alone)
  c) Use in familial hypercholesterolaemia
2 Clofibrate, bezafibrate, gemfibrozil
  a) Isobutyric acid derivatives activating lipoprotein lipase
  b) Reduce VLDL (clofibrate also reduces IDL and increases LDL)
  c) Use in type III (esp.) or mixed hyperlipidaemias
3 Nicotinic acid, nicofuranose
  a) Nicotinic acid derivatives inhibiting lipolysis
  b) Reduce VLDL predominantly, but also reduce LDL and IDL
  c) Use in hypertriglyceridaemia or as adjunctive therapy
4 Probucol — use with anion-exchange resins in hypercholesterolaemia
5 Mevinolin, synvinolin, lovastatin, simvastatin
  a) HMG CoA reductase (cholesterol synthesis) inhibitors
  b) Also enhance LDL receptor activity
  c) Use in hypercholesterolaemia
6 Fish oils, e.g. eicosapentoic acid
  a) Substitute for essential fatty acids in cell membranes
  b) Metabolized by cyclo-oxygenase pathway to prostaglandins
  c) Reduce platelet aggregation and plasma lipid levels (see below)

Side-effects of hypolipidaemic therapy

1 Cholestyramine/colestipol

a) Constipation (usual), abdominal distension (common), steatorrhoea (only with large doses)
b) Nausea, vomiting
c) Reduced absorption of digoxin, thyroxine, warfarin, folate and fat-soluble vitamins (A,D,E,K)
2 Clofibrate/bezafibrate/gemfibrozil
a) Nausea, abdominal discomfort
b) Gallstones, cholecystitis
c) Transaminitis
d) Loss of libido, alopecia, weight gain
e) Myopathy (esp. if hypoalbuminaemic or azotaemic)
f) Potentiation of warfarin
3 Nicotinic acid
a) Flushing; headaches
b) Pruritus, pigmentation
c) Nausea, abdominal pain, diarrhoea
d) Hepatotoxicity; cholestasis
e) Gout, glucose intolerance

FISH OIL

Observations suggesting cardiovascular benefits of fish oil
1 Fish oils, esp. those containing the omega-3-polyunsaturated acids eicosapentaenoic acid (EPA) and docosahexaenoic acid (DHA), are abundant in the diet of populations with little coronary disease, e.g. Eskimos and Japanese
2 An elevated platelet membrane omega-3:omega-6 fatty acid ratio is associated with reduced incidence of coronary disease
3 Dietary omega-3-polyunsaturated fatty acids are associated with the following alterations in atherogenic risk factors:
a) Reduced plasma cholesterol and triglycerides
b) Reduced VLDL and LDL, increased HDL
c) Reduced blood pressure
4 Dietary omega-3-polyunsaturated fatty acids are associated with the following alterations in thrombogenic risk factors:
a) Increased bleeding time (reduced platelet aggregation)
b) Reduced platelet thromboxane A_2
c) Increased vascular prostacyclin
d) Reduced platelet reactivity to ADP, adrenaline, thrombin

Other diseases reportedly responsive to fish oil supplements
1 Rheumatoid arthritis
2 Psoriasis
3 Migraine

Fish oil: putative mechanisms of action
1 Antiatherogenic action ($\rightarrow \downarrow$ coronary artery disease) — $\downarrow$ cholesterol, LDL/VLDL, triglycerides; $\uparrow$ HDL
2 Antithrombotic action ($\rightarrow \downarrow$ incidence of vascular 'events') — competitive inhibition of arachidonic acid
— Cyclo-oxygenase inhibition
— $\downarrow$ Thromboxane A_2-mediated platelet aggregation

3 Anti-inflammatory action ($? \rightarrow \downarrow$ severity of arthritis, migraine) — competitive inhibition of arachidonic acid
$\rightarrow$Lipo-oxygenase inhibition; $\downarrow$IL-1; $\downarrow$ TNF
$\rightarrow \downarrow$ Leukotriene B4-mediated neutrophil chemotaxis

HYPERTENSION

Differential diagnosis of hypertension
'RECAP'
1 'R' — Renal
a) Renal artery stenosis
b) Chronic renal failure with fluid overload
c) Unilateral parenchymal renal disease
d) Polycystic kidneys
2 'E' — Essential
Endocrine
a) Phaeochromocytoma
b) Primary hyperaldosteronism
c) Cushing's syndrome
d) Thyrotoxicosis
e) Acromegaly
f) Hyperparathyroidism
3 'C' — Collagen-vascular diseases (e.g. polyarteritis nodosa)
Cerebral (e.g. raised intracranial pressure)
Contraceptive pill
Clonidine withdrawal
4 'A' — Alcohol
Aortic coarctation
Acute intermittent porphyria
5 'P' — Pregnancy-associated hypertension
Polycythaemia rubra vera

Causes of malignant phase
1 Essential hypertension
2 Rapidly progressive glomerulonephritis
3 Pregnancy-associated hypertension
4 Other
a) Renovascular (may be acute if haemorrhage occurs into atheromatous plaque, or if aortic aneurysm expands over renal artery origin)
b) Polyarteritis; scleroderma
c) Phaeochromocytoma
d) Iatrogenic
— Interaction with MAO inhibitor
— Clonidine withdrawal

Postural hypotension in the hypertensive patient
1 Iatrogenic
a) e.g. prazosin, diuretics, methyldopa
b) Haemodialysis
2 Phaeochromocytoma
3 Hyponatraemic hypertensive syndrome (may be seen in renovascular hypertension of recent origin)

Non-pharmacological management of mild hypertension
1 Stop smoking (reduces morbidity; does not reduce BP)
2 Ideal body weight
3 Low salt diet

4 Alcohol restriction
5 Biofeedback/relaxation/hypnotherapy
6 Regular exercise

Efficacy of antihypertensive treatment

1 Therapy is effective in reducing mortality from *moderate/severe* hypertension
2 Therapy is less effective in *mild* hypertension or in *elderly* patients
3 Therapy reduces risk of stroke but **not** of myocardial infarction
4 Therapy is not effective in *reversing* ischaemic heart disease or peripheral vascular disease
5 Continued smoking may *negate* benefits of antihypertensive therapy

Indications for antihypertensive treatment of mild hypertension (<180/95) in elderly patients

1 History of coronary or cerebrovascular disease
2 Retinopathy (grade III or IV); S_4
3 Elevated serum creatinine
4 ECG — left ventricular hypertrophy/strain; CXR — cardiomegaly

A general approach to antihypertensive prescribing

1 Commence with a thiazide
2 If uncontrolled, add a β-blocker and increase as necessary
3 If still uncontrolled, add a third-line agent
  a) Prazosin
  b) Nifedipine
  c) Captopril
4 If still uncontrolled — investigate

RENOVASCULAR HYPERTENSION

Hypertension: indications for further investigation*

1 Age <35
2 Associated postural hypotension
3 Hypertensive retinopathy
4 Abnormal urinalysis (proteinuria/haematuria/glycosuria)
5 Hypokalaemia without diuretic therapy, esp. if marked
6 Azotaemia (esp. if recent onset)
7 Severe hypertension poorly controlled by multiple drugs

*NB: Availability of experienced radiologists and vascular surgeons is a prerequisite

Investigational modalities in renovascular hypertension

1 Plasma renin activity ± captopril 'challenge'
2 Pre-and postcaptopril renal isotopic uptake of $^{99}Tc^m$-DTPA (↓ in stenosed kidney, ↓ ↓ postcaptopril)
3 Rapid-sequence intravenous pyelography
4 Venous digital subtraction angiography
5 Selective venous sampling for renal vein renins
6 Renal arteriography ± immediate angioplasty (best approach)

Varieties of renovascular disease

1 Fibromuscular dysplasia (→age <30 years)
2 Atheromatous (→age >60 years)

Diagnostic potential of arteriography in hypertension

1 Renal artery stenosis
2 Aortic coarctation
3 Polyarteritis nodosa
4 Phaeochromocytoma

NB Severe uncontrolled hypertension contraindicates elective angiography

Abnormal plasma renin activity: differential diagnosis

1 Elevated, no hypertension
  a) Addison's disease
  b) Haemorrhage
  c) Liver disease
  d) Pregnancy
  e) Bartter's syndrome
  f) Drugs
    — Diuretics, vasodilators
    — Oestrogens
    — Sympathomimetics; lithium
2 Elevated, hypertensive
  a) Malignant hypertension
  b) 'Essential' hypertension (in 15% of cases)
  c) Renovascular disease or end-stage renal failure
  d) Haemangiopericytoma (reninoma)
3 Low, no hypertension
  a) Old age
  b) Drugs
    — β-blockers
    — Clonidine, methyldopa; guanethidine
4 Low, hypertensive
  a) Essential hypertension (85%, esp. if elderly)
  b) Conn's/Cushing's syndromes
  c) Congenital adrenal hyperplasias
    — 11-hydroxylase deficiency
    — 17-hydroxylase deficiency
  d) Drugs — corticosteroids

Therapeutic options in 'renal' hypertension

1 Salt and fluid restriction
2 Drug therapy
  —ACE inhibitors (e.g. captopril)
  —β-blockers (e.g. metoprolol)
  —Vasodilators (e.g. prazosin)
3 If refractory, consider treating 'operable' renovascular disease by
  —Percutaneous angioplasty
  —Vascular surgery
4 If refractory to medical therapy, and no operable extrarenal vascular lesion identified — consider nephrectomy (± bilateral) (a desperation measure)

Surgical intervention in renovascular hypertension: indications

1 Percutaneous transluminal angioplasty
  a) Fibromuscular dysplasia
  b) Single discrete atheromatous plaque in renal arterial midportion
  c) Intrarenal arterial stenosis inaccessible to surgery
  d) Transplant artery stenosis

e) Contraindication to surgery
2 Surgical revascularisation
  a) Ostial lesions
  b) Extensive atheromatous plaques

Renovascular hypertension: predictors of surgical cure
1 Young patient
2 Recent onset of hypertension
3 Normal serum creatinine
4 Homolateral: contralateral renal vein renin ratio >1.5:1.0
5 Captopril challenge → ↓ ↓ BP, ↑ ↑ plasma renin activity

Drug regimens for severe acute hypertension
1 For hypertensive encephalopathy or dissecting aortic aneurysm — sodium nitroprusside 50–100 mg/L infusion regulated by indwelling arterial pressure monitor
2 For less urgent indications
  a) Labetalol infusion 100 mg/h (esp. for clonidine rebound)
  b) Hydralazine 10 mg i.m.i.
  c) Clonidine 75 μg i.m.i.
  d) Prazosin 5 mg orally
  e) Nifedipine 5–10 mg sublingually

OESTROGENIC STATES AND CARDIAC DISEASE

Cardiac conditions commonly exacerbated by pregnancy
1 Mitral stenosis
2 Aortic stenosis
3 Aortic coarctation
4 Pulmonary hypertension — primary
5 Pulmonary hypertension — Eisenmenger's syndrome

Treatment options in pregnancy-associated hypertension
1 Methyldopa
2 Hydralazine
3 β-blockers (beware of fetal bradycardia/hypoglycaemia)
4 Low-dose aspirin (→ ↓ TXA_2 : PGI_2)

Metabolic alterations in oral contraceptive users
1 ↑ Fibrinogen/plasminogen/FDPs/factors VII, VIII, X
2 ↓ Antithrombin III; ↓ albumin, haptoglobin
3 ↑ Transferrin, caeruloplasmin (→ ↑ *total* serum iron, copper)
4 ↑ Triglycerides (VLDL), insulin, aldosterone, cortisol (↓ renin, ACTH)

PULMONARY HYPERTENSION

Mechanisms of pulmonary hypertension
1 Increased pulmonary blood flow — left-to-right shunt
2 Elevated pulmonary venous pressure — mitral stenosis

3 Obliteration of vascular bed
  a) Pulmonary emboli
  b) Emphysema
  c) Primary pulmonary hypertension
  d) Collagen-vascular diseases

Diseases involving pulmonary arteries
1 Primary pulmonary hypertension
2 Churg-Strauss syndrome (cf. PAN)
3 Wegener's granulomatosis
4 Takayasu's arteritis
5 Systemic sclerosis

Associations of primary pulmonary hypertension
1 Raynaud's phenomenon, SLE*, scleroderma
2 Mitral valve prolaps
3 Familial
4 Pregnancy
5 Iatrogenic: oral contraceptives, metformin
6 Ingestion of aminorex or crotolaria alkaloids

Diagnosis of primary pulmonary hypertension
1 CXR
  a) Peripheral oligaemia ('pruning' of peripheral vasculature)
  b) Proximal dilatation of pulmonary arteries ('deer's antlers')
  c) Pulmonary arterial calcification if long-standing
2 Pulmonary angiography
  a) No emboli
  b) No peripheral arterial stenosis
  c) No intracardiac shunt
  d) Normal PCWP (excludes mitral stenosis, cor triatriatum)
3 Open lung biopsy
  a) Plexogenic pulmonary arteriopathy
  b) Pulmonary veno-occlusive disease
  c) Vasculitis

VENOUS THROMBOSIS

General predispositions to venous thrombosis
1 History of thrombosis or embolism
2 Hypomobility
  a) Cerebrovascular accident
  b) Myocardial infarction, cardiac failure
  c) Post-operative, esp. hip/pelvic/abdominal
3 Hypovolaemia
  a) Nephrotic syndrome
  b) Dehydration, esp. in elderly
4 Hypercoagulability
  a) Malignancy
  b) Cigarette smoking
  c) Oestrogens, puerperium
5 Homocystinuria, Behçet's syndrome

Haematological conditions associated with thromboembolism
1 Lupus anticoagulant (anticardiolipin antibody)
2 Paroxysmal nocturnal haemoglobinuria
3 Polycythaemia vera, essential thrombocythaemia

---

*Esp. if anticardiolipin antibody positive.

4 'Warm' autoimmune haemolytic anaemia
5 Sickle-C disease
6 Hereditary hypercoagulability
  a) Antithrombin III deficiency
  b) Protein C (or S) deficiency
  c) Heparin co-factor II deficiency

'Postphlebitic syndrome': pathogenesis, features and diagnosis
1 Previous venous thrombosis irreversibly damages venous valves (esp. in perforating veins) and thus distorts drainage
2 Gradual onset of symptoms worsened by upright posture
  a) Tense ankle oedema (implies deep vein incompetence)
  b) Calf pain, esp. on exercise ('venous claudication')
  c) Cyanosis, pigmentation, induration and ulceration
3 Essentially a diagnosis of exclusion:
  a) Negative venogram (misleading if thrombus has organized)
  b) Negative impedance plethysmography
  c) Negative radiofibrinogen scan
  d) Doppler — deep venous reflux

The swollen calf
1 Deep venous thrombosis
2 Ruptured plantaris
3 Ruptured Baker's cyst
4 Popliteal artery aneurysm (incl. mycotic)
5 Haematoma (e.g. in patient on anticoagulants)

Techniques of detecting thrombi
1 Venography
  a) Advantages — quick, accurate
  b) Disadvantages
    — May be painful and/or cause phlebitis
    — Risk of contrast hypersensitivity
    — Radioactivity exposure
    — False-negative: re-canalized thrombus
2 Duplex β-mode ultrasound
  a) Advantages — quick, painless, non-invasive and cheap
  b) Disadvantages
    — Insensitive for calf thrombi
    — False-negative: non-occlusive proximal thrombi; false-positive in CCF
3 ^{125}I-labelled fibrinogen scanning
  a) Advantages
    — Non-invasive, painless
    — Accurate for actively extending calf thrombi

b) Disadvantages
  — Slow (results take 24—72 h) and expensive
  — Radioactivity exposure
  — Insensitive for iliofemoral thrombus
  — False-negative: non-extending thrombus
  — False-positives: haematoma or inflammation
4 Impedance plethysmography
  a) Advantages
    — Non-invasive, painless, no radioactivity
    — Sensitive for proximal occlusive thrombi
  b) Disadvantages
    — May require serial studies
    — Insensitive for calf thrombi
    — False-negative: non-occlusive proximal thrombi
    — False-positive: cardiac failure
5 Thermography
  a) Advantages
    — Non-invasive, no radioactivity
    — Sensitive for calf thrombi
  b) Disadvantages — false-positives with any inflammation

PERIPHERAL ARTERIAL DISEASE

Cardiogenic sources of systemic emboli
1 Mitral stenosis
2 Postinfarct
3 Atrial fibrillation (alone), esp. if intermittent
4 Prosthetic valve
5 Other
  a) Sick sinus syndrome
  b) Mitral valve prolapse
  c) Infective endocarditis
  d) Left atrial myxoma

Digital gangrene with normal pulses
1 Diabetes mellitus
2 Vasculitis
3 Thromboembolism
4 Hyperviscosity
5 Iatrogenic
  a) Excess ergot or dopamine
  b) Intra-arterial thiopentone or adrenaline

Claudication of the upper limb
1 Buerger's disease
2 Takayasu's arteritis
3 Severe atherosclerosis
4 Proximal coarctation
5 Thoracic outlet syndrome
6 Polymyalgia rheumatica

Reviewing the Literature: Cardiology

2.1 Brown M S, Kovanen P T, Goldstein J L 1981 Regulation of plasma cholesterol by lipoprotein receptors. Science 212: 628–635

Nobel prize-winning work which helped clarify the interaction between LDL receptors and apolipoprotein B, thus shedding light on the genetic basis for atherosclerosis

Rajput-Williams J et al 1988 Variation of apolipoprotein-B

gene is associated with obesity, high blood cholesterol levels, and increased risk of coronary heart disease. Lancet ii: 1442–1445

Linkage study of a random sample of 290 males indicating that inherited variations of the apolipoprotein-B gene affect the phenotypic features underlying ischaemic heart disease

2.2   Pell S, Fayerweather W E 1985 Trends in the incidence of myocardial infarction and in associated mortality and morbidity in a large employed population 1957–83. New England Journal of Medicine 312: 1005–1015

Study which revealed a 20–30% decline in the incidence of ischaemic heart disease over the last 25 years in the USA, a finding which has more recently been reproduced in Australia

Krombout D et al 1985 The inverse relationship between fish ingestion and 20 year mortality from coronary heart disease. New England Journal of Medicine 312: 1205–1209

Demonstration of lower cardiovascular mortality in habitual fish eaters, suggesting antiatherogenic effects of fish oil

Jensen T et al 1989 Partial normalization by dietary cod-liver oil of increased microvascular albumin leakage in patients with insulin-dependent diabetes and albuminuria. New England Journal of Medicine 321: 1572–1557

Fish oil caused increased HDL and reduced VLDL, triglycerides and blood pressure, while olive oil reduced LDL but increased VLDL and triglycerides. No effect was seen on plasma glucose or urinary albumin excretion

Reis G J 1989 Randomised trial of fish oil for prevention of restenosis after coronary angioplasty. Lancet ii: 391–393

Study pouring cold water on fish oil, showing that no benefit could be demonstrated vis-à-vis rates of restenosis following coronary recanalization

2.3   Lipid Research Clinics Program 1984 The relationship of reduction in incidence of coronary heart disease to cholesterol lowering. Journal of the American Medical Association 251: 351–374

Four thousand men with asymptomatic hypercholesterolaemia were randomized to receive cholestyramine in addition to a low-cholesterol diet. Full compliance with therapy led to a 25% reduction in total cholesterol which was in turn accompanied by a 50% reduction in coronary heart disease

Rabelink A J et al 1988 Effects of simvastatin and cholestyramine on lipoprotein profile in hyperlipidaemia of nephrotic syndrome. Lancet ii: 1335–1338

Crossover trial of 10 patients suggesting that simvastatin, one of the new class of HMG CoA-reductase inhibitors, was both significantly more effective and better tolerated than the traditional cholesterol-lowering agent, cholestyramine

Pollare T et al 1989 A comparison of the effects of hydrochlorothiazide and captopril on glucose and lipid metabolism in patients with hypertension. New England Journal of Medicine 321: 868–873

Thiazide treatment caused glucose intolerance, increased LDL-cholesterol and VLDL-triglyceride levels, while captopril improved glucose sensitivity and didn't affect lipids or lioproteins

2.4   Samuelsson O et al 1987 Cardiovascular morbidity in

relation to change in blood pressure and serum cholesterol levels in treated hypertension; results from the Primary Prevention Trial in Goteborg, Sweden. Journal of the American Medical Association 258: 1768–1776

In addition to antihypertensive therapy, reduction in cholesterol was required to reduce coronary artery disease in this study. Moreover, lowering blood pressure below 150/85 appeared to be deleterious

2.5   Medical Research Council Working Party 1985 MRC trial of treatment of mild hypertension: principal results. British Medical Journal 291: 97–104

The conclusions were: (a) cessation of smoking is more important than drug treatment, (b) antihypertensive therapy does not reduce coronary events, (c) thiazides should always be tried prior to β-blockers, and (d) non-pharmacological antihypertensive treatment should be tried prior to drug treatment

2.6   Shaper A G et al (British Regional Heart Study) 1988 Alcohol and mortality in British men: explaining the U-shaped curve. Lancet ii: 1267–1272

Prospective study of 7735 middle-aged men suggesting that the previously reported 'protective' effect of moderate alcohol consumption on cardiovascular mortality is an artefact of pre-existing cardiovascular disease, i.e. that the apparently higher death rate among non-drinkers arises from cessation of alcohol following diagnosis of cardiac disease

Intersalt Co-operative Research Group 1988 An international study of electrolyte excretion and blood pressure. British Medical Journal 297: 319–328

Study of 10 079 patients from 52 centres showing strong correlation between alcohol intake and blood pressure, but no overall correlation between salt intake and hypertension

2.7   CASS (Coronary Artery Surgery Study) Investigators 1985 A randomized trial of coronary artery bypass surgery: survival of patients with low ejection fraction. New England Journal of Medicine 26: 1665–1672

In contrast to the earlier CASS reports, this study suggested that coronary artery surgery did indeed improve outcome in a subgroup of patients with triple-vessel disease and impaired ejection fractions. The overall conclusion of the study was that patients with mild symptoms, coronary artery disease and normal left ventricular function should be managed medically until symptoms become refractory to conservative measures

2.8   Pedersen T R et al 1985 Six-year follow-up of the Norwegian multicentre study on timolol after acute myocardial infarction. New England Journal of Medicine 313: 1055–1058

The originally reported 30–40% reduction in postinfarct mortality was maintained, but no additional benefit was seen following continuation of β-blockade for longer than 18 months

ISIS-1 Collaborative Group 1986 Randomized trial of intravenous atenolol among 16 027 cases of suspected acute myocardial infarction. Lancet ii: 57–66

15% reduction in postinfarct mortality using atenolol; very few patients were excluded from β-blockade due to contraindications

2.9   ISIS-2 (2nd International Study of Infarct Survival)

Collaborative Group 1988 Randomized trial of intravenous streptokinase, oral aspirin, both, or neither among 17 187 cases of suspected acute myocardial infarction: ISIS-2. Lancet ii: 349–360

Streptokinase and aspirin treatment each significantly improved cardiovascular mortality, and the combination of both was superior to that of either one administered alone

GISSI Study Group (final report) 1987 Long-term effects of intravenous thrombolysis in acute myocardial infarction. Lancet 2: 871–874

Italian study of 11 712 patients treated with streptokinase. A 23% reduction in mortality was seen in patients treated within 3 hours of symptoms. These conclusions were later supported by the Netherlands' trial

Anglo-Scandinavian Study of Early Thrombolysis (ASSET) group 1988 Trial of tissue plasminogen activator for mortality reduction in acute myocardial infarction. Lancet ii: 525–530

Thrombolytic therapy with tPA was associated with a 26% reduction in mortality within the month following infarction

Goldhaber S Z et al 1988 Randomized controlled trial of recombinant tissue plasminogen activator versus urokinase in the treatment of acute pulmonary embolism. Lancet ii: 293–298

Randomized controlled trial of 45 patients showing that pulmonary emboli were lysed within 2 hours in 82% of

tPA-treated patients, but only in 48% of urokinase-treated patients. tPA was also associated with less morbidity. Lung scan appearances at 24 hours were, however, identical in the two groups

2.10 Cairns J A, Gent M, Singer J et al 1985 Aspirin, sulfinpyrazone, or both in unstable angina. New England Journal of Medicine 313: 1369–1375

Canadian multicentre trial of 555 patients suggesting that aspirin was beneficial in unstable angina but that sulphinpyrazone was ineffective. On the basis of this study the FDA recommended use of aspirin in the postinfarction period

Theroux P et al 1988 Aspirin, heparin or both to treat acute unstable angina. New England Journal of Medicine 319: 1105–1111

Randomized double-blind placebo-controlled trial of 479 patients from Quebec, showing major reduction of acute myocardial infarction in patients treated with either aspirin or heparin or both

Physicians' Health Study Research Group 1988 Preliminary report: findings from the aspirin component of the ongoing Physicians' Health Study. New England Journal of Medicine 318: 262–264

Randomized study of 22 071 healthy male physicians aged 40 to 84: aspirin-treated (325 mg alternate days) patients incurred 47% fewer myocardial infarcts, but also experienced more haemorrhagic strokes

CHAPTER 3

Endocrinology

Physical examination protocol 3.1 You are asked to assess a patient for clinical evidence of hypopituitarism

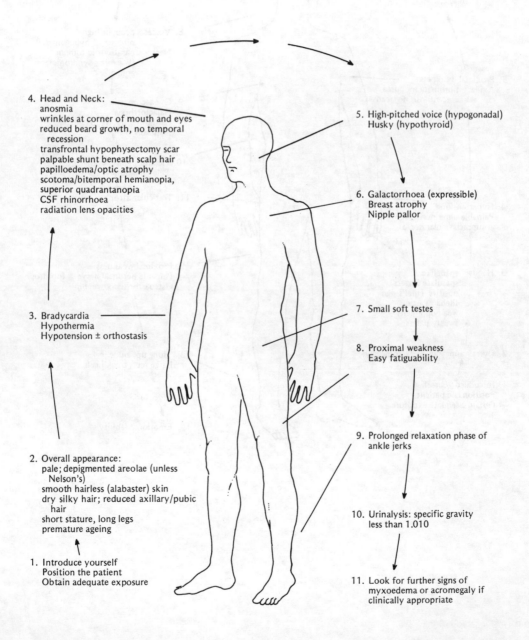

4. Head and Neck:
   anosmia
   wrinkles at corner of mouth and eyes
   reduced beard growth, no temporal recession
   transfrontal hypophysectomy scar
   palpable shunt beneath scalp hair
   papilloedema/optic atrophy
   scotoma/bitemporal hemianopia, superior quadrantanopia
   CSF rhinorrhoea
   radiation lens opacities

5. High-pitched voice (hypogonadal)
   Husky (hypothyroid)

6. Galactorrhoea (expressible)
   Breast atrophy
   Nipple pallor

3. Bradycardia
   Hypothermia
   Hypotension ± orthostasis

7. Small soft testes

8. Proximal weakness
   Easy fatiguability

9. Prolonged relaxation phase of ankle jerks

2. Overall appearance:
   pale; depigmented areolae (unless Nelson's)
   smooth hairless (alabaster) skin
   dry silky hair; reduced axillary/pubic hair
   short stature, long legs
   premature ageing

10. Urinalysis: specific gravity less than 1.010

1. Introduce yourself
   Position the patient
   Obtain adequate exposure

11. Look for further signs of myxoedema or acromegaly if clinically appropriate

Physical examination protocol 3.2 You are asked to examine a patient who has recently noticed increasing hat size

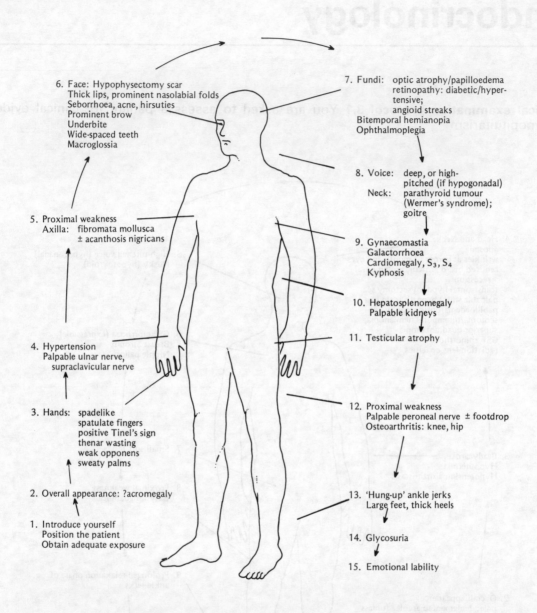

6. Face: Hypophysectomy scar
   Thick lips, prominent nasolabial folds
   Seborrhoea, acne, hirsuties
   Prominent brow
   Underbite
   Wide-spaced teeth
   Macroglossia

5. Proximal weakness
   Axilla: fibromata mollusca
   ± acanthosis nigricans

4. Hypertension
   Palpable ulnar nerve,
   supraclavicular nerve

3. Hands: spadelike
   spatulate fingers
   positive Tinel's sign
   thenar wasting
   weak opponens
   sweaty palms

2. Overall appearance: ?acromegaly

1. Introduce yourself
   Position the patient
   Obtain adequate exposure

7. Fundi: optic atrophy/papilloedema
   retinopathy: diabetic/hyper-
   tensive;
   angioid streaks
   Bitemporal hemianopia
   Ophthalmoplegia

8. Voice: deep, or high-
   pitched (if hypogonadal)
   Neck: parathyroid tumour
   (Wermer's syndrome);
   goitre

9. Gynaecomastia
   Galactorrhoea
   Cardiomegaly, S_3, S_4
   Kyphosis

10. Hepatosplenomegaly
    Palpable kidneys

11. Testicular atrophy

12. Proximal weakness
    Palpable peroneal nerve ± footdrop
    Osteoarthritis: knee, hip

13. 'Hung-up' ankle jerks
    Large feet, thick heels

14. Glycosuria

15. Emotional lability

Physical examination protocol 3.3 You are asked to examine a patient with recent onset of lethargy and cold intolerance

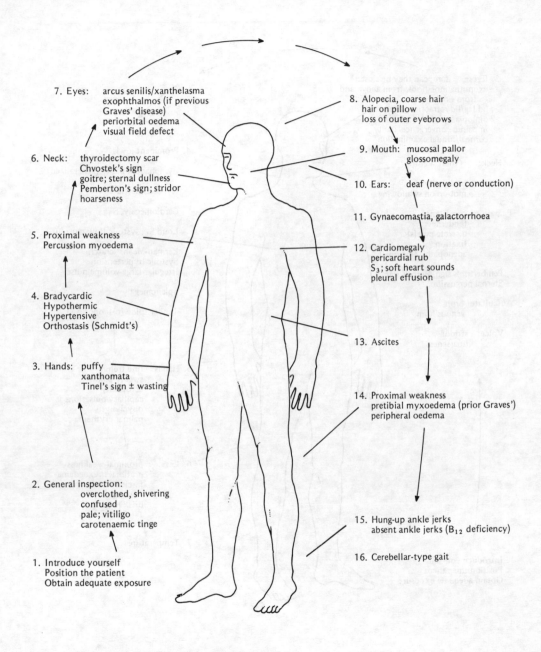

7. Eyes: arcus senilis/xanthelasma
   exophthalmos (if previous Graves' disease)
   periorbital oedema
   visual field defect

6. Neck: thyroidectomy scar
   Chvostek's sign
   goitre; sternal dullness
   Pemberton's sign; stridor
   hoarseness

5. Proximal weakness
   Percussion myoedema

4. Bradycardic
   Hypothermic
   Hypertensive
   Orthostasis (Schmidt's)

3. Hands: puffy
   xanthomata
   Tinel's sign ± wasting

2. General inspection:
   overclothed, shivering
   confused
   pale; vitiligo
   carotenaemic tinge

1. Introduce yourself
   Position the patient
   Obtain adequate exposure

8. Alopecia, coarse hair
   hair on pillow
   loss of outer eyebrows

9. Mouth: mucosal pallor
   glossomegaly

10. Ears: deaf (nerve or conduction)

11. Gynaecomastia, galactorrhoea

12. Cardiomegaly
    pericardial rub
    S_3; soft heart sounds
    pleural effusion

13. Ascites

14. Proximal weakness
    pretibial myxoedema (prior Graves')
    peripheral oedema

15. Hung-up ankle jerks
    absent ankle jerks (B_{12} deficiency)

16. Cerebellar-type gait

Physical examination protocol 3.4 You are asked to begin by examining the neck of a patient who looks possibly thyrotoxic

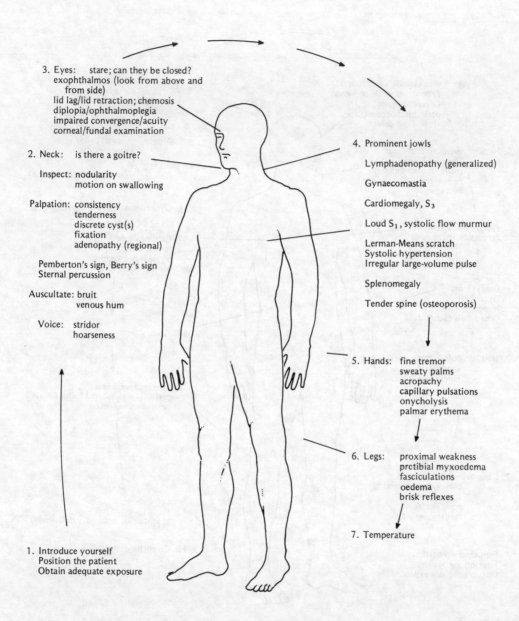

3. Eyes: stare; can they be closed?
exophthalmos (look from above and
   from side)
lid lag/lid retraction; chemosis
diplopia/ophthalmoplegia
impaired convergence/acuity
corneal/fundal examination

2. Neck: is there a goitre?

Inspect: nodularity
motion on swallowing

Palpation: consistency
tenderness
discrete cyst(s)
fixation
adenopathy (regional)

Pemberton's sign, Berry's sign
Sternal percussion

Auscultate: bruit
venous hum

Voice: stridor
hoarseness

4. Prominent jowls

Lymphadenopathy (generalized)

Gynaecomastia

Cardiomegaly, S_3

Loud S_1, systolic flow murmur

Lerman-Means scratch
Systolic hypertension
Irregular large-volume pulse

Splenomegaly

Tender spine (osteoporosis)

5. Hands: fine tremor
sweaty palms
acropachy
capillary pulsations
onycholysis
palmar erythema

6. Legs: proximal weakness
pretibial myxoedema
fasciculations
oedema
brisk reflexes

7. Temperature

1. Introduce yourself
Position the patient
Obtain adequate exposure

Physical examination protocol 3.5 You are asked to examine a patient who is known to have diabetes mellitus

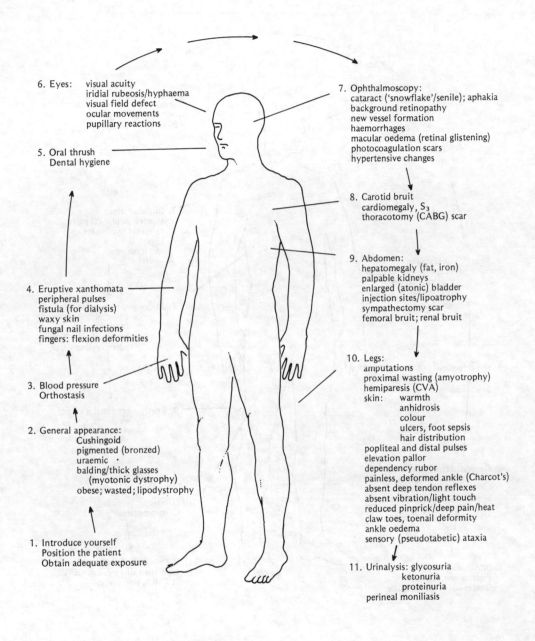

6. Eyes: visual acuity
   iridial rubeosis/hyphaema
   visual field defect
   ocular movements
   pupillary reactions

5. Oral thrush
   Dental hygiene

4. Eruptive xanthomata
   peripheral pulses
   fistula (for dialysis)
   waxy skin
   fungal nail infections
   fingers: flexion deformities

3. Blood pressure
   Orthostasis

2. General appearance:
   Cushingoid
   pigmented (bronzed)
   uraemic
   balding/thick glasses
      (myotonic dystrophy)
   obese; wasted; lipodystrophy

1. Introduce yourself
   Position the patient
   Obtain adequate exposure

7. Ophthalmoscopy:
   cataract ('snowflake'/senile); aphakia
   background retinopathy
   new vessel formation
   haemorrhages
   macular oedema (retinal glistening)
   photocoagulation scars
   hypertensive changes

8. Carotid bruit
   cardiomegaly, S_3
   thoracotomy (CABG) scar

9. Abdomen:
   hepatomegaly (fat, iron)
   palpable kidneys
   enlarged (atonic) bladder
   injection sites/lipoatrophy
   sympathectomy scar
   femoral bruit; renal bruit

10. Legs:
    amputations
    proximal wasting (amyotrophy)
    hemiparesis (CVA)
    skin: warmth
             anhidrosis
             colour
             ulcers, foot sepsis
             hair distribution
    popliteal and distal pulses
    elevation pallor
    dependency rubor
    painless, deformed ankle (Charcot's)
    absent deep tendon reflexes
    absent vibration/light touch
    reduced pinprick/deep pain/heat
    claw toes, toenail deformity
    ankle oedema
    sensory (pseudotabetic) ataxia

11. Urinalysis: glycosuria
                ketonuria
                proteinuria
    perineal moniliasis

Physical examination protocol 3.6 You are asked to examine a patient suspected of having Cushing's syndrome

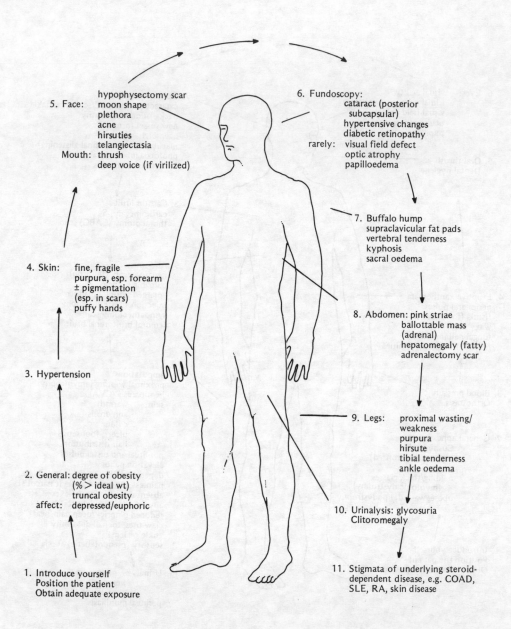

5. Face: hypophysectomy scar
           moon shape
           plethora
           acne
           hirsuties
           telangiectasia
   Mouth: thrush
           deep voice (if virilized)

6. Fundoscopy:
           cataract (posterior
             subcapsular)
           hypertensive changes
           diabetic retinopathy
   rarely: visual field defect
           optic atrophy
           papilloedema

4. Skin: fine, fragile
           purpura, esp. forearm
           ± pigmentation
           (esp. in scars)
           puffy hands

7. Buffalo hump
   supraclavicular fat pads
   vertebral tenderness
   kyphosis
   sacral oedema

3. Hypertension

8. Abdomen: pink striae
            ballottable mass
            (adrenal)
            hepatomegaly (fatty)
            adrenalectomy scar

2. General: degree of obesity
            (% > ideal wt)
            truncal obesity
   affect: depressed/euphoric

9. Legs: proximal wasting/
           weakness
           purpura
           hirsute
           tibial tenderness
           ankle oedema

10. Urinalysis: glycosuria
    Clitoromegaly

1. Introduce yourself
   Position the patient
   Obtain adequate exposure

11. Stigmata of underlying steroid-
    dependent disease, e.g. COAD,
    SLE, RA, skin disease

Diagnostic pathway 3.1 This patient has a goitre. What is the differential diagnosis?

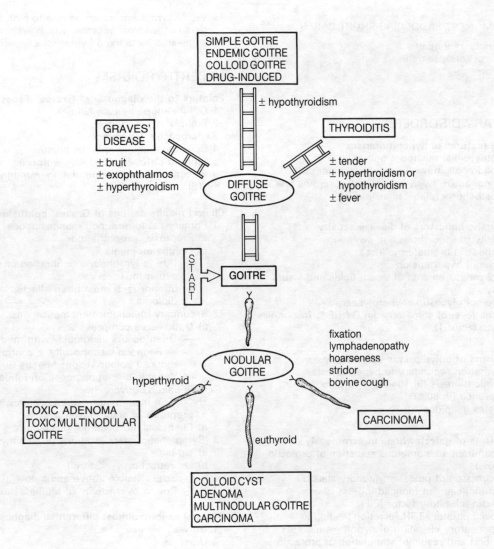

SIMPLE GOITRE
ENDEMIC GOITRE
COLLOID GOITRE
DRUG-INDUCED

± hypothyroidism

GRAVES'
DISEASE

± bruit
± exophthalmos
± hyperthyroidism

THYROIDITIS

± tender
± hyperthroidism or
  hypothyroidism
± fever

DIFFUSE
GOITRE

START

GOITRE

NODULAR
GOITRE

fixation
lymphadenopathy
hoarseness
stridor
bovine cough

hyperthyroid

TOXIC ADENOMA
TOXIC MULTINODULAR
GOITRE

CARCINOMA

euthyroid

COLLOID CYST
ADENOMA
MULTINODULAR GOITRE
CARCINOMA

CLINICAL ASPECTS OF ENDOCRINE DISEASE

COMMONEST ENDOCRINE SHORT CASES

1 Diabetic retinopathy
2 Graves' disease/goitre
3 Acromegaly

PITUITARY DISORDERS

Principal features of hypopituitarism

1 Hypothyroidism (without goitre)
2 Hypoadrenalism (with pallor: 'alabaster skin')
3 Hypogonadism (with wrinkled skin: 'crows feet')
4 Hyposthenuria (diabetes insipidus)

Acromegaly: indicators of disease activity

1 Severity of seborrhoea and sweating
2 Number of fibromata mollusca
3 Degree of hypertension
4 Serial measurements of visual fields and visual acuity
5 Degree of glycosuria/hyperglycaemia
6 Plasma level of somatomedin C (IGF-1: insulin-like growth factor-1)

Mechanisms of polydipsia in acromegaly

1 Dehydration secondary to hyperhidrosis
2 Osmotic diuresis (in 10%) due to glucose intolerance (in 50%)
3 Diabetes insipidus

Mechanisms of galactorrhoea in acromegaly

1 Concomitant adenomatous secretion of prolactin (in 30%)
2 Compression of posterior pituitary stalk by adenoma, causing reduced ingress of prolactin-inhibitory factor (PIF)
3 Reduced pituitary TSH secretion leading to compensatory elevation of hypothalamic TRH secretion and resultant stimulation of prolactin release

Prolactinomas: clinical presentations in females

1 Galactorrhoea (in 25% only*)
2 Infertility associated with regular anovulatory menstrual cycles
3 Amenorrhoea due to hypogonadotropic ovulatory failure
4 Dysfunctional uterine bleeding
5 Reduced libido
6 Visual field defect (in 5%) due to macroadenoma (in 30%)

*Conversely, most women presenting with non-puerperal lactation do *not* have hyperprolactinaemia.

Distinguishing features of prolactinomas in males

1 Less common; later age of presentation
2 Galactorrhoea distinctly unusual
3 Hypogonadism in 90%: impotence, obesity, infertility
4 Visual symptoms common due to high frequency (80%) of macroadenomas (which are, in turn, suggested by marked hyperprolactinaemia)

HYPERTHYROIDISM

Pointers to the diagnosis of Graves' disease

1 Ophthalmopathy (see below)
2 Pretibial myxoedema
3 'Acropachy' (clubbing)
4 Splenomegaly, lymphadenopathy
5 Smooth diffuse goitre, esp. with bruit
6 Presence of thyroid-stimulating immunoglobulin (TSI)

Clinical manifestations of Graves' ophthalmopathy

1 Primary ('autoimmune') manifestations
   a) Proptosis, exophthalmos
   b) Ophthalmoplegia
      — Due to lymphocytic infiltration of external ocular muscles
      — Inferior recti most often affected → vertical diplopia
2 Secondary (mechanical) complications
   a) Optic nerve compression
      — Often occurs insidiously with *mild* proptosis
      — → Reduced visual acuity ± central scotoma; reduced colour vision; Marcus-Gunn pupil
      — Variable disc appearance on fundoscopy
   b) Impaired convergence
   c) Corneal ulceration — often occurs with *marked* proptosis of acute onset
   d) Chemosis, lid oedema, glaucoma
3 'Sympathetic' manifestations (**if** also thyrotoxic)
   a) Lid-lag
   b) Lid retraction (→ 'stare')
      — Sclera visible above and below iris
      — Due to overactivity of Müller's muscle

Bilateral exophthalmos: differential diagnosis

1 Graves' disease
2 Uraemia
3 Alcoholism
4 Malignant hypertension
5 Carcinomatosis
6 Chronic lung disease and/or superior vena caval obstruction

Unilateral exophthalmos: differential diagnosis

1 Graves' disease (commonest cause)
2 Contralateral Horner's syndrome (i.e. misdiagnosis)
3 Cavernous sinus pathology
   a) Cavernous sinus thrombosis
   b) Caroticocavernous fistula (pulsating)
   c) Rhinocerebral mucormycosis
4 Intraorbital pathology
   a) Histiocytosis X

b) Wegener's granulomatosis
c) Riedel's thyroiditis with pseudotumour oculi
d) Tumour (e.g. optic nerve glioma)

Neuromyopathies in thyroid disease
1 Proximal myopathy
  a) Seen in thyrotoxicosis, less commonly in hypothyroidism
  b) Affects upper limbs esp.; reverts on becoming euthyroid
2 Hypokalaemic periodic paralysis
  a) Seen in association with toxic multinodular goitre
  b) Commonest in Asian males, esp. in hot season; R_x propranolol
3 Myasthenia gravis
  a) Occurs in 5% of Graves' patients; suspect if bulbar weakness
  b) Exacerbated by coexisting thyrotoxicosis or hypothyroidism
4 Graves' ophthalmoplegia
  a) Seen also in euthyroid patients
  b) Predominant weakness of upward and lateral gaze
5 Hoffmann's syndrome
  a) Pseudomyotonia of hypertrophied (weak) muscles in myxoedema
  b) Manifests with muscle aching following exertion

HYPOTHYROIDISM

Signs suggesting severe hypothyroidism
1 Hoarseness
2 Profound bradycardia or hypothermia
3 Mental confusion or coma
4 Markedly prolonged relaxation phase of deep tendon reflexes

Differential diagnosis of 'hung-up' tendon jerks
1 Myxoedema
2 Other (rare) causes
  a) Diabetes mellitus
  b) Sarcoidosis
  c) Syphilis
  d) Profound hypothermia
  e) Postpartum
  f) Anorexia nervosa
  g) β-blockade

Factors favouring secondary (pituitary) hypothyroidism
1 No goitre
2 No soft-tissue (myx)oedema
3 Other stigmata of hypopituitarism (pale areolae, hyposthenuria)
4 Normal plasma cholesterol
5 Enlargement of sella turcica
6 TSH not elevated despite low free T_4

Pathogenetic mechanisms of thyroid enlargement
1 Thyroiditis (Hashimoto's)
2 TSI (Graves')

3 TSH (multinodular goitre)
4 Tumour

DIABETES MELLITUS

Abdominal pain in diabetic patients
1 Gastric dilatation
  a) Acute (ketoacidosis)
  b) Chronic (autonomic neuropathy)
2 Pancreatitis
  a) Acute (follows development of type IV hyperlipidaemia)
  b) Chronic (precedes development of diabetes)
3 Infarction
  a) Mesenteric
  b) Myocardial (painless in autonomic neuropathy)
4 Genitourinary
  a) Urinary tract infection
  b) Bladder retention (painless in early stages)
5 Hepatobiliary
  a) Cholecystitis
  b) Hepatic capsular distension due to fatty infiltration, esp. in poorly controlled patients receiving high insulin dosages
6 Thoracolumbar radiculopathy (nerve root ischaemia)

Clinical features of diabetic amyotrophy
1 Acute onset in a poorly-controlled type II (non-insulin-dependent) diabetic with markedly elevated HbA_{1c} but without microvascular disease
2 Initially manifests with asymmetric weakness of hip/knee movement
3 Radicular pain and/or other sensory symptoms may be associated; almost always accompanied by hyporeflexia
4 Often complicated by development of contralateral pelvic girdle weakness, wasting, weight loss, incontinence and impotence
5 Occasionally associated with extensor plantar response and/or elevated CSF protein
6 Excellent long-term prognosis: at least partial recovery usually within 1–2 years, though recurrence not uncommon

The diabetic foot: factors contributing to morbidity
1 Ischaemia (macro- or microvascular disease)
2 Neuropathy ($\rightarrow$ trauma)
3 Poor wound healing
4 Predisposition to infection (ulcers, osteomyelitis, 'wet' gangrene)
5 Reduced visual acuity ($\rightarrow$ poor foot care)

Patterns of fetal morbidity in gestational diabetes
1 Mild (newly dignosed) diabetes: macrosomia ($\rightarrow$ dystocia)
2 Severe (known microvascular disease): small-for-dates
3 Spontaneous abortions (incidence reduced if tightly controlled blood glucose levels in first trimester): intrauterine fetal death
4 Malformations (esp. anencephaly): increased with maternal ketosis

5 Neonatal morbidity
  a) Jaundice, respiratory distress
  b) Hypoglycaemia (←recent maternal hyperglycaemia)

DIABETIC EYE DISEASE

Differential diagnosis of ocular pain
1 Third nerve palsy
2 Iridial rubeosis
3 Mucormycosis
4 Secondary glaucoma
5 Poor visual acuity → eyestrain

Characteristics of a diabetic third nerve palsy
1 Sudden onset
2 Painful
3 Pupillary sparing
4 Probably reflects microvascular disease of vasa nervorum
5 Diplopia usually improves within 12 months

Common causes of impaired visual acuity
1 Macular oedema in acute hyperglycaemia
2 Retinopathy impinging on macula
3 Retinal detachment or vitreous haemorrhage
4 Hyphaema secondary to iridial rubeosis
5 Cataract (classical albeit rare 'snowflake' type in insulin-dependent diabetes)
6 Cerebrovascular accident

Diabetic retinopathy: characterizing the lesions
1 Maculopathy (commonest cause of diabetic blindness)
  a) Macular oedema
  b) Macular exudates
  c) Macular ischaemia
2 Background retinopathy (visual acuity 6/6 or better)
  a) Microaneurysms
  b) Haemorrhages (dot and blot)
  c) Hard exudates (lipid deposits)
  d) Soft exudates (cotton wool spots; 'preproliferative' infarcts)
  e) Changes in venous calibre: beading/looping/sheathing/dilatation
  f) Arteriolar changes: narrowing/tortuosity/opacity, a-v nipping
3 Proliferative retinopathy (commoner in insulin-dependent diabetes)
  a) New vessels (arising from disc or periphery)
  b) Fibrous patches
  c) Vitreous haemorrhage
  d) Retinal detachment
  e) Rubeosis iridis

COMPLICATIONS OF DIABETES

Prognostic variables in vascular complications
1 Major predictive factors in *macrovascular* complications
  a) Patient's age
  b) Disease duration

2 Major predictive factors in *microvascular* complications
  a) Severity of hyperglycaemia
  b) Disease duration
3 *Retinopathy* appears worsened by smoking particularly
4 *Nephropathy* appears worsened by uncontrolled hypertension particularly
5 *Neuropathy/amyotrophy* appears worsened by (recent) uncontrolled hyperglycaemia particularly (correlates best with HbA_{1c} level)

Clinical presentation of nephropathy
1 Worsening of hypertension
2 Development of nocturia
3 Apparent reduction of glycosuria (i.e. 'threshold' elevation)
4 Increase in microalbuminuria
5 Decrease in insulin requirement
6 Increase in hypoglycaemic frequency

Predispositions to recurrent hypoglycaemia
1 Inappropriate insulin regimen (e.g. 'sliding scale' urinalysis in patient with 'renal' glycosuria; Somogyi effect; i.m. injections)
2 Insulin sensitivity
  a) Renal failure
  b) Coeliac disease
  c) Hypothyroidism
3 Alcohol abuse
4 Hypoadrenalism (±hypopituitarism) Autonomic neuropathy β-blockade (esp. non-selective) } Neuroglycopenia in absence of systemic 'warning signs'
5 Factitious hyperinsulinism or sulphonylurea administration

Causes of premature death in insulin-dependent diabetes
1 Macrovascular disease:
  a) Ischaemic heart disease (35%)
  b) Cerebrovascular disease (15%)
2 Microvascular disease — renal failure (25%)
3 Ketoacidosis (20%)
4 Hypoglycaemia (5%)

Causes of apparent insulin resistance in treated diabetics
1 Common
  a) Poor compliance with (exogenous) insulin regimen
  b) Obesity (→ 'down regulation' of endogenous receptors)
2 Acute
  a) Acidaemia (e.g. in ketoacidosis)
  b) Profound hypokalaemia
3 Circulating antagonist — acromegaly, Cushing's, pregnancy
4 Rare
  a) Insulin receptor abnormalities type A, B with acanthosis nigricans
  b) *Pathogenic* insulin antibodies
5 Iatrogenic, e.g. thiazide administration

CLINICAL DIAGNOSIS OF ADRENAL DISORDERS

Cushing's syndrome: features of discriminative value
1 Cushing's disease
  a) Atrophic livid striae (skin atrophy)
  b) Proximal myopathy (→*truncal* obesity: 'lemon-on-sticks')
  c) Spontaneous purpura
  d) Osteoporosis (in males or premenopausal females)
2 Adrenal carcinoma
  a) Childhood onset
  b) Hirsutism/virilism/acne
  c) Abdominal mass
3 Ectopic ACTH
  a) Hypokalaemia → weakness
  b) Pigmentation *if* duration of survival sufficient (e.g. thymoma, carcinoid)
4 Iatrogenic
  a) Posterior subcapsular cataracts
  b) Aseptic necrosis of bone
  c) Glaucoma; papilloedema (pseudotumour)
5 Simple obesity/polycystic ovaries
  a) Pale striae
  b) Generalized (± massive) obesity
  c) 'Buffalo hump'
  d) Oligomenorrhoea
  e) Hypertension, glucose intolerance

    } i.e. *poor* discriminative value

Hypoadrenalism: primary or secondary?
1 Primary (adrenal failure)
  a) Pigmentation
  b) Eosinophilia
  c) Hyperkalaemia
  d) Metabolic acidosis
2 Secondary (pituitary failure)
  a) Depigmented areolae
  b) Despite normal aldosterone secretion, symptomatic hypovolaemia *may* still occur due to vomiting/diarrhoea or diabetes insipidus
  c) Similarly, hyponatraemia *may* still occur due to concomitant hypothyroidism or SIADH
3 The above may be formally distinguished by
  a) A reliable ACTH assay
  b) A tetracosactrin (Synacthen) test, unless *long-term* pituitary failure is suspected (i.e. with supervening adrenal atrophy)

Differential diagnosis of grossly elevated plasma ACTH
1 Addison's disease
2 Nelson's syndrome
3 Ectopic (neoplastic) ACTH production

PHAEOCHROMOCYTOMA

Common sites of extra-adrenal phaeochromocytoma
1 Organ of Zuckerkandl (aortic bifurcation)
2 Paraspinal sympathetic ganglia
3 Bladder wall (→ symptoms on micturition)
4 Spermatic cord
5 Glomus jugulare (usually non-secreting tumours)

Clinical aspects of phaeochromocytoma
1 **H**eadache
  Hypertension (non-paroxysmal in 50%, may paradoxically worsen following β-blockade)
  Hypotension (orthostatic) in 50%
  Heartbeat awareness (palpitations)
  Hyperhidrosis
2 10% are malignant (histology not predictive)
  10% are extra-adrenal (greater risk of malignancy)
  10% are familial (often bilateral): usually non-secretory
  10% are multiple (30% in children)
3 Noradrenaline-secreting type
  a) May mimic essential hypertension
  b) Absent tachycardia
  c) Pallor
  d) *Angor animi*
4 Adrenaline-secreting type
  a) May mimic acute anxiety attacks
  b) Orthostasis
  c) Flushing *may* follow initial upper body pallor
5 Aspects distinguishing diagnosis from carcinoid syndrome
  a) Pallor > flushing
  b) Hypertension > hypotension
  c) Constipation > diarrhoea
  d) Cardiomyopathy > valve defects
6 Complications
  a) **C**onstipation
  b) **C**ardiomyopathy
  c) **C**erebral haemorrhage
  d) **C**holelithiasis
  e) **C**hronic renal failure
  f) **C**arcinoma (medullary) of thyroid (Sipple's syndrome)
  g) **C**ushing's syndrome (ACTH secretion by tumour)

DISORDERS OF GROWTH AND SEXUAL DEVELOPMENT

Presentations of congenital adrenal hyperplasia
1 21-hydroxylase deficiency (commonest type; gene frequency 1: 50)
  a) Primary ↓ aldosterone/cortisol → hypotension/salt-wasting, ↑ plasma renin activity
  b) Secondary ↑ ACTH → ↑ androgens, incl. testosterone
    — → Precocious puberty in males (despite small testes)
    — Virilization in females
  c) ↑ urinary 17-hydroxysteroids
2 3-β-hydroxysteroid dehydrogenase deficiency
  a) Primary ↓ cortisol/aldosterone → hypotension/salt-wasting
  b) Primary ↓ testosterone → male pseudohermaphroditism
  c) Secondary ↑ ACTH → ↑ DHEA (weak androgen) → female virilization
  d) ↑ urinary 17-ketosteroids
3 11-β-hydroxylase deficiency
  a) Primary ↓ cortisol/aldosterone → ↑ ACTH

→ ↑ androgens → sexual phenotype similar to 21-hydroxylase deficiency
  b) Secondary ↑ desoxycorticosterone → *hypertension*
  c) ↑ urinary 17-hydroxy- and 17-ketosteroids
4 17-hydroxylase deficiency
  a) Primary ↓ cortisol → mineralocorticoid excess → hypertension and hypokalaemia
  b) Primary ↓ testosterone → male pseudohermaphroditism primary amenorrhoea
  c) Urinary 17-hydroxysteroids and 17-ketosteroids
5 18-hydroxylase deficiency (very rare)
  a) Primary ↓ aldosterone → salt-wasting/↑ plasma renin activity
  b) Normal cortisol → normal ACTH/androgens; no genital defects
  c) Normal 17-hydroxysteroids and 17-ketosteroids

Phenotypes of abnormal sexual development

1 Klinefelter's syndrome
  a) Karyotype: XXY (due to chromosomal non-disjunction)
  b) Eunuchoid male with small firm (hyalinized) testes
2 Turner's syndrome
  a) Karyotype: XO (due to chromosomal non-disjunction)
  b) Prepubertal female with streak (vestigial) ovaries
3 True hermaphroditism
  a) Karyotype: XX/XY (due to dizygotic fusion)
  b) Ambiguous genitalia with ovary and testis (or ovotestis)
4 Male pseudohermaphroditism: testicular feminization syndrome
  a) Karyotype: XY (X-linked defective androgen receptor)
  b) High testosterone levels (end-organ insensitivity)
  c) Breasts, short vagina (absent uterus/oviducts), minimal axillary and genital hair, impalpable prostate/testes
  d) Presents with inguinal herniae in childhood, primary amenorrhoea in adolescence/adulthood
  e) Castration indicated after puberty to prevent malignancy
5 Male pseudohermaphroditism: 5-α-reductase deficiency
  a) Karyotype: XY (autosomal recessive, expressed in males only)
  b) Failure to activate testosterone to dihydrotestosterone
  c) Gives rise to 'penis-at twelve' syndrome, i.e. masculinizes at puberty due to large increase in testosterone secretion
  d) Prepubertal phenotype: male with hypospadias/epispadias or vagina, impalpable prostate/testes
6 Female pseudohermaphroditism:
  a) Karyotype: XX
  b) Seen in congenital adrenal hyperplasia: 21-hydroxylase, 11-β-hydroxylase or 3-β-dehydrogenase deficiency
  c) Partial enzyme defects may manifest only with hirsutism or menstrual irregularities

Differential diagnosis of dwarfism

1 Dwarfism with normal limb proportions
  a) Growth hormone deficiency (e.g. hypopituitarism)
  b) Severe systemic disease
2 Dwarfism with disproportionately short limbs
  a) Achondroplasia
  b) Ellis van Creveld syndrome
  c) Hereditary hypophosphatasia

INVESTIGATING ENDOCRINE DISEASE

THE PITUITARY AND HYPOTHALAMUS

Tests of hypothalamic integrity
1 Insulin tolerance test
  a) ↑ Cortisol (CRF, ACTH), GH (GHRF), somatostatin, dopamine
  b) In long-standing hypoadrenalism, give depot tetracosactrin (*synthetic ACTH*: 'Synacthen') for two weeks beforehand to prevent false-positives
2 Clomiphene stimulation — ↑ LH, ↑ FSH (GnRH)
3 Metyrapone (11-β-hydroxylase inhibitor) test:
  a) ↑ ACTH (CRF), ↑ urinary 17-hydroxysteroids
  b) Exaggerated response in (pituitary) Cushing's disease
4 Water deprivation test — ↑ ADH (synthesized in hypothalamus)

Contraindications to insulin tolerance testing
1 Hypoadrenalism (unless premedicated with dexamethasone)
2 Ischaemic heart disease
3 Epilepsy

Tests of pituitary reserve post-hypophysectomy
1 TRH stimulation → ↑ TSH; ↑ prolactin
2 GnRH stimulation → ↑ LH > ↑ FSH
3 Arginine vasopressin stimulation → ↑ growth hormone (GH) in children
4 Tetracosactrin/ACTH stimulation → ↑ serum cortisol (indirectly confirming normal long-term ACTH release by excluding gross adrenal atrophy)

Investigating pituitary function
1 Screening — serum levels of target hormones — e.g. T_4, cortisol
2 Serum levels of pituitary hormones — e.g. TSH, prolactin
3 Pituitary hormone suppression (if excess suspected), e.g.
  a) Dexamethasone suppression (ACTH: Cushing's disease)
  b) Glucose tolerance test (GH: acromegaly)
4 Pituitary hormone stimulation (if deficiency suspected) — e.g. 'Synacthen' test, GnRH stimulation (see below)

Common endocrine deficiencies post-hypophysectomy
1 ↓ GH increment on stimulation (80%)
2 ↓ FSH/LH (75%)

3 ↓ ACTH/TSH (40%): *always* signifies need for replacement

Imaging the pituitary gland
1 Lateral skull X-ray with coned views of the pituitary fossa
  a) Sellar enlargement (pituitary tumour, empty sella)
  b) Double floor of dorsum sellae (may be normal variant)
  c) Erosion of posterior clinoid processes
  d) Suprasellar calcification (craniopharyngioma)
2 High-resolution coronal-plane CT with contrast
  a) Obviates need for pneumoencephalography to demonstrate suprasellar tumour extension
  b) Concomitant metrizamide cisternography excludes empty sella
3 Magnetic resonance imaging

Differential diagnosis of an enlarged sella turcica
1 Pituitary tumour
2 Primary hypothyroidism (hyperplasia of TSH-secreting cells)
3 Pregnancy
4 Empty sella syndrome (classically occurring in obese hypertensive multipara)

Factors against the diagnosis of empty sella syndrome
1 Hyperprolactinaemia (or other endocrine abnormality)
2 Visual field defect
3 Erosion of posterior clinoid processes or dorsum sellae on SXR

Laboratory diagnosis of acromegaly
1 Serological
  a) Failure to suppress plasma GH with oral glucose load
  b) Grossly elevated fasting a.m. GH (10% false-negative rate)
  c) Elevated plasma somatomedin C (IGF-1) level
  d) Coexisting elevation of prolactin (in 30%)
2 Radiological
  a) Enlarged sella turcica (in 90%)
  b) Enlarged frontal sinuses; increased skull thickness
  c) Macrognathia, underbite, wide-spaced teeth
  d) 'Arrowhead' tufting of fingertips; ↑ joint space
  e) Heelpads > 22 mm thick (female), > 25 mm thick (male)
3 Histological — eosinophilic pituitary adenoma

THYROID FUNCTION TESTS

Indications for TRH stimulation
1 *Exclusion* of thyrotoxicosis in patients with undetectable plasma TSH
2 Unexplained proptosis in a euthyroid TSI-negative patient
3 Documentation of adequate thyrotropin (TSH) reserve following pituitary irradiation and/or surgery

4 Documentation of adequate surgical excision (TRH → ↓ GH) in acromegaly (TRH → ↑ GH)
5 Documentation of adequate surgical excision (TRH → ↑ prolactin) of prolactinoma (TRH → no change in serum prolactin)
6 Investigation of hypogonadism with borderline gonadotrophin levels: delayed puberty (TRH → ↑ prolactin) vs hypogonadotropic hypogonadism (TRH → no change in serum prolactin)

Abnormalities of the TRH stimulation test
1 'Flat'
  a) Thyrotoxicosis
  b) Hypopituitarism
  c) Euthyroid patients with
    — Ophthalmic Graves' disease
    — Functioning adenoma
    — Recently treated toxicosis
    — Multinodular goitre
  d) Miscellaneous — acromegaly, Cushing's syndrome, L-DOPA use
2 Exaggerated or prolonged TSH rise
  a) Primary hypothyroidism
  b) Hypothalamic disease
  c) Pregnancy

A quick approach to excluding thyroid dysfunction
1 Suspected thyrotoxicosis?
  a) Free T_4, plus
  b) Free T_3
2 Suspected hypothyroidism?
  a) Free T_4, plus
  b) TSH

Thyrotoxicosis with low radioactive iodine uptake
1 Thyroiditis (see p. 98)
  a) Subacute granulomatous (de Quervain's) thyroiditis
  b) Subacute lymphocytic ('silent') thyroiditis
    — postpartum painless thyroiditis
    — spontaneously resolving hyperthyroidism
  c) Chronic lymphocytic thyroiditis ('Hashitoxicosis')
2 Iatrogenic
  a) Recent iodine administration (Jod-Basedow phenomenon)
  b) Incompletely radioiodine-treated Graves' disease
  c) Thyrotoxicosis factitia (self-administration of thyroxine)
3 Neoplastic
  a) *Struma ovarii*
  b) Functioning metastases from follicular thyroid carcinoma
  c) Extrinsic compression of normal gland by tumour mass

Clinical spectrum of thyroid dysfunction
1 T_3-toxicosis
  a) Clinically toxic
  b) ↑ T_3, normal free thyroxine index (FTI)
  c) Commoner
    — In iodine-deficient communities
    — In toxic adenomas
    — Following ablative therapy for toxicosis

2 T_3-euthyroidism
   a) Clinically euthyroid
   b) ↓ FTI, normal/↑ T_3
   c) Occurs in
      — 'Compensated' (early) hypothyroidism
      — Subclinical gland autonomy (ophthalmic Graves', functioning adenoma)
3 T_4-toxicosis
   a) Clinically toxic in 50% ('sick hyperthyroid')
   b) ↑ FTI, ↓ T_3
4 Sick euthyroid
   a) Clinically euthyroid (albeit sick)
   b) ↓ T_3, ↑ rT_3 (reverse-T_3)
   c) ↓ FTI (often), normal TSH
5 Euthyroid hyperthyroxinaemia
   a) Clinically euthyroid
   b) ↑ T_4 (total or free): variable TBG and total T_3
   c) Normal fT_3; normal fT_4 by equilibrium dialysis
   d) Normal TSH rise in response to TRH stimulation

Differential diagnosis of euthyroid hyperthyroxinaemia
1 Elevated thyroid-binding globulin (any cause)
2 Familial dysalbuminaemic hyperthyroxinaemia
3 Hyperemesis gravidarum
4 Iatrogenic
   a) Iodine-rich drugs, e.g. amiodarone
   b) High-dose propranolol (blocks $T_4 \rightarrow T_3$)

INVESTIGATING THE DIABETIC PATIENT

Indications for a glucose tolerance test
1 Pregnancy
   a) Glycosuria
   b) Risk factors for diabetes mellitus
2 Non-diagnostic elevation of blood glucose (random or fasting) ± glycosuria
3 Investigation of peripheral neuropathy

Abnormalities of the glucose tolerance test
1 Pronounced glycaemia: diabetes mellitus
2 'Flat'
   a) Malabsorption
   b) Addison's disease
3 'Lag storage' curve
   a) Postgastrectomy
   b) Thyrotoxicosis
   c) Chronic liver disease

Indications for home blood glucose monitoring
1 Initial stabilization of any young and/or insulin-dependent diabetic
2 Gestational diabetes
3 Abnormal renal threshold for glucose (e.g. renal failure)
4 Impaired colour vision (e.g. due to retinopathy ± photocoagulation; prevents accurate urinalysis interpretation)
5 Unexplained symptoms of sleep disturbance, anxiety attacks, angina or epilepsy

Factors tending to elevate the glycosylated haemoglobin level
1 Hyperglycaemia (previous 8–12 weeks), esp. ketoacidosis

2 Hypertriglyceridaemia
3 Pregnancy (first and second trimester)
4 Renal failure
5 Iron deficiency
   Hereditary spherocytosis (postsplenectomy)
   Elevated HbF (e.g. thalassaemia): mimics HbA_{1c}
6 Aspirin/alcohol ingestion

Factors tending to depress the glycosylated haemoglobin level
1 Reticulocytosis (e.g. haemolysis, haemorrhage) ± anaemia
2 Pregnancy (third trimester)
3 Assay performed in hot environment

HYPOGLYCAEMIA

Nocturnal hypoglycaemia
1 Clinical
   a) Nocturnal distress, nightmares
   b) Mental dullness/depression
   c) Morning headaches and/or hypothermia
   d) Onset of idiopathic epilepsy
2 Waking urinalysis: glucose *and* ketones ('Somogyi effect')
3 Overnight voided urine sample:
   ↑ cortisol/creatinine ratio
4 Confirmation of hypoglycaemia with 3 a.m. (in-hospital) blood sugar
5 Distinguish 'dawn effect' (greater endogenous insulin requirement in morning) from Somogyi effect (where hyperglycaemia occurs due to *reactive* — rather than circadian — excess of counter-regulatory hormones)
6 Avoid by giving intermediate-acting insulin at bedtime instead of with the evening meal

Recurrent hypoglycaemia in the insulin-dependent diabetic?
1 Excessive or inappropriate dosage schedule
2 Low renal threshold in patient monitoring dose with urinalysis
3 Coexisting hypoadrenalism or hypopituitarism (e.g. following hypophysectomy for retinopathy, or in Sheehan's syndrome)
4 Gastrointestinal precipitants
   a) Coeliac disease
   b) Diabetic gastroparesis
5 Non-compliance or manipulative behaviour (esp. in adolescents)

Hypoglycaemia without hyperinsulinaemia: differential diagnosis
1 Postprandial
2 Alcohol ingestion
   a) Inhibits hepatic gluconeogenesis (as does lactic acidosis)
   b) Usually presents as hypothermic coma in semi-starved alcoholics with depleted hepatic glycogen
3 Starvation; prolonged exercise; sepsis (esp. *P. falciparum*)
4 Non-islet cell tumours (release IGF-II)
   a) Bulky mesenchymal tumours (e.g. fibrosarcoma, mesothelioma)

b) Hepatoma, adrenal carcinoma
5 Iatrogenic
  a) Oral hypoglycaemics
  b) Postpolya gastrectomy (late dumping)
  c) Salicylism (in children)
  d) Propranolol (inhibits hepatic glycogenolysis)

Insulinoma: making the diagnosis
1 Clinical
  a) Symptoms (esp. syncope, amnesia) induced by fasting or exercise
  b) Symptoms accompanied by demonstration of low plasma glucose
  c) Symptoms relieved by glucose
2 Screening test: 3 overnight 16-hour fasts
  a) Blood sugar abnormally low in 90% of insulinomas
  b) Non-suppression of insulin (> 6 μU/ml) and C-peptide
  c) Low C-peptide/proinsulin suggests factitious hypoglycaemia
3 Supporting tests
  a) Elevated fasting insulin : glucose ratio
  b) High proinsulin (> 20% total insulin)
  c) Stimulation of insulin secretion by calcium infusion
4 Insulin (or tolbutamide) tolerance test:
  a) Non-suppression of proinsulin and/or C-peptide
  b) Non-suppression excludes postprandial hypoglycaemia
5 Tumour localization and biopsy

NB: paradoxically, insulinoma may be associated with postprandial *hyperglycaemia*, since the normal postprandial increase in insulin secretion may be suppressed.

Factitious hypoglycaemia
1 Clinical: recurrent hypoglycaemic episodes in a paramedically employed patient or member of diabetic patient's family
2 Grossly elevated plasma insulin during attacks
3 Low proinsulin levels and/or C-peptide levels (cf. insulinoma)
4 Insulin antibodies may be assayed if porcine insulin used
5 *Sulphonylurea abuse* may lead to elevated insulin and C-peptide levels, normal proinsulin levels, and positive urine/serum drug screens

NB: most iatrogenic hypoglycaemia is inadvertent; cf. thyrotoxicosis factitia

DIAGNOSING DIABETES AND ITS COMPLICATIONS

Rapid assessment of glucose tolerance using single plasma levels
1 Random glucose <8 mmol/l
  Fasting glucose <6 mmol/l } — normal
2 Random glucose 8–11 mmol/l
  Fasting glucose 6–8 mmol/l } — impaired glucose tolerance
3 Random glucose >11 mmol/l
  Fasting glucose >8 mmol/l } — diabetes mellitus

Assessing diabetic treatment using glycosylated haemoglobin
1 HbA_{1c} normal range — 5–8.5%
2 HbA_{1c} < 10% — reasonable control
3 HbA_{1c} 11–14% — control can be improved ?compliance ?regimen
4 HbA_{1c} > 15% — treatment plan needs major overhaul

Hyperosmolar coma: making the diagnosis
1 Blood glucose level > 50 mmol/l, serum osmolality < 340 mosmol
2 Minimal or absent ketonuria and acidosis
3 Azotaemia and hypernatraemia not infrequent (correlate with biological severity)
4 Plasma insulin usually detectable; lactate/alcohol usually not

Indications for renal biopsy in diabetes mellitus
1 Red cell casts, or persistent (micro)haematuria with sterile urine
2 Unusually early (e.g. no retinopathy) or rapid development of renal dysfunction

INVESTIGATING ADRENAL DISEASE

Diagnostic sequence in suspected Cushing's syndrome
1 Overnight dexamethasone suppression screening test
2 24-hour urinary free cortisol
3 Plasma ACTH
4 8 a.m. and midnight cortisol level
5 CT scanning of sella and/or adrenals

NB: no single test should be relied upon

Causes of false-positive dexamethasone suppression tests
1 Simple obesity (cf. false-negatives: *rare*)
2 Non-compliance (check dexamethasone level)
3 Depression
4 Alcoholism
5 Iatrogenic
  a) Oestrogens
  b) Antiandrogens: spironolactone, cyproterone acetate
  c) Phenytoin

Aetiological clues in established Cushing's syndrome
1 Pituitary Cushing's ('disease')
  a) High-dose (8 mg/day) dexamethasone → cortisol suppression
  b) Metyrapone test — normal rise in ACTH (in 90%)
2 Primary adrenal adenoma
  a) Metyrapone test: no rise in ACTH
  b) Selenium-75 scanning (lateralizes lesion for surgery)
3 Primary adrenal carcinoma
  a) Urinary cortisol excretion may exceed 5000 nmol/24 hr
  b) Metyrapone test : no rise in ACTH
  c) ↑ DHEA/urinary 17-ketosteroids; ↑ testosterone in females
  d) Selenium-75 scanning if lesion not visible on CT*

4 Ectopic ACTH secretion
  a) Absolute plasma ACTH level may exceed 500 ng/l
  b) Urinary cortisol excretion may exceed 5000 nmol/24 hr
  c) Metyrapone test: no further rise in ACTH
5 Alcohol- or depression-induced pseudoCushing's syndrome — insulin hypoglycaemia test
  a) No insulin resistance
  b) Normal cortisol rise

Conn's syndrome (primary hyperaldosteronism): diagnosis
1 Suggestive presentations
  a) Unexpected occurrence of *severe* hypokalaemia in a mild hypertensive on diuretic therapy
  b) *Untreated* hypertensive with hypokalaemia and urinary postassium excretion > 30 mmol/24 h (NB: untreated renovascular or 'malignant' hypertension may also be associated with hypokalemia due to *secondary* hyperaldosteronism)
2 Proposed screening tests
  a) High-salt diet → persistent hypokalaemia
  b) Lack of aldosterone suppressibility (plasma/24 hour urine) despite
     — High-salt diet or intravenous sodium loading
     — Oral fludrocortisone or captopril
  c) Aldosterone elevation following IV metoclopramide
  d) Plasma aldosterone : renin ratio >30: 1
3 Dexamethasone suppression test if screening test positive (suppressibility in this context constitutes a contraindication to laparotomy): diagnostic of glucocorticoid-suppressible hyperaldosteronism
4 Tests definitively distinguishing aldosterone-producing adenomas from idiopathic hyperaldosteronism (bilateral hyperplasia)
  a) Venous catheterization and effluent analysis
  b) Surgical biopsy (± preceding CT evidence of adenoma/hyperplasia)

Bartter's syndrome (primary hyperreninaemia): diagnosis
1 Usually presents in childhood with failure to thrive, enuresis (due to potassium-depletion nephropathy), and weakness
2 *Normal* blood pressure (due to intravascular hypovolaemia); *no* oedema
3 Low serum potassium, elevated urinary potassium Hypochloraemic metabolic alkalosis
4 Elevated urinary chloride; cf. diuretic abuse, laxative abuse, surreptitious vomiting (bulimia)
5 Insensitivity to i.v. angiotensin or vasopressin Hypersensitivity to i.v. saralasin (an angiotensin II inhibitor) or captopril (an ACE inhibitor)
6 Therapeutic response to indomethacin

---

* Adrenal nodular hyperplasia may occur in pituitary-dependent Cushing's disease; hence, visualization of an adrenal nodule is not diagnostic of a primary adrenal tumour

Liddle's syndrome (pseudohyperaldosteronism): diagnosis
1 Hypertension
2 *Low* aldosterone levels
3 Responsive to sodium restriction or triamterene administration

Phaeochromocytoma: how to diagnose your first
1 24-hour urinary free catecholamines/VMA/meta-adrenalines
2 Plasma adrenaline/noradrenaline: sample taken at rest via an indwelling needle inserted 30 minutes previously
3 Pentolinium (or clonidine) catecholamine suppression tests
4 Whole-body ^{131}I-MIBG (metaiodobenzylguanidine) scanning
5 Abdominal CT scanning
6 Selective venous sampling, or angiography (premedicate with the α-blocker phenoxybenzamine for three days beforehand)

NB: no single investigation excludes the diagnosis

DISORDERS OF SEXUAL FUNCTION

Approach to investigation of amenorrhoea
1 Measure urinary HCG to exclude pregnancy
2 ↑ FSH
  a) Proceed to karyotyping if 'primary' amenorrhoea
  b) Consider diagnosis of premature menopause
3 ↓ FSH: perform
  a) Serum prolactin
  b) Thyroid function tests (esp. TSH)
  c) Skull X-ray ± coronal CT/visual field mapping
4 ↓ FSH and ↑ LH: perform GnRH stimulation to confirm Stein-Leventhal syndrome (→ exaggerated LH response)
5 ↑ Testosterone: consider
  a) Testicular feminization
  b) 5α-Reductase deficiency (cf. 17-ketoreductase deficiency → ↓ testosterone)

Laboratory features of anorexia nervosa
1 ↓ FSH/LH/17β-oestradiol/DHEA
2 Normal serum prolactin
3 'Sick euthyroid' (q.v.)
  Delayed peak following TRH- and GnRH-stimulation
4 ↑ GH/ACTH/cortisol
5 Hyposthenuria

Hirsutism: principles of investigation
1 ↑ ↑ Plasma DHEA/urinary 17-ketosteroids: adrenal origin (e.g. tumour)
2 ↑ ↑ Testosterone/androstenedione: ovarian origin (e.g. Sertoli-Leydig cell tumour; 'arrhenoblastoma')
3 Pelvic mass(es)
  a) ↑ Pregnanetriol/LH/GnRH response } Stein-Leventhal syndrome
  b) ↑ Free testosterone }

Investigation of males with abnormal sexual phenotype

1 Small (firm) testes
  Hypogonadal $\left.\right\}$ Proceed to karyotyping
  ↑ FSH
2 Small testes $\left.\right\}$ Screen for congential adrenal
  Virilized hyperplasia using
  17-OH-progesterone
3 Normal testicular size $\left.\right\}$ Untreatable testicular
  ↑ FSH malfunction with
  azoöspermia (e.g. tubular
  hyalinization)
4 Normal testicular size $\left.\right\}$ Epididymal/vas obstruction
  Azoöspermia (e.g. Young's syndrome),
  Normal FSH Varicocoele
5 Normal testicular size $\left.\right\}$ Exclude pituitary tumour
  Azoöspermia, ↓ FSH
6 Absent pubic hair — investigate for gonadal failure (cf. in females; absent pubic hair implies adrenal failure)

Criteria for normal semen analysis

1 Ejaculate volume — 1.5–6 ml
2 Number — $>20 \times 10^6$/ml
3 Motility — >60% active forward progression
4 Morphology — >60% normal oval shapes
5 Count must be performed 3 times over a 6–12 week period

Laboratory characterization of amenorrhoea

1 ↑ FSH: ovarian failure ($1^0/2^0$)
2 ↑ LH, ↓ FSH: polycystic ovary (Stein-Leventhal) syndrome
3 ↑ LH, normal FSH — pregnancy
4 ↓ FSH, ↓ LH — hypopituitarism
5 ↓ FSH, ↑ prolactin — hyperprolactinaemia ± prolactinoma

Investigating infertility in the menstruating female

1 Check ovulation
  a) Chart basal body temperature for several months
  b) Measure midluteal phase serum progesterone
2 Serum prolactin
3 Laparoscopy in secretory phase with diagnostic curettage
  a) Diagnosis
    — Endometriosis
    — Polycystic ovaries
    — Unruptured luteinized follicles
  b) Therapy — hydrotubation

MANAGING ENDOCRINE DISEASE

Pituitary tumours: therapeutic considerations

1 Trans-sphenoidal microadenomectomy
  a) Encouraging results reported in Cushing's disease, esp. in children
  b) May be complicated by postoperative CSF rhinorrhoea or diabetes insipidus
2 Transfrontal hypophysectomy
  a) Remains the treatment of choice for most patients with macroadenomata and visual symptoms or signs
  b) Usual first-line treatment for craniopharyngioma
3 Radiotherapy (incl. yttrium-90 implantation, etc.)
  a) Reduction of adenoma size and function may take years
  b) Inappropriate for patients with visual symptoms or infertility
  c) High incidence of subsequent hypopituitarism
  d) Occasionally complicated by (late) pituitary apoplexy
  e) Defined place in general management remains controversial
4 Medical management — bromocriptine administration may lead to shrinkage of prolactin- or GH-secreting macroadenomata and has been used for this purpose in the first instance
5 Mechanical (rather than oral) contraception should be used in prolactinoma patients not desiring pregnancy in view of the risk of oestrogen-induced tumour expansion

Replacement therapy in panhypopituitarism

1 Cortisone acetate 25 mg *mane* 12.5 mg *nocte*
2 Thryoxine 100–150 μg/day
3 Intranasal dDAVP 2–6 times per day
4 Conception not desired
  a) Females: daily combined oral contraceptive pill
  b) Males: intramuscular testosterone enanthate every 2–3 weeks
5 Conception desired — short-term administration of FSH *or* HCG *or* low-dose pulsatile GnRH analogues

GOITRE

Non-toxic multinodular goitre: management considerations

1 Reduction of nodule size using T_4 suppression (150–200 μg/day), if undertaken, can be expected to be less effective if
  a) Goitre is long-standing
  b) TRH-stimulation test is 'flat' (i.e. subclinical autonomous T_4 production)
2 Biopsy and/or thyroidectomy should be undertaken if there has been no shrinkage within 3 months of conservative therapy
3 Carcinoma occurs with greater frequency in multinodular goitre

Approach to thyroid nodules

1 Clinical: multiple nodules? fixed? nodes? bruit? euthyroid?
2 ^{99}Tc scan
  a) 'hot' nodule (1% cancer risk)
  b) 'cold' nodule (20% cancer risk)
3 Ultrasound — smooth thin-walled cyst has lower cancer risk
4 Trial of T_4-suppressive therapy (for up to 3 months)
5 Needle biopsy — proceed directly to this if clinical suspicion high; negative cytology does not exclude malignancy
6 Thyroidectomy — partial or total, pending frozen section and operative findings

Complications of thyroidectomy
1 Short-term
  a) 'Thyroid storm' (if thyrotoxic pre-op.)
  b) Hypocalcaemia (hypoparathyroidism)
  c) Recurrent laryngeal nerve palsy; haemorrhage
2 Long-term — hypothyroidism (may present insidiously many years postoperatively)

THERAPY OF THYROTOXICOSIS

Thyroid storm: approach to management
1 Prevention
  a) Treat possible precipitating factors (e.g. sepsis)
  b) Render euthyroid prior to elective surgery
2 IV fluids as required to maintain BP; tepid sponge, fan
3 Propylthiouracil (PTU) 200 mg p.o. q 6 h
4 Potassium iodide 200 mg i.v. over 15 mins (give 1 hour after PTU)
5 Propranolol 1 mg i.v., then 2 mg i.v. q 4 h p. r. n. (*not* contraindicated in thyrocardiac failure of suspected rate-dependent origin)
6 Dexamethasone in supraphysiological ('shock') dosage

Rationâle of dexamethasone therapy in thyroid storm
1 Prevents possible Addisonian crisis, e.g. in patients with associated (albeit unrecognized) autoimmune hypoadrenalism
2 Inhibits glandular release of T_4
3 Inhibits peripheral conversion (activation) of $T_4 \rightarrow T_3$

Drugs inhibiting glandular release of thyroxine
1 Dexamethasone
2 Lithium
3 Iodine (cf. the *Wolff-Chaikoff effect,* where iodine administration leads to transient inhibition of organification/coupling)

Pharmacological actions of propylthiouracil
1 Inhibits organification of tyrosine
2 Inhibits coupling of MIT (monoiodotyrosine) and DIT
3 Inhibits peripheral conversion (activation) of $T_4 \rightarrow T_3$

Elective management of thyrotoxicosis
1 Antithyroid drugs (carbimazole/methimazole, PTU)
  a) Usually given for 12–18 month therapeutic trial
  b) 60% patients relapse (100% of toxic adenoma patients)
  c) Occasionally used long-term in elderly patients
2 Radioiodine (^{131}I)
  a) Takes 2–3 months to achieve response
  b) Teratogenic; contraindicated if pregnancy possible
  c) *Not* carcinogenic (cf. low-dose external thyroid radiation)
  d) No longer contraindicated in young patients
  e) 30% will still be thyrotoxic after a single treatment
  f) 60% will become hypothyroid within 20 years of treatment
3 Subtotal thyroidectomy
  a) Undertaken only after thyrotoxicosis controlled,

e.g. after 6 weeks carbimazole + 1 week's iodine ± propranolol
  b) 30% will become hypothyroid within 10 years of treatment
  c) Losing popularity now to I^{131}

Key clinical monitors of response to antithyroid therapy
1 Slowing of heart rate
2 Weight gain
3 Goitre shrinkage

Factors predictive of prolonged remission to thionamides
(methimazole/carbimazole, propylthiouracil)
1 Small goitre
2 Reduction in goitre size on treatment
3 Mild thyrotoxicosis
4 T_3-toxicosis
5 Low or absent TSI titre
6 HLA-DRw3 negative

Relative indications for PTU rather than methimazole/carbimazole
1 Thyroid storm
2 Pregnancy
3 Puerperium

Potential indications for β-blockers
1 Rapid control of symptoms during initial treatment (e.g. thionamides)
2 Thionamide hypersensitivity or toxicity (temporary measure)
3 Preparation for surgery

Relative indications for ablative therapy in Graves' disease
1 Elderly patient
2 Poor compliance
3 Large goitre
4 Nodular change in goitre
5 Recurrent disease despite conservative therapy

Relative indications for radioiodine therapy
(NB: patients should be *rendered euthyroid* prior to ^{131}I therapy)
1 Thyrotoxic patient aged > 45 years*
2 Thyrotoxic patient relapsing following thionamide therapy
3 Thyrotoxic patient relapsing following thyroidectomy
4 Thyrotoxic patient normally treatable with surgery (e.g. toxic adenoma) but unfit for anaesthesia

Indications for total thyroidectomy
1 Medullary thyroid carcinoma
2 Anaplastic thyroid carcinoma
3 Differentiated (papillary or follicular) thyroid carcinoma involving both lobes

---

*In recent years it has become more popular to treat younger patients with ^{131}I (see ref. 3.9)

Indications for subtotal thyroidectomy in thyrotoxicosis

1 Thyrotoxic patient with large symptomatic goitre (e.g. SVC obstruction, thoracic outlet syndrome)
2 Young thyrotoxic patient unable to tolerate thionamide therapy
3 Young thyrotoxic woman desiring pregnancy

Graves' disease in pregnancy: management considerations

1 The plancenta is crossed by
   a) TSI (but not T_4)
   b) Methimazole, carbimazole (> PTU): → fetal goitre, teratogenic
   c) [131]I (causes cretinism; teratogenic)
   d) Propranolol (→ fetal bradycardia)
2 Neonatal hyperthyroidism (suggested by persistent fetal tachycardia) poses a greater risk than hypothyroidism in the immediate postnatal period
3 Thyrotoxic maternal Graves' disease may be treated with the *smallest possible* dose of thionamide and/or propranolol
4 Neonates may require thionamide therapy for up to 2 months postpartum even if maternal antithyroid treatment has led to fetal euthyroidism at delivery (since TSI may passively persist in the neonate)

Therapeutic approach to severe Graves' ophthalmopathy

1 Assess severity
   a) Clinical examination (p. 82)
   b) CT scanning
2 Conservative therapy
   a) Lubricating eyedrops
   b) Fresnel prisms (for diplopia)
3 Corticosteroids
   a) Retro-orbital
   b) Systemic
4 Surgery
   a) Lateral tarsorrhaphy (for corneal protection)
   b) Muscle transposition (for ophthalmoplegia)
   c) Orbital decompression (for optic nerve compression)
5 Non-surgical measures
   a) Cyclosporin A
   b) Cytotoxic immunosuppression
   c) Orbital radiotherapy
   d) Plasmapheresis

HYPOTHYROIDISM

Management of myxoedema in the patient with ischaemic heart disease

1 Begin replacement with low-dose L-thyroxine (e.g. 25 μg/day: probably safer than T_3 in this context)
2 Increase dose by approximately 25 μg/day every 2 weeks; monitor symptoms (of angina, arrhythmia or failure) and ECG
3 Reduce digoxin if toxicity suspected despite 'therapeutic' level
4 Avoid β-blockers if bradycardic or borderline CCF

Common perioperative complications in the hypothyroid patient

1 Intraoperative
   a) Hypotension
   b) Cardiac failure (esp. during cardiac surgery)
2 Postoperative
   a) Lack of fever despite documented infection
   b) Constipation, ileus
   c) Neuropsychiatric disorder, esp. confusion

MANAGEMENT OF DIABETIC KETOACIDOSIS

Potential hazards in ketoacidosis

1 Insulin-induced hypophosphataemia may enhance oxygen-haemoglobin affinity and thereby aggravate tissue hypoxia; presumptive phosphate supplementation is not, however, of proven value
2 Severe acidaemia may
   a) Impair cardiac function
   b) Reduce ventricular threshold to fibrillation
   c) Increase ventilatory work
   d) Lead to insulin resistance
3 Rapid correction of acidaemia with intravenous bicarbonate may be associated with the following hazards:
   a) Development of alkalaemia, as correction of CSF acidosis (which controls ventilatory rate) 'lags' behind periphery
   b) Paradoxical worsening of CSF acidosis as CO_2 (but not HCO_3) equilibrates across the blood-brain barrier
   c) Subsequent development of CSF hyperosmolality leading to cerebral oedema
   d) Exacerbation of tissue hypoxia due to Bohr effect, i.e. rapid correction of acidosis leads to an immediate increase in oxyhaemoglobin affinity, accompanied by a slower increase in red cell 2,3-DPG
4 Intracellular potassium depletion may result if supplements not prescribed when K^+ <5.0 mmol/l

An approach to managing diabetic ketoacidosis

1 Insulin
   a) Administer via pump at 0.1 U/kg/h initially
   b) Aim to lower blood glucose by 3 mmol/l/h
   c) Increase rate by 2 U/h if no improvement after 2 hours
2 Potassium
   a) Generally need to give about 20 mmol/h if K^+ <6 mmol/l
   b) Withhold if anuric *or* K^+> 6 mmol/l *or* ECG signs of ↑K^+
   c) If serum K^+ <3 mmol/l, give 30–40 mmol/h
   d) Aim to maintain K^+ >4 mmol/l during insulin infusion
3 Fluids
   a) Must be clinically assessed
   b) A typical regimen in an averagely dehydrated DKA patient might be: normal saline 1 litre i.v. stat, 1 litre over 1 hour, 1 litre over 2 hour, then 1 litre q 4 h as needed

4 Bicarbonate — consider giving 50 mmol $NaHCO_3^-$ if pH <7.0
5 Tapering off — when blood glucose <10 mmol/l, change fluids from saline to 5% dextrose; monitor blood glucose and potassium hourly

Managing the acutely ill diabetic: a few tips
1 An acutely ill insulin-dependent diabetic generally needs to *increase* (rather than reduce) his/her insulin dose
2 Even if meals have been missed due to illness, elevated blood or urine glucose indicates an increase in insulin dosage
3 *Vomiting* may indicate severe ketosis, therefore requiring urgent insulin supplementation
4 Heavy ketonuria and/or severe vomiting constitute indications for hospitalization in any ill diabetic patient

INNOVATIONS IN INSULIN

Continuous subcutaneous infusion of insulin: therapeutic benefits
1 Lowering of blood glucose and HbA_{1c} to near-normal levels
2 Lowering of serum lipids
3 Regression of retinopathy after two years treatment (sometimes associated with initial worsening)
4 Reduction in microalbuminuria after two years treatment
5 Improvement of motor, autonomic and painful neuropathies

NB: risk of diabetic ketoacidosis may be *increased*

Indications for using recombinant human insulin
1 Newly diagnosed diabetes
2 Lipoatrophy at porcine insulin injection sites
3 Proven allergy to porcine insulin
4 Diabetic pregnancy (? prevents fetal pancreatic insulitis)
5 Insulin resistance due to antibody production (rare)

RETINOPATHY

Diabetic retinopathy: indications for photocoagulation
1 Proliferative retinopathy — esp. new vessels within one disc diameter of the optic disc
2 Fresh haemorrhages — esp preretinal vitreous haemorrhages
3 Maculopathy
   a) *Focal* photocoagulation controls early *exudative* maculopathy
   b) *Peripheral* ('panretinal') photocoagulation is needed to control maculopathy due to *oedema* or *ischaemia*

Efficacy of retinal laser photocoagulation
1 Laser photocoagulation renders hypoxic retina anoxic, thus preventing further secretion of the putative neovascularising factor(s)

NB: human insulin use is associated with less warning of developing hypoglycaemia (see ref. 3.4)

2 Central visual acuity remains normal if therapy undertaken early, but visual fields constrict and night vision worsens
3 New vessels atrophy within a month of treatment
4 In general, argon laser is better suited for focal photocoagulation, while xenon laser is better suited for peripheral photocoagulation

Indications for fluorescein angiography
1 To evaluate and follow up patients with significant retinopathy evident on fundoscopy
2 To evaluate patients with known retinopathy in whom visual deterioration occurs
3 To evaluate major changes in fundoscopic signs
4 To direct laser treatment in patients with maculopathy or proliferative retinopathy

NB: fluorescein angiography is *not* indicated in patients without fundoscopic abnormality.

Potential indications for vitrectomy
1 Retinitis proliferans
2 Bilateral vitreous haemorrhages with visual acuity <6/60
3 Failure of laser photocoagulation to preserve visual acuity

SURGERY IN THE DIABETIC PATIENT

Perioperative management of insulin-dependent diabetes
1 Admit at least two days pre-op. to assess glycaemic control
2 Cease long-acting insulin and stabilise on short-acting and intermediate-acting insulin
3 Schedule operation for first thing in the morning
4 On day of operation, commence infusion of dextrose, soluble insulin (1–2 U/h at first) and potassium at least 1 hour pre-op.
5 Measure blood glucose q 2 h initially; aim for 5–10 mmol/1 level; measure serum potassium q 6 h
6 Post-op, continue insulin infusion until first meal, recommence preprandial subcutaneous soluble insulin in lieu of infusion, and commence intermediate-acting insulin prior to evening meal

Perioperative management of sulphonylurea-treated diabetics
1 Omit tablets on morning of surgery
2 If preoperative blood glucose > 15 mmol/l, cancel surgery and reschedule while stabilization underway
3 If preoperative blood glucose >12 mmol/l, commence 'sliding scale' insulin titrated against regular blood/urine glucose
4 If glucose drops below 10 mmol/l while receiving insulin, commence dextrose infusion
5 Cease insulin when euglycaemic
6 Once eating, recommence tablets if and when hyperglycaemia recurs

ORAL HYPOGLYCAEMICS

Postulated mechanisms of section of oral hypoglycaemic agents

1 Sulphonylureas
   a) Initial effect: stimulate pancreatic insulin release
   b) Chronic effect: increase number of insulin receptors
2 Biguanides (metformin)
   a) Increase peripheral glucose utilization by increasing availability of insulin receptors
   b) Increase anaerobic glycolysis (hence lactic acidosis risk)
   c) Reduce intestinal glucose absorption
   d) Reduce hepatic gluconeogenesis
   e) Induce anorexia (and hence weight loss)

Clinical problems with sulphonylurea therapy

1 High failure rate
   a) 80–90% overall
   b) 40% failure within first 3 months
   c) Of those 'successfully' controlled, 25% per annum will need to be changed to insulin
   d) Of those successfully controlled in the longer term, 50% can cease drug treatment if challenged
2 Hypoglycaemia (cf. metformin), esp. with chlorpropamide
3 Leucopenia/thrombocytopenia
4 Cholestasis
5 Photosensitivity

Clinical associations of oral hypoglycaemia therapy

1 Drugs undergoing predominant renal excretion
   a) Chlorpropamide
   b) Metformin
   Drugs undergoing predominant hepatic metabolism
   a) Glibenclamide
   b) Tolbutamide
2 Drugs with long half-life (once-daily administration) — chorpropamide*
   Drugs with medium half-life (once- to twice-daily administration) — glibenclamide
   Drugs with short half-life (up to three times daily)
   a) Tolbutamide
   b) Metformin
3 Effects on water metabolism
   a) Chlorpropamide → ↑ ADH sensitivity (mimics SIADH)
   b) Tolbutamide → SIADH (infrequently)
   c) Glibenclamide → diuretic effect
4 Chlorpropamide → alcohol-induced flushing; associated with
   a) Positive family history of non-insulin-dependent diabetes
   b) Reduced incidence of microangiopathic complications
5 Metformin-induced lactic acidosis: commoner if

a) Renal failure
b) Perioperative (or other cause of relative hypoxia)
c) >2 g/day metformin dosage
d) Associated cardiovascular and/or liver disease

MISCELLANEOUS MANAGEMENT MODALITIES IN DIABETES

Principles of dietary management

1 Non-insulin-dependent diabetes
   a) 2000 kCal/day
   b) Regular exercise
2 Insulin-dependent diabetes
   a) Caloric restriction as required to maintain ideal body weight
   b) Balanced diet consisting of a variety of foods normally enjoyed by the patient
   c) Protein intake averaging 1 g/kg/day
   d) Approximately 50% of total caloric intake should consist of complex carbohydrate (high fibre)
   e) Restrict
      — Alcohol
      — Refined sugar
      — Saturated fats
      — Salt
   f) Maintain a regular exercise programme

Useful drugs in diabetic autonomic neuropathy

1 Gustatory facial sweating: tricyclics
2 Gastroparesis: metoclopramide
3 Diarrhoea: tetracycline

Anticipated problems in uraemic diabetics

1 If managed with haemodialysis
   a) Vascular access
   b) Worsening of retinopathy
2 If managed with peritoneal dialysis
   a) Hyperglycaemia
   b) Recurrent peritonitis
3 If managed with transplantation
   a) Steroid-induced worsening of diabetic control
   b) Severe and/or recurrent infections

CUSHING'S DISEASE

Treatment modalities in Cushing's disease

1 Transsphenoidal microadenomectomy is now the treatment of choice for adults
2 Best indicator of surgical cure is post-op. hypocortisolism
3 Bilateral adrenalectomy now routinely indicated only following failed transsphenoidal microadenomectomy in women desiring pregnancy
4 Nelson's syndrome (ACTH-secreting pituitary tumour) occurs in 10% of adults and 30% of children undergoing bilateral adrenalectomy
5 ^{60}Co (heavy-particle) pituitary irradiation is used primarily in children; ocular nerve palsies may result
6 Medical management alone (e.g. with cyproheptadine) has been reported to be effective

---

*Drugs with long half-lives are most likely to cause hypoglycaemia. Drugs with short half-lives are therefore particularly suitable for elderly patients

PREGNANCY

Diseases often improved by pregnancy
1 Rheumatoid arthritis
2 Graves' disease
3 Sarcoidosis
4 Migraine

Diseases often exacerbated by pregnancy
1 SLE (esp. in puerperium)
2 Diabetes mellitus (glucose tolerance and microvascular disease may both deteriorate)
3 Rheumatic heart disease
4 Epilepsy
5 Sickle-cell anaemia
6 Multiple sclerosis (esp. in puerperium)
7 Nerve entrapment syndromes — CTS, meralgia paraesthetica
8 Intracranial lesions
   a) Pituitary macroadenoma, esp. prolactinoma
   b) Suprasellar meningioma   } all may enlarge
   c) Arteriovenous malformation

'Test-tube' pregnancies: what's the success rate?
1 In vitro fertilization (IVF): 10–15% per operation
2 Gamete intrafallopian transfer (GIFT): 15–20% per operation
3 Zygote intrafallopian transfer (ZIFT): 20–25% per operation

ORAL CONTRACEPTIVES

Beneficial effects of combined oral contraceptives
1 Contraception (incl. fewer ectopic pregnancies; cf. IUDs)
2 Less dysmenorrhoea or menorrhagia; less endometriosis
3 Less benign breast disease
4 Fewer follicular and luteal ovarian cysts
5 Lower risk of endometrial and ovarian cancer

Patient evaluation prior to (oestrogenic) oral contraception
1 Past history of neoplasia
   a) Breast cancer
   b) Endometrial cancer
   c) Hydatidiform mole
   d) Uterine leiomyomata (fibroids)
   e) Hepatic tumours
   f) Prolactinoma
2 History of disorder worsening during pregnancy
   a) Pruritus
   b) Jaundice
   c) Herpes gestationis
   d) Otosclerosis
3 History of vascular disorder
   a) Thromboembolism
   b) Cardio- or cerebrovascular problem
   c) Hypertension (incl. pulmonary)
   d) Cigarette smoking
   e) Migraine (esp. 'classical', focal, basilar, ophthalmoplegic)

4 Examination
   a) Weight, urinalysis, blood pressure
   b) Breasts, liver, fundi
   c) Vaginal examination
5 Baseline investigations
   a) Cervical smear
   b) Urine HCG
   c) Serum lipids (fasting)
   d) Liver function tests
   e) ECG if indicated

Drug interactions with oral contraceptives (OCs)
1 Drugs reducing OC efficacy due to hepatic enzyme induction:
   a) Rifampicin (contraindicated in OC users); griseofulvin
   b) Phenytoin, carbamazepine, barbiturates
2 Drugs reducing OC efficacy by disrupting enterohepatic recirculation:
   a) Tetracycline, ampicillin; purgatives
3 Hepatic enzyme inhibition by OCs → drug potentiation:
   a) Imipramine
   b) Barbiturates
   c) Chlordiazepoxide; pethidine
4 Reduction of epileptic threshold by OCs — i.e. seizure activity may worsen despite increased plasma anticonvulsant levels

GONADOTROPHIN-RELEASING HORMONE

Indications for pulsatile (stimulatory) GnRH therapy
(mainly LHRH agonists, e.g. buserelin, goserelin, leuprolide)
1 Anovulatory infertility
2 Male hypogonadotrophic hypogonadism
3 Initiation of puberty

Potential indications for continuous (suppressive) GnRH therapy
1 Endometriosis
2 Polycystic ovary syndrome
3 Uterine fibroids
4 Dysfunctional uterine bleeding
5 Premenstrual syndrome
6 Contraception (male and female)
7 Precocious puberty
8 Metastatic prostate cancer
9 Premenopausal metastatic breast cancer

SEX HORMONE REPLACEMENT THERAPY

Undisputed indications for oestrogen replacement
1 Gonadal dysgenesis
2 Premature menopause (e.g. Wertheim's hysterectomy)

Proven benefits of postmenopausal low-dose oestrogen replacement
1 Reduced morbidity and mortality from osteoporotic fractures
2 Reduced cardiovascular mortality

3 Prevention/reversal of urogenital atrophy (atrophic vaginitis)
4 Improvement of perimenopausal vasomotor instability (hot flushes)

Neoplastic hazards of postmenopausal low-dose oestrogen replacement

1 Endometrial cancer
  a) Absolute risk 1% per year; relative risk about six-fold
  b) Risk reduced by concomitant progestogen therapy (similar protective effect of combined therapy claimed for ovarian cancer)
2 Hepatic adenoma ($\pm$ intraperitoneal haemorrhage)
3 Breast cancer
  a) Long-term oestrogens increase risk
  b) Progestogens may further increase risk

SEXUAL DISORDERS AND DRUG THERAPY

Treatment options in idiopathic hirsutism

1 Mild hirsutism — reassurance
2 Moderate hirsutism Pregnancy desired ⎱ Shaving, waxing, depilatory creams, electrolysis
3 Moderate hirsutism Pregnancy not desired ⎱ Combined oral contraceptive ($\rightarrow$ ↓ FSH/LH)
4 Severe hirsutism Pregnancy desired ⎱ Dexamethasone 0.25 mg nocte ($\rightarrow$ ↓ adrenal androgens)
5 Severe hirsutism Pregnancy not desired ⎱ Cyproterone acetate (an anti-androgen) or spironolactone

Major drug classes causing male sexual dysfunction
(loss of libido; impotence; ejaculatory impairment)
1 Alcohol/narcotic addiction
2 Oestrogens, corticosteroids
3 'Antiandrogens' — spironolactone, cimetidine
4 Antihypertensives — methyldopa, propranolol
5 Phenothiazines, tricyclics

Anabolic steroids: their clinical relevance

1 Include — oxymethalone, nandrolone decanoate, stanozolol
2 Established use — aplastic anaemia
3 Experimental use — osteoporosis, scleroderma
4 Commonest use — bodybuilding amongst athletes (illicit)
5 Hazards
  a) Testosterone suppression (testicular atrophy, impotence)
  b) Liver tumours (hepatoma, angiosarcoma)

UNDERSTANDING ENDOCRINE DISEASE

Characteristics of hormonal action

1 Steroid and thyroid hormones
  a) Lipid soluble; require plasma carrier protein for cell delivery
  b) Long plasma $t^{\frac{1}{2}}$; easily measured in serum

  c) Actions tend to be gradual in onset (hours to days)
  d) Hormone binding leads to conformational change in nuclear receptor which then acquires increased affinity for specific DNA enhancer sequences
2 Polypeptide hormones and catecholamines
  a) Water soluble; circulate free in plasma and bind to cell membrane receptors
  b) Short plasma $t^{\frac{1}{2}}$; serum measurements may be hard to interpret
  c) Actions tend to be rapid in onset (minutes to hours)
  d) Hormone binding to membrane receptor proteins leads to activation of cytoplasmic 'second messenger' system (cAMP, diacylglycerol, tyrosine kinases, protein kinase C, etc.) which mediates signal transduction to nucleus

Prohormones: hormones requiring activation for maximal function

1 T_4: prohormone for T_3
2 Testosterone — prohormone for dihydrotestosterone
3 (Dietary) vitamin D_2 (ergocalciferol) (Skin) vitamin D_3 (cholecalciferol) ⎱ prohormones for 1,25-dihydroxy vitamin D

Hormones with structural similarities

1 Glycoproteins with identical α-subunits
  a) LH, FSH
  b) TSH
  c) HCG (weak TSH agonism may rarely result in choriocarcinoma patients developing thyrotoxicosis)
2 Large single-chain polypeptides with amino acid homology
  a) Growth hormone (GH)
  b) Prolactin (PRL)
  c) Human placental lactogen (HPL)
  d) Parathyroid hormone (PTH)
3 Melatonin
  Serotonin

Circadian rhythmicity of hormone release

1 Late afternoon: PRL — hence to demonstrate hyperprolactinaemia, test in morning
2 Early phase of sleep — GH
3 Late phase of sleep
  a) ACTH/cortisol
  b) TSH, LH
4 Stress
  a) ACTH/cortisol
  b) ADH
  c) PRL
  d) GH (in lean patients)
  e) Glucagon

Endorphins: their effect on hormone release

1 Stimulation
  a) Growth hormone
  b) Prolactin
  c) TSH

2 Inhibition
  a) ADH
  b) ACTH
  c) Adrenaline/noradrenaline
  d) LH/FSH

Predominant oestrogens in the human life cycle
1 E_1 (oestrone) — postmenopausal
2 E_2 (oestradiol) — child-bearing period
3 E_3 (oestriol)
  a) Pregnancy
  b) Fetal life

Diseases caused by end-organ resistance to hormones
1 Testicular feminization syndrome — defective receptors for testosterone/dihydrotestosterone
2 Pseudohypoparathyroidism — resistance to PTH
3 X-linked nephrogenic diabetes insipidus — resistance of distal nephron to ADH
4 Type II vitamin D-dependent rickets — end-organ resistance to 1,25 dihydroxy-vitamin D
5 Laron dwarfism — absence of GH receptors preventing somatomedin C (IGF-I) induction; treatable with IGF-I
6 Type A insulin receptor abnormality
  a) Reduced number of insulin receptors
  b) Associated with Stein-Leventhal (polycystic ovary) phenotype

UNDERSTANDING DIABETES

Antibodies detectable in diabetes mellitus
1 Insulin antibodies
  a) Usually seen in patients treated with porcine insulin
  b) IgE type may mediate allergic reactions
  c) *Rarely* associated with insulin resistance
2 Islet cell cytoplasm antibodies — may play a role in pathogenesis of insulin-dependent diabetes
3 Islet cell insulin receptor-blocking antibodies (i.e. Type B insulin receptor abnormality)
  a) IgG-mediated reduction in receptor affinity for insulin
  b) Associated with SLE-like phenotype
4 Islet cell insulin receptor-stimulating antibodies — may play a role in disturbed glucose homeostasis

Anomalies of diabetic adiposities
1 Lipodystrophy — associated with insulin-resistant diabetes, i.e. type A insulin receptor abnormality (see above)
2 Lipoatrophy — occurs at sites of porcine insulin injection; responds to injection of monocomponent insulin
3 Lipohypertrophy — commoner with monocomponent insulin use, esp. if injection sites not rotated

Factors correlating with severity of microvascular disease
1 Duration of diabetes
2 Degree of long-term hyperglycaemia
3 Hypertension

NB: the relationship between glycaemic control and macrovascular disease remains unclear

Infections increased in poorly-controlled diabetics
NB: infection may either complicate or precipitate ketoacidosis
1 Rhinocerebral mucormycosis
2 Emphysematous cholecystitis (*Clostridia* spp.)
3 Necrotising cellulitis/fasciitis (mixed aerobes and anaerobes)
4 Malignant otitis externa (*Ps. aeruginosa*)
5 Oral or vulvovaginal candidiasis
6 Furunculosis (staphylococcal)
7 Abscesses, e.g. perinephric
8 Influenza/*Staph*. pneumonia
9 Tuberculosis

UNDERSTANDING THYROID DISEASE

Clinical varieties of thyroiditis
1 Chronic lymphocytic (Hashimoto's) thyroiditis
  a) Common
  b) Female — male = 20:1
  c) Onset — gradual, transient 'Hashitoxicosis' unusual
  d) Signs — diffuse painless goitre, no bruit
  e) Biopsy — lymphocytic infiltrate, Askanazy cells
  f) Associations — thyroid autoantibodies, HLA DR5; painless
  g) Sequelae — persistent hypothyroidism in 80%
2 Subacute granulomatous (de Quervain's) thyroiditis
  a) Uncommon
  b) Female — male = 2:1
  c) Onset — acute, transient thyrotoxicosis usual
  d) Signs — small goitre, extremely tender
  e) Biopsy — giant cell infiltrate, granulomata
  f) Associations — viral infection, malaise; painful gland
  g) Sequelae — transient hypothyroidism in 10%
3 Subacute lymphocytic ('silent') thyroiditis
  a) Common
  b) Female — male = 5:1
  c) Onset — acute (often postpartum), transient thyrotoxicosis usual
  d) Signs — goitre usually absent
  e) Biopsy — similar to Hashimoto's
  f) Associations — thyroid autoantibodies, HLA DR5; painless
  g) Sequelae — transient hypothyroidism in 25%
4 Chronic fibrosing (Riedel's) thyroiditis
  a) Rare
  b) Onset — gradual
  c) Signs — woody (ligneous) indurated thyroid
  d) Biopsy — widespread fibrosis
  e) Associations — retroperitoneal fibrosis, sclerosing cholangitis, fibrosing mediastinitis, Peyronie's disease
  f) Sequelae — persistent hypothyroidism in 50%

Cardiac manifestations of thyroid disease
1 Hypothyroidism
  a) Hypercholesterolaemia, ischaemic heart disease
  b) Pericarditis, pericardial effusion

c) Cardiomyopathy, cardiac failure
d) Hypotension or hypertension
e) Bradycardia; low-voltage ECG
2 Thyrotoxicosis
a) Sinus tachycardia; atrial fibrillation ± thromboembolism
b) Bounding pulse, widened pulse pressure
c) Angina, myocardial infarction
d) High-output CCF; cardiomyopathy, focal myocarditis
e) Sudden death (presumed VF)

POLYGLANDULAR ENDOCRINE DISORDERS

Multiple endocrine adenomatosis: the clinical spectrum
1 Multiple endocrine adenomatosis type I (Wermer's syndrome)
a) Hyperparathyroidism (90%) — adenomatous or hyperplastic
b) Pituitary adenoma (60%)
c) Islet cell tumour (e.g. gastrinoma)
d) Other — lipomata, carcinoids, thymoma
2 Multiple endocrine adenomatosis type IIa (Sipple's syndrome)
a) Phaeochromocytoma
b) Medullary carcinoma of the thyroid
c) Parathyroid hyperplasia (50%) — generally subclinical
d) Gliomas, meningiomas
3 Multiple endocrine adenomatosis type IIb (mucosal neuroma syndrome)
a) Similar to IIa, though hyperparathyroidism rare
b) Marfanoid habitus
c) Mucosal neuromata, protuberant lips, intestinal ganglioneuromatosis

Other polyglandular endocrine syndromes
1 Schmidt's syndrome
a) Addison's + Hashimoto's
b) ± Hypoparathyroidism
c) Primary gonadal failure
d) Diabetes mellitus
2 Candidiasis/endocrinopathy syndrome
a) Hypoparathyroidism
b) Addison's disease
c) Pernicious anaemia
3 Lipodystrophies
a) Diabetes mellitus
b) Stein-Leventhal syndrome
c) Acromegaly, Cushing's
4 Albright's syndrome
a) Precocious puberty in girls (predominantly)
b) ± Cushing's syndrome, acromegaly
5 Pinealoma
a) Diabetes insipidus (ectopic location)
b) Precocious puberty in boys (only about 10%)

Endocrine causes of proximal weakness
1 Thyroid dysfunction
a) Thyrotoxicosis (myopathy or periodic paralysis)
b) Hypothyroidism
2 Adrenal dysfunction
a) Cushing's disease

b) Corticosteroid therapy (esp. dexamethasone, triamcinolone)
c) Nelson's syndrome
d) Addison's disease
3 Acromegaly
4 Primary hyperparathyroidism
5 Primary hyperaldosteronism
6 Vitamin D deficiency (osteomalacia)

DRUG INTERACTIONS IN ENDOCRINE DISORDERS

Alcohol abuse and glucose homeostasis
1 Hypoglycaemia may occur due to
a) Prolonged fasting
b) Reduced hepatic glycogen storage capacity
c) Impaired gluconeogenesis due to high NADH levels
d) 'Reactive' to high-carbohydrate diet (i.e. → ↑ ↑ insulin release)
e) Potentiation of insulin- and tolbutamide-/glibenclamide-induced hypoglycaemia with acute ingestion
2 Hyperglycaemia may occur due to
a) Obesity
b) Chronic pancreatitis
c) Insulin resistance due to elevated free fatty acid levels
d) Induced hepatic metabolism of tolbutamide/glibenclamide with chronic ingestion (i.e. worsening of diabetic control)

β-blockers and glucose homeostasis
1 May predispose to hypoglycaemia due to prevention of catecholamine-induced hepatic glycogenolysis
2 May lead to potentiation and prolongation of (say) sulphonylurea-induced hypoglycaemia due to secondary lack of negative feedback on insulin release (esp. if α-agonism, e.g. labetalol)
3 Impair awareness of developing (systemic) hypoglycaemia, with attendant risk of profound neuroglycopaenia; this effect is most marked with use of non-selective β-blockade

Drug-induced gynaecomastia and/or galactorrhoea
1 Drugs causing gynaecomastia alone (± impotence; normal prolactin)
a) Alcohol (± chronic liver disease)
b) Androgens/progestogens (converted to oestrogens); HCG
c) Antiandrogens
— Cyproterone acetate
— Spironolactone
— Cimetidine
d) Weak oestrogens
— Digoxin
— Griseofulvin
— Marijuana
2 Drugs causing gynaecomastia and/or galactorrhoea (↑ prolactin)
a) Methyldopa, reserpine
b) Heroin, morphine

c) Tricyclics, haloperidol, phenothiazines, metoclopramide

d) Oestrogens (only rarely cause galactorrhoea)

Drug-induced azoöspermia: causes
1 Cytotoxics (esp. MOPP, alkylators)
2 Sex steroids (incl. high-dose androgens; → ↓ FSH)
3 'Anti-androgens':

a) Danazol, stanozolol (anabolic steroids → ↓ LH → ↓ testosterone)
b) Cimetidine
c) Spironolactone
4 Sulphasalazine
5 Colchicine, phenytoin, nitrofurantoin; major tranquillizers
6 Alcohol, marijuana

Reviewing the Literature: Endocrinology

3.1 Kroc Collaborative Study Group 1984 Blood glucose control and the evolution of diabetic retinopathy and albuminuria. New England Journal of Medicine 311: 365–372

Randomized trial of 70 patients with low-C-peptide diabetes. Continuous insulin infusion was associated with improvement of proteinuria, but was also associated with initial deterioration of retinopathy and a tendency to ketoacidosis

McCance D R et al 1989 Long-term glycaemic control and diabetic retinopathy. Lancet ii: 824–826

Recent study supporting the view that tight sugar control *is* important in reducing the incidence of microvascular diabetic complications after all

3.2 Feldt-Rasmussen B et al 1986 Kidney function during 12 months of strict metabolic control in insulin-dependent diabetic patients with incipient nephropathy. New England Journal of Medicine 314: 655–670

Feldt-Rasmussen B et al 1986 Effect of two years of stict metabolic control on progression of incipient nephropathy in insulin-dependent diabetes. Lancet ii: 1300–1303

Danish studies of 36 patients showing that continuous-infusion insulin can significantly reduce proteinuria and glycosylated Hb; improvement of the renal lesion took two years to become evident

3.3 Assan R, Feutren G et al 1985 Metabolic and immunological effects of cyclosporin in recently diagnosed type I diabetes mellitus. Lancet i: 67–71

Of 12 recently-diagnosed insulin-dependent diabetics, 4 experienced a complete remission and 4 a partial remission following 2–8 months cyclosporin A therapy

Feutren G et al 1986 Cyclosporin increases the rate and length of remissions in insulin-dependent diabetes of recent onset. Lancet ii: 119–123

Double-blind placebo-controlled trial of 122 patients over 9 months. 65% of cyclosporin patients went into remission, compared with 29% of controls

3.4 Berger W et al 1989 Warning symptoms of hypoglycaemia during treatment with human and porcine insulin in diabetes mellitus. Lancet i: 1041–1043

Heine R J et al 1989 Responses to human and porcine insulin in healthy subjects. Lancet ii: 946–948

Two studies documenting that human insulin causes fewer sympathoadrenergic (but not neuroglycopaenic) symptoms than does porcine for a given level of hypoglycaemia

3.5 Dornhorst A et al 1985 Aggravation by propranolol of hyperglycaemic effect of hydrochlorothiazide in type II diabetes without alteration of insulin secretion. Lancet i: 123–126

Small study of 14 male patients: both drugs together caused a 56% elevation of blood glucose and a 15% increase in Hb_{A1c}

3.6 Haffner S M et al 1988 Increased insulin concentrations in nondiabetic offspring of diabetic parents. New England Journal of Medicine 319: 1297–1301

Cohort study of 1500 non-diabetic Mexicans showing that hyperinsulinaemia was predictive of subsequent non-insulin-dependent diabetes, supporting the notion that this disorder may arise primarily from insulin resistance

3.7 Lever E, Jaspan J B 1983 Sodium bicarbonate therapy in severe diabetic ketoacidosis. American Journal of Medicine 75: 263–268

In this retrospective study of 95 patients, the use of intravenous bicarbonate (given either as a 'push' or as an infusion) was found to be associated neither with increased morbidity nor with improved therapeutic efficacy

3.8 Graham G D, Burman K D 1986 Radioiodine treatment of Graves' disease: an assessment of potential risks. Annals of Internal Medicine 105: 900–905

The authors of this study conclude that radioiodine is 'a safe treatment, except during (and 6 months before) pregnancy

3.9 Styne D M, Grumbach M M, Kaplan S L et al 1984 Treatment of Cushing's disease in childhood and adolescence by trans-sphenoidal microadenomectomy. New England Journal of Medicine 310: 889–893

A high success rate is reported in this series which relied on direct operative visualization for tumour localization; radiographic studies were found to be unhelpful

3.10 Krenning E P et al 1989 Localisation of endocrine-related tumours with radioiodinated analogue of somatostatin. Lancet i: 242–244

Yet another use for the somatostatin analogue octreotide (SMS 201–995) which is already popularly used in therapy of carcinoid syndrome, VIPoma and glucagonoma

CHAPTER 4

Gastroenterology

Physical examination protocol 4.1 You are asked to examine the gastrointestinal system

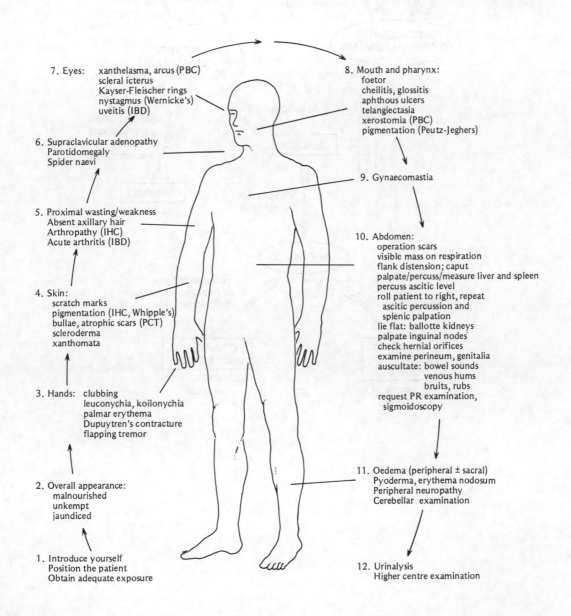

7. Eyes: xanthelasma, arcus (PBC)
scleral icterus
Kayser-Fleischer rings
nystagmus (Wernicke's)
uveitis (IBD)

6. Supraclavicular adenopathy
Parotidomegaly
Spider naevi

5. Proximal wasting/weakness
Absent axillary hair
Arthropathy (IHC)
Acute arthritis (IBD)

4. Skin:
scratch marks
pigmentation (IHC, Whipple's)
bullae, atrophic scars (PCT)
scleroderma
xanthomata

3. Hands: clubbing
leuconychia, koilonychia
palmar erythema
Dupuytren's contracture
flapping tremor

2. Overall appearance:
malnourished
unkempt
jaundiced

1. Introduce yourself
Position the patient
Obtain adequate exposure

8. Mouth and pharynx:
foetor
cheilitis, glossitis
aphthous ulcers
telangiectasia
xerostomia (PBC)
pigmentation (Peutz-Jeghers)

9. Gynaecomastia

10. Abdomen:
operation scars
visible mass on respiration
flank distension; caput
palpate/percuss/measure liver and spleen
percuss ascitic level
roll patient to right, repeat
ascitic percussion and
splenic palpation
lie flat: ballotte kidneys
palpate inguinal nodes
check hernial orifices
examine perineum, genitalia
auscultate: bowel sounds
venous hums
bruits, rubs
request PR examination,
sigmoidoscopy

11. Oedema (peripheral ± sacral)
Pyoderma, erythema nodosum
Peripheral neuropathy
Cerebellar examination

12. Urinalysis
Higher centre examination

Diagnostic pathway 4.1 The patient is jaundiced. Why do you think this might be?

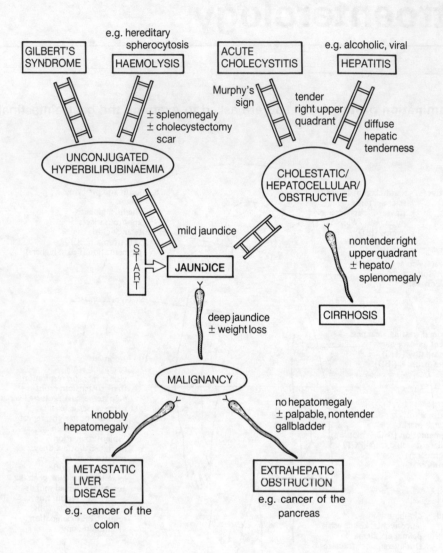

Diagnostic pathway 4.2 This patient is noted to have hepatomegaly. What is your provisional diagnosis?

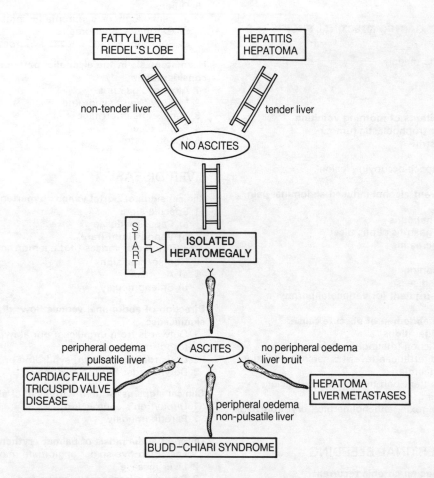

CLINICAL ASPECTS OF GASTROINTESTINAL DISEASE

COMMONEST GASTROINTESTINAL SHORT CASES

1 Hepatosplenomegaly
2 Ascites
3 Jaundice

Common precipitants of morning vomiting
1 Pregnancy or trophoblastic tumour
2 Alcoholic gastritis
3 Migraine
4 Intracranial space-occupying lesion

Causes of recurrent alcohol-induced abdominal pain
1 Common
  a) Alcoholic hepatitis
  b) Alcoholic gastritis/peptic ulcer
  c) Acute pancreatitis
2 Classical
  a) Lead poisoning
  b) Hodgkin's disease
  c) Acute intermittent (or variegate) porphyria

Recurrent acute abdomen of obscure cause: diagnostic considerations
1 Narcotic addiction (malingering)
2 Familial Mediterranean fever ($\pm$ narcotic addiction)
3 Sickle-cell anaemia
4 Acute intermittent porphyria; C1-INH deficiency
5 Lead poisoning
6 Iatrogenic (digoxin, anticholinergics, erythromycin)

GASTROINTESTINAL BLEEDING

Local lesions causing chronic recurrent gastrointestinal bleeding
1 Angiodysplasia
  a) Often multiple
  b) Tend to affect right colon
  c) Higher incidence in elderly patients and in aortic stenosis
  d) Rarely visible macroscopically; angiography often required
2 Haemangioma
  a) Tend to affect stomach, small bowel, or rectum
  b) Typically gross (visible) lesions; cf. angiodysplasia
3 Telangiectasia — e.g. hereditary haemorrhagic telangiectasia
4 Diverticulitis — incl. Meckel's

Systemic diseases causing recurrent gastrointestinal bleeding
1 Polycythaemia rubra vera
2 Vasculitis — PAN, Henoch-Schönlein
3 Behçet's syndrome
4 Amyloidosis

5 Inherited collagenoses
  a) Pseudoxanthoma elasticum
  b) Type IV Ehlers-Danlos syndrome
  c) Degos disease
6 Other
  a) Peutz-Jegher's syndrome ($\pm$ intussusception)
  b) Gardner's syndrome
  c) Blue rubber bleb naevus syndrome

Haematemesis in the alcoholic: pathogenetic considerations
1 Alcoholic gastritis
2 Mallory-Weiss syndrome
3 Variceal haemorrhage
4 Peptic ulcer
5 Coagulopathy

LIVER DISEASE

Clinical signs of portal venous hypertension
1 Specific signs
  a) Caput medusae
  b) Venous hum (rare)
  c) Anorectal varices (not haemorrhoids)
2 Non-specific signs
  a) Ascites
  b) Splenomegaly

Direction of abdominal venous flow: diagnostic significance
1 Outwards from umbilicus: portal hypertension (caput medusae)
2 Upwards: Budd-Chiari syndrome or IVC thrombosis
3 Downwards: SVC obstruction

Clinical signs associated with alcohol abuse
1 Dupuytren's contracture
2 Parotidomegaly

Differential diagnosis of palmar erythema/spider naevi
1 Less than five spider angiomata may be normal
2 Liver disease
3 Pregnancy/oral contraceptive use
4 Thyrotoxicosis
5 Rheumatoid arthritis

Massive hepatomegaly: some causes
1 Fatty infiltration
2 Metastatic liver disease
3 Polycystic disease

Hepatomegaly and heart failure
1 Right ventricular failure $\pm$ tricuspid incompetence
2 Constrictive pericarditis
3 Alcoholic cardiomyopathy with fatty liver
4 Haemochromatosis
5 Amyloidosis
6 Carcinoid syndrome

Conditions which may cause splenomegaly without portal venous hypertension
1 Chronic active hepatitis
2 Alcoholic hepatitis
3 Idiopathic haemochromatosis
4 Primary biliary cirrhosis

Helpful clinical features in characterizing chronic liver disease

1 Fever
  Ascites
  Oedema
  Dupuytren's
  Parotidomegaly } — Alcoholic cirrhosis

2 Pigmentation
  Marked hepatomegaly
  Testicular atrophy and
    hypogonadism
  Gynaecomastia
  MCP arthropathy
  Cardiac failure
  Glycosuria
  Usually male } — Haemochromatosis (jaundice/ascites uncommon)

3 Splenomegaly (often without
    other signs of portal
    hypertension)
  Prominent spider naevi
  Often young (15–30) } — Chronic active hepatitis (pigmentation uncommon)

4 Scratch marks
  Xanthelasma
  Pigmentation
  Usually female } — Primary biliary cirrhosis (ascites/oedema unusual)

LIVER FAILURE

Features of hepatic encephalopathy

1 Grade I
  a) Fluctuating confusion ± euphoria/depression
  b) Inversion of sleep pattern
  c) Slow, slurred speech
2 Grade II (signs of hepatic precoma)
  a) Drowsiness, inappropriate behaviour
  b) Fetor hepaticus
  c) Flapping tremor
  d) Constructional apraxia
3 Grade III
  a) Incoherent
  b) Sleeps all day, but rousable
  c) Hyperreflexia, myoclonus, extrapyramidal signs
4 Grade IV
  a) Unrousable (comatose)
  b) Extensor plantar responses

The flapping tremor: differential diagnosis

1 Hepatic precoma
2 Uraemia
3 CO_2 narcosis

ASCITES

Ascites: sudden worsening in stable cirrhosis

1 'Spontaneous' bacterial peritonitis (e.g. coliforms, *Flavobacterium* spp., TB)
2 Hepatic vein thrombosis (Budd-Chiari syndrome)
3 Hepatoma
4 Acute deterioration of hepatocellular function (e.g. due to sepsis, alcoholic binge, gut haemorrhage)
5 Rupture of dilated abdominal lymphatics
  (→ chylous ascites)

Differential diagnosis of chylous ascites

1 Intra-abdominal lymphoma or carcinoma
2 Hepatic cirrhosis
3 Nephrotic syndrome
4 Tuberculosis
5 Trauma (incl. surgery, e.g. distal splenorenal shunt)

Further examination of the patient with ascites

1 Abdominal signs suggesting primary liver disease
  a) Ballottable spleen
  b) Caput medusae, venous hum, testicular atrophy
2 Signs suggesting intra-abdominal malignancy
  a) Absent ankle oedema
  b) Palpable supraclavicular nodes
  c) Hepatic bruit
  d) Palpable tumour (e.g. on rectal examination)
3 Signs suggesting cardiac aetiology
  a) Elevated jugular venous pressure ± 'v' waves
  b) Pulsatile tender hepatomegaly
  c) Cardiomegaly, S_3, tricuspid murmur
  d) Pulsus paradoxus, rapid 'y' descent in JVP (constrictive pericarditis)
4 Signs suggesting hepatic vein/proximal inferior vena caval thrombosis
  a) Ascites > oedema
  b) Absent hepatojugular reflux (i.e. even with patient lying flat)
  c) Upward-draining lower abdominal wall veins
  d) Non-pulsatile tender hepatomegaly

INTESTINAL DISEASES

Chronic diarrhoea: factors favouring primary (organic) bowel pathology

1 Nocturnal diarrhoea (interrupting sleep)
2 Passage of blood per rectum
3 Faecal incontinence
4 Weight loss; fever; anaemia
5 Age of symptom onset > 50 years

Inflammatory bowel disease: indicators of severity

1 Extent of colonic disease (may not be able to be determined during acute exacerbation)
1 Number of stools/day — <4 = mild, >8 = severe (esp. if bloody)
2 Constitutional — fever, tachycardia, pain, distension
3 Weight loss >5 kg
4 Blood count — ↓ Hb; ↑ WCC/platelets/ESR
5 Biochemistry — ↓ K^+/albumin
  Acute phase reactants — ↑ CRP/orosomucoid
6 AXR
  a) Transverse colonic diameter >6.5 cm
  b) Subdiaphragmatic free gas (may be asymptomatic if on steroids)
  c) Mucosal 'islands' (pseudopolyps)

Common presentations of irritable bowel syndrome

1 Chronic or recurrent abdominal distension
2 Abdominal pain relieved by defaecation
3 Feeling of incomplete evacuation
4 Passage of mucus in stool

INVESTIGATION OF GASTROINTESTINAL DISEASE

GASTRO-OESOPHAGEAL DISORDERS

Investigation of oesophageal dysfunction
1 Is reflux present? — best test: 24-hour intraoesophageal pH monitoring (positive if pH <4, esp. during sleep)
2 Are symptoms due to reflux? — best test: acid perfusion, or Bernstein test (correlates well with symptoms, poorly with oesophagitis)
3 Is there a peptic stricture or erosion? — best test: barium swallow (limited usefulness otherwise)
4 Is oesophagitis present? — best test: oesophagoscopy and biopsy
5 Is there a dysmotility syndrome? — best test: oesophageal manometry

Applications of radionuclide oesophageal transit studies
1 May provide a non-invasive alternative to endoscopy in patients (esp. children) with suspected oesophagitis
2 Correlates well with manometry in assessment of dysmotility
3 Supplements findings of ambulatory oesophageal pH monitoring by demonstrating reflux *volume* (and hence severity)

Indications for fasting serum gastrin estimation
1 Family history of peptic ulceration
2 Multifocal peptic ulceration
Peptic ulceration of distal duodenum or jejunum
Recurrent postoperative peptic ulceration
3 Peptic ulceration associated with hypercalcaemia (i.e. ?MEA type I)
4 Intractable watery diarrhoea or steatorrhoea
5 Radiological or endoscopic evidence of gastric rugal hypertrophy

Hypergastrinaemia: differential diagnosis
1 *Gross* elevation (>600 ng/l)
  a) Achlorhydria
  b) Gastrinoma
  c) Renal failure
2 Minor elevation
  a) Failure of patient to fast
  b) Antral G-cell hyperplasia; retained antrum post-gastrectomy
  c) Gastric outlet obstruction and/or gastric ulcer
  d) Small bowel resection and/or Crohn's disease
  e) Hepatic insufficiency
  f) Hypercalcaemia

Gastrinoma: diagnostic confirmation
1 Fasting hypergastrinaemia
2 Paradoxical rise in serum gastrin following secretin infusion
Supranormal rise in serum gastrin following calcium infusion
3 Barium studies

a) Ectopic ulceration (e.g. postbulbar, oesophageal)
b) Rugal hypertrophy, duodenal nodularity
c) Increased secretions; hyperperistalsis
4 Tumour visualization with CT, ultrasound or visceral angiography
5 Percutaneous transhepatic portal venous sampling
6 Biopsy

Associations of achlorhydria
1 Type A atrophic gastritis ± pernicious anaemia
2 Vagotomy
3 Gastric cancer
4 VIPoma, somatostatinoma

DIAGNOSTIC ASPECTS OF LIVER DISEASE

True liver 'function' (as opposed to liver damage) tests
1 Albumin
2 Prothrombin time

Elevated alkaline phosphatase: features favouring liver origin
1 Heat-stable isoenzyme ('bone burns')
2 ↑GGT
3 ↑5'-nucleotidase
4 ↑serum bile acids
5 ↑ LDH-5

Investigation of suspected alcoholic liver disease
1 Gamma-glutamyl transpeptidase (GGT) elevation
  a) Induced by alcohol ingestion
  b) May also reflect intrahepatic obstruction in cirrhosis
2 Blood film
Macrocytosis (round, unless coexisting folate deficiency)
Target cells (non-specific in liver disease)
3 Biochemistry
AST — ALT >2:1 with AST <500 i.u./l (cf. viral hepatitis)
Hyperuricaemia
Hypertriglyceridaemia } — less specific
Hypomagnesaemia
Hypoalbuminaemia
4 Blood alcohol (if drinking within last 24 hours suspected)
5 Plasma AFP, gallium scan (*if* hepatoma suspected)
6 Liver biopsy (see below)

Investigation of unexplained gastrointestinal blood loss
1 Faecal occult blood testing (for confirmation)
2 Endoscopy: gastroduodenoscopy and colonoscopy
3 Angiography (detects angiodysplasias and small bowel bleeding)
4 Barium follow-through, or small-bowel enema via duodenal tube (NB: angiography impossible if barium studies performed first)
5 Radionuclide studies
  a) ^{59}Fe (oral) whole body counting (good for assessing intermenstrual blood loss)
  b) ^{99}Tc^m-labelled sulphur colloid (i.v.); sensitive detection of *active* haemorrhage >0.5 ml/min
  c) ^{51}Cr-RBC or ^{99}Tc^m-RBC labelling (i.v.: 'blood pool

scan'); may also be of value in intermittent bleeding

d) $^{99}Tc^m$ pertechnate (i.v.); lights up ectopic gastric mucosa in Meckel's diverticulum (investigation of choice here)

6 Exploratory laparotomy — a last resort

Laboratory diagnosis of idiopathic haemochromatosis

1 Transferrin saturation >80% (plus increased serum Fe, reduced TIBC)

2 Serum ferritin > 1000 μg/l (best screening test) Serum ferritin increases following desferrioxamine

3 Desferrioxamine-chelatable 24-hour urinary Fe excretion > 7.5 mg Fe

4 Quantitative phlebotomy > 7.5 g Fe

5 Liver biopsy — stainable Fe grade 3 or 4

6 Hepatic Fe quantitation: > 100 μmol/g dry weight (definitive test)

Distinction of haemochromatosis from alcoholic liver disease

1 Ferritin >1000 μg/l (normal range < 300 μg/l; cf. alcoholics → often 300–1000 μg/l)

2 Massive iron overload on liver biopsy (cf. alcohol: moderate)

3 Elevated ferritin levels in first-degree relatives

4 HLA-A3 linkage (not a diagnostic test)

Diagnosis of hepatic vein thrombosis (Budd-Chiari syndrome)

1 Isotope liver scan — selective caudate lobe uptake

2 Liver biopsy — centrizonal venous congestion

3 Hepatic venography — thrombosis (± inferior vena caval thrombosis)

Biochemical characterization of jaundice

1 Conjugated hyperbilirubinaemia
↑↑ GGT/alkaline phosphatase
Bilirubinuria, absent urobilinogen } — common bile duct obstruction

2 Conjugated ± unconjugated hyperbilirubinaemia
AST/ALT>1000 i.u./l
Bilirubinuria ± urobilinogenuria } — acute hepatitis

3 Unconjugated hyperbilirubinaemia
Normal urinary urobilinogen } —Gilbert's, Crigler-Najjar

4 Unconjugated hyperbilirubinaemia
Elevated urinary urobilinogen } — haemolysis

5 Conjugated hyperbilirubinaemia
Elevated urinary urobilinogen } — portal-systemic shunt

HEPATITIS

Serological investigation of monosymptomatic acute hepatitis

1 IgM antiHAV

2 HBsAg and antiHBc

3 EB viral capsid antigen IgM; CMV serology

Hepatitis B serology made easy

1 Presence of HBsAg implies active infection
Appearance of anti-HBs implies recovery and immunity

2 Presence of HBeAg implies patient is infective to others
Appearance of anti-HBe generally (but not invariably; see ref. 4.6) implies loss of infectivity

3 HBcAg (core antigen) cannot be detected in peripheral blood
Presence of high-titre IgM anti-HBc implies acute (and usually severe) hepatitis B; anti-HBc appears after HBsAg disappears

4 Persistence of IgM anti-HBc implies chronic HBV infection, esp. chronic active hepatitis

Investigation of the patient with chronic hepatitis

1 HBsAg
If negative, request anti-HBc and anti-HBs

2 If HBsAg or anti-HBc positive for longer than six months (i.e. chronic hepatitis), request HBeAg and anti-HBe

3 If chronic HBsAg carrier presents with unexplained exacerbation, request delta agent antibody

4 If patient is not proven to have hepatitis B, request
a) Smooth muscle/antimitochondrial/antinuclear antibodies
b) Serum caeruloplasmin, 24-hour urinary copper excretion
c) α_1AT level

5 Liver biopsy is always requested in the initial work-up

The stages of chronic hepatitis B infection

1 Active replicative phase (→acute, or chronic active, hepatitis)
a) HBeAg +, antiHBe −
b) HBV DNA + (most sensitive index)
c) HBV DNA polymerase +
d) ↑ AST/ALT (implies liver necrosis due to cell-mediated immunity)

2 Intermediate phase
a) Cessation of HBV replication
b) Acceleration of hepatocyte damage

3 Integrative phase (→chronic persistence hepatitis, or hepatoma)
a) HBeAg −, antiHBe +
b) HBV DNA −, HBV DNA polymerase −
c) HBsAg remains + usually but not invariably
d) HBV DNA becomes integrated into hepatocyte genome

LIVER BIOPSY

Provisional diagnoses contraindicating liver biopsy

1 Uncorrected coagulopathy

2 Haemangioma, angiosarcoma

3 Amyloidosis with prolonged bleeding time

4 Hydatid disease

5 Extrahepatic biliary obstruction

How to biopsy a chronically diseased liver

1 If prothrombin time, Hb and platelet count are normal, cross-match 2 units of blood and proceed with caution. If abnormal platelet function is suspected, do a bleeding time

2 If prothrombin time abnormal and patient *not* jaundiced, give vitamin K 10 mg/day (i.m.i. for 3 days or orally for 5 days) and repeat prothrombin time; if index <1.3, proceed
3 If prothrombin time abnormal and patient *is* jaundiced, give vitamin K by slow i.v. infusion (with anaphylactic kit ready) and check prothrombin time the next day; if normal, proceed
4 If prothrombin time remains >4 seconds prolonged after vitamin K replenishment (indicating major hepatic parenchymal damage), and if biopsy required urgently, cover with fresh frozen plasma (FFP). Check the prothrombin time
   a) Following completion of FFP infusion
   b) Immediately prior to biopsy
   c) During the postbiopsy observation period (when further FFP may be required)
5 If FFP ineffective, dispense with percutaneous biopsy altogether and opt instead for a transjugular approach using a biopsy catheter

Differential diagnosis of hepatic granulomata
1 Sarcoidosis
2 Primary biliary cirrhosis
3 Infection — TB, syphilis, schistosomiasis, Q fever, brucellosis, histoplasmosis
4 Drug-induced — allopurinol, phenylbutazone, sulphonamides
5 Berylliosis

Liver histology in selected disorders
1 Alcoholic liver disease
   a) Mallory's hyaline (*not* pathognomonic)
   b) Centrilobular necrosis
   c) Giant mitochondria
   d) Ballooning degeneration of hepatocytes
   e) Pericellular fibrosis → 'chicken wire' appearance
2 α_1 AT deficiency: PAS-positive globules within hepatocytes
3 Chronic persistent hepatitis
   a) Preservation of lobular architecture with minimal fibrosis (intact limiting plate)
   b) Mononuclear infiltrate confined to portal tracts
4 Chronic active hepatitis
   a) Disruption of lobular architecture — piecemeal necrosis (erosion of limiting plate); bridging necrosis; 'rosette' and pseudolobule formation
   b) Mononuclear infiltrate extends into lobules
   c) Councilman bodies, Kupffer cell hyperplasia

INVESTIGATING PANCREATOBILIARY DISEASE

Laboratory diagnosis of acute pancreatitis
1 ↑ Serum amylase
   a) Good screening test, but significant false-positive rate
   b) False-negatives may occur if hyperlipidaemia-induced
2 ↑ Serum lipase — most specific test; equally sensitive as amylase

Indicators of poor prognosis in acute pancreatitis
1 Clinical
   a) Age >60; first attack; gallstone aetiology
   b) Hypotension
   c) Grey-Turner's sign: left flank ecchymoses
      Cullen's sign: periumbilical ecchymoses   —in haemorrhagic pancreatitis
2 Ascites, esp. if
   a) High protein level
   b) Frankly haemorrhagic on peritoneal lavage
3 Methaemalbuminaemia (indicates haemorrhagic pancreatitis)
4 ↓ Albumin
   ↓ Ca^{2+} (when corrected for albumin) (NB: elevated calcium? exclude hyperparathyroidism)
5 ↓ Hb, ↑ WCC
6 ↑ Blood glucose
7 ↑ BUN, ↑ AST
8 ↑ Fibrinogen
9 ↓ P_aO_2

Investigations of choice for suspected gallbladder disease
1 Oral cholecystography
   a) Cheap, widely available; assesses both function and anatomy
   b) Used to demonstrate gallstones in anicteric patients when ultrasound unavailable or inconclusive
   c) Also assesses gallstone composition and cystic duct patency
   d) Useful in work-up for gallstone dissolution or lithotripsy
   e) Side-effects frequent — 25% diarrhoea, 10% nausea, 10% dysuria
2 Real-time ultrasonography
   a) Quick, painless, non-invasive; difficult in obese patients
   b) Risk-free: no radiation exposure or contrast hypersensitivity
   c) High sensitivity for cholecystitis (incl. chronic)
   d) Distinguishes obstructive from hepatocellular jaundice by demonstrating bile duct dilatation
   e) May detect unsuspected non-biliary causes of pain
3 $^{99}Tc^m$-HIDA cholescintigraphy*
   a) High sensitivity and specificity for acute cholecystitis: cystic duct obstruction prevents gallbladder visualization
   b) False-positives occur in heavy drinkers, fasting, TPN, hepatitis or pancreatitis
   c) False-negatives occur in acalculous or chronic cholecystitis
4 ERCP
   a) Invasive, expensive; useful in postcholecystectomy jaundice
   b) Helps exclude false-negative ultrasound/cholecystography

---

*DISIDA preferred to HIDA in jaundiced patients

c) Localizes obstruction within pancreatic or common bile duct
5 Percutaneous transhepatic cholangiogram (PTC)
a) Localizes obstruction when intrahepatic ducts dilated
b) Useful for draining bile in inoperable obstruction
c) Contraindicated in gross ascites or coagulopathy
6 Percutaneous gallbladder puncture — useful in diagnosis and treatment of acalculous cholecystitis

Positive findings on oral cholecystography
1 Gallstones
2 Failure to visualize gallbladder despite second dose of contrast

Failure of gallbladder visualization by oral cholecystography: why?
1 Patient non-compliance (tablets and/or contrast not taken)
2 Gastric stasis or outlet obstruction; vomiting
3 Intestinal malabsorption or diarrhoea
4 Liver disease
5 Gallbladder unable to concentrate contrast (e.g. chronic cholecystitis)
6 Mechanical obstruction preventing entry of contrast (e.g. acute cholecystitis)

(NB: In *jaundiced* patients the initial investigation of choice is hepatobiliary ultrasound)

Indications for ERCP
1 Suspected choledocholithiasis (usually postcholecystectomy)
2 Persistent symptoms following biliary surgery
3 Cholestasis without intrahepatic bile duct dilatation (PTC preferred if dilated)
4 For diagnosis (or preoperative assessment) of chronic pancreatitis or pancreatic carcinoma

Indications and contraindications for intravenous cholangiography
1 Sole indication — demonstration of common bile duct calculi/strictures/cysts in cholecystectomized patients with suggestive symptoms
2 Contraindications
a) Bilirubin >50 μmol/l
b) Oral cholecystogram performed within last week
c) Combined liver and renal disease
d) Waldenström's macroglobulinaemia
e) Contrast hypersensitivity

INVESTIGATING INTESTINAL DISEASE

Indications for colonoscopy
1 Bleeding per rectum
2 Persistent colonic symptoms (e.g. changed bowel habit) with normal sigmoidoscopy (see ref. 1.1)
3 Dysplasia monitoring in patients with ulcerative pancolitis of more than 10 years' duration
4 Surveillance for suture line recurrence following surgery for colonic cancer
5 Abnormal barium enema (e.g. stricture, polyp) performed for other indication

Contraindications to colonoscopy
1 Peritonism
2 Toxic megacolon
3 *Any* acute severe inflammatory colonic process
4 Pregnancy
5 Recent (<6/12) history of myocardial infarction

Pros and cons of colonoscopy vis-à-vis double-contrast barium enema (DCBE)
1 Colonoscopy advantages
a) More sensitive than DCBE for tumours >5 mm diameter
b) More accurate than DCBE in assessing sigmoid colon and caecum
c) May detect vascular lesions such as angiodysplasia
d) May be useful in emergency assessment of PR bleeding
2 Colonoscopy disadvantages
a) Inexperienced operator may fail to visualize entire colon in up to 25% of examinations
b) May miss large tumours, esp. in proximal colon and in rectal ampulla
c) More expensive, dangerous, and inconvenient than DCBE
d) Less available than DCBE, esp. in outlying areas

Rectal biopsy: diagnostic value
1 Amyloidosis
2 Tay-Sachs; metachromatic leucodystrophy
3 Amoebiasis (and other infective proctocolitides)
4 Pseudomembranous colitis (though may spare rectum)

GASTROINTESTINAL RADIOLOGY

Radiological features of achalasia
1 Plain film
a) Intrathoracic air-fluid level
b) Absent gastric air bubble
c) Lower zone lung fibrosis (bronchiectasis)
2 Barium swallow
a) Tertiary contractions replacing peristaltic activity at all levels
b) Dilated oesophagus with tapered lower end ('beaked', 'rattail')

Giant gastric rugae: differential diagnosis
1 Malignancy, e.g. lymphoma, leiomyoma
2 Gastrinoma
3 Menètrier's disease (hypoproteinaemic hypertrophic gastropathy)

Jejunal ulcers: differential diagnosis
1 Ulcerative jejunitis (malignant histiocytosis)
2 Coeliac disease, Crohn's disease
3 Gastrinoma
4 Meckel's diverticulitis (usually in boys; 5–10% bleed)
5 Mesenteric ischaemia; polyarteritis
6 Lymphoma
7 Infection — typhoid, bacillary dysentery, syphilis, TB, fungal, actinomycosis
8 Iatrogenic — digoxin, potassium tablets

Syndromes of multiple intestinal polyps
1 Familial polyposis (→ numerous premalignant colonic adenomas)
2 Gardner's syndrome (→ occasional premalignant colonic adenomas)
3 Peutz-Jeghers syndrome (→ small- and large-intestinal hamartomas)

Space-occupying lesions on liver scan: clinical significance
1 Solid tumour(s)
  a) Dx — echodense on liver ultrasound
    — primary tumours commoner in cirrhosis, i.e., in context of patchy parenchymal uptake and increased bone marrow uptake
    — biopsy (laparoscopic or CT/ultrasound-guided) positive; not needed for diagnosis if AFP > 1000 ng/ml
  b) Rx — excision/transplant (early disease), chemotherapy
2 Amoebic liver abscess
  a) Dx
    — thick-walled cavity on liver ultrasound
    — gallium scan negative
    — amoebic serology positive
  b) Rx — metronidazole (small abscesses), aspiration
3 Pyogenic liver abscess
  a) Dx
    — thick-walled cavity on liver ultrasound
    — gallium scan (or indium-111-labelled WBCs) positive
  b) Rx — percutaneous aspiration (ultrasound-guided)
4 Hydatid cyst
  a) Dx
    — thin-walled cyst on liver ultrasound
    — presence of daughter cysts virtually diagnostic
    — serology often inconclusive
  b) Rx
    — open surgical drainage
    — percutaneous aspiration contraindicated

Abdominal imaging techniques: ultrasound or CT?
1 Ultrasound
  a) Advantages
    — No radiation dose
    — Quick and relatively cheap
    — Good resolution of luminal structures (e.g. biliary tree), cysts and abscesses
  b) Disadvantages
    — Difficult in obese patients
    — Less detail than CT
2 CT
  a) Advantages
    — High quality images, incl. in obese patients
    — Excellent delineation of retroperitoneal structures (e.g. pancreas, psoas)
  b) Disadvantages
    — Difficult if lots of bowel gas
    — High radiation dose
    — Time-consuming and expensive

MALABSORPTION

Measurement of fat malabsorption
1 ^{14}C-triolein breath test (indirect test of lipase secretion)
2 Fluorescein dilaurate test (index of esterase secretion)
3 PABA/^{14}C excretion (indirect test of chymotrypsin secretion)
4 3-day faecal fats — now virtually outmoded

Diagnosis of bacterial overgrowth
1 High index of suspicion (Crohn's, post-Polya, hypomotility state)
2 Low B$_{12}$; abnormal Schilling's test following addition of intrinsic factor
3 ^{14}C-bile acid breath test (see below)
4 Duodenal aspiration and culture (>10^5 organisms/ml)
5 Therapeutic trial (e.g. tetracycline)

Diagnosis of lactose intolerance
1 History of milk-related diarrhoea
2 Successful therapeutic trial of milk-free diet
3 Stool: pH <6.5; Benedict's test positive
4 'Flat' lactose tolerance test (rarely used now)
5 Hydrogen breath test following oral lactose (best screen)
6 Small bowel biopsy with lactase quantification (definitive)
  a) Primary alactasia — other disaccharidases normal
  b) Secondary lactose intolerance: all disaccharidases depleted

Breath testing: diagnostic value in malabsorption
1 ^{14}C-glycocholate (bile acid) breath test
  a) Bacterial overgrowth (low faecal ^{14}C)
  b) Ileal insufficiency (excess faecal ^{14}C)
2 Hydrogen breath test (following oral glucose or lactulose)
  a) Bacterial overgrowth
  b) Lactose intolerance (following oral lactose)
  c) Indirect index of small intestinal transit time
3 ^{14}C-triolein breath test — steatorrhoea
4 ^{14}C-galactose breath test — galactosaemia
5 ^{14}C-urea breath test — *Helicobacter pylori* (and other gastric infections)

Small bowel biopsy: diagnostic value
1 Coeliac disease (villous atrophy, crypt hypertrophy, mononuclear infiltrate)
2 Whipple's disease (infiltration or replacement of lamina propria with foamy PAS-positive macrophages; rod-like structures on EM)
3 Nodular lymphoid hyperplasia Hypogammaglobulinaemia (no plasma cells, villous atrophy)
4 A beta lipoproteinaemia (lipid infiltration); eosinophilic gastroenteritis
5 Crohn's; lymphoma; lymphangiectasia; alpha heavy chain disease
6 Parasites (*Giardia, Strongyloides, Coccidia*) or fungal (*Candida, Histoplasma*) infections

Measurement of gut permeability
1 D-Xylose absorption (traditional test) —
false-positive results in
  a) Renal failure
  b) Delayed gastric emptying
2 Alternatives
  a) Polyethylene glycol
  b) ^{51}Cr-EDTA
3 In coeliac disease — lactulose/mannitol absorption
ratio: since increased disaccharide (lactulose) but
decreased monosaccharide (mannitol) absorption is
seen in gluten-induced enteropathy

AN APPROACH TO DIARRHOEA

Watery diarrhoea: is it secretory?
1 Stool volume — compare volume on normal diet
with volume determined after 24-hour nil by mouth
with i.v. fluids only; volumes are similar in
secretory (cholera-like) diarrhoea
2 Stool electrolytes — in secretory diarrhoea, faecal
Na^+ and Cl^- are similar to plasma levels, faecal
HCO_3^- and K^+ are 2–5 times plasma levels
3 Stool osmolality — virtually isotonic with plasma if
secretory

Investigating suspected laxative abuse
1 Hypokalaemia
2 Urinary phenolphthalein
3 Stool volumes/electrolytes/osmolality
4 Endoscopy
  a) Melanosis coli (if anthracene laxatives used)
  b) Absent mucosal damage
5 Locker search during hospital admission

**Indications for stool culture in the patient with
diarrhoea**
1 History
  a) Recent return from developing country
  b) Recent ingestion of undercooked meat/shellfish,
    unpasteurized milk, tank/stream water
  c) Immunosuppressed
2 Symptoms
  a) Bloody diarrhoea
  b) Fever
  c) Abdominal pain
3 Duration — >5 days
4 Severity — >10 bowel movements/day
5 Faecal leucocytes on stool microscopy

Diagnosis of giardiasis
1 Stool examination
  a) Trophozoites (in unformed stools)
  b) Cysts (in formed stools)
2 Peroral jejunal fluid sampling (duodenal
intubation/aspiration)
3 Jejunal biopsy using Crosby capsule
4 Therapeutic trial of metronidazole or tinidazole
(commonest test)

Bloody diarrhoea: microbiological differential diagnosis
1 *Shigella* spp.

2 Enterotoxigenic *E.coli*
3 *Campylobacter jejuni*
4 *Salmonella* spp.
5 *Entamoeba histolytica* (if recent travel)
6 *Yersinia enterocolitica*
7 *Clostridium difficile* (if recent antibiotics)

INFLAMMATORY BOWEL DISEASE

Histological hallmarks of inflammatory bowel disease
1 Ulcerative colitis
  a) Crypts reduced in number; irregular; branched
  b) Cryptabscesses +++
  c) Loss of goblet cells
  d) Paneth cell metaplasia +++
  e) Thickening of muscularis mucosae
  f) Mucosal infiltration with polymorphs,
    lymphocytes, eosinophils and plasma cells
2 Crohn's disease
  a) Transmural involvment, fissuring
  b) Glandular pattern relatively undisturbed
  c) Non-caseating granulomata
  d) Focal inflammation
  e) Goblet cell preservation
  f) Infiltration with lymphocytes, macrophages and
    histiocytes
  g) Cryptabscesses infrequent
  h) Paneth cell metaplasia rare

Radiological hallmarks of inflammatory bowel disease
1 Ulcerative colitis
  a) Fine, spiculating superficial tiny ulcers, fuzzy
    contour
  b) 'Collarstud' ulcers
  c) 'Pseudopolyps' (luminal filling defects —
    inflamed mucosal islands between ulcer craters
    in severe disease)
  d) Featureless tubular
    'hosepipe' colon (loss of
    haustration pattern)
  e) Shortened and narrowed
    colon   } Indicative of
  f) Widening of retrorectal   disease *chronicity*
    space on lateral
    radiography >2 cm
  g) Barium reflux through
    patulous ileocaecal valve
2 Crohn's disease
  a) Early lesions
    — Thickening of valvulae coniventes
    — Aphthoid ulceration
  b) Late lesions
    — 'Cobblestoning'
    — 'Rose-thorn' and 'collarstud' ulcers
    — *Transmural* fissuring
    — 'Skip lesions' (i.e. involved segments)
  c) Complications
    — Fistulae and sinuses
    — Segmental stenosis and dilatation
    — Evidence of severe colonic ulceration/oedema
    may be visible on plain films

3 Ischaemic colitis
   a) Large asymmetric 'thumbprint' deformities (due to intramural haemorrhage and oedema), esp. at splenic flexure
   b) Toxic dilatation

Stricture in Crohn's disease: differential diagnosis
1 Transient bowel spasm
2 Inflammatory stenosis
3 Ischaemic fibrosis
4 Pericolic abscess
5 Carcinoma

MANAGING GASTROINTESTINAL DISEASE

OESOPHAGEAL DISEASE

Therapeutic measures in oesophageal reflux
1 Minor disease
   a) Weight reduction, elevate bedhead
   b) Avoid alcohol/nicotine/caffeine/fat
   c) Preprandial metoclopramide (↑ gastric emptying/LOS tone)
   d) Postprandial antacids
   e) Nocturnal H_2-receptor antagonists
2 Major disease (incl. CREST, scleroderma)
   a) Omeprazole
   b) Nissan fundoplication

Indications for surgery in oesophageal reflux
1 Severe symptoms refractory to medical treatment
2 Any penetrating ulcer unresponsive to medical treatment
3 Severe oesophageal bleeding
4 Any severe stricture requiring frequent dilatation

Management of severe recurrent pain due to oesophageal spasm ('nutcracker' oesophagus)
1 Exclude ischaemic heart disease/gallstones/peptic ulcer
2 Nifedipine
3 Nitrates

MANAGEMENT OF PEPTIC ULCERATION

Medical modalities available for peptic ulcer
1 Antacids
   a) Sodium bicarbonate (absorbed; may→alkalosis, fluid overload)
   b) Magnesium salts, esp. trisilicate (tend to cause diarrhoea)
   c) Aluminium salts, hydroxide/silicate (tend to constipate)
2 Cytoprotective agents ('coat' musosa; no antacid properties)
   a) Colloidal bismuth: also bactericidal to *Helicobacter pylori*
   b) Sucralfate (complex of aluminium hydroxide and sucrose); good for stress ulcer prophylaxis
   c) Carbenoxolone, deglycirrhinized liquorice (rarely used)
3 Antisecretory agents

   a) H_2-receptor antagonists
      — Cimetidine
      — Ranitidine
      — Famotidine
   b) H^+/K^+-ATPase inhibitors
      — Omeprazole
4 Antisecretory *and* cytoprotective agents — prostaglandin E_1/E_2 derivatives: misoprostol
5 Proton pump inhibitors (investigational)

Ranitidine or cimetidine for peptic ulcer?
1 Ranitidine is 5–8 times more potent on a molar basis
2 Ranitidine has more prolonged action (less frequent dosage: b.d.)
3 Ranitidine binds less avidly to cytochrome P_{450} (fewer drug interactions)
4 Ranitidine has lower affinity for androgen receptors (minimal antiandrogenic effects)
5 Ranitidine rarely causes confusional states (unlike cimetidine)

Adverse effects of cimetidine
1 Antiandrogenic effects — gynaecomastia, impotence, oligospermia ($\rightarrow \downarrow$ E_2 metabolism)
2 Confusion — esp. in elderly, renal/liver failure, or i.v. therapy
3 Reversible rise in serum creatinine and transaminases
4 Reversible decline in WCC and/or platelet count
5 Inhibition of drug metabolism
   a) Propranolol, labetalol
   b) Warfarin
   c) Phenytoin
   d) Theophylline
   e) Quinidine/procainamide

Omeprazole: what is its place in peptic ulcer management?
1 Treatment of choice in Zollinger-Ellison syndrome (gastrinoma)
2 Far more potent acid inhibitor than ranitidine (by decreasing gut acidity, omeprazole improves its own absorption/bioavailability)
3 Longer duration of action than ranitidine (once-daily dosing)
4 More rapid ulcer healing than ranitidine
5 More effective in advanced oesophagitis than ranitidine

Efficacy of antiulcer therapies
1 H_2-receptor antagonists — 80% ulcers 'heal' within 6 weeks (healing mediated primarily by nocturnal acid inhibition)
2 50–75% of healed ulcers will relapse within 12 months of ceasing therapy with H_2-receptor antagonists, esp. in smokers
3 Nocturnal maintenance cimetidine 400 mg reduces relapse rates to 40% in the first year, while ranitidine 150 mg reduces it to 20%
4 Relapse rates following single-course treatment with colloidal bismuth are superior to those seen with single-course H_2-receptor antagonists, esp. for the subset of patients in whom *H. pylori* is cleared from the gastric mucosa

5 Although maintenance ranitidine appears to offer the lowest overall relapse rates, it is approximately 6 times more expensive than single-course colloidal bismuth

6 Highly selective vagotomy is associated with a 10% relapse rate and a 1% incidence of significant side-effects

POST-GASTRECTOMY SYNDROMES

Anaemia following gastric surgery: mechanisms

1 Iron deficiency (→anaemia in 50%)
   a) Recurrent bleeding (e.g. stomal ulcers, gastritis)
   b) Malabsorption due to hypochlorhydria (Fe^{2+}→ less soluble Fe^{3+})
   c) Malabsorption due to duodenal bypass (Polya)

2 B_{12} deficiency (→anaemia in 5%)
   a) Reduction in parietal cell mass (esp. in total gastrectomy)
   b) Bacterial overgrowth due to
      — Blind loop (Polya): commonest cause
      — Hypochlorhydria
      — Reduced motility (vagotomy)

3 Folic acid deficiency (→anaemia in 1%)

Mechanisms of post-Polya malabsorption

1 Inadequate luminal mixing of food and digestive secretions due to intestinal hurry (leading to steatorrhoea)

2 Duodenal bypass leading to reduced or delayed stimulation of biliary and pancreatic secretions

3 Stagnant loop syndrome

4 Inadvertent gastroileostomy

5 'Unmasking' of gluten sensitivity/alactasia/pancreatic insufficiency

6 Stomal ulceration leading to formation of gastrocolic fistula

Possible significance of stomal ulcer development

1 Inadequate vagotomy/gastrectomy ('retained antrum')

2 Inadvertent gastroileal (-colic) anastomosis

3 Gastrinoma

Other complications of gastric surgery

1 Dumping ('early', 'late'); R_x octreotide

2 Biliary vomiting, biliary gastritis; alkaline reflux oesophagitis

3 Osteomalacia, osteoporosis

4 Protein-losing enteropathy (cause unknown); protein malnutrition (due to poor intake and absorption); diarrhoea

5 Reactivation of TB (cause unknown)

6 Development of malignancy in gastric remnant

UPPER GASTROINTESTINAL HAEMORRHAGE

General measures in managing upper gastrointestinal haemorrhage

1 Patients with known or suspected liver disease
   a) Correction of coagulopathy
   b) Encephalopathy regimen

2 Haemodynamic homeostasis
   a) Adequate transfusion (maintain Hb >10 g/dl)
   b) iv fluid and electrolyte balance (central line if needed)

3 Medical management
   a) High-dose continuous intragastric antacids
   b) *No* evidence for benefit from H_2-receptor antagonists

4 Emergency surgery, e.g.
   a) Oversewing of Mallory-Weiss tear
   b) Partial gastrectomy ± vagotomy for bleeding peptic ulcer
   c) Total gastrectomy for severe erosive gastritis (last resort)

Endoscopic management of bleeding peptic ulcers

1 Uni- or multipolar electrocoagulation (diathermy)

2 Thermal coagulation using heater probe

3 Direct injection of adrenaline or absolute alcohol

4 Nd-YAG laser photocoagulation

Bleeding oesophageal varices: specific therapeutic options

1 Continuous infusion
   a) Somatostatin
   b) Vasopressin/glypressin/terlipressin

2 Balloon tamponade (Sengstaken-Blakemore tube)
   a) Short-term measure only; must be removed within 24 hours
   b) Justified only if decision made to attempt variceal ablation on removal

3 Endoscopic injection sclerotherapy
   a) Proven value in acute bleeding, but not in prophylaxis
   b) Potential complications — sepsis, oesophageal ulceration

4 Staple-gun oesophageal transection — ± oesophagogastric devascularization

5 Portocaval shunting
   a) Proven value in prophylaxis, not in acute bleeding
   b) 50% mortality in emergency shunting

HAEMOCHROMATOSIS

Long-term therapeutic strategies in presymptomatic haemochromatosis

1 Prevention of complications by *screening* first-degree relatives of index cases using
   a) ↑ Serum ferritin
   b) ↑ Transferrin saturation (> 55%)

2 Confirmation of suspected positives using:
   a) Liver biopsy
   b) ± Quantitative phlebotomy, HLA-A3 phenotype

3 Venesection of affected patients until Hb = 10 g/dl

4 Annual monitoring of these patients
   a) Keep male ferritin levels < 350 μg/l
   b) Keep female ferritin levels < 200 μg/l

5 This approach effectively prevents development of liver disease, cardiac disease, and skin bronzing

Benefits and limitations of therapy for established haemochromatosis

1 Benefits — prolongs life in symptomatic patients

2 Limitations
  a) *Arthropathy* fails to improve
  b) *Insulin requirement* in established diabetics is rarely eliminated (although control may be improved)
  c) *Hypogonadotrophic hypogonadism* (impotence, premature menopause) seldom if ever improves; moreover, androgen therapy for impotence greatly increases hepatoma risk
  d) *Risk of hepatoma* is unaffected by therapy in patients with established cirrhosis

MANAGEMENT OF ASCITES

An approach to the management of ascites in chronic liver disease
1 Mild, minimally symptomatic ascites
  a) Outpatient management
  b) Spironolactone
  c) Low-salt diet
2 Tense, symptomatic ascites in patients with associated *oedema*, normal renal function, and serum sodium >130 mmol/l
  a) Hospital admission
  b) Large-volume (5–10 litre) paracentesis
  c) Early discharge following stabilization on diuretic therapy and arrangement for outpatient follow-up
3 Tense, symptomatic ascites in patients *without* oedema, or in patients with renal impairment or serum sodium <130 mmol/l
  a) Hospital admission
  b) Large-volume paracentesis *plus* albumin infusion
  c) Early discharge following stabilization on diuretic therapy and arrangement for outpatient follow-up
4 Rapid recurrence of ascites following paracentesis and diuretics
  a) Culture ascites (bacteria, AFB)
  b) Sudan III stain if fluid opalescent (chylous ascites)
  c) Cytology (malignant cells)
  d) Plasma AFP (hepatoma)
  e) Liver scan (hepatoma, hepatic vein thrombosis)
5 Intractable ascites without identifiable reversible cause — peritoneovenous (LeVeen) shunt

Complications of peritoneovenous shunting
1 Disseminated intravascular coagulation (clinical or subclinical)
2 Sepsis
3 Shunt blockage (major long-term problem)
4 Intravascular fluid overload ($\rightarrow$ pulmonary oedema)
5 Peritoneal fibromatosis (foreign body reaction)

HEPATIC ENCEPHALOPATHY

Inpatient monitoring of the patient in hepatic precoma
1 Higher centres — regular close questioning by staff and relatives
2 Constructional apraxia
  a) Handwriting chart
  b) Five-pointed star chart
  c) Reitan trail test (consecutive number connection)
3 Plasma ammonia (sampled from large vein without tourniquet); CSF glutamine
4 EEG (see p. 227)

Hepatic encephalopathy: management of the 'at-risk' patient
1 Prevention/correction of hypothermia/hypokalaemia/hypomagnesaemia
2 Witholding/withdrawal of loop diuretics/sedation/alcohol
3 Active exclusion of sepsis
4 Prompt treatment of gastrointestinal bleeding
5 Avoidance of surgery and general anaesthesia if possible
6 Diet
  a) High-calorie (incl. i.v. dextrose if necessary)
  b) Low-protein (< 50 g/day; vegetable preferable to meat)
7 Magnesium sulphate enema
8 Gut sterilization ($\pm$ malabsorption of putative neurotoxin)
  a) Routine prophylaxis — oral neomycin
  b) Acute encephalopathy — neomycin plus metronidazole
  c) Long-term therapy } —ampicillin (obviates risk
     Renal failure   } of ototoxicity)
9 Lactulose (or lactilol) to acidify gut lumen, thus converting liposoluble (absorbable) NH_3 to NH_4^+ (watersoluble; excreted in urine) as well as promoting bowel washout

Relative contraindications to portal-systemic shunting
1 Age > 50 years
2 Previous episode(s) of encephalopathy
3 Jaundice
4 Ascites
5 Profound hypoalbuminaemia
6 High IQ required for livelihood

Potential complications of portal-systemic shunting
1 Perioperative death ($\rightarrow$50% of 'poor-risk' patients)
2 Precipitation of hepatic encephalopathy
3 Development of hepatic nephropathy (hepatorenal failure)

DRUG-INDUCED LIVER DISEASE

Primary liver diseases mimicked by iatrogenic biopsy abnormalities
1 Viral hepatitis — halothane, isoniazid, ketoconazole
2 Alcoholic hepatitis — perhexiline maleate
3 Reye's syndrome — aspirin, valproate
4 Acute fatty liver of pregnancy — tetracycline
5 Cryptogenic cirrhosis
  a) Long-term methotrexate; amiodarone
  b) Vitamin A intoxication, vinyl chloride monomer
6 Primary biliary cirrhosis — chlorpromazine
7 Chronic active hepatitis — methyldopa, isoniazid, nitrofurantoin, dantrolene
8 Granulomatous (hypersensitivity) hepatitis — allopurinol

9 Budd-Chiari syndrome — synthetic oestrogens
10 Veno-occlusive disease — 6-thioguanine ± irradiation (for childhood malignancies)

Halothane hepatitis: occurrence and outcome
1 Incidence of clinically evident hepatitis: 1 in 10 000
  Incidence of asymptomatic ↑ AST/ALT — 10–25%
2 70% of affected patients are female
  50% of affected patients are obese
3 More than 80% of patients have had at least 2 exposures
  Initial exposure is often followed by unexplained fever
  Toxic re-exposure usually occurs within a month
4 Fever is seen in 75% of established hepatitis cases
  Eosinophilia is seen in 30% of cases
5 The mortality of established halothane hepatitis is 50%

Chronic active hepatitis: eligibility criteria for steroid therapy
1 Symptoms causing reduced quality of life, *plus*
2 Severe histologic abnormalities on biopsy, *plus*
3 HBsAg *and* anti-HBc negativity, *plus*
4 Exclusion of reversible aetiology
  a) Drug-induced chronic active hepatitis
  b) Wilson's disease
  c) α_1 Antitrypsin deficiency

LIVER TRANSPLANTATION

Principal indications for liver transplantation
1 In children
  a) Congenital biliary atresia with persistent cholestasis despite Kasai procedure (1-year survival >90%)
  b) Metabolic disorders — Wilson's disease, α_1-antitrypsin deficiency, galactosaemia, Crigler-Najjar syndrome, hypercholesterolaemia
2 In adults with end-stage (but stable; not in ICU!) liver disease
  a) Primary biliary cirrhosis
  b) Sclerosing cholangitis
  c) Budd-Chiari syndrome (hepatic vein thrombosis)
  d) Cryptogenic cirrhosis, chronic active hepatitis
3 Neoplasms (disappointing results so far)
  a) *Small* hepatocellular carcinomas without grossly elevated AFP
  b) Fibrolamellar tumours, haemangioendotheliomas
  c) Occasional carcinoid or APUDoma metastases (esp. if solitary)
4 Fulminant hepatic failure; hepatorenal syndrome

Therapeutic outcome in liver transplantation
1 Overall 12-month survival — 70%
2 Primary biliary cirrhosis — 12-month survival 90%
3 Other causes of cirrhosis — 12-month survival 60%
4 Hepatitis B-induced liver disease — 12-month survival 50%
5 Hepatoma — 12-month recurrence-free survival 30%
6 Liver disease patients alive at 12 months — 80% 5-year survival

Contraindications to liver transplantation
1 Common
  a) Liver disease too far advanced
  b) Patient unfit for surgery
  c) No suitable donor
2 Absolute
  a) Active alcoholism
  b) Systemic or biliary infection (incl. AIDS)
  c) Extrahepatic malignancy
3 Relative
  a) Age >50 years
  b) Portal vein thrombosis
  c) Portocaval shunt (→ uncontrollable operative bleeding)
  d) Intrapulmonary AV shunting (>50%)
  e) Multiple previous laparotomies
  f) HBeAg/HBV DNA +; delta agent infection

Complications of liver transplantation
1 Death — affects up to 30% within 3 months of transplant
2 Hepatic artery thrombosis
  a) Occurs in up to 20%; may cause graft infarction, necessitating immediate retransplantation
  b) May also manifest as biliary peritonitis (bile duct infarct)
3 Infection — esp. *Pseudomonas, Candida,* CMV
4 Acute rejection
  a) Almost invariable (day 4–10 post-transplant)
  b) Treated with steroids, cyclosporin A, antilymphocyte globulin or OKT3 (CD3) mouse monoclonal antihuman T-cell antibody
5 Chronic rejection
  a) In 10–20% patients
  b) Manifests as 'vanishing bile duct syndrome' (jaundice)
  c) May respond to OKT3 antibody or retransplantation
6 Cyclosporin A toxicity
  a) Nephrotoxicity
  b) Hypertension
  c) CNS syndrome — confusion, cortical blindness, pyramidal lesions, ± peripheral neuropathy

GALLSTONE DISSOLUTION THERAPY

Pharmacology and rationale of gallstone dissolution
1 Cheno- and ursodeoxycholic acid (CDCA, UDCA) inhibit HMG-CoA reductase, thus reducing biliary cholesterol concentration
2 Treatment is most helpful in patients unfit for cholecystectomy
3 Treatment does not dissolve pigment (radio-opaque) stones
4 Treatment usually → ↑ plasma cholesterol, ↓ triglycerides
5 Treatment may be antagonized by phenobarbitone
6 CDCA is metabolized to lithocholic acid, a hepatotoxin, resulting in frequent transaminase elevation during treatment

Prerequisites for dissolution therapy
1 Functioning gallbladder (patent cystic duct) on cholecystography

2 Radiolucent (cholesterol) stones (successful therapy likely if cholecystogram shows stones floating within gallbladder, since this implies hypodense stones with relatively large surface area for dissolution)
3 Stone diameter(s) <1.5 cm
4 No common bile duct stones
5 No history of liver or pancreatic dysfunction
6 Not pregnant or morbidly obese

Clinical aspects of gallstone dissolution
1 Main problems with this treatment are
   a) Expense
   b) Stringent patient eligibility criteria
   c) Diarrhoea
2 In *highly-selected patients* dissolution rates of up to 80% are achievable within 12 months of therapy *Overall* 12-month dissolution rates in patients with functioning gallbladders and radiolucent stones average 40%
3 *Recurrence rates* in successfully treated patients approximate 50% over 5–10 years
4 Treatment of hypercholesterolaemic females (in conjunction with a low-cholesterol diet) has yielded the best results (concomitant NSAID therapy has been associated with fewer relapses)
5 Advantages of UDCA over CDCA
   a) Less diarrhoea and nausea
   b) Less transaminitis
   c) More potent reduction of biliary cholesterol secretion
   d) More rapid onset of dissolution
   Disadvantage of UDCA: may → 'rim' calcification of gallstones, inhibiting dissolution
6 Patients remaining symptomatic after 6 months medical therapy should be considered for surgery

OTHER ALTERNATIVES TO CHOLECYSTECTOMY

Endoscopic sphincterotomy: when should it replace cholecystectomy?
1 Elderly patients, *plus*
2 Patent cystic duct, *plus*
3 Common duct stone(s)

Therapy of gallstones without recourse to cholecystectomy
1 Oral dissolution using CDCA or UDCA
2 Endoscopic sphincterotomy
3 T-tube stone extraction using Dormia basket
4 T-tube solvent infusion
   a) Bile acids/EDTA for calcium-containing stones
   b) Methyl tertiary butyl ether for cholesterol stones
5 Nasobiliary or transhepatic catheter with solvent perfusion
6 Extracorporeal ultrasonic lithotripsy

Prerequisites for extracorporeal lithotripsy
1 History of biliary colic (i.e. patient *must* be symptomatic)
2 Solitary radiolucent gallstone < 3 cm diameter (or <3 stones with equivalent combined mass)

3 Functioning gallbladder on oral cholecystography
4 No recent history of cholecystitis/cholangitis, clotting defect, NSAID therapy, pregnancy

LAXATIVE THERAPY

Indications for prescribing laxatives
1 Short-term therapy of constipation/painful defaecation associated with illness
2 Long-term therapy of elderly or debilitated patients with chronic abdominal/perineal muscular weakness
3 Prevention of iatrogenic constipation
4 Bowel preparation prior to investigation or surgery

Classifying laxatives
1 Bulking agents — bran, ispaghula husk, sterculia, methylcellulose
2 Faecal softeners — paraffin, docusate sodium
3 Osmotic laxatives — magnesium salts, lactulose, glycerol supp.
4 Stimulant laxatives — senna, bisacodyl, danthron, phenolphthalein

Individualizing laxative treatment
1 Therapy of predominantly rectal discomfort
   a) Glycerol suppositories
   b) Bisacodyl suppositories
2 Long-term therapy of constipation
   a) Ispaghula husk
   b Sterculia
   c) Methylcellulose
3 Short-term therapy of constipation — senna
4 Second-line therapy of constipation
   a) Magnesium hydroxide
   b) Lactulose (expensive)
5 Approach to refractory symptoms — investigate to clarify diagnosis

ANTIDIARRHOEAL THERAPY

Infectious diarrhoea: indications for antibiotics
1 Always
   a) Giardiasis
   b) Amoebiasis *if* symptomatic
   c) Severe bacillary dysentery
2 Usually: pseudomembranous (antibiotic-associated) colitis*
3 Occasionally
   a) Campylobacter enterocolitis
   b) 'Traveller's diarrhoea' — therapy or prophylaxis

Antibiotics of relevance to pseudomembranous colitis
1 Frequent causes
   a) Ampicillin
   b) Clindamycin/lincomycin
   c) Metronidazole (occasionally)
2 Therapy
   a) Vancomycin (oral)
   b) Bacitracin

---

*Relapses may be due to loss of aerobic flora, and may respond to *Bacteroides* instillation

c) Metronidazole
(Non-antibiotic therapy using cholestyramine — to bind the toxin — is also effective)

INFLAMMATORY BOWEL DISEASE

Indications for surgery
1 Crohn's disease
  a) Acute appendicitis; perforation
  b) Persistent bowel obstruction
  c) Enteric fistulae with complications
  d) Perirectal suppuration
  e) Obstructive hydronephrosis
  f) Selected instances of growth retardation (e.g. refractory to home parenteral nutrition)
2 Ulcerative colitis
  a) Severe colitis with failure to stabilize on intensive in-hospital medical therapy (e.g. five days of i.v. steroids)
  b) Acute complications, e.g. toxic megacolon, life-threatening bleeding, perforation
  c) Severe dysplasia
  d) Development of carcinoma (colonic or cholangiocarcinoma)
  e) Unacceptable treatment side-effects
  f) Intractable pararectal or extraintestinal complications

Colectomy: its effect on complications of ulcerative colitis
1 Complications *responsive* to colectomy
  a) Peripheral arthropathy (p. 296)
  b) Pyoderma gangrenosum
  c) Para-rectal disease (NB: uncommon in ulcerative colitis)
2 Complications *resistant* to colectomy
  a) Ankylosing spondylitis
  b) Sclerosing cholangitis

Mechanisms of debility
1 Anaemia — normochromic, iron deficiency
2 Hypoalbuminaemia (protein-losing enteropathy)
3 Portal pyaemia
4 Liver disease
5 Fistulae (malabsorption)

Therapeutic role of sulphasalazine
1 Effective in inducing remission in active ulcerative colitis and Crohn's disease, and in preventing flare-ups from quiescence in ulcerative colitis
2 Drug consists of sulphapyridine (sulphonamide) moiety and 5-acetylsalicylic acid joined by azo-bond
3 Very little drug is absorbed in the small intestine
4 Azo-linkage is lysed in colon and unabsorbed (topical) 5-ASA is felt to exert prime therapeutic effect
5 Dose-related toxicity is maximal in slow acetylators and is felt to be due to the sulphapyridine moiety (see ref. 4.10)

Side-effects of sulphasalazine
1 Anorexia, nausea, vomiting
2 Headaches
3 Haemolysis, methaemoglobinaemia, agranulocytosis, folate deficiency
4 Male infertility — oligospermia and reduced motility
5 Peripheral neuropathy, tinnitus, vertigo
6 Hepatitis; nephrotic syndrome
7 Sulphonamide hypersensitivity reactions
8 Depression

Crohn's disease: approach to management
1 Acute ileitis: *steroids* are effective in inducing remission
  Cyclosporine may be effective in steroid-resistance or intolerance
2 Acute colitis: *sulphasalazine* ± steroids is effective in inducing remission
3 Fistulae ⎫
  Perianal disease ⎬ — anecdotal efficacy of *metronidazole*
  Colonic disease ⎭
4 Maintenance prophylaxis — no firmly established regimen (cf. ulcerative colitis)
5 Cholorrheic enteropathy (i.e. diarrhoea due to ileal malabsorption of bile acids leading to colonic irritation): diagnose with faecal bile acid estimation, treat with *cholestyramine*
6 Extensive ileal resection (>100 cm) with frank steatorrhoea: treat with medium-chain triglyceride (MCT) diet and parenteral vitamin supplements (A,D,E,K,B_{12}); low oxalate ± low lactose diet
7 Bacterial overgrowth — may be responsible for apparently refractory disease; treat with broad-spectrum antibiotics
8 Postsurgical disease recurrence — typically occurs proximal to anastomoses. Minimal surgical intervention is favoured
9 Malignancy — typically occurs in surgically excluded segments (due to increased duration of disease in such segments), but routine surveillance not indicated; an excess of right-sided colonic carcinoma is also recognized in Crohn's
10 Other problems
  a) Osteopenia ⎫
   ⎬ may be steroid- or disease-related.
  b) Growth retardation ⎭
  c) Gallstones
  d) Renal (oxalate) stones
  e) Ureteric obstruction
  f) Psoas abscess
  g) Amyloidosis
  h) Aphthous ulcers
  i) Thromboembolism

Continent ileorectal reservoirs ('Kock's ileostomy'): progress and problems
1 Continence achievable in 80–95% patients
2 Anastomotic strictures occur in about 10%
3 Pouch failure occurs in 2–5%
4 Faecal stasis may lead to anaerobic overgrowth with 'pouchitis' manifesting as diarrhoea; responds to metronidazole
5 'Primary' ileostomy diarrhoea may respond to the long-acting somatostatin analogue SMS–201–995
6 If pouch requires dismantling, this may entail further bowel shortening with exacerbation of pre-existing short bowel syndrome

UNDERSTANDING GASTROINTESTINAL DISEASE

GUT HORMONES

Classification of regulatory peptides coexisting in gut and CNS

1 Paracrine (locally acting) — somatostatin
2 Neurotransmitters — VIP, substance P, bombesin, endorphins
3 Endocrine (distantly acting) — cholecystokinin (CCK), neurotensin

(NB: all other gut peptides mentioned below exhibit predominantly *endocrine* mode of action)

Gut peptides exhibiting structural similarities

1 Gastrin
  CCK
  Insulin
2 Secretin
  (Entero)glucagon
  VIP
  GIP
3 Bombesin
  Substance P

Physiology of gut regulatory peptides

1 Gastrin
  a) Location — gastric antrum (also jejunum)
  b) Released by
    — Vagal stimulation (esp. gastric distension)
    — Protein meals; alcohol
    — Bombesin
  c) Effects
    — Stimulates gastric acid and pepsin secretion
    — Inhibits gastric emptying
    — Trophic to gastric mucosa
    — Increases lower oesophageal sphincter tone
  d) Clinical
    — Zollinger-Ellison (gastrinoma) syndrome
    — Achalasia (gastrin hypersensitivity → ↑ lower oesophageal sphincter tone)
2 Cholecystokinin (CCK; 'hormone of satiety')
  a) Location — duodenum and jejunum
  b) Released by — protein/fat ingestion
  c) Effects
    — Stimulates gallbladder contraction and relaxes sphincter of Oddi
    — Releases pancreatic proteolytic enzymes
    — Trophic to pancreas
  d) Clinical — analogues used to assess pancreatic and gallbladder function
3 Secretin ('physiological antacid')
  a) Location — duodenum and jejunum
  b) Released by — entry of acid into duodenum
  c) Effects — stimulates pancreatic bicarbonate secretion
  d) Clinical — ↓ secretion in coeliac disease
4 Vasoactive intestinal polypeptide (VIP)
  a) Location — postganglionic gut nerve cells
  b) Released by — direct neural mediation (*not* by meals)
  c) Effects
    — Inhibits gastric acid secretion
    — Stimulates pancreatic bicarbonate secretion
    — Stimulates gut secretion and insulin release
    — Induces vasodilatation and hypotension
  d) Clinical
    — VIPoma
    — ↓ secretion in Chagas' and Hirschprung's
    — ↑ secretion in Crohn's disease
    — Implicated in postgastrectomy 'dumping'
5 Substance P
  a) Location — gut nerve cells
  b) Released by — unknown stimuli
  c) Effects
    — Inhibits pancreatic bicarbonate/amylase release
    — Inhibits biliary secretion
    — Inhibits insulin, stimulates glucagon release
    — Stimulates salivation, vasodilatation, smooth muscle contraction, and natriuresis
  d) Clinical — implicated in nociception, asthma
6 Bombesin
  a) Location — gut nerve cells
  b) Released by — unknown stimuli
  c) Effects
    — Stimulates gastrin/gastric acid secretion
    — Stimulates pancreatic enzyme secretion
  d) Clinical — frequently secreted in small-cell lung cancer, but *no* recognized paraneoplastic syndrome
7 Glucose-dependent insulinotrophic polypeptide (formerly, gastric inhibitory polypeptide; GIP)
  a) Location — throughout gut, esp. duodenum and jejunum
  b) Released by — *oral* glucose
  c) Effects
    — Stimulates insulin release (such that glucose administered orally leads to greater insulin release than does parenteral glucose, per unit glycaemia)
    — Inhibits gastric acid secretion
  d) Clinical: ↓ secretion in coeliac disease
8 Motilin ('hormone of diarrhoea')
  a) Location — duodenum and jejunum
  b) Released by — meals (including drinking water, i.e. by vagally-mediated gastric distension; also by fat)
  c) Effects
    — Stimulates gastric emptying
    — Stimulates small intestinal motility
    — Mediates gastrocolic reflex
  d) Clinical
    — ↑ In infective diarrhoeas
    — ↑ In inflammatory bowel disease
    — ↑ In carcinoid syndrome
9 Neurotensin
  a) Location — ileum
  b) Released by — entry of food (esp. fat) to ileum
  c) Effects
    — Inhibits gastric emptying and acid secretion
    — Stimulates intestinal secretion
    — Induces hypotension
  d) Clinical — implicated in postgastrectomy 'dumping'
10 Enteroglucagon

a) Location — ileum and colorectum
b) Released by — meals
c) Effects
   — Trophic to small intestinal mucosa
   — Inhibits gastric emptying and acid secretion
d) Clinical
   — ↑↑ Secretion in remaining functional gut following bowel resection or bypass
   — ↑↑ Secretion in coeliac disease/cystic fibrosis
   — Implicated in post-gastrectomy 'dumping'

11 Pancreatic polypeptide ('hormone of indigestion'; PP)
   a) Location — pancreas
   b) Released by
      — Vagal stimulation
      — Protein meals
   c) Effects — inhibits pancreatic and biliary secretion
   d) Clinical — secreted coincidentally in many gut endocrine tumour syndromes esp: VIPoma (75%), glucagonoma (50%), gastrinoma (25%), carcinoid syndrome

12 Somatostatin ('growth hormone release inhibiting hormone')
   a) Location — pancreas ('D' cells), and throughout gut
   b) Released by — diverse stimuli
   c) Effects
      — Stimulates gastric emptying
      — Inhibits almost everything else: gastric acid/pepsin secretion; pancreatic and biliary secretions; coeliac blood flow; release of GH, TSH, insulin, glucagon, gastrin, secretin, PP, GIP, motilin, enteroglucagon
   d) Clinical — synthetic analogues have been successfully used in VIPoma diarrhoea control, gastrinoma, insulinoma, glucagonoma and acromegaly; tumour size sometimes reduced; used also in GI haemorrhage and pancreatitis

NB: *no* abnormality of gut hormones has yet been characterized in irritable bowel syndrome

GUT ENDOCRINE TUMOUR SYNDROMES

General features of gut endocrine tumour syndromes

1 *All* may be due to malignant tumours, and metastasis is frequently demonstrable at presentation (see below)
2 *Most* may cause diarrhoea (see p. 120–121)
3 *Many* may be associated with secretion of other peptides (such as calcitonin, ACTH/CRH, PTH, adrenaline, noradrenaline, VMA) and clinical evolution from (say) VIPoma to insulinoma may occur
4 *Any* may be associated with multiple endocrine adenomatosis (MEA #I, Wermer's syndrome) – this possibility should be periodically excluded by measuring plasma Ca^{2+} (+ PTH if Ca^{2+} elevated) and performing lateral skull X-ray (and assaying pituitary hormones where indicated)
5 Streptozotocin may be used to palliate unresectable disease, but response rates are very variable (typically about 25%)

Gastrinoma: features

1 Primary G-cell tumours, usually found in pancreatic body/tail
2 50% have, or develop, parathyroid/pituitary adenoma (MEA #I) (ask about family history of renal stones, pituitary tumour or hypoglycaemia)
3 50% manifest with diarrhoea or steatorrhoea (see below)
4 95% present with duodenal ulceration, classically
   a) Young patient without risk factors (unless MEA #I)
   b) Multiple large, deep ulcers
   c) Ectopic position (postbulbar, jejunal, oesophageal)
   d) Associated with pyloric stenosis or oesophageal stricture
   e) Prone to perforation or haemorrhage, esp. postoperatively
   f) Healing resistant to normal-dose H^2-receptor antagonists
5 Management
   a) Medical
      — Omeprazole (an H^+/K^+-ATPase inhibitor), or
      — *High-dose* (up to 5 times normal) H_2-receptor antagonists
      — Addition of anticholinergics (if needed)
      — Pancreatic enzyme supplements, cholestyramine (for steatorrhoea, diarrhoea respectively)
   b) Surgical
      — If hypercalcaemic: assess for parathyroidectomy prior to further intervention
      — If no evidence of metastasis: laparotomy
      — If primary tumour localizable: resection
      — If disease unresectable *and* preoperative ulceration controllable with drugs, close up
      — If disease unresectable *and* difficulties in medical symptom control, consider highly selective vagotomy
      — If disease unresectable *and* symptoms resistant to optimal medical therapy, consider total gastrectomy (a last resort)

VIPoma: features

1 Primary tumours are usually pancreatic in adults; children may develop benign extrapancreatic ganglioneuroblastomas
2 Pancreatic origin (in 80%) is confirmed by coexisting elevation of pancreatic polypeptide
3 Manifests with profuse diarrhoea, dehydration and ↓ K^+
4 Associated
   a) Achlorhydria
   b) Flushing, hypotension (esp. on tumour palpation)
   c) Cholelithiasis and gallbladder dilatation
   d) Hypercalcaemia (with or without MEA #I)
   e) Glucose intolerance (usually subclinical)
5 Management
   a) **S**urgery if feasible
   b) ***S**omatostatin analogues (85% → ↓ VIP → ↓ diarrhoeà)

---

*Drug of choice for symptom control

c) Symptomatic
— Opiates (codeine, loperamide)
— Metoclopramide; indomethacin
— Steroids
— Fluid and electrolyte balance
d) Streptozotocin (cytotoxic) for metastases

Glucagonoma: features
1 Primary α-cell pancreatic tumours, commoner in females
2 Spontaneous symptomatic remissions characteristic
3 Sequelae
a) Diarrhoea (see below); hypercatabolic weight loss
b) Stomatitis, glossitis, vulvovaginitis, nail dystrophy
c) Thromboembolism
d) Necrolytic migratory erythema (transient bullous or crusting rash, often involving perineum and leaving residual pigmentation)
e) Glucose intolerance (often clinical)
f) Hypocholesterolaemia
4 Management
a) Somatostatin analogues (for diarrhoea)
b) Insulin if required (for diabetes)
c) Oral zinc (for rash)
d) Anticoagulant prophylaxis (for thromboembolism)
e) Tumour resection (for operable disease)
f) Streptozotocin (for inoperable disease)

Other gut endocrine tumours: features
1 Somatostatinoma (D-cell tumour; rare)
a) Diarrhoea, steatorrhoea (see below)
b) Achlorhydria; dyspepsia
c) Cholelithiasis, dilated gallbladder
d) Glucose intolerance (usually subclinical)
2 Enteroglucagonoma (very rare)
a) Small intestinal hypomotility
b) Massive villous hypertrophy on jejunal biopsy
c) Oedema due to protein loss (see below)
3 PPoma/neurotensinoma (very rare): these appear to be the only gut endocrine tumours which present with symptoms and signs of invasion or metastasis rather than of endocrine sequelae

Malignant potential of gut endocrine tumours
1 Insulinoma — 5–10% are metastatic at presentation
2 Gastrinoma — 30% are metastatic at presentation
3 Glucagonoma ⎫
4 VIPoma   ⎬ — >50% are metastatic at presentation
5 Somatostatinoma ⎭
6 Carcinoid syndrome — >98% are metastatic at presentation (cf. carcinoid tumours without syndrome — <10% metastasize)

CARCINOID SYNDROME

Symptoms and signs of carcinoid syndrome
1 *Acute* symptoms (induced by 5HT, kinins, etc.) include
a) Upper body flushing ± lacrimation, facial oedema
b) Pruritic wheals, serpentine flush (if histamine-secreting)

c) Wheezing; hypotension; fever; tachycardia
d) Borborygmi, abdominal pain, diarrhoea, vomiting
2 *Chronic* complications indicative of disease duration include
a) Telangiectasia; pellagra-like rash; arthropathy
b) Hepatomegaly* — cirrhosis may also supervene
c) Mesenteric fibrosis ('sclerosing peritonitis')
d) Tricuspid incompetence (chordal fibrosis)
e) Pulmonic stenosis (valvular adhesions)

Benefits of somatostatin analogues (e.g. octreotide, SMS-201-995) in carcinoid syndrome
1 Effective in reducing *diarrhoea*
2 Best available treatment for *flushing* (effective in 90%)
3 Infusion valuable in treating 'carcinoid crisis'

Other treatment modalities in carcinoid syndrome
1 Diarrhoea (serotonin-induced)
a) Non-specific: codeine, loperamide
b) Serotonin antagonists — cyproheptadine (cf. methysergide: contraindicated due to increased risk of fibrotic sequelae)
2 Flushing (due to kinins, substance P, serotonin) — phenoxybenzamine, corticosteroids; ketanserin (serotonin blocker)
Serpentine (histamine-induced) flushing of gastric carcinoids — H_1 and H_2 histamine receptor antagonists
3 Hepatic pain
a) Hepatic embolization
b) Surgical debulking
4 Carcinoid crisis (e.g. perioperative) — corticosteroids
5 Pellagra — nicotinamide supplements
6 Metastases
a) Streptozotocin (limited efficacy)
b) Interferon-α

HUMORAL DIARRHOEA

Characteristics of diarrhoea due to gut endocrine tumours
(NB: *all* may be associated with weight loss and anaemia if symptoms severe and/or disease advanced)
1 Gastrinoma
a) Diarrhoea not caused by hypergastrinaemia per se, but low intestinal pH
b) This leads to pancreatic enzyme denaturation and bile salt precipitation, with consequent ileal bile salt malabsorption and (i) dietary fat malabsorption (steatorrhoea) and/or (ii) colonic irritation by bile salts (watery diarrhoea)
2 VIPoma ('pancreatic cholera')
a) 'Rice-water' (secretory) diarrhoea (1–20 L/day; frequently nocturnal or fasting)
b) Associated with
— Colicky abdominal pain
— Dehydration (± azotaemia)
— Hypokalaemic *acidosis* (achlorhydria leads to predominant loss of alkaline secretions; may be life-threatening)

---

*Rarely, bronchial or ovarian primaries may cause the syndrome in the absence of hepatic metastases

3 Glucagonoma
  a) Diarrhoea, no steatorrhoea
  b) May be associated with hypokalaemic alkalosis
  c) Characteristic rash
  d) Normochromic anaemia
4 Somatostatinoma
  a) Steatorrhoea (reduced biliary secretion and intestinal absorption)
  b) Associated with achlorhydria (reduced gastric acidity)
5 Enteroglucagonoma
  a) Steatorrhoea
  b) No diarrhoea (gut hypomotility)
  c) Protein-losing enteropathy with oedema (due to massive villous hypertrophy)
6 Carcinoid syndrome — profuse secretory diarrhoea (5HT-induced): associated with borborygmi, abdominal pain, nausea

THE UPPER GASTROINTESTINAL TRACT

Pathogenetic mechanisms contributing to reflux oesophagitis
1 ↓ Lower oesophageal sphincter tone, e.g. in scleroderma
2 ↓ Oesophageal clearance of refluxed material, e.g. in oesophageal spasm
3 ↑ Irritant content of refluxed material, e.g. postgastrectomy biliary gastritis, ZES
4 ↑ Volume of gastric contents, e.g. delayed gastric emptying, Menétrier's disease

Barrett's oesophagus* : how important is it?
(*columnar-lined oesophageal metaplasia above cardia)
1 Commoner in males
2 Found in 10% of oesophagoscopic biopsies for oesophagitis
3 Found in 40% of patients with chronic peptic strictures
4 Carcinoma risk
  a) Probably predisposes to 5% of all oesophageal cancer
  b) Lifetime risk in a given patient is probably about 5%
  c) This represents a 30-fold increase in relative risk compared to the general population
5 30% of patients presenting with carcinoma in Barrett's oesophagus have no prior history of reflux symptoms
6 Other carcinomas (e.g. colonic) may occur with increased frequency in patients with Barrett's oesophagus

Approach to managing the patient with Barrett's oesophagus
1 Antireflux therapy (no evidence of metaplastic regression)
2 Endoscopic surveillance
3 If multiple foci of high-grade dysplasia develop, resection may be indicated

Clinical features of hypertrophic gastropathies
1 Menétrier's disease
  a) Male predominance (3:1)
  b) Presents with epigastric pain and peripheral oedema
  c) Giant gastric rugae with antral sparing
  d) Achlorhydria (5% develop carcinoma)
  e) Protein-losing enteropathy
2 Schindler's disease
  a) Giant gastric rugae
  b) Acid hypersecretion
  c) Normal protein balance

HEPATITIS

Hepatitis in pregnancy
1 HBV is most likely to be vertically transmitted if acutely acquired in the third trimester
2 HBeAg-positive mothers have an 85% chance of transmission; anti-HBe-positive mothers have a 25% chance of transmission
3 Delta agent may also be transmitted at delivery
4 Caesarean section may reduce the risk of HBV transmission (controversial)
5 Neonates at risk should be commenced immediately on both active and passive immunization
6 50% of vertically-infected male children die of cirrhosis or hepatoma

The delta agent ('hepatitis D'): clinical significance
1 A defective RNA virus which requires HBV to replicate (i.e. minimally infective to normal, HBsAg-negative patients); the delta antigen is coated with HBsAg
2 Main reservoirs
  a) Drug addicts
  b) Polytransfused patients, esp. haemophiliacs
  c) South Americans, Middle Easterns, Africans and Italians
  d) Sexual partners of these people
  (NB: relatively infrequent among homosexual HBsAg carriers)
3 Clinical scenarios
  a) Co-primary infection with HBV (low morbidity)
  b) Infection superimposed on chronic HBV (high morbidity)
  c) Conversion of chronic persistent to chronic active hepatitis
4 Persistence of anti-delta IgM usually signifies development of chronic active hepatitis or cirrhosis, even though delta agent predominantly infects anti-HBe-positive patients and inhibits HBV replication
5 Superinfection can precipitate progression from minimal liver disease to cirrhosis within 12 months
6 There appears to be no link with hepatoma

Hepatitis C and non-A, non-B hepatitis
1 Hepatitis C virus:
  a) Causes parenterally transmitted non-A non-B hepatitis: post-transfusion, venereal or sporadic; complicates about 1% of transfusions; implicated in 95% of transfusion-related hepatitis cases
  b) Due to recently cloned RNA virus (? a togavirus) for which serology is now available

c) Incubation period intermediate between that of hepatitis A and hepatitis B (about 60 days)
d) Manifests as:
   - Mild anicteric infection which is *subclinical* despite large fluctuations in ALT
   - Progression to *chronic hepatitis* in 50%; of these, 50% will develop CAH and 20% cirrhosis
   - Development of *fulminant hepatitis* in a significant proportion of cases
2 Non-A non-B hepatitis virus:
   a) Causes *enterically transmitted* non-A non-B hepatitis; may mimic sporadic hepatitis A Specifically implicated in *epidemic waterborne non-A* hepatitis reported in India in association with high fetal wastage and mortality in pregnant women
   b) Due to? a calicivirus; not yet definitively identified or serologically recognisable; hence, remains a diagnosis of exclusion
   c) Acute illness indistinguishable from other forms of hepatitis, but *no* chronic sequelae (cf. hep C)

Chronic viral hepatitis: principal causes
1 Hepatitis B virus ± delta agent
2 Non-A, non-B hepatitis (i.e. *not* hepatitis A)

Precipitants of fulminant hepatic failure (80% mortality)
1 Viral hepatitis (responsible for 50% of cases)
   a) Non-A non-B hepatitis (commonest viral cause)
   b) Hepatitis A (esp. in adults)
   c) Acute hepatitis B
   d) Chronic hepatitis B *with* delta agent superinfection
2 Toxicity
   a) Paracetamol overdose (responsible for 40% of cases)
   b) Halothane hepatitis
3 Other
   a) Acute fatty liver of pregnancy
   b) Weil's disease (leptospirosis)
   c) Wilson's disease (in children)

Antigens implicated in pathogenesis of chronic active hepatitis
1 Autoimmune type I ('lupoid') hepatitis — actin
2 Autoimmune type II hepatitis — $P_{450}db1$ (a minor hepatic microsomal P_{450} isozyme)
3 Tienilic acid (ticrynafen)-induced hepatitis — P_{450} isozyme metabolizing tienilic acid

SECONDARY CAUSES OF LIVER DISEASE

Alcohol-induced liver disease
1 Steatosis (fatty infiltration); dose-dependent, reversible
2 Hepatic siderosis
3 Alcoholic hepatitis (10–40% mortality); cirrhosis precursor lesion
4 Micronodular cirrhosis
5 Hepatocellular carcinoma

Hormone-induced liver disease
1 Pregnancy
   a) Benign cholestasis (recurs with subsequent pregnancy or oral contraceptive use)
   b) Acute fatty liver (75% maternal/fetal mortality; does *not* recur)
   c) Hepatic rupture (frequently preceded by minimally symptomatic pre-eclamptic liver disease)
2 Oral contraceptive use
   a) Cholestasis (pruritus ± jaundice)
   b) Cholelithiasis
   c) Hepatic vein thrombosis
   d) Adenoma(s) ± intraperitoneal rupture
   e) Focal nodular hyperplasia
3 Androgens (C-17 substituted testosterones)
   a) Peliosis hepatis
   b) Hepatoma, angiosarcoma
   c) Cholestasis

Cirrhosis
1 Viruses — hepatitis B, non-A non-B
2 Alcohol
3 Prolonged cholestasis (intra- or extrahepatic)
4 Prolonged venous obstruction (Budd-Chiari, constrictive pericarditis)
5 Metabolic
   a) Idiopathic haemochromatosis
   b) Wilson's disease
   c) α_1AT deficiency
6 Drugs — methotrexate, INH, methyldopa, nitrofurantoin, vitamin A, dantrolene, oxyphenisatin

LIVER DISEASE: CLINICAL BACKGROUND

Liver dysfunction in inflammatory bowel disease
1 Cholangitis
   a) Recurrent ascending cholangitis
      — Uncommon
   b) 'Pericholangitis'
      — Common — typically manifests as minimally symptomatic elevation of alk. phos.
   c) Sclerosing cholangitis
      — In ulcerative colitis only — no effective treatment, incl. colectomy; may mimic PBC or cholangiocarcinoma
   Cholangiocarcinoma
   Cholelithiasis: in Crohn's disease
2 Hepatic vein thrombosis
   Hepatic infiltration (fat, amyloid)
   Hepatitis
   a) Chronic active (→ cirrhosis)
   b) Granulomatous
   c) Transfusion-related (e.g. non-A, non-B)

Amoebic liver abscesses
1 Right lobe affected in 90%
   Males affected in 80%
   Single abscess only in 70%
2 Liver function tests usually normal
3 Formed stools may contain cysts (often difficult to

distinguish from leucocytes) and vegetative forms (usually early stages)
4 Secondary bacterial infection in 20%
5 Past history of amoebic dysentery *rare*

PREDISPOSITIONS TO LIVER DISEASE

Hepatitis B surface antigenaemia
1 Male homosexuality
2 Narcotic addiction
3 Haemophilia; haemodialysis; transplantation
4 Polyarteritis nodosa
5 Essential (mixed) cryoglobulinaemia

Predispositions to hepatic vein thrombosis
1 Severe dehydration, esp. in early life
2 Postpartum; oral contraceptive use
3 Paroxysmal nocturnal haemoglobinuria
4 Malignancies, e.g. hepatoma, renal cell carcinoma, polycythaemia vera
5 Inflammatory bowel disease

Fatty liver
1 Alcohol ingestion
2 Diabetes mellitus, esp. if receiving high-dose insulin treatment
3 Pregnancy
   a) Acute (fulminating) type
   b) High-dose intravenous tetracycline therapy (should *never* be used in pregnancy in any case)
4 Thyrotoxicosis, Cushing's syndrome
5 Inflammatory bowel disease
6 Morbid obesity; protein-calorie malnutrition; jejunoileal bypass

HEPATIC ENCEPHALOPATHY

Pathogenesis of hepatic encephalopathy: general mechanisms
1 Hepatic insufficiency →
   —Circulation of undetoxified metabolites (e.g. ammonia, aromatic amino acids) due to urea cycle breakdown
   —Abnormal cerebral metabolism
2 Urea cycle breakdown →
   — ↓ Hepatic gluconeogenesis and insulin release
   — ↓ Uptake/metabolism of potentially toxic branched-chain amino acids by muscle
3 Increased permeability of blood-brain barrier
4 Disturbed neurotransmitter balance
5 Impairment of cerebral Na^+/K^+-ATPase activity

Pathogenesis of hepatic encephalopathy: specific mechanisms
1 ↑ Blood ammonia → ↑ CNS ammonia
2 ↑ CNS ammonia → ↑ CNS (CSF) glutamine
3 ↑ CNS ammonia → abnormal α ketoglutarate metabolism
4 ↑ Blood tryptophan (an aromatic amino acid) → ↑ CNS 5-hydroxytryptamine (serotonin)
5 ↑ Methionine → ↑ mercaptan (→ fetor), ↑ taurine

6 ↓ CNS dopamine/noradrenaline
7 ↑ Accumulation of CNS octopamine (a false neurotransmitter)
8 ↑ Activation of CNS GABA (an inhibitory neurotransmitter)
   (GABA antagonists are currently being tested as therapy)

PATHOPHYSIOLOGY OF INTESTINAL DISORDERS

Predispositions to giardiasis
1 Hypogammaglobulinaemia; selective IgA deficiency
2 Coeliac disease
3 Achlorhydria; postgastrectomy
4 Chronic pancreatitis
5 Homosexuality; institutionalized children

Malabsorptive mechanisms in bacterial overgrowth
1 Invasive mucosal damage (villous atrophy)
2 Mechanical barrier to absorption
3 Nutrient consumption by organisms (incl. B_{12} catabolism)
4 Production of abnormal gut motility
5 Deconjugation of bile acids leading to
   a) Steatorrhoea (jejunoileal malabsorption)
   b) Colonic irritation → diarrhoea

Mechanisms of diarrhoea following ileal resection
1 Rapid transit ('short bowel' syndrome) → sodium/water malabsorption
2 Loss of ileocaecal valve
3 Gastric hypersecretion due to impaired gastrin inactivation
4 Limited or recent resection — cholorrheic diarrhoea due to colonic irritation
5 Extensive resection — frank steatorrhoea due to biliary insufficiency

Gastrointestinal concomitants of panhypogammaglobulinaemia
1 Infections — giardiasis, bacterial overgrowth, viral enteritis, bacterial enteritides
2 Coeliac disease
3 Nodular lymphoid hyperplasia
4 Pancreatic insufficiency
5 Pernicious anaemia, gastric carcinoma

GLUTEN-INDUCED ENTEROPATHY (COELIAC DISEASE)

Clinical presentations of gluten-induced enteropathy
1 Common
   a) Persistent non-specific gastrointestinal upset
   b) Constitutional symptoms
   c) Minor abnormality detected on full blood count, e.g. mild macrocytic anaemia, hyposplenism
2 Classical
   a) Steatorrhoea
   b) Growth retardation

c) Osteomalacia
d) Symptomatic anaemia
3 Unusual
   a) Amenorrhoea, hypogonadism, infertility
   b) Dermatitis herpetiformis
   c) Clubbing, bone pain, tetany
   d) Oedema, nocturia
   e) Aphthous stomatitis
   f) Neuropathy
4 Rare
   a) Fever of unknown origin
   b) Lymphadenopathy
   c) Recurrent pericarditis
   d) Thrombocytosis
   e) Gastrointestinal lymphoma or adenocarcinoma
5 Proctalgia fugax

Diagnostic criteria in gluten-induced enteropathy

1 Best screening tests
   a) Red cell folate (↓ in 70%)
   b) Howell-Jolly bodies on blood film (high specificity in clinical context)
2 Definitive diagnosis (always justified if lifelong gluten-free diet under consideration)
   a) Subtotal villous atrophy on small bowel biopsy, *plus*
   b) Symptomatic resolution on gluten-free diet, *plus*
   c) Symptomatic and histological relapse on gluten re-challenge
3 D-Xylose absorption ⎤ high incidence of
  3-day faecal fats   ⎬ false-negatives despite
                       ⎦ confirmed 'flat' biopsy

NB: Often *poor* correlation between symptomatic, biochemical and histological improvement following instigation of gluten-free diet (biopsy appearances in particular may take months to improve)

Composition of the gluten-free diet

1 Excluded
   a) Wheat
   b) Rye
   c) Barley
   d) Oats
   e) Malt
2 Not excluded
   a) Rice
   b) Corn
   c) Soybean

Efficacy of the gluten-free diet

1 90% of patients will achieve *clinical* remission on this diet
2 Only 70% will have full '*biochemical*' remission (e.g. normalization of red cell folate)
3 Only 50% will have achieved '*mucosal*' remission on rebiopsy

Failure of clinical remission with gluten-free diet

1 Inadequate dietary compliance
2 Undiagnosed problem
   a) Lactose intolerance
   b) Hypogammaglobulinaemia
   c) Bacterial overgrowth
   d) Pancreatic insufficiency
   e) Tropical sprue

3 Development of collagenous sprue (treatable with steroids)
4 Development of small bowel lymphoma

INFECTIVE DIARRHOEAS: RECENT OBSERVATIONS

Features of Campylobacter enteritis (*C. jejuni, C. coli*)

1 Probable animal reservoir (asymptomatic carrier state *rare*)
  Primarily affects older children and young adults (cf. rotavirus)
2 Rapid onset; duration less than one week; relapses in 25%
3 Abdominal pain and fever (may simulate acute abdomen)
  Myalgia, backache
4 Bloody diarrhoea in 60% ⎤
  Toxic megacolon may   ⎥ may simulate
  occur   ⎬ inflammatory bowel
  Reactive arthritis, esp. ⎥ disease, incl.
  if B27+   ⎦ sigmoidoscopy and biopsy
5 Culture requires special conditions (↑ CO_2, ↓ O_2)
6 Antibiotics usually not indicated

Features of viral gastroenteritis

1 Rotavirus (DD_x = *Pestivirus*)
   a) Affects infants and young children (6 months – 2 years old)
   b) Incubation period 1-3 days
   c) Illness duration ~ 1 week
   d) Mucosal IgA production confers *lifelong* immunity
   e) Vomiting prominent
2 Parvoviruses (esp. Norwalk virus)
   a) Affects all ages (esp. older children and adults)
   b) Typically produces winter epidemics ('winter vomiting disease')
   c) Fever, vomiting, abdominal pain common
   d) Illness duration ~ 48 hours; incubation period 1–2 days
   e) No predictable development of immunity
   f) Asymptomatic carriage may occur (cf. *Campylobacter*)
   g) Frequently transmitted via shellfish ingestion

PSEUDO-OBSTRUCTION

Chronic intestinal pseudo-obstruction: aetiopathogenesis

1 Familial neuromyopathies
   a) Familial myenteric plexus degeneration
   b) Familial dysautonomia (Riley-Day syndrome)
   c) Familial amyloidosis with autonomic neuropathy
   d) Myotonic dystrophy
   e) Acute intermittent porphyria
2 Acquired neuromyopathies
   a) Systemic sclerosis (smooth muscle replaced by fibrosis)
   b) Polymyositis
   c) Parkinson's disease
   d) Lead poisoning
   e) Pelvic irradiation

3 Endocrinopathies
   a) Diabetes mellitus ($\to$ ↓ delayed gastric emptying)
   b) Myxoedema
   c) Phaeochromocytoma (long-standing)
   d) Congenital hypoparathyroidism
4 Anticholinergic drugs
   a) Phenothiazines
   b) Tricyclics
   c) Antiparkinsonian medication

MECHANISMS UNDERLYING GASTROINTESTINAL DISEASE

Gynaecomastia in alcoholic cirrhosis
1 Increased sex-hormone binding globulin (SHBG) levels leading to reduced free testosterone levels
2 Hypothalamopituitary axis suppression leading to reduced total testosterone levels
3 Increased oestrogen production from precursors (e.g. DHEA) despite *normal* oestrogen **clearance**

Anaemia in alcoholic liver disease
1 Hepatic insufficiency per se depresses erythropoiesis
2 Alcohol per se depresses erythropoiesis
3 Folate deficiency
4 Hypersplenism
5 Bleeding (see below)

Bleeding tendency in alcoholic cirrhosis
1 Reduced synthesis of coagulation factors } see
  Reduced activation of coagulation factors } below
2 Platelet function defect
   a) Cirrhosis-induced von Willebrand's-type defect
   b) Separate alcohol-induced platelet function defect
3 Thrombocytopenia
   a) Hypersplenism
   b) Marrow suppression
4 Local factors
   a) Varices
   b) Peptic ulceration
   c) Gastritis
   d) Mallory-Weiss

Coagulopathy in cirrhosis
1 Synthesis of *all* clotting factors except VIII may be reduced
2 Jaundiced patients may malabsorb vitamin K $\to$ reduced activation (carboxylation) of factors II, VII, IX, X, and proteins C and S
3 Prolongation of prothrombin time reflects reduced levels of factors II, V, VII, and X (cf. vitamin K dependence)

4 Since the half-life of factor VII is only 6 hours, the prothrombin time is a sensitive index of hepatic function
5 Marked prolongation of both thrombin time and reptilase clotting time despite normal levels of fibrinogen antigen may reflect presence of abnormal fibrinogen (dysfibrinogenaemia; associated with hepatoma)

Ascitic tendency in cirrhosis
1 Excessive hepatic lymph formation
2 Reduced hepatic degradation of aldosterone (prob. minor significance)
3 Activation of renin-angiotensin-aldosterone axis (leading to impaired salt and water excretion) due to
   a) ↑ Renal sympathetic tone
   b) ↓ 'Effective' central blood volume
      — Dilatation of splanchnic vascular bed
      — Peripheral vasodilatation associated with arteriovenous shunting
      — High portal venous pressure
      — Low serum albumin

Familial non-haemolytic hyperbilirubinaemias
1 Gilbert's syndrome (autosomal dominant)
   a) Affects 2–5% of the population
   b) $\to$ (Mild) unconjugated hyperbilirubinaemia
   c) Precipitated by fasting (e.g. GTT), stress (e.g. surgery), or alcohol ingestion
   d) Liver function and histology normal
   e) Commoner in slow acetylators
   f) Due to minor deficiency of UDP-glucuronyl transferase $\to$ ↓ conjugation and uptake (± shortened RBC survival)
   g) Phenobarbitone confers effective prophylaxis
2 Crigler-Najjar syndrome type II
   a) Rare, relatively benign autosomal dominant condition
   b) $\to$ Unconjugated hyperbilirubinaemia
   c) Due to major deficiency of UDP-glucuronyl transferase
   d) Phenobarbitone useful in management (cf. type I)
3 Dubin-Johnson syndrome
   a) Conjugated hyperbilirubinaemia
   b) Exacerbated by pregnancy, oral oestrogens
   c) BSP elimination: biphasic (late 2° rise)
   d) Failure of oral i.v. cholecystography
   e) Abnormal urinary coproporphyrin excretion
   f) Biopsy — black centrilobular pigment
   g) Due to defective canalicular excretion
4 Rotor's syndrome
   a) Conjugated hyperbilirubinaemia
   b) Normal cholecystogram, biopsy, BSP test
   c) Abnormal urinary coproporphyrin excretion

Reviewing the Literature: Gastroenterology

4.1 Wood S M et al 1985 Treatment of patients with pancreatic endocrine tumours using a new long-acting somatostatin analogue: symptomatic and peptide responses. Gut 26: 438–444

Successful therapy of VIPoma, gastrinoma, glucagonoma and malignant carcinoid syndrome using somatostatin analogue SMS 201–995

4.2   Marshall B J et al 1988 Prospective double-blind trial of duodenal ulcer relapse after eradication of *Campylobacter pylori*. Lancet ii: 1438–1442

Randomized double-blind study of 100 patients from the Western Australian group, showing that eradication of *C. pylori* (best achieved using colloidal bismuth subcitrate plus tinidazole) was strongly correlated with prolonged ulcer healing, while persistence of *C. pylori** (seen particularly with short-course cimetidine) was associated with ulcer relapse.

4.3   Nyren O et al 1986 Absence of therapeutic benefit from antacids or cimetidine in non-ulcer dyspepsia. New England Journal of Medicine 314: 339–343

Controlled trial of 159 patients suggesting that only patients with proven peptic ulcers should be treated with antacids or H2-receptor antagonists

Walan A et al 1989 Effect of omeprazole and ranitidine on ulcer healing and relapse rates in patients with benign gastric ulcer. New England Journal of Medicine 320: 69–75

Double-blind trial of 609 Swedish patients with gastric or prepyloric ulcers treated with omeprazole or ranitidine; omeprazole proved significantly more effective in healing ulcers

4.4   Groll A, Simon J B, Wigle R D et al 1986 Cimetidine prophylaxis for gastrointestinal bleeding in an intensive care unit. Gut 27: 135–140

Placebo-controlled double-blind randomized study of 221 patients; no significant difference was found between the two groups. The identical mortality suggests no indication for prophylactic use of cimetidine in GI bleeding

Levy M et al 1988 Major upper gastrointestinal tract bleeding: relation to the use of aspirin and other non-narcotic analgesics. Archives of Internal Medicine 148: 281–285

Patients taking aspirin at least every other day had a 15-fold increase in frequency of upper gastrointestinal haemorrhage

4.5   Cello J P, Grendell J H, Crass R A et al 1987 Endoscopic sclerotherapy vs portocaval shunt in patients with severe cirrhosis and acute variceal haemorrhage. New England Journal of Medicine 316: 11–15

Study confirming that endoscopic sclerotherapy is now the treatment of choice for acute variceal bleeding

Panes J et al 1987 Controlled trial of endoscopic sclerosis in bleeding peptic ulcers. Lancet ii: 1292–1294

Spanish study of 113 patients. 5% of those receiving endoscopic injection of adrenaline-based sclerosant mixture re-bled, compared with 43% of those treated with cimetidine alone

4.6   Fagan E A, Davison F, Smith P M, Williams R 1986 Fulminant hepatitis B in successive female sexual partners of two anti-HBe-positive males. Lancet ii: 538–540

Molecular hybridization studies demonstrated presence of HBV DNA in semen and saliva of two males who were anti-HBe-positive, DNA polymerase-negative, and seronegative for HBV DNA; this suggests that presence of anti-HBe does *not* necessarily indicate lack of infectivity as traditionally believed

Carman W F et al 1989 Mutation preventing formation of hepatitis B 'e' antigen in patients with chronic hepatitis B infection. Lancet ii: 588–590

Identification of a mutation which prevents transcription of HBeAg, thus causing spurious HBeAg-negativity in a cohort of actively infected patients

Thiers V et al 1988 Transmission of hepatitis B from hepatitis-B-seronegative subjects. Lancet ii: 1273–1275

HBV DNA was detected in a cohort of infectious seronegative patients using the polymerase chain reaction (PCR), suggesting that PCR may be useful in demonstrating mutant HBV genomes in patients labelled 'non-A non-B'

4.7   Alter H J et al 1988 Photochemical decontamination of blood components containing hepatitis B and non-A, non-B virus. Lancet ii: 1446–1449

Successful sterillization of blood products using psoralen photosensitization followed by long-wave UV irradiation

Lok A S F et al 1988 Long-term follow-up in a randomised controlled trial of recombinant α-2-interferon in Chinese patients with chronic hepatitis B infection. Lancet ii: 298–301

Study of 72 Chinese patients showing disappointing results for α-2-interferon in chronic hep B; sustained clearance of HBeAg was seen in 15% of treated patients, but HBsAg remained positive in all patients

Thyagarajan S P, Subramanian S, Thirunalasundari T, Venkateswaran P S, Blumberg B S 1988 Effect of *phyllanthus amarus* on chronic carriers of hepatitis B virus. Lancet ii: 764–766

Treatment with this HBV DNA polymerase inhibitor led to disappearance of HBsAg in 60% of patients, compared with 4% of placebo-treated controls

4.8   Quintero E, Gines P O, Arroyo V et al 1985 Paracentesis vs diuretics in the treatment of cirrhotics with tense ascites. Lancet ii: 611–612

Controlled randomized trial showing that the average length of hospital stay was 12 days for patients treated with paracentesis and albumin infusion, compared with 34 days for diuretics alone. No difference in complication rates was found. This study helped dispel the long-standing bogey surrounding therapeutic paracentesis in cirrhotic ascites

Pockros P J, Reynolds T B 1986 Rapid diuresis in patients with ascites from chronic liver disease: the importance of peripheral oedema. Gastroenterology 90: 1827–1835

This study suggested that oedematous patients being treated for cirrhotic ascites can safely lose 2 kg/day

4.9   Neoptolemos J P et al 1988 Controlled trial of urgent endoscopic retrograde cholangiopancreatography and endoscopic sphincterotomy versus conservative treatment for acute pancreatitis due to gallstones. Lancet ii: 979–983

Early ERCP and sphincterotomy was associated with reduced mortality and shorter hospital stay for patients with severe gallstone-associated pancreatitis when compared with a matched cohort receiving conventional conservative therapy

4.10 Bondesen S et al 1987 5-aminosalicylic acid in the treatment of inflammatory bowel disease. Acta Medica Scandinavica 221: 227–242

Review of trials showing 5-ASA (oral or enema) to be as effective as sulphasalazine in IBD management, but without the toxicity of the (presumably inactive) sulphonamide moiety

---

C. pylori is now called *Helicobacter pylori*

CHAPTER 5

Haematology

Physical examination protocol 5.1 You are asked to examine the patient for signs of haematological disease

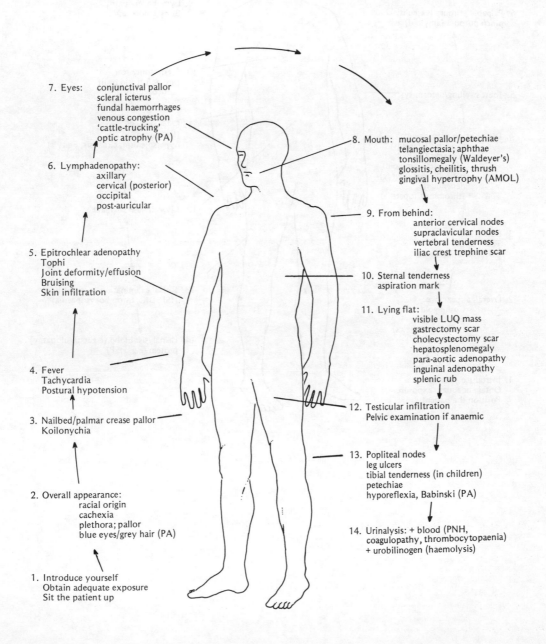

7. Eyes: conjunctival pallor
scleral icterus
fundal haemorrhages
venous congestion
'cattle-trucking'
optic atrophy (PA)

6. Lymphadenopathy:
axillary
cervical (posterior)
occipital
post-auricular

5. Epitrochlear adenopathy
Tophi
Joint deformity/effusion
Bruising
Skin infiltration

4. Fever
Tachycardia
Postural hypotension

3. Nailbed/palmar crease pallor
Koilonychia

2. Overall appearance:
racial origin
cachexia
plethora; pallor
blue eyes/grey hair (PA)

1. Introduce yourself
Obtain adequate exposure
Sit the patient up

8. Mouth: mucosal pallor/petechiae
telangiectasia; aphthae
tonsillomegaly (Waldeyer's)
glossitis, cheilitis, thrush
gingival hypertrophy (AMOL)

9. From behind:
anterior cervical nodes
supraclavicular nodes
vertebral tenderness
iliac crest trephine scar

10. Sternal tenderness
aspiration mark

11. Lying flat:
visible LUQ mass
gastrectomy scar
cholecystectomy scar
hepatosplenomegaly
para-aortic adenopathy
inguinal adenopathy
splenic rub

12. Testicular infiltration
Pelvic examination if anaemic

13. Popliteal nodes
leg ulcers
tibial tenderness (in children)
petechiae
hyporeflexia, Babinski (PA)

14. Urinalysis: + blood (PNH,
coagulopathy, thrombocytopaenia)
+ urobilinogen (haemolysis)

Physical examination protocol 5.2 You are asked to examine a patient who has presented with bruising

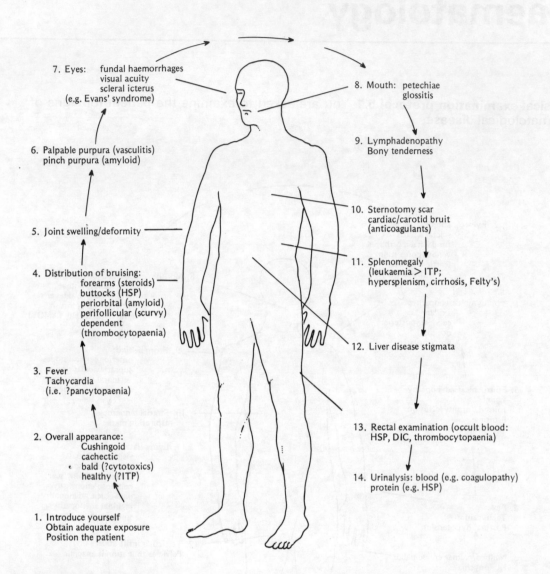

7. Eyes: fundal haemorrhages
            visual acuity
            scleral icterus
            (e.g. Evans' syndrome)

6. Palpable purpura (vasculitis)
   pinch purpura (amyloid)

5. Joint swelling/deformity

4. Distribution of bruising:
   forearms (steroids)
   buttocks (HSP)
   periorbital (amyloid)
   perifollicular (scurvy)
   dependent
   (thrombocytopaenia)

3. Fever
   Tachycardia
   (i.e. ?pancytopaenia)

2. Overall appearance:
   Cushingoid
   cachectic
   bald (?cytotoxics)
   healthy (?ITP)

1. Introduce yourself
   Obtain adequate exposure
   Position the patient

8. Mouth: petechiae
           glossitis

9. Lymphadenopathy
   Bony tenderness

10. Sternotomy scar
    cardiac/carotid bruit
    (anticoagulants)

11. Splenomegaly
    (leukaemia > ITP;
    hypersplenism, cirrhosis, Felty's)

12. Liver disease stigmata

13. Rectal examination (occult blood:
    HSP, DIC, thrombocytopaenia)

14. Urinalysis: blood (e.g. coagulopathy)
    protein (e.g. HSP)

Physical examination protocol 5.3 You are asked to examine a patient who has been found to have an enlarged spleen

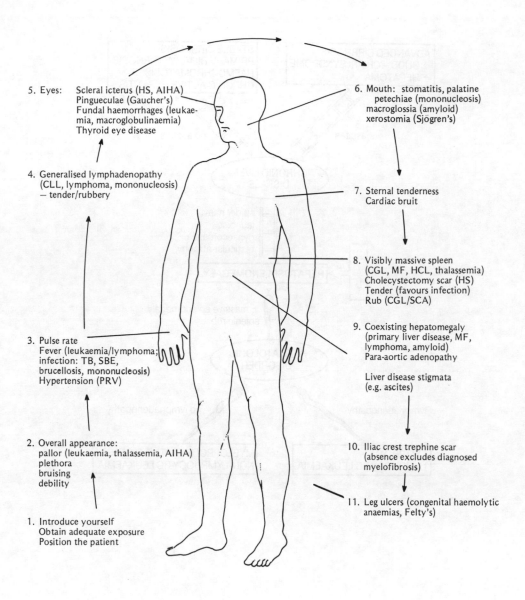

5. Eyes: Scleral icterus (HS, AIHA)
Pingueculae (Gaucher's)
Fundal haemorrhages (leukae-
mia, macroglobulinaemia)
Thyroid eye disease

4. Generalised lymphadenopathy
(CLL, lymphoma, mononucleosis)
— tender/rubbery

3. Pulse rate
Fever (leukaemia/lymphoma;
infection: TB, SBE,
brucellosis, mononucleosis)
Hypertension (PRV)

2. Overall appearance:
pallor (leukaemia, thalassemia, AIHA)
plethora
bruising
debility

1. Introduce yourself
Obtain adequate exposure
Position the patient

6. Mouth: stomatitis, palatine
petechiae (mononucleosis)
macroglossia (amyloid)
xerostomia (Sjögren's)

7. Sternal tenderness
Cardiac bruit

8. Visibly massive spleen
(CGL, MF, HCL, thalassemia)
Cholecystectomy scar (HS)
Tender (favours infection)
Rub (CGL/SCA)

9. Coexisting hepatomegaly
(primary liver disease, MF,
lymphoma, amyloid)
Para-aortic adenopathy

Liver disease stigmata
(e.g. ascites)

10. Iliac crest trephine scar
(absence excludes diagnosed
myelofibrosis)

11. Leg ulcers (congenital haemolytic
anaemias, Felty's)

Diagnostic pathway 5.1 This patient has presented with hepatosplenomegaly. What underlying disorders might be responsible?

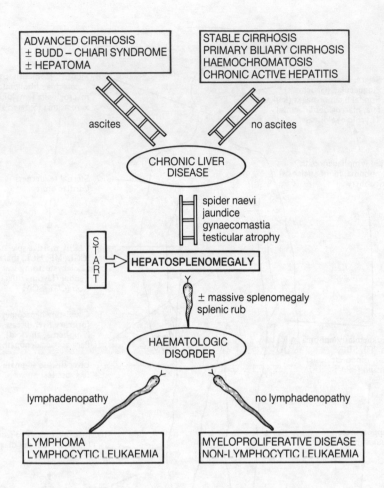

CLINICAL ASPECTS OF HAEMATOLOGICAL DISEASE

> **COMMONEST HAEMATOLOGICAL SHORT CASES**
>
> 1 Splenomegaly
> 2 Cervical lymphadenopathy

PRESENTATIONS OF HAEMATOLOGICAL DISEASE

Abdominal pain in the haematological patient
1 Biliary colic (e.g. hereditary spherocytosis)
2 Splenic infarct (e.g. chronic granulocytic leukaemia)
3 Vaso-occlusive crisis (sickle-cell anaemia)
4 Acute intermittent porphyria
5 Paroxysmal nocturnal haemoglobinuria
6 Hodgkin's disease (alcohol-induced pain)

History of the patient presenting with anaemia
1 Duration of symptoms
2 Past history — e.g. ulcer, prosthetic valve, alcoholism
3 Recent medications — e.g. NSAIDs, warfarin, steroids
4 Operations — e.g. gastrectomy, ileal resection
5 Menstrual history — esp. menorrhagia
6 Diet — green vegetables, special restrictions
7 Family history and racial background
8 Recent travel — e.g. to hookworm-endemic areas
9 Toxic exposures — e.g. benzene, radiation

Clinical manifestations of iron deficiency
1 Anaemia
2 Koilonychia
3 Postcricoid web (premalignant)
4 Atrophic glossitis
5 Angular stomatitis
6 Pica
7 Candidiasis

Infections in the leukaemic host: clinical pitfalls
1 Fevers may arise due to non-infectious causes (e.g. disease per se, drugs, transfusion reactions, graft-vs-host disease)
2 Fevers may arise in the context of infection with *multiple* organisms, any of which may be difficult to identify
3 Fever may persist for the duration of neutropenia despite optimal antibiotic therapy
4 Fevers may not occur at all in elderly or immunosuppressed patients with sepsis
5 Conversely, immunosuppressed febrile patients may fail to localize portal of sepsis due to poor inflammatory response (e.g. pyogenic bacterium infecting without pus formation)

6 False-negative serology may occur due to depressed antibody formation

Clinical sequelae of hyperviscosity
1 CNS — lassitude, headache, deafness, nystagmus, convulsions
2 Visual loss — fundal haemorrhages, 'cattle-trucking', papilloedema
3 Increased plasma volume — dilutional anaemia, hypertension/CCF
4 Platelet dysfunction — bleeding, thrombosis, difficult venepuncture
5 Leucocyte dysfunction — sepsis, difficult crossmatch
6 Renal failure

CLINICAL SIGNS OF HAEMATOLOGICAL DISEASE

So why do you think it's a spleen?
1 Can't get above it
2 Descends prominently on inspiration
3 Distinct edge ± medial notch
4 Not ballottable
5 Dull to percussion
6 ± Audible rub

Causes of epitrochlear lymphadenopathy
1 Non-Hodgkin's lymphoma; chronic lymphocytic leukaemia
2 Infectious mononucleosis; secondary syphilis
3 Sarcoidosis
4 Intravenous drug abuse

Widespread retinal haemorrhages: differential diagnosis
1 Malignant hypertension
2 Diabetes mellitus
3 Hyperviscosity syndrome
4 Severe anaemia, severe thrombocytopenia
5 HbSC disease

Clinical evaluation of bleeding tendency
1 Skin petechiae
  Epistaxes
  Purpura after minor trauma
  Mucosal bleeding
  Menorrhagia
  Immediate bleeding after lacerations
  } —Thrombocytopenia or platelet function defect* ($\uparrow$ bleeding time)
2 Widespread intramuscular haematomas
  Spontaneous haemarthroses
  Delayed bleeding after lacerations
  } —Coagulation factor deficiency: 90% males ($\uparrow$ PTTK)

*Incl. heterozygous von Willebrand's disease, even though platelets themselves are normal

POLYCYTHAEMIA

Clinical features common to primary and secondary polycythaemia
1 Thrombotic tendency (esp. cerebral)
2 Hypertension
3 Headaches
4 Visual disturbances
5 Engorged retinal veins

Clinical features suggestive of polycythaemia vera
1 Splenomegaly
2 Aquagenic pruritus
3 Bleeding (esp. gastrointestinal)
4 Gout
5 Peptic ulcer
6 Disease termination in myelofibrosis or leukaemia (10%)

HODGKIN'S DISEASE

Clinical presentations of Hodgkin's disease
1 'B' symptoms
  a) Fevers (> 38°C)
  b) Sweats (drenching; usually at night)
  c) Weight loss (>10% over last 6 months)
2 Pruritus (*not* a 'B' symptom)
3 Pel-Ebstein (cyclical) fever: classical but *rare*
4 Alcohol-induced pain at sites of disease (incl. abdomen)
5 Infection (see p. 166)

Features of specific histological subtypes
1 Lymphocyte predominant
  a) Best prognosis
  b) Usually early-stage (I, II) disease
2 Nodular sclerosing
  a) Indolent, chemosensitive but relapsing disease
  b) Tends to affect young women; may cause bulky mediastinal nodes
  c) Spreads by contiguity (*cf.* lymphocyte depletion: disseminates)
  d) Good prognosis *unless* bulky mediastinal disease
3 Mixed cellularity
  a) Often associated with occult splenic involvement
  b) Intermediate prognosis
4 Lymphocyte depletion
  a) 'B' symptoms (e.g. fever of unknown origin)
  b) Adenopathy typically more widespread than other subtypes
  c) May present with visceral involvement, e.g. marrow fibrosis, osteoblastic bony disease ('ivory vertebrae')
  d) Worst prognosis

INVESTIGATING HAEMATOLOGICAL DISEASE

THE PERIPHERAL BLOOD FILM

Diagnoses suggested by blood film alone (± normal blood count)
1 'Aleukaemic' leukaemia (circulating blasts, leucoerythroblastosis)

2 Compensated 'warm' autoimmune haemolysis (spherocytosis, polychromasia)
3 Dysproteinaemias (rouleaux, bluish background)
4 Disseminated intravascular coagulation
   Microangiopathic haemolysis } —red cell fragments
5 Infection
  a) Infectious mononucleosis (atypical lymphocytes)
  b) *Mycoplasma pneumoniae* (autoagglutination)
  c) Malaria (*P. vivax/ovale* →. Schüffner's dots)
6 Hereditary spherocytosis
   Thalassaemia trait (microcytosis, teardrops, targets)
   Hb C disease (target cells in abundance)

Features of the postsplenectomy blood film
1 Howell-Jolly bodies
2 Pappenheimer bodies
3 Target cells
4 Spur cells, spherocytes
5 Thrombocytosis ± leucocytosis

Leucoerythroblastic blood film: diagnostic significance
1 **M**yelofibrosis
2 **M**arrow infiltration
  a) **M**etastatic cancer (esp. breast/prostate/small-cell lung) } — Common
  b) **M**alignant lymphoma (± circulating lymphoma cells)
  c) **M**yeloma (+ rouleaux ± circulating plasma cells)
3 **M**arble bone disease (osteopetrosis) } — Uncommon
4 **M**etabolic — Gaucher's disease

Infectious diseases mimicking leukaemic blood films
1 Infectious mononucleosis — may mimic ALL
2 Pertussis, mycoplasma — may mimic CLL

Clues to underlying sepsis on the peripheral blood film
1 Neutrophilia
2 'Left shift' — bandforms, (meta)myelocytes
3 Toxic granulation
4 Döhle bodies

Differential diagnosis of the dimorphic blood film
1 Sideroblastosis
2 Postsplenectomy
3 Posttransfusion
4 Iron loss combined with B$_{12}$/folate malabsorption
  a) Postgastrectomy
  b) Pernicious anaemia with gastric cancer
  c) Coeliac disease and/or intestinal lymphoma
  d) Crohn's disease, Whipple's disease
5 Iron loss combined with hyposplenism
  a) Coeliac disease
  b) Radical gastrectomy (incorporates splenectomy)

Pathological significance of red cell inclusions
1 Howell-Jolly bodies
   Cabot's rings — seen in hyposplenic states, esp. postsplenectomy } — Nuclear remnants
2 Heinz bodies: denatured globin chains in RBC

periphery — seen in unstable Hb, e.g. Hb Zürich, Hb Köln, G6PD deficiency

3 Pappenheimer bodies: iron granules in siderocytes
   a) Positive Prussian blue reaction
   b) Seen postsplenectomy and in lead poisoning
4 Basophilic stippling: implies dyserythropoiesis
   a) Seen in lead poisoning (coarse stippling)
   b) Also seen in thalassaemia, 5'-nucleotidase deficiency

Abnormal erythrocyte morphology: aetiologic significance

1 Target cells
   a) Chronic liver disease
   b) Thalassaemia; Hb C; Hb E
   c) Hyposplenism
   d) Iron deficiency
2 Teardrop poikilocytes
   a) Myelofibrosis
   b) Dyserythropoiesis, e.g. thalassaemia, megaloblastosis
3 Schistocytes
   a) Microangiopathic haemolytic anaemia (e.g. TTP)
   b) Disseminated intravascular coagulation
4 Spur cells (acanthocytes)
   a) Chronic liver disease (esp. Zieve's syndrome)
   b) Abetalipoproteinaemia
   c) Renal failure, hyposplenism

IRON-DEFICIENCY ANAEMIA

Abnormalities of plasma iron studies in haematological disease

1 $\downarrow$ Fe, $\uparrow$ TIBC, $\downarrow$ ferritin — iron deficiency
2 $\downarrow$ Fe, $\downarrow$ TIBC, $\uparrow$ ferritin — chronic disease
3 $\uparrow$, Fe, $\downarrow$ TIBC, $\uparrow$ ferritin — chronic haemolysis

Temporal sequence of iron deficiency

1 Iron depletion
   a) Reduced marrow stainable iron
   b) Low stainable sideroblast ferritin
   c) Increased red cell protoporphyrin
2 Iron deficiency
   a) Absent marrow stainable iron
   b) $\downarrow$ Fe, $\uparrow$ TIBC
   c) Transferrin saturation <15%
3 Iron deficiency anaemia
   a) Hypochromic microcytic film; $\uparrow$ RDW
   b) Low Hb

Microcytosis disproportionate to anaemia: causes

1 Thalassaemia (incl. trait)
2 Venesected polycythaemia vera

Investigation of unexplained hypochromic microcytic anaemia

1 Blood film
   a) Red cell morphology
   b) Reticulocyte count
2 Iron studies
   a) Serum iron, TIBC, transferrin saturation
   b) Serum ferritin
3 Exclusion of gastrointestinal (or uterine) bleeding
   a) Faecal occult blood testing and/or endoscopy

b) Angiography; ^{99}Tc-labelled red cells
4 Marrow aspiration
   a) Stainable iron stores
   b) Ring sideroblasts
5 Urinary haemosiderin — chronic intravascular haemolysis (e.g. PNH)
6 Hb EPG
   a) HbA$_2$ level ($\uparrow$ $\rightarrow$ β-thal trait)
   b) Supravital staining 'golf-ball' red cells with HbH inclusions (α-thal)

Failure of microcytic anaemia to respond to iron supplements

1 Wrong diagnosis
   a) Thalassemia trait
   b) Sideroblastosis (congenital)
2 Persistent bleeding
3 Malabsorption
   a) Blind loop
   b) Gastrectomy
4 Non-compliance

MEGALOBLASTIC ANAEMIAS

Macrocytosis: clues to underlying megaloblastosis on blood film

1 *Oval* macrocytes (esp. if >3%)
2 Markedly elevated MCV (>115 fl)
3 Hypersegmented (>5 lobes) neutrophils
4 Marked poikilo-/anisocytosis; mild basophilic stippling
5 No target/spur cells, round macrocytes (cf. liver disease)
   No polychromatophilic macrocytes (cf. haemolysis)

Clinicopathological correlations in folate metabolism

1 Red cell folate levels more accurately reflect tissue levels than do serum estimations
2 Partial *haematological* responses may be seen in (pure) B$_{12}$ deficiency treated inadvertently with pharmacologic (i.e. supraphysiological 5–15 mg/day) doses of folate (cf. primary folate deficiency, where maximal reticulocytosis follows physiological — 200 μg/day — doses of folate)
3 Catastrophic progression of *neurological* deficit may be seen in B$_{12}$-deficient patients treated inadvertently with folate
   Hence, if in doubt always give both B$_{12}$ *and* folate
4 Folate (and/or B$_{12}$) deficiency may manifest as azoöspermia or subfertility
5 The aetiology of folate deficiency in patients taking anticonvulsants is controversial; proposed mechanisms have included reduced intestinal absorption, competitive inhibition, and poor nutrition

Clinicopathological correlations in B$_{12}$ deficiency

1 The microbiological assay remains the 'gold standard' in determining B$_{12}$ levels. The radioimmunoassay, though cheaper and more widely used, has a higher false-negative and (occasionally) false-positive rate with respect to B$_{12}$ deficiency — often due to uncorrected abnormalities in R-protein quantification

2 In B_{12} deficient patients, *serum* folate (and iron) levels are often elevated ('normal' levels may indicate coexisting folate — or iron — deficiency), while *red cell* folate levels may be reduced; this occurs due to the 'folate trap' mechanism

3 Neurological degeneration may occur in the absence of anaemia

4 Transient ileal mucosal changes (analogous to macrocytosis) may, misleadingly, lead to failure of normalization of the Schilling test following oral intrinsic factor in patients with pernicious anaemia treated for less than (say) six weeks

5 *Mean* corpuscular volume may be normal in patients with coexisting iron deficiency (e.g. Crohn's, coeliac disease, pernicious anaemia with gastric cancer) or thalassaemia trait

6 Blood transfusion is generally best avoided in initial management of severe megaloblastic anaemia due to risk of fluid overload

Investigations distinguishing primary B_{12} from folate deficiency (i.e. if *both* B_{12} and folate levels low)

1 Deoxyuridine suppression test
  a) Deoxyuridine and tritiated thymidine added to patient's bone marrow in vitro
  b) Megaloblastic marrow takes up more thymidine than normal
  c) Abnormality corrects upon adding B_{12} (in primary B_{12} deficiency) or methyltetrahydrofolate (in primary folate deficiency)

2 24-hour urinary methylmalonic acid excretion
  a) 10 g valine given as an initial loading dose
  b) Methylmalonic acid excretion raised in primary B_{12} deficiency *only*

Molecular regulation of B_{12} metabolism

1 Intrinsic factor (IF)
  a) Synthesized by gastric parietal cells
  b) Binds and transports dietary cobalamin (B_{12})
  c) B_{12}-IF complex attaches to specific ileal receptors

2 R-proteins
  a) Incl. transcobalamin (TC) I, III; synthesized by leucocytes
  b) Compete with IF for intragastric binding of cobalamin
  c) Bind B_{12} more avidly than IF at low gastric pH
  d) Facilitate hepatic storage and excretion of cobalamin
  e) Degraded in proximal small bowel by pancreatic enzymes; cf. IF resists proteolysis and binds liberated B_{12}

3 TC II
  a) Plasma protein synthesized by liver
  b) Binds newly absorbed B_{12} in portal blood
  c) Transports B_{12} to target tissues

Abnormalities of transcobalamin metabolism

1 ↓ TC-II — hereditary, leads to vitamin B_{12} deficiency

2 ↑ TC-I — occurs in CGL/polycythaemia vera; may cause ↑ B_{12} levels

3 ↑ TC-III — occurs with benign leucocytosis (e.g. leukaemoid reaction); no change in B_{12} levels

4 ↑ TC-II — occurs with macrophage activation (e.g. SLE, Gaucher's, sarcoid, AMOL); no change in B_{12} levels

Some causes of vitamin B_{12} deficiency

1 Pernicious anaemia
2 Gastrectomy (see p. 113)
3 Bacterial overgrowth (*E. coli, B. fragilis*)
4 Ileal resection (usually > 1 metre)
5 Pancreatic exocrine insufficiency (↓ R-protein proteolysis)
  Gastrinoma (low pH inactivates pancreatic proteases)
6 Imerslund's disease
  Diphyllobothrium latum } —Endemic in Finland
  infestation

Significance of symptomatic B_{12} deficiency in Crohn's disease

1 Bacterial overgrowth
2 Fistula
3 Ileal resection

NB: Major B_{12} deficiency is unusual in uncomplicated Crohn's

Differential diagnosis of an abnormal Schilling test

1 Corrects with addition of intrinsic factor — pernicious anaemia

2 Does not correct with intrinsic factor } — Bacterial overgrowth
  ↑ Faecal bile acids

3 Does not correct with intrinsic factor } — Ileal insufficiency
  Faecal bile acids

4 Does not correct with intrinsic factor } — Renal failure*
  Normal faecal bile acids

*(i.e. renal failure spuriously reduces Schilling test yield; *plasma* B_{12} levels are normal throughout)

Indicators of response following B_{12} replenishment

1 Erythroblastosis (bone marrow) within 12 hours
  Reticulocytosis — begins at 48 hours; maximal after 1 week
2 ↑ serum alkaline phosphatase
3 ↑ Urate
4 ↓ K^+ (may be profound)
5 ↓ Folate; ↓ iron (usually subclinical)

Megaloblastic anaemias with normal B_{12}/folate levels

1 Antimetabolite therapy (p. 26)
2 Erythroleukaemia
3 Hereditary orotic aciduria (uridine-responsive)
  Lesch-Nyhan syndrome (?adenine-responsive)

Aetiology of non-megaloblastic macrocytosis

1 Alcohol ± liver disease
  Liver disease ± alcohol
2 Hypothyroidism (exclude coexisting pernicious anaemia)
3 Acquired sideroblastosis (cf. congenital sideroblastosis: usually microcytic)
4 Reticulocytosis (any cause)
  Auto-agglutination (→ *artefactual* ↑ MCV), e.g. in cold haemagglutinin disease

5 Aplastic anaemia
6 Paroxysmal nocturnal haemoglobinuria

AUTOIMMUNE HAEMOLYTIC ANAEMIA

Investigation of suspected haemolysis
1 Aetiological clues on blood film:
   a) Spherocytes (autoimmune haemolysis, hereditary spherocytosis)
   b) Schistocytes, helmet cells (microangiopathic haemolysis)
   c) Sickled cells
2 Signs of marrow compensation:
   a) Polychromatophilic macrocytes
   b) Reticulocytosis ('warm' > 'cold' haemolysis)
   c) Occasional nucleated red cells
3 Confirmation of red cell lysis:
   a) Mild unconjugated (direct) hyperbilirubinaemia
   b) Urinalysis: urobilinogen +, bilirubin −
   c) ↓ Haptoglobin (NB: false-negatives in acute phase reactions, false-positives in liver disease)
   d) ↓ Haemopexin
   e) ↓ Folate (secondary, esp. in pregnancy)
4 Confirmation of marrow compensation — erythroid hyperplasia
5 Signs of intravascular haemolysis
   a) Haemoglobinaemia/-uria (→ pink serum; cf. myoglobinuria)
   b) Haemosiderinuria (implies chronicity; ± coexisting iron deficiency)
   c) Methaemalbuminaemia (Schumm's test) — implies severe haemolysis
6 Further aetiological investigations
   a) Coombs' and Ham's tests
   b) Cold agglutinins, Donath-Landsteiner antibody
   c) Hb EPG; Heinz body prep; RBC G6PD levels
   d) ^{51}Cr-RBC survival and sequestration study

Coombs tests: what do they do?
1 Direct Coombs antiglobulin test (DAT)
   a) Used to investigate *haemolysis*
   b) i.e. Do the **patient's red cells** have antibody/C3 on them?
2 Indirect Coombs antiglobulin test (IAT)
   a) Used in blood *crossmatching*
   b) i.e. Does the intended **recipient's serum** contain antibodies to the planned red cell transfusion?

Autoimmune haemolysis: diagnostic aspects
1 'Warm' type
   a) IgG-mediated extravascular (intrasplenic) haemolysis — +DAT, +IgG
   b) Progressive anaemia, mild jaundice, splenomegaly
   c) Blood film — spherocytes, marked reticulocytosis
   d) Frequently arises secondary to SLE, CLL, Hodgkin's, drugs
   e) Often responds to steroids/azathioprine or splenectomy
   f) Transfusion may be lifesaving
2 'Cold' type
   a) IgM-κ-mediated intravascular (intrahepatic) haemolysis — +DAT, +C$_3$

   b) Autoagglutination on blood film
   c) Occurrence of symptoms depends on *height of thermal amplitude* rather than absolute titre
   d) May herald development of lymphoma, macroglobulinaemia, infection
   e) Treatment is best directed at the underlying condition
   f) Transfusion should be avoided if possible; if absolutely necessary, warm blood and transfuse slowly

Features of drug-induced autoimmune haemolysis
1 'Methyldopa' (autoimmune) type
   a) → Mild (rarely significant) extravascular haemolysis
   b) +DAT, +IAT (i.e. Coombs+ without drug present), -C3
   c) May remain Coombs + for *years* after drug ceased
2 'Penicillin' (hapten) type
   a) IgG directed against drug (a hapten) which adsorbs to red cell following prolonged high-dose treatment
   b) → Extravascular haemolysis
   c) +DAT, −IAT (i.e. Coombs+ only in presence of drug)
3 'Quinine' (immune complex) type
   a) → Immediate intravascular haemolysis on second or subsequent exposure (so-called 'innocent bystander' mechanism)
   b) IgM-(or IgG) mediated complement activation
   c) Drug-antibody complex dissociates from red cells leaving only C$_3$
   d) +DAT, +C$_3$

OTHER ANAEMIAS

Significance of abnormal reticulocyte counts in anaemia
1 Reticulocytosis
   a) Blood loss/haemorrhage (up to 15% reticulocytes)
   b) Haemolysis (up to 30%)
   c) Response phase of iron/B$_{12}$/folate deficiency (up to 50%)
2 Reticulocytopenia
   a) Aplastic anaemia
   b) Chronic disease, e.g. uraemia

Hypersplenism: diagnostic criteria
1 Cytopenia
2 Splenomegaly
3 Marrow hypercellularity
4 Cytopenia abolished by splenectomy

Anaemia of chronic disease: laboratory features
1 Normocytic ± hypochromic; normal RDW Reticulocytopenia
2 Iron studies — ↓ Fe/TIBC/TF saturation; ↑ ferritin
3 ↓ Red cell survival
    ↓ Erythropoietin activity
    ↑ Red cell protoporphyrin
4 Bone marrow
   a) Absent sideroblasts (RBC precursors)
   b) ↑ Iron stores

Diagnosis of hereditary spherocytosis
1 Family history (in 80%)
2 Clinical picture
  a) Recurrent mild jaundice of unconjugated type
    $(DD_x$ = Gilbert's)
  b) ± Splenomegaly, anaemia, gallstones
3 *Numerous* microspherocytes on blood film
  Negative Coombs test
4 ↑ MCHC (35–38 g%); normal MCV
5 Increased RBC osmotic fragility (high-salt lysis)
  Positive autohaemolysis test, correcting with
  glucose (cf. 'immune' spherocytosis)
6 Reduced $_{51}$Cr-RBC survival; sequestered in spleen

Causes of a grossly abnormal ESR
1 >100 mm/h
  a) Myeloma
  b) Carcinomatosis, esp. active Hodgkin's
  c) Sepsis, esp. florid TB
  d) Active vasculitis, esp. giant-cell
  e) Uraemia
  f) Profound anaemia
2 <3 mm/h (NB: 95% of these will be *normal*)
  a) Polycythaemia rubra vera
  b) Sickle cell anaemia
  c) Massive leucocytosis (e.g. in CLL)
  d) Hypofibrinogenaemia (hereditary or DIC-induced)
  e) High-dose steroids or salicylates

NORMAL AND ABNORMAL HAEMOGLOBINS

Factors improving tissue oxygenation by red blood cells (i.e. reducing Hb affinity for oxygen; right shift of dissociation curve)
1 Acidosis, hypercapnia (via Bohr effect)
2 Hypoxia, anaemia
  Thyrotoxicosis   — via increased red cell
  Pregnancy   2,3-DPG
  Renal failure
3 Increased blood temperature
4 Low-affinity Hb (see below)

Diagnostic value of haemoglobin electrophoresis
1 Hb S (sickle cell)
2 HbA_2 (elevated in β-thal trait, esp.)
3 Hb C, D, E

Haemoglobins with abnormal oxygen affinity: clinical significance
1 High-affinity haemoglobins
  a) e.g. Hb Yakima, Hb Chesapeake, Hb Rainier, Hb Köln
  b) Usually asymptomatic with benign course
  c) Often detected as unexpected polycythaemia on routine testing
2 Low-affinity haemoglobins
  a) e.g. Hb Kansas, Hb Seattle, Hb Hammersmith
  b) Presents as congenital cyanosis
  c) Differential diagnosis: genetic methaemoglobinaemia ('Hb M')
3 Unstable haemoglobins
  a) 'Heinz-body anaemias'
  b) Respond to splenectomy

HAEMATOLOGICAL MALIGNANCIES

Diagnostic priorities in bone marrow examination
1 Aspiration more important
  a) Acute leukaemias
    Chronic granulocytic leukaemia (for chromosomal studies)
    Myelodysplastic syndromes
  b) Megaloblastosis
    Sideroblastosis
  c) Thrombocytopenia
    Leucopenia
2 Trephine more important
  a) Non-contributory aspirate — 'dry' or 'blood' tap,
    e.g.: Myelofibrosis
           Hairy cell leukaemia
           Metastatic carcinoma
           Aplastic anaemia
  b) Chronic lymphocytic leukaemia

Laboratory features of myelodysplastic syndromes
1 Film
  a) Hypersegmented neutrophils, *or*
  b) Hyposegmented neutrophils (Pelger-Huet-like anomalies)
2 NAP score — low
3 Hb electrophoresis — increased HbF (often)
4 Marrow
  a) Hypercellular
  b) Scarcity of mature forms
  c) Slight excess of blasts

Common cytogenetic aberrations in haematological malignancies
1 Ph^1 (= reciprocal 9 : 22 translocation of *c-abl* oncogene)
2 Blastic transformation of CGL
  a) Ph^2 (i.e. second Philadelphia chromosome)
  b) Aneuploidy
  c) Trisomy 8, isochromosome 17
3 8:14 translocation (of *c-myc* — lymphomas, esp. Burkitt's)
4 15:17 translocation — acute promyelocytic leukaemia
5 5q- — refractory anaemia
6 Deletions of 5 and/or 7 — iatrogenic leukaemia

MULTIPLE MYELOMA

Minimal diagnostic criteria
1 Marrow aspirate suggestive of myeloma using combined quantitative, morphological and immunofluorescent data
2 Demonstration of multiple lesions (e.g. by repeated aspirations, skeletal survey, bone scan)

NB: Although in the vast majority of cases the diagnosis will be *supported* by the demonstration of a serum and/or urine paraprotein, such a finding is not sufficient for diagnosis; given the occurrence of non-secretory myeloma, it is not even strictly necessary. Also, development of amyloidosis may be accompanied by paraproteinaemia

Independent prognostic variables
1 Presence of renal impairment
2 Response to therapy

INVESTIGATING MYELOPROLIFERATIVE DISEASE

Thrombocytosis: factors favouring myeloproliferative disease
1 Splenomegaly
2 Platelet count $>1000 \times 10^9/l$
3 Giant platelets on film
4 Abnormal platelet aggregation studies; prolonged bleeding time
5 Associated basophilia, neutrophilia; high NAP score, B_{12} and urate
6 Complicated by haemorrhage and/or thrombosis (note that splenic vein thrombosis may manifest as a sudden further increment in platelet count)

Laboratory features suggestive of polycythaemia vera
1 Coexisting leucocytosis and/or thrombocytosis
2 HbO_2 saturation $>92\%$
3 ↑ NAP score
4 ↑ B_{12}

CHRONIC GRANULOCYTIC LEUKAEMIA

Diagnosis of chronic granulocytic leukaemia
1 Clinical
   a) Splenomegaly ± pain/rub (infarct)
   b) Haemorrhagic or thrombotic phenomena, e.g. priapism
   c) No increased propensity to infection (normal leucocyte function)
2 Blood film
   a) WCC often $>100 \times 10^9/l$
   b) Predominant cells — neutrophils and myelocytes
   c) Left shift
   d) Basophilia (± eosinophilia)
   e) Normochromic anaemia ± thrombocytosis
3 Low NAP score (often zero)
   ↑ B_{12} (↑ TC-I), ↑ urate
4 Bone marrow
   a) < 10% myeloblasts (cf. blastic transformation)
   b) M:E ratio > 10:1 (usually)
   c) Rarely: Gaucher cells, sea-blue histiocytes
5 Philadelphia chromosome ($\rightarrow$>90%)
   a) Generally unaffected by cytotoxic therapy (i.e. persists despite treatment and morphological 'remission')
   b) Constitutes primary rationale for performing marrow examination

Signs of acute transformation
1 Refractoriness to busulphan →
   ↑ WCC/platelets/splenomegaly
2 Lymphadenopathy, fever, bone pain
3 Rising NAP score
4 Appearance of circulating TdT+ or cALLA+ blasts (in 30%; implies lymphoblastic transformation, better short-term prognosis)

5 Bone marrow
   a) >10% blasts
   b) New cytogenetic aberrations (see p. 136)

Differential diagnosis of normal or high NAP score in CGL
1 Partial remission
2 Intercurrent infection (or other stress)
3 Pregnancy
4 Development of myelofibrosis
5 Blastic transformation
6 Leukaemoid reaction (i.e. misdiagnosis)

Characteristics of Philadelphia chromosome-negative CGL
1 Younger onset (< 5 years old — 'juvenile' CGL)
2 Smaller spleen
3 Lower WCC
4 Higher lysozyme and HbF
5 Poorer prognosis

CHRONIC LYMPHOCYTIC LEUKAEMIA (CLL)

Significance of anaemia in CLL
1 Marrow suppression ('chronic disease') in 95%
2 Haemolysis (5%)
3 Hypersplenism (rare)

Immunological considerations in CLL
1 50% of patients have hypogammaglobulinaemia (esp. ↓ IgM) with consequent impairment of humoral immunity
2 Cell-mediated immunity is (also) usually impaired The CD4:CD8 (helper:suppressor) ratio may be inverted
3 Administration of i.v. gammaglobulin to hypogammaglobulinaemic CLL patients appears effective in reducing the incidence of bacterial infections (see ref. 5.10). Steroid therapy increases the risk of infectious complications
4 Hypogammaglobulinaemia may also respond to chemotherapy
5 5% of patients will be found to have a paraprotein; 5–10% will have a positive direct antiglobulin (Coombs) test
6 Less than 5% will have significant haemolysis/thrombocytopenia Occurrence of thrombocytopenia usually indicates marrow failure

OTHER LEUKAEMIAS

Clinicopathologic hallmarks of selected leukaemic subtypes
1 Acute promyelocytic leukaemia (M3)
   a) Clinical — DIC (± cerebral haemorrhage)
   b) Film — Auer rods (see below)
   c) t(15:17) chromosomal translocation
2 Acute (myelo)monocytic leukaemia (M4, M5)
   a) Extramedullary disease:
      — Gingival hyperplasia
      — CNS involvement
   b) Lysozymuria; hypokalaemia

3 B-cell (Burkitt's-type) leukaemia (L3)
   a) t(14:18) translocation (i.e. same as Burkitt's lymphoma)
   b) Poor prognosis
4 T-cell leukaemia/lymphoma:♂>♀
   a) Mediastinal mass
   b) Poor prognosis
5 Prolymphocytic leukaemia (PLL): ♂>♀
   a) Massive splenomegaly
   b) Absent lymphadenopathy
   c) Marked anaemia and leucocytosis
6 Chronic lymphocytic leukaemia: ♂>♀
   a) 'Smudge' cells and/or 'basket' cells on film
   b) Degree of peripheral lymphocytosis may be the only distinction between CLL and well-differentiated lymphocytic lymphoma
   c) May transform to PLL or diffuse lymphoma
7 Hairy cell leukaemia: ♂>♀
   a) Massive splenomegaly (DD$_x$: CGL, myelofibrosis)
   b) Thrombocytopenia (mainly due to hypersplenism)
   c) Anaemia/leucopenia (mainly due to marrow fibrosis/failure)

Laboratory characterization of leukaemias and lymphomas
1 Light microscopy
   a) Auer rods (visible within circulating blasts) — AML (esp. M3)
   b) Reed-Sternberg cells — Hodgkin's disease
   c) Pautrier microabscesses — mycosis fungoides
2 Electron microscopy
   a) Cerebriform nuclei — Sézary syndrome
   b) May distinguish diffuse lymphoma from undifferentiated carcinoma
3 Monoclonal antibodies
   a) Anti-CALLA (defines good-prognosis ALL subtype)
   b) OKT4, Leu 3a (defines helper T-cell phenotype): Sézary syndrome
   c) Anti-light chain (κ, λ) antibodies — may define monoclonality (and thereby malignant nature) of lymphocytes within effusions or CSF, or plasma cells within marrow
4 Cytochemistry
   a) PAS — ALL
   b) Peroxidase/Sudan black — AML
   c) TdT
      — ALL (except rare B-cell subtype)
      — Lymphoblastic transformation of CGL
   d) Acid phosphatase
      — T-cell ALL
      — Hairy cell leukaemia
5 Lysozyme — (myelo)monocytic leukaemia
6 Cytogenetics

LEUKAEMIAS: CLASSIFICATION, STAGING AND PROGNOSIS

Acute non-lymphocytic leukaemia: the FAB classification
1 M1 — acute myeloblastic leukaemia, undifferentiated (common)
2 M2 — acute myeloblastic leukaemia with maturation (common)
3 M3 — acute promyelocytic leukaemia
4 M4 — acute myelomonocytic leukaemia (common)
5 M5 — acute monocytic leukaemia
6 M6 — erythroleukaemia

Poor prognostic signs in acute lymphoblastic leukaemia
1 Adult onset
2 Male sex
   a) Associated with T-cell leukaemia and mediastinal mass
   b) Increased testicular relapse
3 cALLA negative (T-cell, B-cell, null-cell)
4 Presentation with
   a) Initial WCC >100 × 10^9/l
   b) Massive extramedullary disease
   c) CNS leukaemia
5 Philadelphia chromosome-positive (cf. CGL: *better* prognosis)

CLL staging: modified Rai criteria
1 Stage 1 — lymphocytosis only (>15 × 10^9/l; >40% in marrow)
2 Stage 2 — lymphocytosis + lymphadenopathy
3 Stage 3 — lymphocytosis + hepato/splenomegaly
4 Stage 4 — lymphocytosis + anaemia/thrombocytopenia

Life expectancy from diagnosis in CLL
1 Stage 1 disease — 15 years
2 Stage 2 disease — 9 years
3 Stage 3 disease — 6 years
4 Stage 4 disease — 1–2 years

LYMPHOMAS

Arguments in favour of staging laparotomy in Hodgkin's disease
1 Remains the only way of accurately detecting splenic involvement and, hence, of determining need for chemotherapy in some cases
2 Detects unsuspected disease in liver (large core biopsy obtained) and abdominal lymph nodes
3 Improves WBC and platelet counts (occasionally) following splenectomy, thus improving treatment tolerance
4 Reduces morbidity of radiotherapy by obviating need for splenic irradiation, thus preventing irradiation of left kidney, left lung base, and cardiac apex
5 Enables preservation of fertility in young women requiring pelvic irradiation (since oöphoropexy can be performed at laparotomy)

Hodgkin's disease and the spleen: the facts
1 Absence of splenomegaly does not imply lack of splenic disease
2 Splenomegaly does not necessarily imply splenic involvement
3 20% of patients with clinical stage II disease (i.e. including normal abdominal CT) will be found to have abdominal disease if staging laparotomy undertaken

4 Nonetheless, many oncologists now choose to forego staging laparotomy in stage IA/IIA patients (esp. those with lymphocyte predominant disease), treating instead with radiotherapy and following closely for relapse outside the irradiated field

Staging of Hodgkin's disease: simplified Ann Arbor criteria
1 Stage 1 — involvement of a single lymph node region
2 Stage 2 — involvement of more than one lymph node region on the same side of the diaphragm
3 Stage 3 — involvement of nodes on both sides of the diaphragm
4 Stage 4 — extranodal disease
5 'A' = asymptomatic
6 'B' = fevers > 38°C; sweats; >10% weight loss in last 6 months

Non-Hodgkin's lymphomas: modified Kiel histological subtypes
1 Indolent
   a) Follicular (nodular)
      — Centrocytic
      — Centroblastic
   b) Diffuse small-cell
      — Lymphocytic (WDLL, CLL-like)
      — Centrocytic
      — Immunocytic (lymphoplasmacytoid)
2 Aggressive — diffuse large cell
   a) Lymphoblastic (T-cell or Burkitt-type)
   b) Centroblastic
   c) Immunoblastic

Assessing prognosis in lymphoma
1 Hodgkin's disease — prognosis (treated or untreated) determined by disease *stage*,* e.g.
   a) Stage IA/IIA disease → 90% cure
   b) Stage IIIB/IV disease → 30% cure
2 Non-Hodgkin's lymphoma — prognosis (untreated) mainly determined by disease *histology,* e.g.
   a) Indolent histology → median survival 5 years
   b) Aggressive histology → median survival 12 months
   c) Paradoxically, however, chemocurability is greatest in those tumours with more aggressive (diffuse large-cell) histology

HYPERCOAGULABLE STATES

Indications for investigation of hypercoagulability
1 Family history of venous thrombosis
2 Recurrent venous thrombosis or pulmonary embolism
3 Single episode of venous thrombosis in a young patient
4 Unusual site of thrombosis
   a) Retinal vein thrombosis
   b) Renal vein thrombosis
   c) Hepatic vein thrombosis
   d) Arterial thrombosis

---

*Note that *older* patients with Hodgkin's disease have a markedly worse prognosis than do *young* patients with the same disease stage

Laboratory characterization of suspected hypercoagulability
1 Exclude hyperviscosity
   a) Hb/PCV (polycythaemia), platelets (thrombocytosis)
   b) Paraproteinaemia
   c) Whole blood viscosity
2 Exclude defective fibrinolysis
   a) FDPs, hypofibrinogenaemia (DIC), schistocytes (TTP, DIC)
   b) Euglobulin clot lysis time (tPA deficiency/inhibitor)
   c) Factor XII deficiency
   d) Abnormal fibrinogen or plasminogen
3 Exclude primary deficiency of endogenous anticoagulation
   a) Antithrombin III
   b) Protein C; protein S
   c) Heparin cofactor II
4 Acquired inducers of hypercoagulability
   a) Lupus anticoagulant
   b) Acid haemolysis test (PNH)
   c) Fibrin monomers/fibrinopeptide A (malignancy)

Antithrombin III deficiency: causes
1 Hereditary
2 Oestrogens— (pregnancy, OCs, Ca prostate)
3 Liver disease
4 Nephrotic syndrome
5 Disseminated thrombosis (since heparin acts via AT-III, massive thrombosis may be associated with relative heparin resistance)
6 Heparin therapy

HAEMOSTATIC DISORDERS

Investigation of thrombocytopenia
1 Check automated count by direct vision to exclude spurious result due to sample clotting
2 Film
   a) Schistocytes (DIC, TTP)
   b) Blasts (acute leukaemia)
3 Coagulation screen — helps further exclude DIC
4 Marrow aspirate
   a) Hypoplastic aetiology
   b) Abundant megakaryocytes — ITP, hypersplenism

Prolonged PT, APTT and thrombocytopenia: causes
1 Disseminated intravascular coagulation
2 Liver disease with hypersplenism
3 Heparin therapy

Platelet function tests: clinical correlations
1 von Willebrand's disease
   a) Normal aggregation *in vitro*
   b) Defective ristocetin aggregation }—Corrected by addition of normal plasma
   c) Defective endothelial adhesion
2 Glanzmann's thrombasthenia
   a) Defective aggregation *in vitro* (i.e. to ADP, adrenaline, collagen)

b) Normal ristocetin aggregation
c) Normal endothelial adhesion
3 Bernard-Soulier (giant platelet) syndrome
  a) Normal aggregation
     in vitro
  b) Defective ristocetin
     aggregation   —Not corrected by
  c) Defective endothelial   addition of normal
     adhesion   plasma
  d) Thrombocytopenia
  e) Glycoprotein 1B
     deficiency
4 Aspirin ingestion — defective aggregation in vitro
  (impaired release reaction to ADP)
5 Dysproteinaemia
  Myeloproliferative
  disease   —Defective aggregation
  Uraemia, liver disease   and adhesion

Haemophilia A: levels of severity

1 >50% F VIII_c — normal haemostasis
2 20–40% F VIII_c — excess bleeding after major trauma
3 5–20% F VIII_c — excess bleeding after surgery or minor trauma
4 2–5% F VIII_c — moderate haemophilia; severe post-traumatic and occasional spontaneous bleeding
5 <2% F VIII_c — severe haemophilia; frequent spontaneous bleeds into muscles and joints

Diagnosis of haemophilia

1 Low F VIII_c
2 Normal or increased F VIII_{Ag}
3 Normal F VIII_{VWF} (cf. von Willebrand's disease — low)
4 Normal bleeding time
5 Carrier status? $VIII_c:VIII_{Ag}$ <70%

THE PORPHYRIAS

The acute porphyrias: what do they have in common?
(acute intermittent porphyria; variegate porphyria; hereditary coproporphyria)
1 All three are autosomal dominant
2 All three are frequently precipitated by drugs
3 All three are potentially life-threatening

Rational approach to investigation of suspected acute porphyria

1 Urinary PBG absent   }—Excludes acute
                                  presentation
2 Urinary PBG absent   }—Excludes both acute and
  Faecal screen negative   latent porphyria
3 Urinary PBG present   }—Acute intermittent
  Faecal screen negative   porphyria (in acute or
                                  latent phase)
4 Urinary PBG present   }—Variegate porphyria in
  Faecal screen positive   acute phase
5 Urinary PBG absent   }—Variegate porphyria in
  Faecal screen positive   latent phase

(NB: urinary PBG and/or ALA are the hallmarks of porphyria-induced neurological disease)

Investigation of suspected porphyria-induced photosensitivity

1 Urinary PBG absent
  Red cell screen negative}—Excludes porphyric
  Faecal screen negative   aetiology
2 Urinary PBG present   }—Variegate porphyria
  Faecal screen positive
3 Urinary PBG absent
  Red cell screen negative}—Porphyria cutanea tarda
  Faecal screen positive   Variegate porphyria
4 Urinary PBG absent
  Red cell screen positive}—Erythropoietic
  Faecal screen negative   coproporphyria
5 Urinary PBG absent
  Red cell screen positive}—Erythropoietic
  Faecal screen positive   uroporphyria
                             Erythropoietic
                             protoporphyria

'Safe' drugs in patients with porphyria
1 Aspirin, paracetamol, codeine
2 Penicillin; low-dose chloroquine*
3 Chlorpromazine, metoclopramide; sodium valproate
4 Propranolol, labetalol; digoxin
5 Insulin

MANAGING HAEMATOLOGICAL DISEASE

PRINCIPLES OF CELL SUPPORT

The leucopenic patient: principles of management
1 Assume any fever is infective in origin until proven otherwise
2 Take urine and blood cultures if febrile
3 If prolonged leucopenia anticipated, perform
  a) Baseline HSV/CMV/toxoplasma titres
  b) Regular swabs of throat/axillae/nose/perineum
  c) Removal of IUD
4 Clinically monitor chest and perineum for sepsis
5 Avoid pelvic examinations unless indispensable

Granulocyte transfusions
1 Prophylaxis — not indicated
2 Sole potential indication — fever persisting >48 hour in a severely neutropenic patient (<500 cells/μl) receiving optimal antimicrobial therapy, esp. if
  a) Positive blood cultures, esp. *Ps. aeruginosa*
  b) Imminent (<1 week) marrow recovery considered unlikely
3 Problems
  a) Questionable benefit
  b) Expense
  c) Poor leucocyte function if obtained by filtration rather than centrifugation
  d) Transfusion reactions
  e) Sensitization, e.g. preventing increments to transfused platelets (alloimmunization)
  f) Possible transmission of CMV
  g) Development of pulmonary infiltrates (intravascular leucostasis)

* NB: *high-dose* chloroquine may precipitate porphyria cutanea tarda, whereas low-dose is therapeutic

h) Risk of graft-versus-host disease if cells not irradiated prior to transfusion

NB: Granulocyte transfusion appears to be less important than prompt prescription of broad-spectrum antibiotics

Massive stored blood transfusions: morbidity

1 Hepatitis (non-A non-B, hepatitis B, CMV); AIDS (HIV)
2 Coagulopathy (low in factors V, VIII and platelets)
3 Citrate toxicity → metabolic alkalosis with hypocalcaemia (usually subclinical)
4 Low 2,3-DPG → tissue hypoxia (reversible after 24 hours)
5 Hyperkalaemia and/or metabolic acidosis (low pH of stored blood), esp. if coexisting renal impairment impairment
6 Fever, fluid overload, haemolysis, DIC

Therapeutic indications for quantitative phlebotomy

1 Polycythaemia rubra vera
2 Idiopathic haemochromatosis
  Sideroblastosis with iron overload
3 Porphyria cutanea tarda
4 Polycythaemia (Hb >20.0 g/dl) secondary to chronic lung disease or cyanotic congenital heart disease; aim to keep haematocrit at 65% (controversial)

SPLENECTOMY

Splenectomy: common indications in haematological disease

1 Hereditary spherocytosis
2 Chronic ITP
3 Hairy cell leukaemia
4 Occasional indications
  a) Hodgkin's disease (staging lap)
  b) Idiopathic 'warm' autoimmune haemolytic anaemia
  c) Massive enlargement: pain, hypersplenism (e.g. in myelofibrosis or thalassemia)

Management of the splenectomy patient

1 Patient selection — *avoid* splenectomy if possible in children, esp. if age <5 years (this age group is at greatest risk of subsequent life-threatening sepsis with encapsulated micro-organisms)
2 Children requiring splenectomy — prophylactic oral penicillin V until adulthood
3 All patients — pneumococcal vaccination

AUTOIMMUNE HAEMOLYTIC ANAEMIA

Management of warm autoimmune haemolytic anaemia

1 Exclude drug-induced cause
2 Exclude B-cell malignancy (bone marrow, EPG)
3 Treat underlying autoimmune disease if present
4 *Avoid* transfusion if possible
5 Trial of medical therapy

a) Steroids (prednisolone 60 mg/day)
b) Folate 5 mg/day
c) ± Azathioprine
5 Consider splenectomy if
  a) Steroids ineffective or unacceptable
  b) DAT → IgG only (no C_3)
  c) ^{51}Cr-RBC studies confirm spleen as site of sequestration
6 Investigational therapy
  a) Danazol
  b) High-dose intravenous IgG
  c) Cyclosporin A

Management of cold autoimmune haemolytic anaemia

1 Keep patient warm
2 Exclude *Mycoplasma pneumoniae,* infectious mononucleosis
3 Exclude B-cell malignancy
4 Avoid steroids and splenectomy (they generally don't work)
5 If transfusion absolutely necessary
  a) Use packed cells (less complement than whole blood); washed packed cells are ideal
  b) Infuse via blood warmer (or at least get the blood up to room temperature)
6 Investigational therapy
  a) High-dose i.v. methylprednisolone
  b) Plasmapheresis/plasma exchange

MANAGING HAEMATOLOGICAL MALIGNANCIES

Treatment options in acute lymphoblastic leukaemia

1 Induction/consolidation (95% → complete remission)
  a) Vincristine/prednisone
  b) L-Asparaginase, daunorubicin
  c) Cytosine arabinoside
2 Maintenance (50% → cure) — methotrexate/6-MP
3 Routine CNS prophylaxis*
  a) Cranial irradiation
  b) Intrathecal methotrexate
4 Marrow transplant
  a) In second remission
  b) In first remission if poor prognosis ALL

Treatment options in acute myeloblastic (non-lymphocytic) leukaemia

1 Induction/consolidation (70% → complete remission) — cytosine arabinoside, plus daunorubicin, ± 6TG (thioguanine) or VP-16
2 Marrow transplant — in first remission
3 Promyelocytic leukaemia (M3) — pre-cytotoxic heparinization
4 Maintenance chemotherapy, late intensification, and CNS prophylaxis are all of doubtful value in AML

Therapeutic approach to chronic lymphocytic leukaemia (CLL)

1 Stage I/II disease — usually observe

---

*NB: Some centres also advocate prophylactic testicular irradiation, while others monitor this potential sanctuary site for relapse by regular testicular biopsy

2 Stage III/IV disease — chlorambucil ±. vincristine/prednisone (CVP)
3 Immune haemolysis/thrombocytopenia — steroids
4 Recurrent infections — gammaglobulin (i.v.)

Specific indications for cytotoxic therapy in CLL
1 Symptomatic lymphadenopathy
2 Refractory constitutional symptoms
3 Non-immune cytopenia

Therapeutic approach to chronic granulocytic leukaemia (CGL)
1 Chronic phase
   a) Busulphan (intermittent), hydroxyurea (daily)
   b) Bone marrow transplantation
2 Myeloblastic transformation (75%) — no effective treatment known
3 Lymphoblastic transformation (25%) — vincristine/prednisone

Management modalities in hairy cell leukaemia
1 Splenectomy (improves pancytopenia, may improve survival)
2 α-Interferon
3 Deoxycoformycin
4 ± Chlorambucil, leucapheresis

Managing polycythaemia vera
1 Mild disease
  Young patient } — Phlebotomy
  Preoperative
2 Thrombocytosis — ^{32}P, chlorambucil

Managing the dysproteinaemias
1 Myeloma
   a) Melphalan ± prednisone; cyclophosphamide; doxorubicin/BCNU/vincristine
   b) Apheresis for hyperviscosity
   c) Prophylactic long bone internal fixation as required
2 Macroglobulinaemia
   a) Chlorambucil, CVP
   b) Plasmapheresis

Management options in cutaneous lymphoma*
1 Topical nitrogen mustard
2 Electron beam therapy
3 PUVA
4 Oral steroids
5 Combination cytotoxic therapy
6 Cyclosporin A; interferon-α

Approach to the management of non-Hodgkin's lymphomas
1 General — treatment determined more by histological subtype than by stage
2 Low-grade (indolent, usually nodular)
   a) CVP and/or local irradiation
   b) Treated with palliative intent
3 High-grade (aggressive, usually diffuse)
   a) CVP + doxorubicin (CHOP)

*None is regularly effective

   b) Treated with curative intent
4 Lymphoblastic lymphoma — treated as for T-cell ALL (incl. CNS prophylaxis)
5 Refractory end-stage disease — total body irradiation (purely palliative)

Approach to the management of Hodgkin's disease
1 General — treatment determined more by *stage* than by histological subtype
2 Clinical stage IA/IIA — ?staging laparotomy (see p. 138)
3 Pathological stage IA — local irradiation
   Pathological stage IIA (above diaphragm) — 'mantle' irradiation (supradiaphragmatic/upper paraaortic nodes)
   Pathological stage IIA (below diaphragm) — 'inverted Y' (all paraaortic, iliac and pelvic nodes)
4 Pathological stage III or IV
   Bulky disease (irrespective of stage)   } —Combination chemotherapy, e.g. MOPP, ABVD
   'B' symptoms (irrespective of stage)
   'E' (extranodal) disease

Toxicity of therapy for Hodgkin's disease
1 Induced by radiotherapy (e.g. mantle)
   a) Hypothyroidism
   b) Lhermitte's phenomenon (radiation myelitis)
   c) Radiation pneumonitis/pericarditis
   d) Reduced haemopoietic reserve
2 Induced by chemotherapy (e.g. MOPP)
   a) 25% chemoresistance — esp.
      — 'B' symptoms
      — Nodular sclerosing histology (frequent relapses)
   b) Sterility (esp. in males)
   c) Second malignancies (esp. if prior radiation)

Tumour lysis syndrome: features and clinical significance
1 Typically occurs within days of initial chemotherapy for sensitive tumours, esp.
   a) Burkitt's lymphoma
   b) ALL
   c) Germ-cell tumours
2 Metabolic effects
   a) Hyperuricaemia ± urate nephropathy
   b) Hyperphosphataemia ± reciprocal hypocalcaemia
   c) Hyperkalaemia (esp. if azotaemic or acidotic)
3 Complications
   a) Renal failure (typically irreversible; may be fatal)
   b) Arrhythmias, cardiac arrest (due to hyperkalaemia)
   c) Tetany, weakness, paralytic ileus (hypocalcaemia)
   d) Severe metabolic acidosis
4 Prevention
   a) Pretreatment allopurinol
   b) Forced alkaline diuresis
5 Treatment of established syndrome — haemodialysis

BONE MARROW TRANSPLANTATION

Indications for bone marrow transplantation
1 Established indications
  a) Aplastic anaemia (preferably untransfused)
  b) ALL (good prognosis) in second remission
  c) ALL (poor prognosis) or AML in first remission
  d) CGL in chronic phase
  e) Severe combined immunodeficiency (SCID)
2 Occasional indications
  a) Refractory lymphoma
  b) Neuroblastoma
  c) β-thalassaemia major
  d) Osteopetrosis
  e) Hurler's syndrome
  f) Chronic granulomatous disease
  g) Wiskott-Aldrich syndrome
  h) Paroxysmal nocturnal dyspnoea (severe)

Prerequisites for marrow transplantation
1 HLA- and MLC-compatible sibling
2 Recipient's age less than 40 years (preferably less than 20)

Complications of bone marrow transplantation
1 High-dose cyclophosphamide
  a) Cystitis
  b) Cardiomyopathy
2 Total body irradiation
  a) Pancreatitis
  b) Pneumonitis
  c) Parotitis
  d) Hepatic veno-occlusive disease
  e) Cataracts
3 Combined toxicity — sterility
4 Other
  a) Infection
  b) Disease relapse
  c) Graft failure
  d) Graft-versus-host disease

Graft-versus-host disease (GVHD): presentation and management
1 Acute GVHD (mediated by cytotoxic T-cells)
  a) Dermatitis (bullous, scarlatiniform, morbilliform)
  b) Hepatitis; abnormal LFTs →→ liver failure
  c) Enterocolitis → diarrhoea
2 Chronic GVHD
  a) Dermatitis (sclerodermatous, lichen planus-like)
  b) Conjunctivitis, stomatitis, oesophagitis
  c) Wasting, recurrent infections (bacterial, zoster)
  These affect 30% of long-term survivors, esp. if older
3 Interstitial pneumonitis is also a major hazard to survival in the post-transplant period, but appears to be caused by CMV or radiation rather than GVHD
4 Patients who have survived an episode of graft-versus-host disease have a significantly lower risk of leukaemic relapse, suggesting that GVHD exerts an antileukaemic effect
5 Prophylaxis
  a) Cyclosporin A (agent of choice in aplastic anaemia)
  b) ± Methotrexate
  c) ± Autologous marrow purging with anti-T-cell (OKT3) monoclonal antibodies
6 Established disease
  a) Symptomatic treatment
  b) Steroids, azathioprine

Differential diagnosis of CXR infiltrates in bone marrow transplants
1 CMV pneumonia
2 GVHD
3 Radiation pneumonitis

THROMBOCYTOPENIA

Points to remember in managing the thrombocytopenic patient
1 Precautions on the ward
  a) No aspirin
  b) No intramuscular injections
  c) No routine blood pressure measurements
2 Precautions at the bedside
  a) Inspect skin and oral mucosa daily
  b) Examine fundi daily
  c) Remove IUD if prolonged thrombocytopenia anticipated
3 Precautions in the laboratory — check coagulation screen (esp. to exclude DIC)

Predictors of response to splenectomy for ITP
1 Age <60 years
2 Short history of ITP (i.e. not chronic)
3 Initial promising response to steroids
4 Postoperative platelet count $>500 \times 10^9$/L

Failed splenectomy for ITP?
1 Look at the blood film; absence of Howell-Jolly bodies suggests presence of an accessory spleen
2 Short-term control measures
  a) Intravenous gammaglobulin (esp. if recent onset of ITP)
  b) Vincristine or vinblastine
  c) Plasmapheresis
3 Long-term control measures
  a) Cyclophosphamide
  b) Azathioprine
4 Experimental control measures
  a) Colchicine
  b) Danazol

Post-transfusion (thrombocytopenic) purpura
1 Occurs in susceptible 2–3% of population lacking Pl^{A1} antigen
2 Prior sensitization required (e.g. transfusion, pregnancy)
3 Most commonly occurs in older women 2–10 days post-transfusion
4 Widespread purpura and mucosal bleeding — 10% mortality
5 Diagnosis may be confirmed by direct detection of anti-Pl^{A1}
6 Management:

a) Pl^{A1}-negative transfusions
b) High-dose i.v. IgG
c) Steroids, plasmapheresis if necessary

Features of heparin-associated thrombocytopenia
1 General
   a) Overall incidence is about 1%
   b) Incidence is not dose-dependent
2 Early-onset type
   a) Occurs within one week of heparin commencement
   b) Rarely associated with bleeding
   c) May resolve with continued heparin therapy
3 Late-onset type
   a) Typically occurs 1–4 weeks after heparin commencement
   b) More severe thrombocytopenia which may cause bleeding
   c) Major complication is paradoxical thromboembolism in 40%
   d) Mediated by heparin-induced IgG → platelet aggregation
   e) Diagnosed by platelet aggregometry studies
   f) Treatment — cease heparin and commence warfarin

HAEMOPHILIA

Long-term complications of haemophilia A
1 AIDS
2 Chronic hepatitis (esp. non-A non-B)
3 Arthropathy
4 Narcotic addiction
5 F VIII antibodies (inhibitors: seen in 10%)

Replacement factor levels required in haemophilia
1 Minor haemarthrosis — 10–20%
2 Dental extraction
  Major joint/muscle bleed } —20–50% (may need multiple transfusions)
3 Surgery, major trauma (esp. cranial) — 50–100%

Management of bleeding in patients with factor VIII inhibitors
1 Plasmapheresis, or extracorporeal passage of patient's plasma over protein A/Sepharose (for *serious* haemorrhage or pre-operatively)
2 Porcine factor VIII, or alternate-day human factor VIII 'desensitisation' (if inhibitor levels *low*)
3 Activated prothrombin complex concentrates (APCCs) if inhibitor levels *high*
4 *Megadose* factor VIII plus APCCs
5 Recombinant activated factor VII (*factor VIIa*)
6 Combined therapy (protein A/Sepharose plasma passage *plus* intravenous IgG *plus* cyclophosphamide *plus* regular factor VIII)

ANTICOAGULATION

Duration of therapeutic anticoagulation: a rough guide
1 Prosthetic heart valve
  Arterial emboli associated with mitral valve disease or atrial fibrillation
  Recurrent thromboses or emboli } —Treat forever
2 Life-threatening pulmonary embolism
  Extensive proximal DVT } —Treat for at least 12 months
3 Uncomplicated pulmonary embolus
  Localized proximal DVT
  Carotid TIA in a female } —Treat for at least 6 months
4 Uncomplicated calf DVT —Treat for at least 3 months

Mechanisms of antithrombotic drugs
1 Heparin — AT III-dependent inhibition of fibrin formation from fibrinogen; antagonism of factor Xa
2 Warfarin — prevents activation of vitamin K, thereby inhibiting γ-carboxylation of factors II VII IX X
3 Streptokinase/urokinase
  Tissue plasminogen activator } —Activate plasminogen

Mechanisms of antiplatelet drugs
1 Reduced thromboxane A$_2$ synthesis
   a) Aspirin — irreversibly acetylates cyclo-oxygenase
   b) Sulphinpyrazone — reversibly acetylates cyclo-oxygenase
2 Increased platelet cAMP
   a) Prostacyclin (PGI$_2$) — activates adenyl cyclase
   b) Dipyridamole — inhibits phosphodiesterase

Mechanisms of warfarin potentiation
1 ↑ Catabolism of coagulation factors — fever, thyrotoxicosis, postoperative
  ↓ Hepatic drug metabolism — liver disease, cardiac failure, acute alcoholic binge
  ↓ Renal excretion — renal failure, old age
2 ↑ Bleeding tendency (independent of coagulation): aspirin, indomethacin, phenylbutazone
3 Potentiation of hypoprothrombinaemia
   a) Aspirin
   b) Quin(id)ine
   c) Tetracycline, chloramphenicol (↓ bacterial vitamin K synthesis)
   d) Latamoxef
4 Drugs inhibiting hepatic metabolism — antibiotics (isoniazid, chloramphenicol, metronidazole, sulphonamides); amiodarone; cimetidine; allopurinol; dextropropoxyphene; valproate; phenylbutazone (selectively inhibits S-enantiomer metabolism)
5 Other mechanisms (e.g. plasma protein displacement) — clofibrate

Drugs inducing hepatic metabolism of warfarin
1 Phenytoin, phenobarbitone, carbamazepine
2 Chronic alcohol ingestion; cigarette smoking
3 Rifampicin; griseofulvin

'Safe' drugs in warfarinized patients
1 Analgesics — paracetamol
2 Sedatives, anticonvulsants — benzodiazepines
3 Antibiotics — penicillins, cephalosporins, aminoglycosides

NB: Caution must *always* be exercised when *changing* therapy of patients stabilized on warfarin

UNDERSTANDING HAEMATOLOGICAL DISEASE

Clinical varieties of B-cell neoplasms
1 Dysproteinaemias
 a) Benign monoclonal gammopathy
 b) Multiple myeloma, solitary plasmacytoma
 c) Waldenström's macroglobulinaemia
 d) Heavy chain disease (α and γ)
 e) 'Primary' amyloidosis
2 Leukaemias
 a) ALL (most cases)
 b) CLL (98% cases)
 c) Hairy cell leukaemia
3 Lymphomas — most subtypes, incl. Burkitt's

Clinical varieties of T-cell neoplasms
1 Mycosis fungoides
2 Sézary syndrome
3 T-cell leukaemia/lymphoma
4 Lymphoblastic lymphoma

The myelodysplastic syndromes ('pre-leukaemias')
1 Classification
 a) Idiopathic refractory sideroblastic anaemia — 30%
 b) Refractory anaemia — 40%
 c) Refractory anaemia with excess blasts — 30%
 d) Chronic myelomonocytic leukaemia* — 1%
2 Acute leukaemia (usually myelomonocytic: M4) supervenes in 10%
3 Risk of leukaemia is *not* reliably predicted by marrow features
4 Overall prognosis is inversely proportional to the transfusion requirement (i.e. irrespective of leukaemic transition)
5 Low-dose cytosine arabinoside has been used to 'differentiate' dysplastic marrow precursors

MULTIPLE MYELOMA

Relative incidence of myeloma subtypes
1 IgG — 50%
2 IgA — 25%
3 Light-chain (BJP) only — 20–25%
4 IgD — 1%
5 Non-secretory
 Biclonal   —<1% altogether
 IgM

Mechanisms of renal failure in myeloma
1 Intratubular precipitation of Bence-Jones protein ($\rightarrow$ adult Fanconi's syndrome)
2 Prerenal (e.g. dehydration with IVP)
3 Sepsis (e.g. pyelonephritis) $\pm$ nephrotoxic antibiotics
4 Amyloid; plasma cell infiltration
5 Hypercalcaemia, urate nephropathy
6 Hyperviscosity

*Consider diagnosis in 'Philadelphia-chromosome-negative CGL'

Mechanisms of anaemia in myeloma
1 Marrow failure (leucoerythroblastic)
2 Marrow failure (iatrogenic)
3 'Chronic disease' ($\pm$ azotaemia)
4 Dilutional
5 Bleeding (reduced platelet number and function)
6 Iatrogenic sideroblastosis (? preleukaemic)

Spectrum of bony involvement in myeloma
1 Lytic lesions esp. ($\rightarrow$ 60%)
 a) Vertebral bodies (cf. carcinoma $\rightarrow$ pedicles)
 b) Skull (usually painless; cf. carcinoma)
 c) Mandible (classical)
2 Diffuse osteoporosis ($\rightarrow$20%)
3 Skeletal survey traditionally regarded as more sensitive than isotope bone scan
 Osteosclerotic lesions are very rare; when present they may be associated with peripheral neuropathy
4 Serum alkaline phosphatase typically *normal*

Neurological manifestations of myeloma
1 Spinal cord compression — usually due to vertebral collapse
2 Confusion
 a) Hyperviscosity
 b) Hypercalcaemia
 c) Steroid-induced
3 Peripheral neuropathy — amyloid
4 Cranial nerve palsies — base of skull lesions

HAEMOLYTIC ANAEMIAS

Paroxysmal nocturnal haemoglobinuria: features
1 Pathogenesis
 a) A clonal stem-cell defect
 b) Red cell subpopulation develops with abnormal affinity and/or sensitivity to complement
 c) May terminate in leukaemia, aplasia, myelofibrosis
2 Clinical features
 a) Episodic 'smoky' urine
 b) Abdominal/back pain
 c) Thrombotic events (e.g. Budd-Chiari syndrome)
3 Laboratory diagnosis
 a) Anaemia
  — Normochromic, $\pm$ macrocytic
  — May be hypochromic
 b) Haemoglobinuria, haemosiderinuria
 c) +Ham's (acid haemolysis) test; sucrose lysis test/sugar-water test now outmoded
 d) ↓ NAP
 e) ↓ Red cell acetylcholinesterase
 f) Bone marrow hypoplastic in 25%
4 Management principles
 a) Transfusion of washed packed red cells
 b) Avoidance of whole blood or iron supplements
 c) $\pm$ Androgens, folate, warfarin

Causes of intravascular haemolysis
1 Paroxysmal nocturnal haemoglobinuria
 Paroxysmal cold haemoglobinuria (IgG-mediated)
 Cold haemagglutinin disease (IgM-mediated)
2 Intracardiac prostheses
 a) Aortic valve replacements

b) Patch repair of ostium primum ASD/endocardial cushion defect
3 Incompatible blood transfusion
   Burns, snake venom, 'march' haemoglobinuria

Causes of microangiopathic haemolytic anaemia
1 Thrombotic thrombocytopenic purpura
   Haemolytic uraemic syndrome
2 Malignant hypertension
   Pregnancy-associated hypertension
3 Mucinous adenocarcinoma
4 Vasculitis
5 Transplant rejection

Thrombotic thrombocytopenic purpura
1 Diagnostic pentad
   a) Thrombocytopenic purpura
   b) Microangiopathic haemolytic anaemia
   c) Bizarre neurological features (cf. haemolytic-uraemic syndrome)
   d) Fever
   e) Renal failure
2 Investigations
   a) Blood film — schistocytes, no spherocytes
   b) Coombs negative
   c) PI, PTTK, FDPs, fibrinogen — usually normal
   d) ANA — negative in 80%
3 Management
   a) Plasma exchange ± FFP and/or antiplatelet therapy and/or steroids
   b) Splenectomy

Disseminated intravascular coagulation
1 Major causes
   a) Sepsis (Gram-negative septicaemia, *P. falciparum*)
   b) Malignancy (promyelocytic leukaemia, prostate cancer)
   c) Obstetric disaster
2 Diagnosis
   a) Film — RBC fragments, thrombocytopenia
   b) ↑ PI, PTTK, TT
   c) ↑ FDPs (→ anticoagulant action: ↓ thrombin, ↓ platelet function)
   d) ↓ Fibrinogen, F V/VIII, AT III
   e) + Ethanol gelation/soluble fibrin monomer complexes
3 Management
   a) Treat underlying condition
   b) Prevention (e.g. heparin prophylaxis in M3 AML)
   c) Symptomatic bleeding
      — Platelets
      — Transfusion
      — Fresh frozen plasma
   d) Use of heparin in *established* DIC remains controversial
      Treatment may be monitored using antithrombin III levels

HAEMOGLOBINOPATHIES

Thalassaemias: basic concepts
1 Thalassaemias are a heterogeneous group of disorders due to abnormal production of globin chains
2 Anaemia in (say) β-thalassaemia results from
   a) Ineffective erythropoiesis (insufficient β-chains)
   b) Haemolysis (precipitation of relative excess RBC α-chains)
3 α-Thalassaemias arise predominantly due to gene deletions on chromosome 16
4 β-Thalassaemias arise due to complex genetic derangements on chromosome 11 resulting, for example, in abnormal globin mRNA

Clinical categorisation of thalassaemias
1 Thalassaemia *trait* — an asymptomatic condition which may only be detected on screening
2 Thalassaemia *minor* — mild anaemia with minimal symptoms
3 Thalassaemia *intermedia*
   a) Moderate anaemia and splenomegaly
   b) e.g. Hb C, Hb Lepore; HbE *plus* β-thal trait
4 Thalassaemia *major* — severe transfusion-dependent anaemia

Features of alpha-thalassaemia
1 αα/α-
   a) α-Thalassaemia trait
   b) Asymptomatic carrier
   c) Low normal MCV
   d) 1–2% Hb Bart's (γ_4) in cord blood
2 α-/α-
   a) Homozygous α + thalassemia (thalassemia minor)
   b) 5–10% Hb Bart's; normal, HbA_2; ± ↓ MCV
3 αα/--
   a) Heterozygous α° thalassaemia (thalassemia minor)
   b) Low MCV, mild anaemia; normal Hb A_2
   c) Blood film — target cells; occasional Hb H (β_4) inclusion bodies (Hb H = 0–1%)
4 α-/--
   a) Hb H disease (thalassaemia major)
   b) Moderate to severe anaemia
   c) Onset of symptoms in adult life; gallstones, splenomegaly
   d) 10–30% Hb H ± ↓ Hb A_2
5 --/-- ($\alpha°$)
   a) Hydrops fetalis (→ stillbirth)
   b) 80% Hb Bart's, 20% Hb Portland (i.e. absent HbA_2)

Features of beta-thalassaemia
1 β-thalassaemia minor
   a) ↓ MCV, ↑ red cell count
   b) Basophilic stippling; targets, poikilocytes on occasion
   c) ↓ Osmotic fragility (cf. spherocytosis)
   d) ↑ Hb A_2 ± ↑ Hb F
   e) Definitive diagnosis by Hb EPG
2 Suspected thalassaemia minor with *normal* Hb A_2
   a) α-Thalassaemia
   b) δβ-Thalassaemia (heterozygous)
3 β-Thalassaemia major
   a) ↑ Hb F (>70%) ± ↑ Hb A_2 (cf. β-thal minor)
   b) β_0-Thalassaemia — no detectable Hb A
      β^+-Thalassaemia — up to 30% Hb A

c) Blood film — numerous teardrops, targets, nucleated red cells

4 Management of thalassaemia major
   a) Hypertransfuse to maintain Hb > 10.0 g/dl
   b) Folate supplements
   c) Splenectomy if indicated for hypersplenism or discomfort
   d) Iron chelation regimen at earliest possible age
   e) Genetic counselling, amniocentesis
   f) Hepatitis B vaccination
   g) Bone marrow transplantation work-up

Approach to the patient with thalassaemia trait
1 Test spouse (or spouse-to-be) for thal trait; refer for genetic counselling if positive
2 Prescribe prophylactic folate supplements at times of marrow stress, e.g. menorrhagia, pregnancy
3 Educate patient against accepting unnecessary oral iron on basis of blood film interpreted by doctors unaware of diagnosis

SICKLE-CELL ANAEMIA

Clinical spectrum of sickle-cell disease
1 Hb AS (sickle trait)
   a) 60% Hb A, 35% Hb S
   b) Normal life expectancy
   c) Hyposthenuria, nocturia ⎱ papillary necrosis
   d) (Micro)haematuria ⎰
   e) Bacteriuria in pregnancy; zinc wasting
   f) Hypoxia (e.g. unpressurized aircraft at high altitude) may precipitate splenic infarction or retinal complications
2 Hb SS (sickle-cell disease)
   a) No Hb A; 85% Hb S, 10% Hb F
   b) Dactylitis, leg ulcers, hyposplenism, cerebrovascular disease, gout, priapism (→ impotence), retinopathy
3 Hb SC (sickle-C disease)
   a) Sickle and target cells on film
   b) Thrombotic tendency

— Proliferative retinopathy
— Aseptic necrosis of femoral head or shoulder
— Haematuria
— Complications during pregnancy

Hepatic manifestations of sickle-cell anaemia
1 Complications related to transfusion
   a) Haemochromatosis
   b) (Chronic) hepatitis B/non-A non-B
2 Complications related to chronic haemolysis — gallstones
3 Complications related to repeated vascular occlusion
   a) Hepatic fibrosis or infarction
   b) Liver failure

Varieties of sickle cell crises
1 Haemolytic crises
   a) May signify sepsis or associated G6PD deficiency
   b) Relatively uncommon; transfusion not routinely indicated
2 Aplastic crises
   a) May signify parvovirus infection or folate deficiency
   b) Low reticulocyte count (cf. haemolytic crisis)
3 Thrombotic (vaso-occlusive, painful) crises
   a) Commonest; may affect abdomen, lung, brain
   b) Infarcts precipitated by tissue hypoxia
   c) May be accompanied by fever, fits, dyspnoea
   d) α HBD may be elevated
   e) Complications include
      — Autosplenectomy (hyposplenism)
      — Aseptic necrosis of bone
      — Permanent brain damage
      — Renal failure
4 Sequestration crises
   —Most serious, esp. in infants (due to hypovolaemia)
   —Presents with rapid-onset hepato/splenomegaly

NB: it is generally adequate to maintain Hb levels at 7–10 g/dl (since HbS has a relatively low oxygen affinity)

Reviewing the Literature: Haematology

5.1 Estrov Z et al 1986 Detection of residual acute lymphoblastic leukaemia cells in cultures of bone marrow obtained during remission. New England Journal of Medicine 315: 538–542

Of 13 patients in remission from ALL, 4 out of 6 with positive marrow colony-culture assay relapsed, while 7/7 negative remained in remission. The assay may therefore be useful in predicting need for more chemotherapy, or for timing of bone marrow transplantation

5.2 Gomez G A et al 1984 Staging laparotomy and splenectomy in early Hodgkin's disease: no therapeutic benefit. American Journal of Medicine 77: 205–210

Study concluding that stage I/II patients derived no survival benefit from being subjected to routine staging laparotomy

5.3 Martin P J et al 1985 Efficacy of T-cell depletion of allogeneic marrow. Blood 66: 664–672

First report showing that donor marrow could be successfully purged of T-cells ex vivo using monoclonal antibodies, thus raising the prospect of avoiding graft-vs-host disease in the future

5.4 Hochberg J et al 1983 CNS lymphoma related to Epstein-Barr virus. New England Journal of Medicine 309: 745–748

Discovery of EBV DNA and antibodies in cerebral lymphomas of immunosuppressed patients

5.5 Chessels J M et al 1986 Bone marrow transplantation has a limited role in prolonging second marrow remission in childhood lymphoblastic leukaemia. Lancet i: 1239–1241

About 40% (5/13) ALL children treated with HLA-compatible sibling bone marrow transplant survived, as did 16/40 (40%) ALL children treated with conventional chemotherapy. Length of first remission was the best predictor of second remission duration; the biggest problem in successfully transplanted patients was marrow relapse of original disease.

5.6 Baranski B et al 1988 Epstein-Barr virus in the bone marrow of patients with aplastic anaemia. Annals of Internal Medicine 109: 695–704

Study showing presence of EBV in bone marrow of six patients with aplastic anaemia, raising the prospect of a pathogenetic role for this virus. Hybridization analysis suggested that the EBV DNA was dissimilar to that normally seen in infectious mononucleosis.

5.7 Weiden P L, Sullivan K M, Flournoy N, Storb R, Thomas E D 1981 Antileukaemic effect of chronic graft-versus-host disease. New England Journal of Medicine 304: 1529–1533

This report documented improved survival and decreased relapse rate in allogeneic marrow transplant recipients with chronic graft-versus-host disease

5.8 Freeman A P, Giles R W, Berdoukas V A, Walsh W F, Choy D, Murray P C 1983 Early left ventricular dysfunction and chelation therapy in thalassaemia major. Annals of Internal Medicine 99: 450–454

Subclinical radionuclide left ventricular abnormalities were demonstrable on exercise in 18 of 23 patients; normalization of the ventricular exercise response was seen in four of these patients following 12 months intensive DFO chelation therapy

5.9 Newland A C, Treleaven J G, Minchinton R M, Waters A H 1983 High-dose intravenous IgG in adults with autoimmune thrombocytopenia. Lancet i: 84–77

Pooled IgG infusions led to the elevation of platelet counts which were only sustained if followed by splenectomy

Co-operative Group for the Study of Immunoglobulin in CLL 1988 Intravenous IgG for the prevention of infection in CLL. New England Journal of Medicine 319: 902–907

Randomized double-blind trial of 84 CLL patients with either hypogammaglobulinaemia, a history of recent infections, or both. Patients receiving high-dose i.v. IgG experienced far fewer bacterial infections than did placebo-treated patients, though the frequency of non-bacterial infections was similar

5.10 Dallenbach F E, Stein H 1989 Expression of T-cell receptor β-chain in Reed-Sternberg cells. Lancet ii: 828–829

Study indicating that most Hodgkin's disease is T-cell-derived (as is the enigmatic Reed-Sternberg cell itself), with the apparent exception of the lymphocyte-predominant subtype which appears to be B-cell-derived on the basis of these data

CHAPTER 6

Immunology

Physical examination protocol 6.1 You are asked to examine a patient suspected of having a collagen-vascular disease

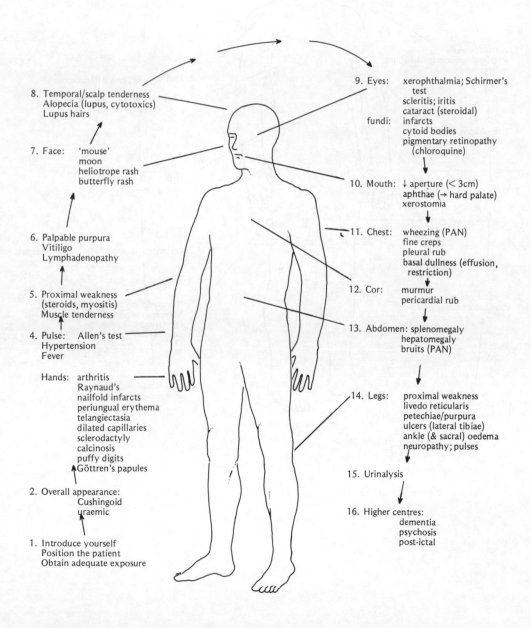

8. Temporal/scalp tenderness
   Alopecia (lupus, cytotoxics)
   Lupus hairs

7. Face: 'mouse'
          moon
          heliotrope rash
          butterfly rash

6. Palpable purpura
   Vitiligo
   Lymphadenopathy

5. Proximal weakness
   (steroids, myositis)
   Muscle tenderness

4. Pulse: Allen's test
   Hypertension
   Fever

   Hands: arthritis
           Raynaud's
           nailfold infarcts
           periungual erythema
           telangiectasia
           dilated capillaries
           sclerodactyly
           calcinosis
           puffy digits
           Göttren's papules

2. Overall appearance:
   Cushingoid
   uraemic

1. Introduce yourself
   Position the patient
   Obtain adequate exposure

9. Eyes: xerophthalmia; Schirmer's
           test
           scleritis; iritis
           cataract (steroidal)
   fundi: infarcts
           cytoid bodies
           pigmentary retinopathy
           (chloroquine)

10. Mouth: ↓ aperture (< 3cm)
            aphthae (→ hard palate)
            xerostomia

11. Chest: wheezing (PAN)
            fine creps
            pleural rub
            basal dullness (effusion,
            restriction)

12. Cor: murmur
            pericardial rub

13. Abdomen: splenomegaly
             hepatomegaly
             bruits (PAN)

14. Legs: proximal weakness
            livedo reticularis
            petechiae/purpura
            ulcers (lateral tibiae)
            ankle (& sacral) oedema
            neuropathy; pulses

15. Urinalysis

16. Higher centres:
            dementia
            psychosis
            post-ictal

Physical examination protocol 6.2 You are asked to examine a patient suspected of having Sjögren's syndrome

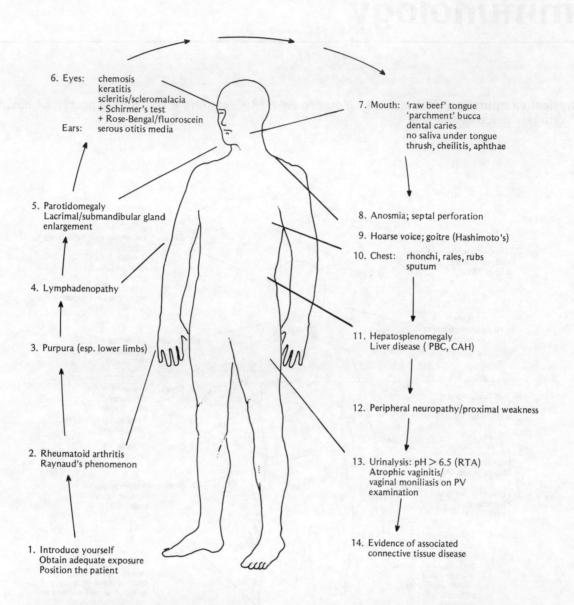

6. Eyes: chemosis
   keratitis
   scleritis/scleromalacia
   + Schirmer's test
   + Rose-Bengal/fluoroscein

   Ears: serous otitis media

5. Parotidomegaly
   Lacrimal/submandibular gland
   enlargement

4. Lymphadenopathy

3. Purpura (esp. lower limbs)

2. Rheumatoid arthritis
   Raynaud's phenomenon

1. Introduce yourself
   Obtain adequate exposure
   Position the patient

7. Mouth: 'raw beef' tongue
   'parchment' bucca
   dental caries
   no saliva under tongue
   thrush, cheilitis, aphthae

8. Anosmia; septal perforation

9. Hoarse voice; goitre (Hashimoto's)

10. Chest: rhonchi, rales, rubs
    sputum

11. Hepatosplenomegaly
    Liver disease (PBC, CAH)

12. Peripheral neuropathy/proximal weakness

13. Urinalysis: pH > 6.5 (RTA)
    Atrophic vaginitis/
    vaginal moniliasis on PV
    examination

14. Evidence of associated
    connective tissue disease

Physical examination protocol 6.3   You are asked to examine a patient with Raynaud's phenomenon and oesophageal reflux

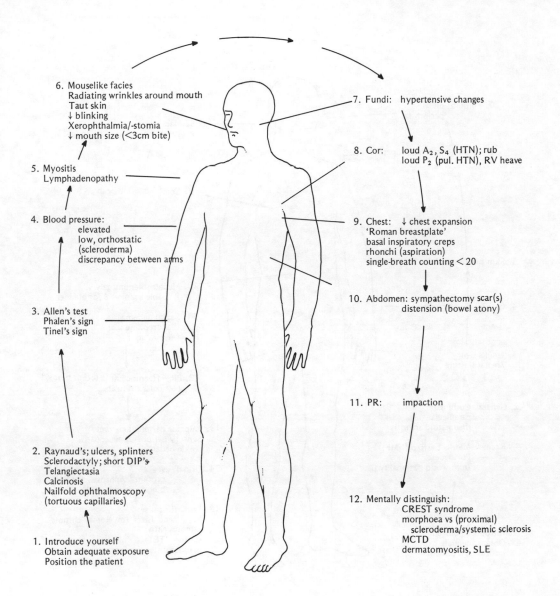

6. Mouselike facies
   Radiating wrinkles around mouth
   Taut skin
   ↓ blinking
   Xerophthalmia/-stomia
   ↓ mouth size (<3cm bite)

5. Myositis
   Lymphadenopathy

4. Blood pressure:
   elevated
   low, orthostatic
   (scleroderma)
   discrepancy between arms

3. Allen's test
   Phalen's sign
   Tinel's sign

2. Raynaud's; ulcers, splinters
   Sclerodactyly; short DIP's
   Telangiectasia
   Calcinosis
   Nailfold ophthalmoscopy
   (tortuous capillaries)

1. Introduce yourself
   Obtain adequate exposure
   Position the patient

7. Fundi: hypertensive changes

8. Cor: loud A_2, S_4 (HTN); rub
            loud P_2 (pul. HTN), RV heave

9. Chest: ↓ chest expansion
            'Roman breastplate'
            basal inspiratory creps
            rhonchi (aspiration)
            single-breath counting < 20

10. Abdomen: sympathectomy scar(s)
             distension (bowel atony)

11. PR: impaction

12. Mentally distinguish:
    CREST syndrome
    morphoea vs (proximal)
       scleroderma/systemic sclerosis
    MCTD
    dermatomyositis, SLE

Physical examination protocol 6.4 You are asked to examine a patient for stigmata of amyloidosis

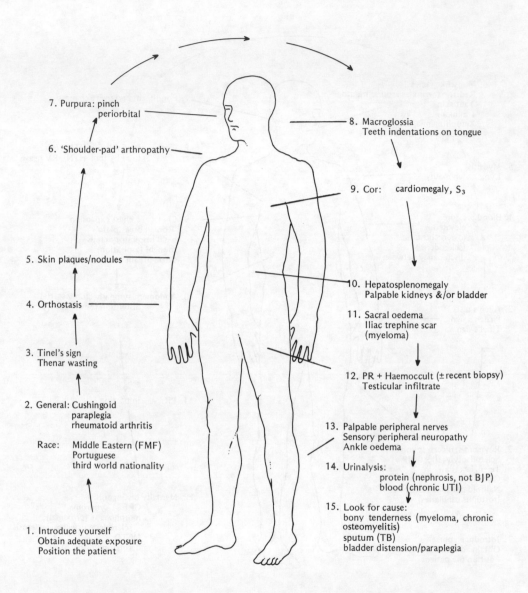

7. Purpura: pinch periorbital

6. 'Shoulder-pad' arthropathy

5. Skin plaques/nodules

4. Orthostasis

3. Tinel's sign
   Thenar wasting

2. General: Cushingoid
   paraplegia
   rheumatoid arthritis

   Race: Middle Eastern (FMF)
           Portuguese
           third world nationality

1. Introduce yourself
   Obtain adequate exposure
   Position the patient

8. Macroglossia
   Teeth indentations on tongue

9. Cor: cardiomegaly, S_3

10. Hepatosplenomegaly
    Palpable kidneys &/or bladder

11. Sacral oedema
    Iliac trephine scar
    (myeloma)

12. PR + Haemoccult (± recent biopsy)
    Testicular infiltrate

13. Palpable peripheral nerves
    Sensory peripheral neuropathy
    Ankle oedema

14. Urinalysis:
       protein (nephrosis, not BJP)
       blood (chronic UTI)

15. Look for cause:
    bony tenderness (myeloma, chronic osteomyelitis)
    sputum (TB)
    bladder distension/paraplegia

CLINICAL ASPECTS OF IMMUNOLOGICAL DISEASE

COMMONEST IMMUNOLOGICAL SHORT CASES

1 Raynaud's (± scleroderma, CREST, MCTD, SLE etc.)
2 Fibrosing alveolitis

Clinical classification of hypersensitivity reactions

1 Type I (immediate): IgE-mediated — induces vasodilatation and eosinophil chemotaxis, e.g.
   —atopic asthma/hay fever
2 Type II (membrane-bound antigen): IgM/IgG-mediated — induces either (i) cell lysis due to granulocyte and/or complement activation, or (ii) receptor binding (agonistic or antagonistic), e.g.
   a) (Cytotoxic)
      — Transfusion reactions
      — AIHA, ITP, methyldopa haemolysis
      — Anti-GBM disease (Goodpasture's syndrome)
   b) (Blocking antibody)
      — Pernicious anaemia
      — Myasthenia gravis
      — Hashimoto's disease
   c) (Receptor agonism) — Graves' disease
3 Type III (circulating immune-complexes): IgA/IgG-mediated — induces Arthus reaction (if antibody in excess) or serum sickness (if antigen in excess), e.g.
   a) (Arthus)
      — Hypersensitivity pneumonitis
      — Allergic bronchopulmonary aspergillosis
   b) (Serum sickness)
      — Rheumatic fever
      — Postinfectious glomerulonephritis
      — Secondary syphilis
      — Lepromatous leprosy
      — Erythema multiforme
      — Henoch-Schönlein purpura
4 Type IV (delayed): T-cell/macrophage-mediated — induces mononuclear chemotaxis/activation, e.g.
      — Graft rejection, graft-versus-host disease
      — Contact dermatitis
      — Tuberculin reaction; TB gumma/caseation
      — Tuberculoid leprosy

COLLAGEN-VASCULAR DISEASES

Clinical stigmata of vasculitis

1 Leucocytoclastic vasculitis — palpable purpura
2 Non-inflammatory obliterative endarteritis
   a) Nailfold infarcts
   b) Splinter haemorrhages
3 Necrotizing vasculitis
   a) Purpura with skin ulceration
   b) Mononeuritis multiplex
   c) Motor neuropathy
   d) Non-tender aneurysmal dilatations overlying arterial bifurcations

4 Non-specific cutaneous signs sometimes indicating vasculitis
   a) Livedo reticularis
   b) Atrophie blanche
   c) Haemorrhagic bullae/vesicles/ulcers
   d) Panniculitis; pustulonecrotic nodules
   e) Scarring alopecia
   f) Urticarial lesions >24-hour duration
5 Non-cutaneous signs sometimes indicating vasculitis
   a) Hypertension
   b) Microscopic haematuria
   c) Retinal vasculopathy, cytoid bodies

Differential diagnosis of purpura in connective tissue disease

1 Vasculitis (see above)
2 Corticosteroid therapy
3 Thrombocytopenia
   a) Immune (SLE) ± hypersplenism (Felty's)
   b) Iatrogenic (penicillamine, gold)
      Platelet dysfunction (NSAIDs)
4 Amyloidosis
5 Cryoglobulinaemia
6 Factor VIII antibodies (SLE, RA)

Raynaud's phenomenon: features suggesting systemic disease

1 Severe vasospasm with
   a) Digital oedema, ulceration, gangrene
   b) Thumb involvement
   c) Abrupt onset
2 *Avascular areas* associated with tortuous capillaries on nailfold capillaroscopy (far more specific for scleroderma or dermatomyositis than simple capillary dilatation)
3 Abnormal Allen's test
4 Digital artery occlusion on Doppler study; abnormal arteriogram
   Subcutaneous calcinosis on plain X-ray
   Abnormal barium swallow
5 Strongly positive non-organ-specific autoantibody profile (esp. ANA)
   Grossly elevated ESR ± elevated whole blood viscosity
   Hypocomplementaemia (incl. C_7 deficiency)

SCLERODERMA

Criteria for scleroderma diagnosis

1 Major criterion — bilateral skin thickening proximal to MCP joints and associated with Raynaud's phenomenon
2 Supporting clinical findings
   a) Sclerodactyly, pitted fingertip scars, finger pulp loss
   b) Bibasilar pulmonary fibrosis
3 Supporting investigations
   a) Nailfold capillaroscopy: enlarged and distorted capillary loops, reduced in number and associated with haemorrhages
   b) Positive ANA, esp. if nucleolar or centromeric pattern
   c) Abnormal oesophageal motility on barium swallow

Differential diagnosis of scleroderma
1 'Overlap' syndrome
   a) Mixed connective tissue disease
   b) CREST syndrome (strictly, a subtype of scleroderma)
   c) Dermatomyositis, SLE
2 Eosinophilic fasciitis
   a) Spares hands and feet (no Raynaud's)
   b) No visceral complications
   Morphoea
   a) Localized sclerodermatous plaques
   b) No systemic features
3 Sclerosant exposure, e.g. bleomycin, silica, vinyl chloride
4 Carcinoid syndrome
5 Graft-versus-host disease
6 Amyloidosis

Spectrum of pulmonary disease in scleroderma
1 Interstitial fibrosis ± (secondary) pulmonary hypertension
2 Primary pulmonary arterial hypertension, esp. in CREST variant
3 Pleurisy
4 Aspiration pneumonitis
5 Restriction of chest wall expansion
6 Bronchioloalveolar cell carcinoma

Mechanisms of cardiac failure in scleroderma
1 Left ventricular failure
   a) Severe hypertension
   b) Diffuse myocardial fibrosis (scleroderma cardiomyopathy)
   c) Reperfusion necrosis (?due to myocardial Raynaud's)
2 Right ventricular failure — pulmonary hypertension (primary or secondary)
3 Pericarditis
   a) Tamponade (acute)
   b) Constriction (chronic)
4 Arrhythmias

Differential diagnosis of anaemia in scleroderma
1 Normocytic ('chronic disease' ± uraemia)
2 Microcytic (oesophagitis, telangiectasia)
3 Macrocytic (bacterial overgrowth)
4 Microangiopathic (renal involvement with severe hypertension)

Gastrointestinal presentations of scleroderma
1 Epigastric pain
   Dysphagia
   Regurgitation
2 Postprandial 'bloating'
   a) Gastric dilatation/delayed emptying
   b) Malabsorption
3 Steatorrhoea
   a) Bacterial overgrowth (due to gut hypomotility)
   b) Lymphatic fibrosis
4 Anaemia
   a) Severe oesophagitis ± peptic ulceration; telangiectasia
   b) Bacterial overgrowth
5 Constipation
   a) Chronic intestinal pseudo-obstruction
   b) Faecal impaction; barium impaction

Oesophageal abnormalities in the scleroderma patient
1 Distal hypoperistalsis (in 70%)
2 Reflux (in 60%)
3 Oesophageal dilatation (in 50%)
4 Absent lower oesophageal sphincter tone (in 40%)
5 Positive Bernstein (acid perfusion) test (in 30%)
6 Hiatus hernia (in 20%)
7 Stricture (in 10%)

Radiology of the lower gastrointestinal tract in scleroderma
1 Plain abdominal film
   a) Fluid levels, dilated loops of bowel
   b) Pneumoperitoneum (pneumatosis intestinalis with cyst rupture)
2 Small bowel series
   a) Flocculated barium ('moulage' sign)
   b) Close-packed valvulae coniventes ('hidebound' or 'accordion' appearance)
   c) Dilatation of second and third parts of duodenum
3 Barium enema
   a) Megacolon; pneumatosis intestinalis
   b) Widemouthed diverticulae on antimesenteric border
   c) Reduced motility, slow transit time

SYSTEMIC LUPUS ERYTHEMATOSUS

Clinical associations of SLE
1 IgA deficiency
2 C_2 deficiency (and other complement components)
3 $\alpha_1 AT$ deficiency
4 Thymoma
5 Porphyria cutanea tarda
6 Klinefelter's syndrome

Adverse prognostic indicators in SLE
1 High-titre dsDNA Ab
2 Marked hypocomplementaemia (esp. C_3)
3 Active urinary sediment (esp. red cell casts)
4 Azotaemia, heavy proteinuria
   Renal biopsy; diffuse proliferative or membranous
5 +Sm Ab (favours development of renal disease)
   +IgG 'lupus band' on (uninvolved) skin biopsy (cf. IgM/A); cryoglobulinaemia
6 Clinical evidence of CNS involvement

Features of drug-induced SLE
1 Older patients than primary SLE
   More frequently male (40% vs 10% in primary disease)
2 Lung, joint and serosal (esp. pleural) involvement common
3 Renal and skin manifestations relatively uncommon
4 CNS disease rare
5 ANA
   a) When positive, typically directed against histones (homogeneous pattern)
   b) Double-stranded DNA antibodies typically absent
6 Complement levels normal
7 Slow acetylation status usual (incidence approaches 100% in hydralazine-induced lupus); less marked association in primary SLE

8 HLA association — DR4 (cf. primary SLE: DR2, DR3)
9 Incidence increases with dosage and duration of drug therapy
10 Symptoms usually persist for 2–6 months after drug ceased

Features of neonatal SLE
1 *Cutaneous* type
  a) Commoner in female neonates (75%)
  b) Transient photosensitive skin eruptions, often discoid
  c) May be associated with thrombocytopenia, hepatomegaly, abnormal liver function tests
2 *Cardiac* type
  a) Commoner in male neonates
  b) Manifests with perinatal complete heart block in 95%
  c) Anti-Ro antibody is present in virtually 100%, and is thought to be pathogenic
  d) 20% of affected neonates will need pacemaker insertion
  e) 15% will die of associated myocarditis
  f) Pathology reveals endomyocardial fibrosis leading to AV nodal obliteration
3 *Mothers* of affected neonates
  a) 70% are asymptomatic at time of neonatal diagnosis
  b) 90% will develop a connective tissue disease (usually SLE or scleroderma) within 10 years
  c) Presence of anti-Ro antibody in a pregnant woman is an indication for fetal monitoring using echocardiography
  d) Documentation of fetal myocarditis is an indication for high-dose dexamethasone (not inactivated by placenta) or plasmapheresis

SJÖGREN'S SYNDROME

Clinical concomitants of Sjögren's syndrome
1 Dry mouth and eyes; also nose, throat, trachea, skin
2 Secondary otitis, bronchitis, pneumonitis
3 Dental caries
4 Vulvovaginitis — dyspareunia, pruritus vulvae
5 Atrophic gastritis
6 Recurrent parotidomegaly
7 Lymphadenopathy, splenomegaly; 'pseudolymphoma'
8 Lymphoma, thymoma
9 Cryoglobulinaemia
  Waldenström's macroglobulinaemia
  Benign hyperglobulinaemic purpura of Waldenström
10 Pulmonary atelectasis (esp. postoperative)
  Renal tubular acidosis (esp. postpartum)
11 Drug hypersensitivity
12 Autoimmune disease, esp. PBC, Raynaud's, Hashimoto's

Distinction of primary from secondary Sjögren's syndrome
1 No other clinically evident connective tissue disease
2 ANA more commonly positive (90% vs 50%) similarly, Ro (SS-A) antibodies (80% vs 50%)

3 La (SS-B) antibodies positive in 50% (vs 10%)
4 Antisalivary duct antibodies *less* common (15% vs 60%)
5 Associated with HLA-DR3 (cf. secondary type: HLA DR4)

NB: rheumatoid factor is positive in almost 100% of *both* primary and secondary Sjögren's syndrome

Diagnosis of Sjögren's syndrome
1 Clinical sicca syndrome ± connective tissue disease (usually RA)
2 Positive Schirmer's test — <15 mm in 5 minutes
  Rose-Bengal stain — punctate uptake in conjunctival/corneal erosions
  Slit-lamp examination — reduced tear film; erosions
3 High-titre rheumatoid factor/ANA
4 Sialography; scintigraphy
5 Salivary/labial gland biopsy
  a) Lymphocytic infiltrate
  b) Acinar atrophy
  c) Myoepithelial islands

OTHER CONNECTIVE TISSUE DISEASES

Diagnosis of polymyositis
1 Clinical
  a) Proximal weakness > wasting
  b) Muscle tenderness
  c) Heliotrope rash, Göttren's papules
2 Laboratory
  a) CPK
  b) EMG
  c) Muscle biopsy

Diagnosis of polyarteritis nodosa
1 Clinical
  a) Hypertension
  b) Mononeuritis multiplex
  c) Asthma (suggests Churg-Strauss variant)
2 Laboratory
  a) Neutrophilia, eosinophilia (suggests Churg-Strauss variant), ↑ ESR
  b) Biopsy of clinically involved tissue
  c) Angiography (e.g. coeliac axis) → aneurysms

Diagnosis of 'mixed connective tissue disease'
1 Clinical
  a) Raynaud's; puffy fingers/hands (scleroderma-like)
  b) Arthralgias/itis; lymphadenopathy (SLE-like)
  c) Myositis, serositis, pneumonitis (polymyositis-like)
  d) Renal involvement rare
2 Laboratory
  a) High-titre (>1:1024) speckled ANA
  b) High-titre (cf. SLE) anti-RNP Ab
  c) Negative dsDNA Ab; negative Sm Ab
  d) Normal complement levels
  e) Polyclonal hypergammaglobulinaemia
  f) Abnormal upper (polymyositis-like) and/or lower (scleroderma-like) oesophageal motility
  g) ↓ DL_{co}
3 Therapy
  a) Steroid-responsive features

— Myositis
— Pleurisy
— Depression
b) Steroid-resistant features
— Interstitial lung fibrosis, pulmonary hypertension
— Oesophageal dysmotility
4 Clinical course
a) *Not* as benign as previously thought; 5–10% 10-year mortality
b) Indiscriminate steroid use may cause osteoporosis and other cushingoid side-effects

Clinical significance of mixed connective tissue disease (MCTD)
1 Although the existence of a distinct clinical entity remains controversial, the diagnosis of MCTD is important because it implies the presence of *myositis*
2 Myositis is an indication for *steroids* even in cases with only *mild* symptoms
3 Even in cases with only mild symptoms, initial steroid therapy should be *aggressive* (e.g. prednisone 1 mg/kg) where myositis is present

AMYLOIDOSIS

Clinical significance of amyloid components
1 AL
a) Amyloid L-(light-chain) component
b) Denotes amyloidosis of monoclonal immunocytic origin
c) Derived from light-chain (BJP) fragments, $\lambda > \kappa$ (cf. most paraproteins, and normal immunoglobulins: $\kappa > \lambda$)
d) Occurs in
— 10% Myeloma cases (overall)
— 25% BJP-only myeloma
— 5% Benign monoclonal gammopathy
2 AA
a) Amyloid A-component
b) Denotes amyloidosis of reactive systemic origin
c) Derived from the acute phase plasma protein SAA
d) Occurs in
— Familial Mediterranean fever (may present with amyloid)
— *Long-standing* (>10 y):
rheumatoid arthritis (10%)
juvenile chronic arthritis (5%)
Hodgkin's disease (5%)
TB, leprosy, osteomyelitis
3 AP
a) Amyloid P-component
b) Pathogenetic significance unknown
c) Related to the acute phase reactant C-reactive protein
d) Occurs in association with all known amyloid subtypes *except* cerebral amyloid

Classification of clinical amyloidosis variants
1 Monoclonal immunocytic dyscrasia (AL-amyloidosis) — include myeloma-associated and 'primary' amyloidosis

2 Reactive systemic amyloidosis (AA-amyloidosis) — includes FMF-associated and 'secondary' amyloidosis
3 Endocrine amyloid (affects APUD cells) — derived from calcitonin-related fibrils in medullary thyroid carcinoma; from insulin-derived fibrils in islets
4 Senile amyloid (affects heart, joints, seminal vesicles) — amyloid composed of prealbumin ASc_1 (from plasma prealbumin)
5 Haemodialysis-associated amyloid (affects bones and kidneys) — amyloid derived from plasma β_2-microglobulin
6 Cerebral amyloid (in Alzheimer's, Down's, senile dementia) — amyloid from β-protein (coded on chromosome 21), A4 precursor
7 Hereditary cerebral amyloid ($\rightarrow$ cerebral haemorrhage) — autosomal dominant; amyloid from γ-trace protein (cystatin C)
8 Hereditary neuropathic amyloid (e.g. Portuguese amyloid) — autosomal dominant; amyloid derived from plasma prealbumin
9 Hereditary nephropathic amyloid (familial Mediterranean fever) — autosomal recessive; colchicine prophylaxis effective

AL- ('primary') vs AA- ('secondary') amyloidosis
1 Common in AL-amyloidosis — *mesenchymal* tissue deposition
a) Neuropathy
— Peripheral (incl. carpal tunnel syndrome)
— Autonomic
b) Cardiomyopathy — restrictive
c) Arthropathy — large joints, e.g. 'shoulder-pads'
d) Macroglossia
e) Acquired factor X deficiency } Highly specific for AL-amyloidosis
f) Purpura
— 'pinch' (non-thrombocytopenic) purpura
— postproctoscopic periorbital purpura
g) Hyposplenism
2 Common in AA-amyloidosis — *parenchymal* tissue deposition
a) Nephrotic syndrome
b) Hepatosplenomegaly
c) Goitre

Diagnosis of amyloidosis
1 Paraproteinaemia
2 Biopsy (Congo red stain)
a) Routinely biopsied site (e.g. marrow in myeloma)
b) Affected site (e.g. kidney in nephrosis*; sural nerve in neuropathy)
c) Deep rectal biopsy
3 Biopsy (polarized light microscopy) — 'apple-green' birefringence
4 Electron microscopy — β-pleated sheets
5 Direct immunofluorescence of bone marrow plasma cells
a) Monoclonality demonstrated with anti-light chain antibodies (monoclonal immunocytic amyloidosis)
b) Polyclonality (e.g. in reactive systemic amyloidosis)

---

*Due to increased risk of bleeding in amyloidosis, suspected renal amyloid is usually considered an indication for *rectal* biopsy

INVESTIGATING IMMUNOLOGICAL DISEASE

B-lymphocytes: laboratory characteristics
1 Phenotype
   a) Surface immunoglobulin (IgM, IgD) present
   b) $\kappa:\lambda$ chains = 2:1
2 Function
   a) IgG, A, M levels
   b) Isohaemagglutinins (IgM)
   c) Antibodies to
      — Pneumococcus (IgM)
      — Tetanus/polio/diphtheria (IgG)
3 In vitro blastogenesis (T-cell dependent) — inducible with pokeweed mitogen
4 Lymph node localization — follicles, medullary cords

T-lymphocytes: laboratory characteristics
1 Phenotype — spontaneous E-rosette formation with sheep RBCs
2 Differentiation antigens
   a) Pan T-cell — CD3 (T3/Leu4)
   b) Helper/inducer (T_H) — normally comprise about 70% T-cells — CD4 (T4/Leu3) = T-cell surface receptor for HIV envelope glycoprotein
   c) Suppressor/cytotoxic (T_S) — normally comprise about 30% T-cells — CD8 (T8/Leu2)
3 Function
   a) Primary response — DNCB sensitization
   b) Lymphokine (MIF, LIF) production
   c) 'Memory' — DTH skin testing to tuberculin, Candida, mumps, trichophyton, tetanus, streptokinase
4 In vitro blastogenesis
   a) Inducible with Con A, PHA
   b) Specific antigen, e.g. herpes simplex type II
5 Lymph node localization — paracortical

$T_H:T_S$ ratios in health and disease
1 Normal $T_H:T_S$ (CD4:CD8) = 1.5–2.0
2 Inverted ratio ($T_H < T_S$):
   a) AIDS (with lymphopaenia)
   b) Common variable hypogammaglobulinaemia* X-linked lymphoproliferative (Duncan's) disease } with normal lymphocyte count
   c) CLL (with lymphocytosis)
3 Exaggerated ratio ($T_H \gg T_S$):
   a) SLE
   b) Juvenile chronic arthritis
4 Relative variations of $T_H:T_S$ ratio:
   a) Leprosy, tuberculoid: $\uparrow T_H:T_S$
      Leprosy, lepromatous: $\downarrow T_H:T_S$
   b) Renal transplant, rejection: $\uparrow T_H:T_S$
      Homograft infection (e.g. CMV): $\downarrow T_H:T_S$
   c) Graft-versus-host disease†, acute: $\uparrow T_H:T_S$
      Graft-versus-host disease, chronic: $\downarrow T_H:T_S$

*$T_H:T_S$ ratio is normal in SCID, WAS, Nezelof's (i.e. despite lymphopaenia)
†Acute GVHD is associated with hypergammaglobulinaemia, chronic GVHD with hypogammaglobulinaemia

d) Active sarcoid**, bronchoalveolar lavage: $\uparrow T_H:T_S$
   Active sarcoid, peripheral blood: $\downarrow T_H:T_S$

INVESTIGATION OF HYPERSENSITIVITY STATES

Radioallergosorbent testing ('RAST'): indications
(= relative contraindications to prick testing)
1 Known high risk of anaphylaxis (e.g. suspected major hypersensitivity to penicillin or insect sting)
2 Dermatitis, extensive skin disease, dermatographia
3 Recent (<72 hours) treatment with antihistamines or sympathomimetics
4 Highly suggestive history (esp. of inhalant allergy) with negative prick test
5 Small children (<5 years)

Elevated IgE: differential diagnosis
1 Metazoan parasitic infestation
   a) Trichinosis
   b) Toxocariasis
   c) Filariasis
   d) Schistosomiasis
2 Pulmonary disease
   a) Atopic asthma
   b) Bronchopulmonary aspergillosis
   c) Churg-Strauss syndrome
   d) Löffler's syndrome
3 Skin disease
   a) Pemphigus
   b) Pemphigoid
4 Rare causes:
   a) Wiskott-Aldrich syndrome
   b) Job's syndrome
   c) Hodgkin's disease
   d) Sézary syndrome
   e) Selective IgA deficiency

NB: IgE is not elevated in the hypereosinophilic syndrome or in extrinsic allergic alveolitis (hypersensitivity pneumonitis)

IgA excess states
1 Elevated serum levels
   a) Wiskott-Aldrich syndrome
   b) Berger's (IgA nephropathy) disease
   c) Henoch-Schönlein purpura
   d) Alcoholic cirrhosis
   e) Wegener's granulomatosis
2 Positive direct immunofluorescence
   a) Extrarenal
      — Coeliac disease
      — Dermatitis herpetiformis
      — Pyoderma gangrenosum
   b) Renal
      — Berger's disease
      — SLE (IgA_1)
      — Henoch-Schönlein } IgA_2
      — Alcoholic cirrhosis

**Bronchoalveolar lavage fluid in active sarcoid is associated with lymphocytosis, while peripheral blood is characterised by lymphopaenia

ABNORMALITIES OF PLASMA PROTEINS

Differential diagnosis of polyclonal hypergammaglobulinaemia
1 Liver disease
2 Autoimmune disease, connective tissue disease
3 Sarcoidosis
4 Chronic infection
5 Hodgkin's disease, angioimmunoblastic lymphadenopathy
6 AIDS

Dominant polyclonal gammopathy in liver disease
1 Primary biliary cirrhosis — IgM
2 Chronic active hepatitis — IgG
3 Alcoholic cirrhosis — IgA (not invariably)

Secondary causes of hypogammaglobulinaemia
1 Myeloma
  Chronic lymphocytic leukaemia
  Non-Hodgkin's lymphoma
2 Some infections (e.g. EBV, rubella)
3 Nephrotic syndrome
4 Protein-losing enteropathy (e.g. intestinal lymphangiectasia)
5 Thymoma
6 Myotonic dystrophy

Paraproteinaemia: differential diagnosis
1 Benign monoclonal gammopathy (diagnosis of exclusion)
2 Myeloma (IgG > A > BJP only > D > non-secretory > M > E)
  Plasmacytoma
3 Macroglobulinaemia
4 Heavy chain disease*†
5 Non-Hodgkin's lymphoma; chronic lymphocytic leukaemia; essential cryoglobulinaemia; cold haemagglutinin disease (IgM)
6 Primary amyloidosis

Benign monoclonal gammopathy: diagnostic criteria
1 No increase with time
2 No immune paresis (i.e. other Ig levels normal)
3 Normal skeletal survey
4 Paraprotein level
  a) <20 g/l (IgG)
  b) <10 g/l (other)
  c) Absent Bence-Jones protein
5 Marrow plasmacytosis <10%

Components of normal serum protein electrophoresis
1 α Band
  a) α_1AT; $\alpha_1$acid glycoprotein (orosomucoid)
  b) αFP
2 α_2Band
  a) Haptoglobin
  b) Caeruloplasmin
  c) AT III
3 β_1Band — transferrin
  β_2Band — C_3

---

* γ-Heavy chain disease — lymphoma-like syndrome in elderly men
† α-Heavy chain disease — malabsorption in young patients of Mediterranean origin

Abnormal electrophoretic patterns: clinical significance
1 α_1Pallor — α_1AT deficiency
2 β Pallor — frozen or stored specimen leading to *in vitro* C_3 activation
3 γPallor — hypogammaglobulinaemia
4 β-γ fusion
  a) IgA paraproteinaemia
  b) FDPs (DIC)
  c) Alcoholic liver disease
  d) Haemoglobinaemia (intravascular haemolysis)
5 ↓ Albumin } Chronic liver disease (any
  ↑ Gammaglobulin } aetiology)
6 ↓ Albumin
  ↑ $\alpha_2$globulins } Nephrosis
  ↓ Gammaglobulin
7 Appearance of discrete band cathodal to gamma region in serum and urine — lysozyme (e.g. in AMOL, CGL)
8 Strong prealbumin bands
  ↑IgG: albumin ratio } In CSF —
  Oligoclonal IgG bands } multiple sclerosis, neurosyphilis, SSPE
9 Urine
  a) ↑ IgG: transferrin clearance
     — Glomerular disease
  b) ↑ $\beta_2$microglobulin: transferrin clearance
     — Tubular disease
  c) Bizarre EPG
     — Bladder cancer
     — Factitious contamination

THE COMPLEMENT CASCADE

Complement abnormalities in disease
1 Acute phase reaction — ↑ C_3 ↑ C_4 ↑ total haemolytic complement (THC)
2 Classical pathway activation — ↓ C_3 ↓ C_4 ↓ THC
3 Alternate pathway activation
  a) ↓ C_3
  b) Normal C_4
  c) Normal or reduced THC
4 Fluid phase activation
  a) Normal C_3
  b) ↓ ↓ C_4 ↓ THC
  c) ↓ C_1-INH in hereditary angioedema
5 Deficiency of classical pathway component — ↓ ↓ THC
6 Poorly collected specimen — ↓ THC ± ↓ $C_{3,4}$
  Idiopathic angioneurotic oedema — *normal* complement profile

The alternate pathway: its pathogenetic significance
1 Function — non-immune antibody-independent host resistance, e.g. via opsonization
2 Activation
  a) Endotoxin
  b) Bacterial lipopolysaccharide
3 Defectiveness — hyposplenism
4 Pathogenicity
  a) Postinfective glomerulonephritis
  b) Mesangiocapillary glomerulonephritis type II

('dense deposit disease') ± partial lipodystrophy/C_3-nephritic factor
c) Paroxysmal nocturnal haemoglobinuria

Phenotypes associated with primary complement deficiencies

1 C_1-esterase inhibitor (C_1-INH) deficiency — hereditary angioneurotic oedema (see below)
2 C_2 deficiency
   a) Commonest complement deficiency (affects 1 in 10 000)
   b) 50% are symptomatic; 40% develop SLE (even heterozygotes)
   c) SLE tends to be atypical or mild
   d) Pneumococcal/*H. influenzae* sepsis, esp. meningitis
3 $C_{1,q,r,s}$, C_2 or C_4 deficiency — mild SLE, vasculitis, glomerulonephritis, Henoch-Schönlein
4 C_3 deficiency
   a) Most serious complement deficiency
   b) Recurrent lifethreatening infections (encapsulated bacteria)
   c) May arise secondary to factor H, factor I, or C_3b inactivator deficiency
5 Factor H deficiency — associated with haemolytic uraemic syndrome
6 C_5 dysfunction (Leiner's syndrome — presents in infancy) — eczema, Gram-negative infections, diarrhoea
7 C_7 deficiency — Raynaud's phenomenon
8 C_{5-9} deficiency — *Neisseria* (meningococcal/gonococcal) infections
NB: Total haemolytic complement may be undetectable in C_{1q} or C_2 deficiency (may be confusing in clinically mild SLE). All homozygous complement deficiencies are rare except for C_1-INH and C_2 deficiencies

Features of hereditary angioneurotic oedema (C_1-INH deficiency)

1 Presentations
   a) Non-pruritic skin swellings lasting at least 48–72 hours
   b) Recurrent abdominal colic
   c) Upper respiratory tract obstruction
   d) Intestinal pseudo-obstruction
   e) Family history of unexplained asphyxiation (glottal oedema)
2 *No* inflammation, itching or urticaria with attacks
   Normal histamine levels during attacks
   Interictal low C_4
3 Acute management
   a) Purified C_1-esterase inhibitor (if available)
   b) Fresh plasma (caution: contains C_2/C_4 which may precipitate or worsen glottal oedema)
   c) Tracheostomy
4 Prophylaxis
   a) Danazol, stanozolol
   b) EACA, tranexamic acid
5 *Acquired* C1-INH deficiency may be associated with B-cell malignancy or glomerulonephritis

PATHOPHYSIOLOGY OF AUTOIMMUNE DISORDERS

Vasculitis: clinicopathological correlations

1 Large arteries — giant cell arteritis — Takayasu's
2 Medium-size arteries and veins — Buerger's disease
   Venules, veins, venae cavae, arteries — Behçet's disease
3 Small-to-medium arteries and veins — Churg-Strauss; Wegener's
4 Small-to-medium arteries — PAN
5 Arterioles, capillaries; postcapillary venules
   a) Hypersensitivity (leucocytoclastic) vasculitis (intradermal capillaries)
   c) Rheumatoid vasculitis
   d) Henoch-Schönlein purpura

Ultrastructural features of the vasculitides

1 Giant-cell arteritis
   a) Absent fibrinoid necrosis
   b) Moderate giant cell infiltrate
   c) Mononuclear infiltration
2 Wegener's granulomatosis*
   a) Marked fibrinoid necrosis
   b) Marked giant cell infiltrate
   c) Polymorph/mononuclear infiltration
3 Churg-Strauss syndrome
   a) Moderate fibrinoid necrosis
   b) Moderate giant cell infiltrate
   c) Eosinophil infiltration
4 Polyarteritis nodosa
   a) Marked fibrinoid necrosis
   b) Absent giant cells
   c) Polymorph/eosinophil infiltration
5 Hypersensitivity vasculitis
   a) Slight fibrinoid necrosis
   b) Absent giant cells
   c) Polymorph/lymphocyte infiltration
6 Miscellaneous
   a) Intercellular cement Ab (pemphigus)
   b) Anticollagen type II (relapsing polychondritis)
   c) Glutamic acid decarboxylase Ab ('stiff-man' syndrome)

AUTOANTIBODIES

Putative pathogenic autoantibodies†

1 AChRAb (acetylcholine receptor antibody in myasthenia gravis)
   Ab to voltage-gated calcium channels (Eaton-Lambert syndrome)
2 AntiGBM Ab (antiglomerular basement membrane antibody in Goodpasture's syndrome)
3 Anti-Ro Ab (SS-A antibody in congenital heart block)
4 Antiphospholipid Ab (in thrombotic tendency in SLE)

---

* The diagnosis of Wegener's may now be serologically supported by demonstrating presence of *antineutrophil cytoplasmic antibody (ANCA)*; the absence of this sensitive marker makes Wegener's unlikely
† i.e. The autoantibody actually causes the phenotype, rather than being simply an epiphenomenal disease marker

5 Endocrinopathies
   a) TSI (Graves' disease)
   b) ACTH receptor Ab (Addison's disease)
   c) Insulin receptor Ab (type B insulin receptor abnormality associated with acanthosis nigricans)

Diagnostic patterns of antinuclear antibodies
1 Rim (peripheral)
   a) Associated with native (double-stranded) DNA antibodies directed against DNA sugar-phosphate backbone
   b) Relatively specific (but not sensitive) for SLE diagnosis — dsDNA antibodies detected in 60% cases
   c) Typically present in SLE with renal involvement
2 Homogeneous (diffuse)
   a) Associated with histone (or single-stranded DNA) antibodies
   b) Typically present in drug-induced SLE (95% cases)
   c) Antibody titre shows correlation with disease activity
3 Nucleolar
   a) Associated with antibodies to nucleolar RNA
   b) Occurs in scleroderma/Sjögren's/overlap syndromes
4 Speckled — associated with antibodies to non-histone antigens
   a) Sm (in 20% SLE cases, esp. with renal involvement and/or hypocomplementaemia)
   b) nRNP (high titre antibody in MCTD)
   c) SCl-70 (topoisomerase I; antibody in 20% scleroderma)
   d) Centromere — presence of anticentromere antibody indicates CREST syndrome, thus indicating relatively good prognosis in scleroderma but relatively unfavourable prognosis in Raynaud's phenomenon (i.e. suggests progression to scleroderma)
   e) Ro (SS-A) — see below
   f) La (SS B); antibody associated with sicca syndrome
   g) Jo-1 (aminoacyl tRNA synthetase) — antibody associated with polymyositis, esp. with pulmonary fibrosis (25% of dermatomyositis patients will have anti-Jo-1; of these, 80% will have both myositis and lung fibrosis)

Features of ANA-negative SLE
1 Subacute presentation
2 Prominent skin involvement (e.g. photosensitive dermatitis)
3 Thrombocytopenia common
4 Renal and CNS disease unusual
5 Lupus band negative
6 Antibodies to Ro (SS-A) frequently positive

Clinical associations of anti-Ro antibodies
1 Neonatal SLE, esp. with congenital heart block
2 Subacute cutaneous SLE (SCLE)
3 ANA-negative SLE
4 SLE due to homozygous C_2 deficiency
5 Sicca syndrome ('primary' Sjögren's syndrome)

ANTIPHOSPHOLIPID ANTIBODIES

Detection of antiphospholipid antibodies
1 Anticardiolipin antibody tests
2 'Lupus anticoagulant' test
3 Reaginic tests for syphilis (biological false-positives)

What are antiphospholipid antibodies?
1 Anticardiolipin antibody — *one* of the family of antibodies which comprise antiphospholipid activity in plasma
2 The lupus anticoagulant
   a) Detectable in about 30% of SLE patients
   b) Closely related to anticardiolipin antibody
   c) Inhibits interaction between phospholipid moiety of prothrombin activator complex and prothrombin
       → Prolonged PTTK uncorrected by addition of normal plasma (i.e. true 'anticoagulant' action in vitro)
   d) Paradoxical thrombosis in vivo usually unassociated with bleeding (see below)
3 False-positive syphilis reagins
   a) Distinct from lupus anticoagulant and anticardiolipin antibody
   b) Structurally unrelated to antibodies seen in 'true' syphilis
   c) Distinguishable serologically from true syphilis reagins

Vascular complications of antiphospholipid antibody syndrome (Note: only 50% cases have SLE)
1 Placental arterial insufficiency
   a) Recurrent abortions (first-trimester infarctions)
   b) Intrauterine fetal death (second- and third-trimester)
2 CNS arterial insufficiency
   a) TIAs; cerebral infarction; multi-infarct dementia
   b) Vascular myelopathy (e.g. anterior spinal artery thrombosis)
   c) Migraine; central retinal artery occlusion
3 Coronary arterial insufficiency
   a) Myocardial infarction
   b) Coronary graft thrombosis
4 Pulmonary arterial insufficiency — recurrent pulmonary emboli
5 Peripheral arterial insufficiency
   a) Aortic arch syndrome
   b) Axillary arterial thrombosis
   c) Mesenteric arterial thrombosis
   d) Peripheral vascular disease (incl. gangrene)
6 Venous thrombosis
   a) Superficial thrombophlebitis
   b) Deep venous thrombosis
   c) Renal vein thrombosis
   d) Retinal vein thrombosis
   e) Budd-Chiari syndrome

NB: arterial insufficiency in this context is *not* mediated by vasculitis, but by bland *intimal thickening*

Varieties of hypertension associated with antiphospholipid antibodies
1 'Primary' pulmonary hypertension

2 Systemic hypertension (typically labile)
3 Portal venous hypertension

Minor manifestations of antiphospholipid antibodies
1 Thrombocytopenia (± positive Coombs test)
2 Chorea
3 Mitral/aortic valve lesions (Libman-Sachs mucinous valve degeneration)
4 Splenomegaly
5 Livedo reticularis

Bleeding in patients with lupus anticoagulant? Exclude:
1 Thrombocytopenia
2 Hypoprothrombinaemia
3 Factor VIII antibodies

'COLD' AUTOANTIBODIES

The cryopathies: clinicopathological background
1 Cryoglobulinaemia
  a) May be monoclonal or polyclonal (usually IgM)
  b) Clinical manifestations arise due to *precipitation* of immunoglobulins at low temperatures (i.e. below 37°C)
  c) Sequelae include
    — Raynaud's (may progress to gangrene)
    — Purpura (esp. legs)
    — Hepatosplenomegaly; abnormal LFTs
    — Arthralgias, fever
    — Confusion, weakness (hyperviscosity)
    — Renal failure, uraemia (glomerulonephritis)
  d) Aetiological associations
    — Connective tissue disease (e.g. SLE)
    — Myelo-/lymphoproliferative disease (e.g. CLL)
    — Infections: e.g. HBsAg-positive liver disease, postinfectious nephritis
2 Cold agglutinins
  a) Clinical manifestations arise following IgM binding to red cells at low temperatures, leading to complement activation on rewarming to 37°C with resultant *haemolysis* (p. 135)
  b) Less commonly, red cell *autoagglutination* may supervene, leading to vascular obstruction (Raynaud's, acrocyanosis)
  c) Aetiological associations
    — *M. pneumoniae* (anti-I; Rh specificity)
    — Infectious mononucleosis (anti-i)
    — Diffuse large-cell lymphoma
    — Waldenström's macroglobulinaemia
3 Paroxysmal cold haemoglobinuria
  a) Clinical manifestations arise due to low-temperature binding of IgG (Donath-Landsteiner antibody) to P antigen of red cell membrane, leading to complement fixation with resultant *intravascular haemolysis* on rewarming to 37°C
  b) Haemoglobinaemia and transient leucopenia may also occur
  c) Aetiological associations
    — Measles, mumps, varicella
    — Congenital syphilis

4 Cryofibrinogenaemia
  a) Clinical manifestations may include cold urticaria (p. 314)
  b) Aetiological associations
    — Diabetes mellitus
    — Prostate cancer

TISSUE TYPING

HLA antigens in health
1 Encoded on short arm of chromosome 6; highly polymorphic genetic markers
2 HLA A, B, and C antigens (**class I antigens**) are found on most nucleated cells (not on RBCs) except trophoblast
Function — involved in presentation of foreign antigen (usually viral) to *cytotoxic T-cells;* hence mediate graft rejection
3 D-related (DR, or **class II**) antigens are found on:
  a) B-cells (basis of pretransplant MLC)
  b) Activated T-cells
  c) Monocytes and macrophages
  d) Sperm, epididymal cells
Function — involved in presentation of foreign antigen to *helper T-cells*; hence mediate immune-responsiveness
4 Incidence of some HLA-antigens in Caucasian populations:
  a) HLA-A3 — 15%
  b) HLA-B8 — 10%
  c) HLA-B27 — 5–10%
  d) HLA-DR4 — 20–40%

HLA antigens: strongest disease associations
1 HLA-DR2
  a) Present in 20% controls
  b) Present in >95% *narcolepsy* cases (50-fold increased relative risk)
  c) Also present in 80% *Goodpasture's syndrome* (anti-GBM disease) cases
2 HLA-B27
  a) Present in 5–10% controls
  b) Present in 90% *ankylosing spondylitis* cases (75-fold increased relative risk)
  c) Also present in 80% *Reiter's syndrome* cases (25-fold increased relative risk)

Other disease associations with HLA antigens
1 A3 — idiopathic haemochromatosis (also B14)
2 B5
  a) Behçet's disease with ocular or colonic involvement
  b) Takayasu's arteritis
3 B12
  a) Behçet's disease
  b) Minimal lesion nephrosis
4 B27
  a) Psoriatic arthritis ± sacroiliitis
  b) Juvenile chronic arthritis with sacroiliitis
  c) Reactive arthritis
  d) Acute anterior uveitis
  e) Chronic balanitis; chronic prostatitis

f) 'Frozen shoulder'
g) Asbestosis
5 B35 — subacute (de Quervain's, viral) thyroiditis
6 Cw6 — psoriasis vulgaris
   DQ — pemphigus vulgaris
7 DR2
  a) Multiple sclerosis
  b) SLE (esp. with C_2 deficiency)
8 DR3 (and B8)
  a) Primary Sjögren's (sicca) syndrome
  b) Coeliac disease/dermatitis herpetiformis
  c) SLE (esp. neonatal or subacute cutaneous SLE)
  d) Addison's disease; Graves' disease
  e) Insulin-dependent diabetes (also DR4, B15)
  f) HBsAg-negative chronic active hepatitis
  g) Myasthenia gravis
  h) Buerger's disease
  i) Membranous nephropathy
9 DR4
  a) Seropositive RA; secondary Sjögren's syndrome
  b) Polyarticular (RA-like) juvenile chronic arthritis
  c) SLE (iatrogenic); pre-eclampsia (familial)
10 DR5
  a) Pernicious anaemia
  b) Hashimoto's thyroiditis
  c) Early-onset systemic (Still's) juvenile chronic arthritis
  d) HIV-associated sicca syndrome

MANAGING IMMUNOLOGICAL DISEASE

THERAPEUTIC INDICATIONS

Indications for plasmapheresis/plasma exchange
1 Established indications
  a) Hyperviscosity syndrome (acute or maintenance)
  b) Non-oliguric anti-GBM disease (Goodpasture's syndrome)
  c) Myasthenia gravis — crisis or prethymectomy
  d) Life-threatening Guillain-Barré syndrome
  e) Homozygous familial hypercholesterolaemia
2 Anecdotal indications
  a) Severe refractory collagen-vascular disease (e.g. SLE, RA)
  b) Essential mixed cryoglobulinaemia
  c) Refractory thrombocytopenic purpura
     — Idiopathic (ITP)
     — Thrombotic (TTP)
     — Post-transfusion (p. 143–144)

Indications for high-dose intravenous IgG
1 Recent-onset ITP
2 Post-transfusion (thrombocytopenic) purpura
3 Symptomatic hypogammaglobulinaemia in CLL

Other indications for immunoglobulin administration
1 Definite
  a) Primary panhypogammaglobulinaemia
  b) IgM deficiency
  c) Passive immunization (p. 187–188)
2 Relative
  a) Symptomatic hypogammaglobulinaemia in

b) Combined IgA/IgG_2 deficiency
c) T-cell defects with low immunoglobulin levels
   — Ataxia telangiectasia
   — Wiskott-Aldrich syndrome
   — Di George syndrome

Indications for transfer factor*
1 Varicella-zoster prophylaxis in childhood leukaemia
2 Wiskott-Aldrich syndrome
3 Chronic mucocutaneous candidiasis (maintenance therapy; exacerbations are best treated with ketoconazole)
4 Cutaneous leishmaniasis
5 Lepromatous leprosy

Indications for hyposensitization
1 Bee/wasp sting anaphylaxis, or
  Severe reaction with strongly positive prick test
2 Severe refractory allergic rhinitis if symptoms due to pollen/grass/housedust-mite hypersensitivity (not in food allergy)
3 (Major) penicillin allergy if essential for management (e.g. life-threatening enterococcal endocarditis)

Therapeutic modalities in allergic rhinitis
1 Prophylaxis
  a) Sodium cromoglycate (mast cell stabilizer)
  b) Ketotifen† (antihistamine/mast cell stabiliser)
2 Antihistamines
  a) Astemizole (mane) for
  b) prophylaxis   } —No sedative or
     Terfenadine (b.d.) for   anticholinergic
     symptoms   effects
3 Associated nasal obstruction? add inhaled beclomethasone
4 Refractory symptoms — consider hyposensitization

IMMUNOMODULATORY THERAPY*

Alternate-day steroids: guidelines for use
1 Benefits
  a) Less growth retardation in children
  b) Possibly less
     — HPA axis suppression
     — Infective complications
     — Cataracts, aseptic necrosis
2 Problems — tend to be ineffective in remission induction
3 Useful in
  a) Polymyositis
  b) Myasthenia gravis
4 Ineffective in
  a) Giant cell arteritis
  b) Severe rheumatoid arthritis
  c) Chronic active hepatitis
  d) Asthma

---

*A non-antigenic dialysable lymphocyte extract which enhances T-cell function
†Other actions include antianaphylactic, anti-PAF (platelet-activating factor) and inhibition of SRS-A (i.e. leukotrienes C_4, D_4, E_4)
**See also page 303

Therapeutic immunomodulation: which modality?

1 Azathioprine
   a) Renal transplantation
   b) HBsAg-negative chronic active hepatitis
   c) SLE
2 Cyclophosphamide
   a) Wegener's granulomatosis, lymphomatoid granulomatosis
   b) PAN, systemic vasculitis, SLE with renal involvement
3 Methotrexate
   a) Severe psoriasis (e.g. pustular)
   b) Reiter's syndrome
   c) Dermatomyositis, pemphigus (steroid-sparing)
4 Cyclosporin A
   a) Bone marrow transplantation (helps prevent graft rejection in aplasia, GVHD in leukaemia)
   b) Immunosuppression in renal transplantation
   c) Anecdotal
      — Insulin-dependent diabetes (early stage)
      — Graves' ophthalmopathy
      — Chronic uveitis (Behçet's, sarcoid)
5 Antilymphocyte (-thymocyte) globulin
   a) Organ transplantation
   b) Aplastic anaemia

Mechanisms implicated in therapeutic immunomodulation

1 Corticosteroids
   a) Polymorphs
      — ↓ Extravascular egress (impaired chemotaxis)
      — Postphagocytic defect (impaired intracellular killing)
   b) Mononuclears
      — Extravascular sequestration (↓ T-cell number and function)
      — Impaired antibody-antigen uptake
      — ↓ Immunoglobulin synthesis
   c) Eosinopaenia
   d) ↓ Interleukin II levels
2 Azathioprine
   a) Prodrug for 6MP (metabolized in liver)
   b) Reduced lymphocyte proliferation
   c) Impaired lymphokine release
   d) Reduced antibody synthesis
3 Cyclosporin A
   a) Fungal cyclic polypeptide; no lympholytic action
   b) No myelosuppression
   c) ↓ Activation of helper and cytotoxic T-cells (↓ IL-2 release)
   d) Depletion of helper T-cell number
   e) ↓ Interleukin I levels
4 Antilymphocyte globulin
   a) Reduction of circulating lymphocyte pool
   b) Suppression of cell-mediated immunity

General indications for cytotoxic immunosuppression

1 Uncontrolled disease despite maximal non-cytotoxic therapy, esp. if major organ involvement occurs (e.g. in vasculitis, sarcoid)
2 Unacceptable steroid side-effects
3 Organ transplantation
4 Wegener's granulomatosis, PAN

Comparative morbidity of immunomodulatory therapy

1 Azathioprine
   a) Neutropenia; impaired cell-mediated immunity
   b) Cholestasis, pancreatitis
   c) Lymphomas; SCC (skin/cervix)
   d) 4-fold increased bioavailability (and thence toxicity) if given with allopurinol (also true for oral 6MP)
2 Cyclophosphamide
   a) Myelosuppression, sterility, alopecia
   b) Cystitis, bladder fibrosis/carcinoma (avoidable with mesna)
   c) AML (?less frequently than chlorambucil)
3 Methotrexate
   a) Hepatotoxicity (liver fibrosis); occurs with longterm treatment, may be reversible
   b) No demonstrated second malignancy rate
4 Cyclosporin A*
   a) Nephrotoxicity — manifests as prolonged post-transplant oliguria
   b) Lymphoma — may regress on dose reduction (?EBV-induced)
   c) Hypertension — even with normal renal function and renin levels; hyperuricaemia, gout
   d) CNS syndrome — cortical blindness, confusion, pyramidal lesions
   e) Hepatotoxicity, hirsutism, gum hypertrophy, tremor, breast lumps
5 Antilymphocyte globulin
   a) Transfusion reactions
   b) CMV viraemia

Patient evaluation prior to glucocorticoid therapy

1 Urinalysis (glycosuria), urine culture
2 Blood pressure
3 Chest X-ray
4 Measurement of intraocular pressure in patients with diabetes, severe myopia or family history of glaucoma

INTERFERONS

Varieties of interferon

1 α-('leucocyte') interferon
   a) Derived originally from human monocytes/macrophages
   b) Now mainly produced using recombinant techniques
2 β-(fibroblast) interferon
   a) Derived from human fibroblasts
   b) 30% amino acid homology with α-interferon
3 γ-('immune') interferon
   a) Derived from human T-cells
   b) No homology with α- or β-interferon

Physiological actions of interferons

1 Inhibit viral replication (e.g. in chronic HBV infection)
2 Activate NK cells and macrophages
3 Increase HLA antigen expression
4 Increase plasma membrane rigidity

---

*Toxicity potentiated by *ketoconazole*

Indications for α-interferon immunotherapy

1 Established indications — hairy cell leukaemia (90% response rate)
2 Investigational indications
   a) Kaposi's sarcoma in AIDS
   b) CGL (chronic phase); cutaneous T-cell lymphomas
   c) Islet cell tumours, esp. VIPoma
   d) Genital warts; juvenile laryngeal papillomatosis

Toxicity of interferon

1 'Flu-like syndrome; lethargy, somnolence
2 Nausea, vomiting, anorexia, diarrhoea
3 Thrombocytopenia and/or neutropenia
4 Dysgeusia, xerostomia
5 Abnormal liver function tests
6 Reversible cardiac dysfunction

TRANSPLANTATION

Renal transplantation: predictors of successful engraftment

1 ABO compatibility
2 Negative cytotoxic crossmatch (MLC) } Essential
3 HLA-B/DR matching (esp. DR)
4 Prior transfusions } Desirable

Bone marrow transplantation: predictors of successful engraftment

1 Negative cytotoxic crossmatch
2 HLA-B/DR matching
3 Satisfactory number of transplanted marrow cells
4 *No* prior transfusions

Clinical hazards of bone marrow transplantation

1 For immunodeficiency (e.g. Wiskott-Aldrich) — graft-versus-host disease (GVHD) especially
2 For aplastic anaemia — graft rejection especially
3 For acute leukaemia — GVHD, rejection and disease relapse constitute approximately equivalent risks to survival

Classification of transplant rejection

1 Hyperacute — complement-fixing antibodies present in recipient serum prior to transplant; → *irreversible* Ag-Ab reaction usually presenting as graft thrombosis
2 Acute — *potentially reversible* reaction due to cell-mediated immunity; tends to occur unpredictably and at any time
3 Chronic — *irreversible* process due to subendothelial antibody deposition and arteriolar narrowing

Post-transplant malignancies

1 Squamous cell carcinoma of skin
2 Squamous cell carcinoma of cervix (usually in situ)
3 Non-Hodgkin's lymphoma
   a) In azathioprine-treated patients → CNS
   b) In cyclosporin-treated patients → GIT/lung
4 Acute myeloblastic leukaemia (NB: *only* occurs in patients treated with alkylators and/or irradiation)

SYSTEMIC LUPUS ERYTHEMATOSUS: THERAPY

Clinical approach to management dilemmas

1 Problem — steroid-dependent SLE patient with known CNS involvement presents with confusion
   Approach — actively exclude opportunistic CNS infection prior to consideration of definitive therapy
2 Problem — steroid-dependent SLE patient with cerebral involvement presents with psychosis
   Approach — in the absence of fever, focal neurological signs or metabolic derangement, steroid dosage may be cautiously increased in the first instance (steroid-induced psychosis is uncommon)
3 Problem — steroid-dependent SLE patient presents with fever and arthralgias
   Approach — elevated C_3, C_4 and C-reactive protein suggest sepsis; low C_3, C_4 and C-reactive protein are consistent with primary disease activity
4 Problem — undiagnosed patient on maintenance phenytoin presents with convulsions; investigations reveal high-titre ANA
   Approach — check serum levels of phenytoin and dsDNA Ab, keeping in mind that iatrogenic LE rarely causes cerebral manifestations or positive dsDNA Abs
5 Problem — patient with clinically mild SLE, normal renal function and normal urinary sediment is noted to have persistently low complement levels
   Approach — check levels of individual complement components to exclude primary deficiency (see p. 159)
6 Problem — patient with SLE develops focal neurological signs
   Approach — exclude cerebral infarction with (serial) CT scans, esp. if lupus anticoagulant present; exclude meningoencephalitis with CSF examination, and neurosyphilis with FTA-ABS (serum); then treat as for cerebral vasculitis
7 Problem — patient with SLE develops DVT, and routine coagulation screen prior to heparinization reveals thrombocytopenia and prolonged PTTK
   Approach — confirm immune aetiology of abnormalities with bone marrow aspirate (→ plentiful megakaryocytes) and lupus inhibitor screen; commence (or increase) steroids to normalize platelet count; then heparinize

Principles of drug therapy in SLE

1 Minimally symptomatic disease — withhold medication
2 Tenosynovitis, arthralgias, pleurisy — NSAIDs (except aspirin: potentially hepatotoxic)
3 Skin disease and/or joint symptoms resistant to NSAIDs — hydroxychloroquine 200 mg/day
4 Refractory arthritis (sepsis excluded)
   Immune leucopenia/thrombocytopenia
   Fevers } —Prednisone 20 mg/day
5 Immune haemolysis
   Pneumonitis, peritonitis —Prednisone 40 mg/day
   Myositis

6 Myopericarditis
Focal glomerulonephritis
Vasculitis, neuropathy
—Prednisone 60 mg/day (considered to prolong survival)

7 Diffuse proliferative glomerulonephritis
Membranous glomerulonephritis
—Pulse i.v. methylprednisolone 120 mg/day, *plus* azathioprine or cyclophosphamide*

8 Cerebral lupus
—Exclude infection, use anticonvulsants, and tailor immunosuppression empirically

NB: If prolonged therapy > 10 mg/day prednisone is required, then azathioprine may be added as a steroid-sparing agent

Incidence, therapy and prognosis of lupus nephritis*
1 40% of SLE patients develop clinical nephritis within 1 year
2 65% of SLE patients develop clinical nephritis within 5 years
3 90% of SLE patients will be found to have an abnormal renal biopsy
4 WHO type II or V — 10–15% progress to renal failure within 5 years
5 WHO type III, IV — 20–30% progress to renal failure within 5 years
6 Pulsed cyclophosphamide is the treatment of choice for patients with WHO type III/IV nephritis and/or nephrotic syndrome

CNS lupus: recent advances
1 Evidence of CNS *vasculitis* is rare; the most common pathology is a non-inflammatory vasculopathy with widespread microinfarcts
2 Vasculitis *may* manifest with extracerebral disease, e.g. cranial nerve palsies, basal meningitis; similar manifestations may be due to antiphospholipid antibodies
3 Recent reports suggest that *antineuronal antibodies* may be present in up to 80% of CSF specimens in patients with clinical CNS lupus
4 Other reports suggest that antibodies to *ribosomal P antigen* in neuronal cytoplasm are detectable in the serum of 90% of psychotic lupus patients
5 The presence of such autoantibodies *may* prove to be useful in distinguishing primary CNS lupus from iatrogenic steroid psychosis

Pathogeneses of CNS disease in SLE
1 Focal CNS pathology
e.g. chorea, cranial nerve palsies, stroke
a) Bland thrombosis due to antiphospholipid antibodies
b) Immune-complex deposition
c) Vasculitis
2 Diffuse CNS pathology

*Considered to delay onset and progression of renal disease, and to prolong survival even when proteinuria established

e.g. seizures, psychosis
a) ?Antineuronal antibodies
b) Iatrogenic (steroid-induced)

Therapeutic modalities in Raynaud's phenomenon
1 Cold avoidance (effective in 50% of all patients)
Other general measures
a) Stop smoking (in Buerger's disease)
b) Cessation of β-blockers, ergotamine
2 Glyceryl trinitrate 2% ointment (works only transiently)
3 Oral nifedipine 30–60 mg/day or diltiazem 120 mg/day (effective in 50% of patients requiring medication)
4 Special circumstances
a) Ketanserin, dazoxiben (serotonin antagonists; more effective than nifedipine in sclerodermatous Raynaud's)
b) Sympathectomy (occasionally used in Raynaud's of the feet; contraindicated in primary Raynaud's disease confined to the hands)
5 Acute management
a) Intra-arterial reserpine
b) Plasma exchange (esp. in cryoglobulinaemia)
c) Haemodilution (for incipient digital necrosis)
6 Experimental therapies
a) Prostacyclin
b) ACE inhibitors
c) Stanozolol (a fibrinolytic steroid)

UNDERSTANDING IMMUNOLOGICAL DISEASE

Idiotypes, anti-idiotypic antibodies, and all that
1 The *class* of an antibody (IgG, IgM, etc.) is its *isotype*
2 A given antibody can be further characterized by the composition of its highly variable heavy and light chain regions, where antigen and antibody combine (i.e. its Fab fragment); these specific variations in antibody structure constitute its *idiotype*
3 The particular antigenic determinants comprising a given idiotype are termed *idiotopes*
4 Any one immunoglobulin contains many idiotopes; it can therefore generate a large number of *anti-idiotypic antibodies* raised against these antigens (cf. rheumatoid factors — antibodies raised against the constant Fc portion of the antibody)
5 It is thought that an individual can generate over 100 million different antibodies. The ability of the immune system to develop its own 'network' of anti-idiotypic (auto)antibodies seems likely to play a key role in the creation of this diversity.
6 High doses of anti-idiotypic antibodies may lead to immediate suppression of a specific antibody reaction
7 Circulating idiotype/anti-idiotype immune complexes have been demonstrated, e.g. in cryoglobulinaemia

8 A reciprocal relationship between idiotypic and anti-idiotypic anti-DNA antibodies has been reported in SLE, with the anti-idiotypes being present in convalescent sera but not in active disease

Regulatory functions of interleukins

1 Interleukin I (IL-1) — following antigen recognition, IL-1 is released by activated macrophages, leading to stimulation of helper (CD4+) T-cells with release of IL-2; also induces proliferation of activated B-cells
2 Interleukin-2 (IL-2, T-cell growth factor, — induces proliferation of T-cells and probably also natural killer (NK) cells; stimulates IFN-gamma production
3 Interleukin-3 (IL-3, multi-CSF) — released by T-cells and other cells; stimulates growth of most haemopoietic stem cells

Lymphocytes: functional aspects

1 B-cells
   a) Defence against extracellular bacteria, protozoa
   b) Prevention of viral reinfection in immune host
2 T-cells
   a) Defence against intracellular bacteria
   b) Defence against viruses (esp. herpesviruses), fungi and protozoa
3 K ('killer') cells
   a) Mediate antibody-dependent cell-mediated cytotoxicity (ADCC), e.g. against measles
4 NK ('natural killer') cells
   a) Non-antigen specific action
   b) Postulated but unproven role in 'tumour surveillance'

CLINICAL IMMUNE DEFECTS

Clinical patterns of lymphocyte dysfunction

1 Ataxia-telangiectasia (Louis-Bar syndrome)
   a) $\downarrow$ IgA
   b) $\downarrow$ Cell-mediated immunity
   c) →Recurrent sinopulmonary infections
   d) May terminate as lymphoma
2 Wiskott-Aldrich syndrome (WAS)
   a) $\downarrow$ IgM; $\uparrow$ IgA/E
   b) $\downarrow$ Cell-mediated immunity
   c) $\downarrow$ Platelets
   d) →Eczema, abscesses, bleeding
   e) May terminate as lymphoma

Infective complications of compromised immunity

1 Defective cell-mediated immunity (sarcoid, Hodgkin's, Nezelof's, CMC)
   a) Intracellular bacteria (TB, *Listeria*)
   b) Candidiasis, cryptococcosis
   c) CMV, HZ
   d) *Pneumocystis,* toxoplasmosis, atypical mycobacteria
2 Hypogammaglobulinaemia (incl. CLL, myeloma)
   a) Extracellular bacteria (pneumococcus, *H. influenzae*, staphylococci); *Mycoplasma* (septic arthritis, pneumonia)
   b) Enteroviral CNS infections (e.g. ECHO, esp. in Bruton's)

c) Warts ($\downarrow$ IgM); giardiasis, *Campylobacter* enteritis
3 Hyposplenism — encapsulated bacteria (pneumococci, *H. influenzae, Salmonella* spp., *Neisseria* spp.); babesiosis
4 Hypocomplementaemia
   a) $\downarrow$ C_3 →recurrent pyogenic infections
   b) $\downarrow$ $C_{6,7,8}$ → *Neisseria*
5 Combined B- and T-cell defects (CLL, SCID, WAS, Louis-Bar)
   a) Recurrent sinopulmonary infections (CMV, Gram-negatives, anaerobes, *S. aureus*)
6 Steroid therapy, aspergillosis, *P. carinii*

PROBLEMS WITH POLYMORPHS

Clinical patterns of leucocyte dysfunction

1 Chédiak-Higashi syndrome
   a) $\downarrow$ Neutrophil number and function ($\downarrow$ intracellular killing)
   b) $\downarrow$ K/NK cell function
   c) Associated with partial oculocutaneous albinism
   d) → Giant lysosomes, defective microtubules, myeloperoxidase deficiency
   e) Treatable with vitamin C
2 Chronic granulomatous disease of childhood (CGDC)
   a) $\downarrow$ Intracellular killing (postphagocytic defect)
   b) $\downarrow$ H_2O_2 generation
   c) +NBT test (diagnostic)
   d) → Staphylococcal/Gram-negative infections
3 Job's/hyper-IgE syndrome
   a) $\downarrow$ Intracellular killing
   b) $\downarrow$ T-cell number
   c) $\uparrow$ IgE
   d) → Recurrent staphylococcal abscesses, *H. influenzae* infections, herpes
4 'Lazy leucocyte' syndrome: $\downarrow$ chemotaxis
5 Leucocyte adhesion deficiency
   a) Defective β-chain of lymphocyte-function-associated Ag (LFA-1)
   b) Associated with neutrophilia, but absent pus formation
   c) Severe bacterial childhood infections (e.g. pneumonia)

Infective complications of neutrophil dysfunction

1 Neutropenia
   a) Pneumonia (enterococci, Gram-negatives, *S. aureus, Aspergillus*)
   b) Perirectal suppuration
   c) Pharyngostomatitis (esp. candidal)
   d) Recurrent bacteraemias
2 Defective neutrophil chemotaxis (steroids, diabetes, alcoholism, burns)
   a) Frequently subclinical
   b) → Abscesses, cellulitis (*S. aureus,* β-haemolytic strep, *Ps. aeruginosa*)
3 Defective intracellular killing (CGDC, Job's, Chédiak-Higashi)
   a) Abscesses (*E. coli, S. aureus*)
   b) Septic arthritis/osteomyelitis (*Salmonella* spp., *Serratia marcescens*)

Neutropenia: strategies for regenerating the white cells

1 G-CSF or GM-CSF therapy
2 Red cell hypertransfusion
3 Lithium carbonate
4 Immunosuppressive therapy (in autoimmune neutropaenia)

IMMUNE-DEFICIENT STATES IN ADULT LIFE

Selective IgA deficiency: clinical features
(surface IgA present *but* B-cells fail to differentiate to plasma cells)

1 Sinopulmonary infections ($\pm$ coexisting $\downarrow$ IgG$_2$)
2 Giardiasis (severe and prolonged)
3 Associated autoimmune diathesis/atopy (e.g. asthma)
4 Anaphylactic reactions triggered by small amounts of IgA in transfusions (blood or plasma) or gammaglobulin

Common variable hypogammaglobulinaemia: complications
(*normal* B-cell number — cf. Bruton's — but failure to differentiate into plasma cells and secrete immunoglobulins)

1 Allergies; autoimmune diathesis
2 Gastrointestinal complications
   a) Giardiasis
   b) Gluten-sensitive enteropathy/dermatitis herpetiformis
   c) Nodular lymphoid hyperplasia
   d) Achlorhydria/atrophic gastritis; 50$\times$ $\uparrow$ gastric cancer
3 Splenomegaly; lung/liver granulomata
4 Polyarthritis (reversible with gammaglobulin therapy)
5 Thymoma, esp. in late-onset disease (i.e. onset after 40 years)

SECONDARY IMMUNE DEFECTS

Aetiology of acquired hyposplenism

1 Splenectomy (the incidence of serious sepsis following splenectomy is 1% in children, 0.1% in adults)
2 Autosplenectomy (repeated infarction in sickle cell disease)
3 Coeliac disease
4 Rare
   a) Ulcerative colitis
   b) Amyloidosis
   c) Sarcoidosis
   d) Thyrotoxicosis
   e) Carcinomatosis

Clinical associations of thymoma

1 Myasthenia gravis (40%)
2 Pure red cell aplasia (*not* corrected by thymectomy)
3 Common variable hypogammaglobulinaemia
4 Chronic mucocutaneous candidiasis
5 Autoimmune disease
   a) Sjögren's syndrome
   b) SLE
   c) Dermatomyositis

d) Hashimoto's/Graves' disease
e) Pemphigus

Predispositions to recurrent candidiasis

1 Steroids (incl. oestrogens); pregnancy
2 Iron deficiency
3 Diabetes mellitus
4 Broad-spectrum antibiotic therapy
5 T-cell defects

Predispositions to recurrent boils

1 Idiopathic
2 Diabetes mellitus
3 Hypogammaglobulinaemia
4 Hypocomplementaemia
5 Job's/hyper-IgE syndrome

Skin infections in immunosuppressed patients

1 'Transplant elbow' — *Staph. aureus*
2 Cellulitis — streptococci
3 Opportunistic bacteria — *Nocardia,* atypical mycobacteria
4 Gram-negative sepsis metastatic to skin
5 Fungi — *Aspergillus, Cryptococcus*
6 Dermatophytes
7 Viruses — HSV, V-Z; HPV

HIV INFECTION AND THE ACQUIRED IMMUNODEFICIENCY SYNDROME

Immunological abnormalities in the AIDS patient

1 T-cells
   a) $\downarrow$ helper (CD4+) T-cell number
   b) $\downarrow$ T-cell function ($\downarrow$ IL-2/IFN-α response to Ag)
   c) $\downarrow$ cytotoxic (CD8+) T-cell response to HIV-infected cells
   d) Cutaneous anergy
2 B-cells
   a) $\downarrow$ function ($\downarrow$ humoral response to vaccination)
   b) Activation/proliferation $\rightarrow$ polyclonal hypergammaglobulinaemia
3 NK cells — $\downarrow$ number and function
4 Monocytes/macrophages — $\downarrow$ function ($\downarrow$ IL-1 production, chemotaxis, Ag presentation)

Clinical spectrum of HIV infection

1 Asymptomatic
2 Mononucleosis-like syndrome (p. 178)
3 AIDS-related complex (persistent generalized lymphadenopathy $\pm$ sweats, fever, weight loss; 'AIDS prodrome')
4 AIDS

High-risk transmission modes for HIV infection

1 *Blood-borne* transmission
   a) Needle sharing, e.g. heroin addicts
   b) Multiple transfusions, esp. haemophiliacs
   c) Transplacental/peripartum neonatal infection
2 *Venereal* transmission
   a) Homosexuals, esp. if practising unprotected receptive anal intercourse
   b) Prostitutes (female or male)
   c) Promiscuous heterosexuals, esp. if uncircumcised or with genital ulceration

Occurrence of Kaposi's sarcoma in HIV-infected cohorts
1 Seen commonly in homosexuals with AIDS
2 Seen occasionally in intravenous drug abusers with AIDS
3 Seen rarely in haemophiliacs with AIDS

NB: Incidence of Kaposi's in homosexuals with AIDS is now reportedly declining

Current status of HIV antibody testing
1 HIV ELISA is the best screen (definitive test? Western blot)
2 ELISA may remain negative for 3–6 months postinfection (i.e. negative test does *not* exclude HIV infection unless *no* risk factors for previous 6 months)
3 ELISA is 99% sensitive if performed > 6 months postinfection
4 ELISA has a significant false-positive rate; hence, all positives need to be confirmed using Western blot
5 ELISA+ neonates of infected mothers are *not* necessarily infected by HIV
6 Some patients with AIDS do not have detectable ELISA antibody; whether all 'true' antibody-positive patients develop AIDS remains uncertain

Commonest infective complications of AIDS
1 CMV
2 *Pneumocystis carinii*
3 *Mycobacterium avium-intracellulare*
4 Cryptococcosis

Infective complications of early HIV infection
1 Oral candidiasis
2 Herpesviruses — herpes zoster, recurrent herpes simplex
3 Staphylococcal leukoplakia
4 Oral hairy leukoplakia (EBV)
5 Antibiotic hypersensitivity reactions

Infective complications of advanced HIV infection
1 *Pneumocystis carinii* pneumonia
2 CMV infection, esp. pneumonitis/retinitis/colitis
3 Invasive mucosal candidiasis, esp. oesophageal
4 Cryptococcosis, aspergillosis
5 Intestinal cryptosporidiosis
6 Disseminated strongyloidiasis
7 Toxoplasmosis, esp. CNS
8 Mycobacterial infections, esp. *avium-intracellulare* (→ marrow depression)

Indirect sequelae of HIV infection
(i.e. precipitated by immunodeficiency per se rather than by HIV)
1 Progressive multifocal leucoencephalopathy (JC virus)
2 Cerebral lymphoma (EBV)
3 Kaposi's sarcoma (?)

Approach to infective complications in the AIDS patient
1 Infections for which effective therapy exists:
   a) *P. carinii* pneumonia — the most frequent opportunistic infection (Rx: cotrimoxazole or pentamidine)
   b) Toxoplasmosis, e.g. cerebral mass lesions (Rx: sulphadiazine + pyrimethamine + leucovorin)
   c) Cryptococcosis, e.g. meningitis or disseminated infection (Rx: amphotericin B alone; 5-FC too myelosuppressive here)
   d) Candidiasis (Rx: topical clotrimazole or nystatin. For refractory or disseminated disease, or for oesophagitis, use ketoconazole or amphotericin B)
2 Infections for which promising experimental therapy exists — CMV: ganciclovir, DHPG (dihydropropoxymethylguanine), foscarnet
3 Infections for which no effective therapy exists:
   a) Cryptosporidiosis
   b) *M. avium-intracellulare* (occurs in up to 40% of patients)

Predictors of poor prognosis
1 Advanced disease, late presentation, poor physical condition
2 Marked anaemia
3 CD4+ lymphocyte count < 100/mm^3
4 Loss of p24 antibody; p24 antigenaemia
5 Female sex (prognosis generally worse than for males)

ZIDOVUDINE (AZT) THERAPY

Benefits of zidovudine therapy in AIDS
1 Improved survival (if treatment commenced early)
2 Improved functional capacity
3 Fewer (and less severe) opportunistic infections
4 Weight gain
5 Improved CD4+ lymphocyte number
6 Reduced HIV p24 antigenaemia

Limitations of zidovudine therapy
1 Inhibits retroviral reverse transcriptase (thus preventing HIV infection of new CD4+ cells) but does *not* eradicate established intracellular HIV
2 Transient efficacy (see ref. 6.3)
3 Toxicity, esp. macrocytic anaemia/neutropenia
4 Short half-life; 4-hourly dosage interval required*
5 Expense

DRUG-INDUCED IMMUNOLOGIC DISORDERS

Pathogenesis of drug fever
1 Hypersensitivity reactions
   a) Penicillins, sulphonamides
   b) Methyldopa; hydralazine (SLE)
   c) D-penicillamine
2 Antituberculosis drugs — INH, PAS, rifampicin, streptomycin
3 Cytotoxics — bleomycin, L-asparaginase
4 Dose-related pyrogens — amphotericin B
5 Thermoregulatory dysfunction

---

*Though this may be prolonged by probenecid

a) Anticholinergics (impaired sweating)
b) Phenothiazines (hypothalamic effect)
6 Overdosage — aspirin; iodine (may induce transient hyperthyroidism)
7 Drug abuse — amphetamines, LSD, barbiturates, i.v. cocaine; laxatives
8 Drug withdrawal — corticosteroids
9 Malignant hyperthermia — anaesthetic agents, esp. inhalational
10 Rare (unlikely) causes
a) Digoxin
b) Chloramphenicol, tetracycline
c) Monocomponent insulin

Anaphylaxis: most frequent iatrogenic causes
1 Penicillins
2 Insulin
3 Streptomycin
4 Intravenous vitamin K
5 Iron dextran infusion

Anaphylactoid reactions: frequent causes
1 Aspirin
2 Codeine, morphine
3 Gammaglobulin administration
4 Anaesthetic agents (e.g. thiopentone)
5 Iodinated contrast agents (esp. in venography)

Cross-reactive drug sensitivity
1 ρ-Aminobenzoates
a) Sulphonamides
b) Sulphonylureas
c) Thiazides
d) Phenothiazines
e) Procainamide
f) Acetazolamide
2 Penicillins
a) Penicillin G
b) Semisynthetic penicillins
c) Penicillamine
d) Cephalosporins
3 Allopurinol-induced maculopapular rash is commoner in patients with past history of ampicillin rash, esp. if renal dysfunction coexists (ampicillin rash is also commoner in allopurinol patients)

Clinical aspects of penicillin hypersensitivity
1 *Allergic* reactions most commonly occur with semisynthetic penicillins; such reactions represent **'major determinant'** (i.e. penicilloyl group of the cleaved β-lactam ring) hypersensitivity mediated by IgG/IgM antibodies
2 True IgE-dependent *anaphylactic* reactions are rare (incidence 0.05%, mortality 0.0002%); such reactions most commonly occur with parenteral administration, esp. of benzylpenicillin, and represent **minor determinant** (penilloate, penicillin, or penicilloic acid), or hapten, hypersensitivity
3 *Fatal* anaphylactic reactions usually occur in patients with *no* known past history of penicillin allergy or atopy. To confirm a suspected past history of anaphylaxis, prick testing is indicated
4 85% of patients with a history of minor reactions can be re-exposed without toxicity, possibly indicating transient sensitization. The only major contraindication is that of true anaphylaxis.
5 Cephalosporin cross-sensitization does occur, but is uncommon
6 Rarely, if penicillin is required for a serious bacterial infection in a patient with a history of penicillin-induced anaphylaxis, temporary desensitization may be undertaken and completed within 4 hours. Desensitization works by raising the cell threshold to IgE; it cannot effectively be performed using steroid or antihistamine cover

Reviewing the Literature: Immunology

6.1 Bolton A E et al 1987 Identification of placental protein 14 as an immunosuppressive factor in human reproduction. Lancet i: 593–595

First reported isolation of the putative physiological immunosuppressant of pregnancy

6.2 Barre-Sinoussi F et al 1983 Isolation of a T-cell lymphotropic virus from a patient at risk from the acquired immunodeficiency syndrome (AIDS). Science 220: 868–870

Initial report from the French group linking HIV retrovirus to AIDS

6.3 Yarchoan R et al 1986 Administration of AZT, an inhibitor of HIV replication, to patients with AIDS. Lancet i: 575–578

Report from the NIH group suggesting therapeutic benefit to AIDS patients from azidodideoxythymidine, an inhibitor of viral reverse transcriptase; the drug prevents new cells becoming infected, but does not eradicate established intracellular HIV infection

Claude Bernard Hospital AZT Study Group 1988 Effects of zidovudine in 365 consecutive patients with AIDS or AIDS-related complex. Lancet ii: 1297–1302

Disappointing results, showing only transient (less than 6 months) benefit for symptomatic HIV-infected patients; initial weight gain and increase in CD4+ cell number were not maintained. Marrow suppression led to interruption of therapy in many patients, and the authors speculate that AZT may in fact be toxic to CD4+ cells

6.4 European Collaborative Study 1988 Mother-to-child transmission of HIV infection. Lancet ii: 1039–1042

Vertical transmission rate of HIV was estimated to be at least 24% (and probably greater) on the basis of this trial of 271 children born to infected mothers. Median age of (passive) antibody loss was 10 months

6.5 Loche M, Mach B 1988 Identification of HIV-infected seronegative individuals by a direct diagnostic test based on hybridization to amplified viral DNA. Lancet ii: 418–21

Laure F et al 1988 Detection of HIV1 DNA in infants and children by means of the polymerase chain reaction. Lancet ii: 538–540

New assays for HIV detection based on recombinant DNA technology

Horsburgh C R et al 1989 Duration of human immunodeficiency virus infection before detection of antibody. Lancet ii: 626—630

Time of HIV infection was determined in this study by PCR of HIV DNA using *gag* and *env* primers, and the interval elapsing before (antibody) seroconversion then calculated. On average, seroconversion occurred within 2 months of exposure (95% within 5 months). Hence, seronegativity for 6 months following 'risk' behaviour appears to indicate lack of infection in the vast majority.

6.6 Hamsten A et al 1986 Antibodies to cardiolipin in young survivors of myocardial infarction: an association with recurrent cardiovascular events. Lancet i: 113–115

More than 20% of 62 young infarct survivors were shown to have anticardiolipin antibody (an antiphospholipid antibody related to both the lupus anticoagulant and chronic false-positive reaginic syphilis serology); the risk for further vascular events correlated with antibody titre

Muller S et al 1988 Presence of antibodies to ubiquitin during the autoimmune response associated with systemic lupus erythematosus. Proceedings of the National Academy of Sciences of the USA 85: 8176–8180

80% of SLE patients possessed ubiquitin antibodies, compared with only 16% of controls

6.7 Balow J E et al 1984 Effect of treatment on the evolution of renal abnormalities in lupus nephritis. New England Journal of Medicine 311: 491–495

Cytotoxic drugs were shown to result in significantly less renal failure than was associated with corticosteroid treatment alone

6.8 Kyle R A et al 1985 Primary systemic amyloidosis: comparison of melphalan/prednisone versus colchicine. American Journal of Medicine 79: 708–716

Prospective crossover trial of 101 patients suggesting that melphalan/prednisone is the most effective therapy for monoclonal immunocytic amyloidosis

6.9 Gustafsson R et al 1989 Cold-induced reversible myocardial ischaemia in systemic sclerosis. Lancet ii: 475–477

Reversible cold-induced defects in myocardial thallium uptake suggests that 'coronary Raynaud's' may indeed contribute to the (often asymptomatic) cardiac fibrosis recognised in scleroderma

6.10 Stark B S et al 1987 Acute and chronic desensitization of penicillin-allergic patients using oral penicillin. Journal of Allergy and Clinical Immunology 79: 523–532

25 of 26 penicillin-allergic patients were successfully desensitized using increasing doses of oral phenoxymethylpenicillin at 15-minute intervals (acute desensitization), and only 12 of these had allergic reactions; in two-thirds of these patients, skin tests for penicillin allergy became negative. 7 patients successfully underwent chronic desensitization using b.d. oral penicillin

CHAPTER 7

Infectious diseases

Physical examination protocol 7.1 You are asked to examine a patient with fever of unknown origin

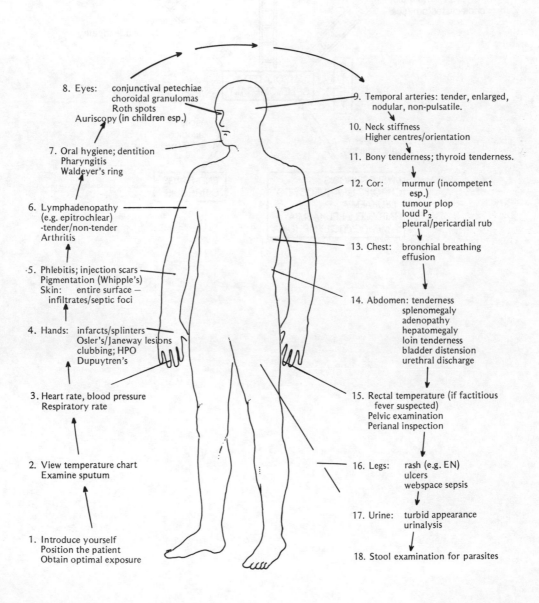

8. Eyes: conjunctival petechiae
            choroidal granulomas
            Roth spots
            Auriscopy (in children esp.)

7. Oral hygiene; dentition
   Pharyngitis
   Waldeyer's ring

6. Lymphadenopathy
   (e.g. epitrochlear)
   -tender/non-tender
   Arthritis

5. Phlebitis; injection scars
   Pigmentation (Whipple's)
   Skin: entire surface —
            infiltrates/septic foci

4. Hands: infarcts/splinters
            Osler's/Janeway lesions
            clubbing; HPO
            Dupuytren's

3. Heart rate, blood pressure
   Respiratory rate

2. View temperature chart
   Examine sputum

1. Introduce yourself
   Position the patient
   Obtain optimal exposure

9. Temporal arteries: tender, enlarged,
   nodular, non-pulsatile.

10. Neck stiffness
    Higher centres/orientation

11. Bony tenderness; thyroid tenderness.

12. Cor: murmur (incompetent
             esp.)
             tumour plop
             loud P_2
             pleural/pericardial rub

13. Chest: bronchial breathing
             effusion

14. Abdomen: tenderness
             splenomegaly
             adenopathy
             hepatomegaly
             loin tenderness
             bladder distension
             urethral discharge

15. Rectal temperature (if factitious
    fever suspected)
    Pelvic examination
    Perianal inspection

16. Legs: rash (e.g. EN)
             ulcers
             webspace sepsis

17. Urine: turbid appearance
             urinalysis

18. Stool examination for parasites

Diagnostic pathway 7.1 The patient has an enlarged spleen. Which aetiologies would you suspect most strongly?

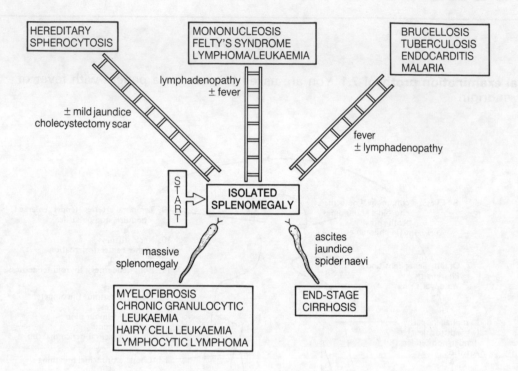

CLINICAL ASPECTS OF INFECTIOUS DISEASE

COMMONEST INFECTIOUS DISEASE SHORT CASES

1 Pneumonia
2 Infective endocarditis

Fever of unknown origin: priorities in history-taking
1 Past medical history
   a) Rheumatic fever
   b) Tuberculosis
   c) Splenectomy
2 Recent drug use
   a) Antibiotics
   b) Alcohol
   c) Intravenous narcotics
3 Recent foreign travel
4 Recent sexual contacts and practices
5 Animal exposure (occupational or domestic)
6 Family history and racial background

Factitious fever: clinical clues
1 Patient's apparent well-being
2 Normal physical examination, cool skin, no sweating
3 No correlation between fever spikes and heart rate
4 Consistently normal rectal temperature
5 Dramatic fluctuations of temperature, often >41°C
6 Absence of normal diurnal variation
7 Normal WCC, ESR
8 Recovery of multiple and/or unusual organisms in blood or urine culture
9 Typical patient profile: young, female, (para)medically trained

Differential diagnosis of night sweats
1 Pulmonary tuberculosis
2 Lymphoma
3 Brucellosis; abscess; endocarditis
4 Alcoholic withdrawal
5 Nocturnal hypoglycaemia
   Nocturnal dyspnoea
   Nightmares

TUBERCULOSIS: CLINICAL

Skin manifestations of TB
1 Primary skin inoculation — ulcer with regional adenopathy
2 Lupus vulgaris — nodules, scarring → face and neck
3 Scrofuloderma — cervical adenopathy, skin fixation
4 Erythema nodosum — signifies onset of Mantoux reactivity
5 Erythema induratum (Bazin's disease) — cyanotic nodules on calves with central necrosis

Manifestations commoner in primary infections
1 Pleurisy and/or large pleural effusion (may follow rupture of peripheral caseous foci). Lower zone infiltrate ±ipsilateral hilar adenopathy
2 Cervical adenopathy
3 Erythema nodosum
4 Phlyctenular conjunctivitis
5 Acute miliary dissemination

Time-course of possible sequelae following untreated primary TB
1 First 3–4 weeks post-inoculation
   a) Positive tuberculin test
   b) Erythema nodosum
   c) Fevers
   d) Phlyctenular conjunctivitis   }—Esp. in children
2 After 4–8 weeks — appearance of primary focus on CXR
3 After 2–6 months — pleural effusion
4 After 3–12 months
   a) Bronchial rupture (erosion by caseating nodes)
   b) Tuberculous meningitis
   c) Miliary TB
5 After 1–3 years — bone and joint involvement
6 After 5 years
   a) Skin involvement
   b) Renal involvement

Potentially misleading clinical presentations of TB
1 Night sweats, hilar adenopathy
   Misdiagnosis — lymphoma
2 PUO, choroidal granulomata, splenomegaly, granulomatous hepatitis, erythema nodosum
   Misdiagnosis — sarcoidosis
3 Right iliac fossa mass and/or ileitis on barium studies
   Misdiagnosis — Crohn's disease, yersiniosis, actinomycosis
4 Ureteric stricture(s)
   Misdiagnosis — idiopathic (steroid-responsive) retroperitoneal fibrosis
5 Headache, nausea, meningism, CSF lymphocytosis with negative Gram-stain
   Misdiagnosis — viral meningitis
6 Constrictive pericarditis
   Misdiagnosis — restrictive cardiomyopathy, attributed to (for example) endomyocardial fibrosis in African migrant
7 Bloodstained ascites
   Misdiagnosis — abdominal malignancy
8 Scrotal (epididymal) mass
   Misdiagnoses — tumour, syphilitic (testicular) gumma

Clinical features of tuberculous meningitis
1 Significance — potentially life-threatening
2 Onset — subacute (days–weeks)
3 Symptoms and signs
   a) Fever
   b) Headache, meningism
   c) Impaired consciousness
4 Complications
   a) Hydrocephalus, cerebral oedema, convulsions
   b) Cranial nerve palsies
   c) Arachnoiditis; hemiparesis
   d) SIADH

NON-TUBERCULOUS MYCOBACTERIA

Pathogenic significance of non-tuberculous mycobacteria
1 Rarely if ever transmitted between humans
2 Clinical pattern of involvement similar to that of TB
3 Positive culture does not necessarily indicate pathogenicity since laboratory contaminants are common; at least two positive cultures should be obtained for diagnosis

Clinical spectrum of non-tuberculous mycobacterial disease
1 Pulmonary
  a) *M. avium-intracellulare*
     — Commonest, most serious pathogen
     — Predilection for diseased lungs or AIDS
     — Resistant to therapy (20% die)
  b) *M. fortuitum/chelonei*
     — Predilection for diseased lungs
     — Responds poorly to therapy
  c) *M. kansasii*
     — Responds well to therapy
  d) *M. xenopi, M. szulgai, M. simiae*
     — Rare
2 Skin/soft tissue
  a) *M. marinum*
     — Swimming-pool granuloma
     — Responds poorly to drug therapy
     — Usually resolves spontaneously
  b) *M. ulcerans*
     — Responds poorly to drug therapy
     — Treat by excision
  c) *M. fortuitum/chelonei*
     — Occurs following trauma or surgery
     — Best treated by initial debridement
3 Lymphadenitis (esp. cervical)
  a) *M. scrofulaceum*
     — Occurs in healthy children
     — Best treated by excision
     — Responds poorly to drug therapy
  b) *M. avium-intracellulare*
     — Treat by excision (see also p. 183–4)

SEXUALLY TRANSMITTED DISEASES

Skin signs of secondary syphilis
1 Symmetric papulosquamous psoriasiform rash extending to involve palms and soles ± paronychia
2 Condylomata lata
3 Mucous patches (buccal)
Mucosal erosions ('snail track' ulcers)
Split papules
4 Leucoderma ('necklace of Venus')
5 Erythema nodosum
6 'Moth-eaten' alopecia

Clinical features of disseminated gonococcal infection
1 Typically occurs in young women or male homosexuals
Symptoms of (primary) gonococcal infection may be absent

Complicates approximately 2% of gonorrhoea cases
2 Symptoms and signs include:
  a) Fever
  b) Arthralgias/arthritis: asymmetrical; polyarticular, upper limb predilection, esp. small joints of hands/wrists (cf. Reiter's); associated with tenosynovitis
  c) Pustular haemorrhagic *skin lesions,* esp. on limbs
  d) Myocarditis may occur, simulating rheumatic fever or gonococcal endocarditis
  e) Hepatitis or perihepatitis (Fitz-Hugh Curtis syndrome; also seen in chlamydial infection) may occur, simulating hepatitis B or cholecystitis; if laparotomy is carried out in error, 'violin-string' adhesions may be seen between the liver and the anterior abdominal wall
3 Laboratory investigations
  a) Routine cultures of urethra, endocervix, rectum, pharynx
  b) Blood and synovial fluid cultures: positivity of one tends to exclude the other; only 25% of clinically involved joints will yield gonococci
  c) Culture of skin lesions (positive only occasionally)
4 Pathogen characteristics
  a) Specific auxotype requires hypoxanthine/uracil for successful culture
  b) Serum-resistant (i.e. resists bactericidal activity of serum antibody/C_3)
  c) Penicillin-sensitive (exquisitely and regularly so)

Vaginal discharges: typical presentations
1 *Candida albicans*
  a) Predispositions
     — Oral contraceptives
     — Antibiotics (esp. tetracyclines)
     — Diabetes mellitus
  b) Presentation
     — Marked pruritus vulvae
     — Perineal erythema
  c) Discharge — scanty, cheesy, little odour
  d) Diagnosis — Gram-stain
2 *Trichomonas vaginalis*
  a) Venereally transmitted
  b) Presentation
     — Foul-smelling discharge
     — Pruritus often absent
     — Variable skin irritation
  c) Discharge — yellow, foamy, offensive; often profuse
  d) Diagnosis — direct microscopy by dark-field illumination
3 *Gardnerella vaginalis*
  a) Venereally transmitted
  b) Presentation
     — Malodorous discharge
     — No skin irritation
  c) Discharge — greyish, foul-smelling ('fishy' odour)
  d) Diagnosis
     — Positive amine test
     — 'Clue cells' on microscopy

4 Gp B streptococci (uterine discharge postpartum)
— Discharge: foul-smelling lochia

ANAEROBIC INFECTION

Common anaerobic infections
1 Dental infections
2 Gynaecological sepsis (e.g. septic abortion)
3 Abscesses: cerebral, lung, liver
4 Aspiration pneumonia
5 Biliary tract sepsis
6 Bite wounds

Factors predisposing to anaerobic infection
1 Mucosal injury
2 Microvascular disease
3 Tissue necrosis
4 Foreign bodies

ZOONOSES

Zoonoses: diseases transmitted to humans by animals
1 Anthrax (*B. anthracis*) — *from goats, sheep*
2 Leptospirosis/Weil's disease (*L. icterohaemorrhagica*) } — from rats
'Plague' (*Y. pestis*)
3 Brucellosis (*B. abortus*)
Q fever (*Coxiella burneti*) } — from cattle
Leptospirosis (*L. hardjo*)
4 Salmonellosis (*Salmonella* spp., esp. *typhimurium* and *enteritidis*) — from cattle, poultry (esp. hens' eggs) (cf. *Shigella* spp.: man is the natural host)
5 Toxocariasis (*Toxocara canis*)
Bite wounds (*Pasteurella multocida*)
Canicola fever (*Leptospira canicola*) } — from dogs
Hydatids (*Echinococcus granulosus*)
DF-2(dysgonic fermenter 2)
6 Toxoplasmosis (*T. gondii*) — from cats
7 Campylobacter enteritis (*C. jejuni, C. coli*)
Yersiniosis (*Y. enterocolitica*) — from several sources: birds, poultry, pigs, dogs, cats
8 Rabies (rabiesvirus; a rhabdovirus)
a) From foxes, bats, small carnivores (in the wild)
b) From infected domestic dogs (or cats) in urban centres

Clinical features of specific zoonoses
1 *Toxocara canis* ('visceral larva migrans')
a) Transmitted to children by dogs
b) Systemic presentation: rash, fever, cough, failure to thrive, eosinophilia; mainly seen at age 1–4 years
c) Retinal presentation: strabismus, unilateral loss of visual acuity, no eosinophilia; affects older children
d) Diagnosis — ELISA or biopsy
e) Treat with thiabendazole (if symptomatic) ± steroids for allergic manifestations

NB: 'cutaneous larva migrans' — caused by *Ancylostoma caninum/braziliense:* treat with topical thiabendazole

2 *Echinococcus granulosus* (hydatid disease)
a) Transmitted to humans by dogs (definitive host) from sheep and cattle (intermediate hosts)
b) Presentation — enlarging cyst(s), esp. in liver and lung
c) Diagnosis — serology, biopsy (Casoni test non-specific)
d) Indications for surgery
— Lung cyst
— Liver cyst > 5 cm } — unless calcified
e) Needle aspiration contraindicated
3 *Toxoplasma gondii*
a) Presentation — most infections subclinical; may present with isolated non-tender adenopathy (DDx: lymphoma)
b) Systemic presentation — malaise, fever, headache, mononucleosis-like syndrome
c) Ocular presentation — posterior uveitis (usually due to reactivation of *in utero* infection)
d) Severe congenital presentations — induced by maternal primary infection during 1st/2nd trimester; may cause thrombocytopenia, hepatosplenomegaly, hydrocephalus
e) Other presentations — CNS toxoplasmosis (e.g. in AIDS)
f) Diagnosis
— Sabin-Feldman dye test (if available)
— IgM antibody (for acute infections only)
g) Treatment — sulphadiazine/pyrimethamine and folinic acid
4 Brucellosis
a) Presentation — back pain, arthralgias, orchitis cough, splenomegaly, endocarditis
b) Diagnosis — blood cultures, bone marrow culture, serology
c) Treatment — rifampicin plus doxycycline
5 Leptospirosis
a) Septicaemic phase — fever, aches and pains, conjunctival injection; renal involvement (pyuria, haematuria); diagnose by finding leptospires in blood and/or CSF
b) 'Immune phase' — meningism, uveitis, rash; diagnose by demonstrating leptospiruria
c) Weil's disease (i.e. severe leptospirosis) — jaundice, renal failure, confusion, cardiovascular collapse; may be seen in any serotype
d) Diagnosis (general) — serology
e) Treatment — parenteral penicillin or doxycycline

NB: efficacy of antibiotics uncertain; penicillin often precipitates Herxheimer reactions

6 Yersiniosis
a) Ileitis/enterocolitis (esp. in children)
b) Ileocaecal mesenteric adenitis (may mimic appendicitis)
c) Reactive polyarthritis
d) Erythema nodosum
e) Diagnosis — stool culture, paired sera
f) Treatment — symptomatic ± tetracycline
7 DF-2 (dysgonic fermenter 2)
a) Slow-growing immotile Gram-negative bacillus; normal in dogs

b) Human infection predisposed to by canine contact (75%) plus either alcoholism (25%), splenectomy (25%), chronic airways disease or immunosuppression (25%)
c) Sepsis → meningitis/pneumonia/endocarditis
d) Treatment — penicillin G (resistant to aminoglycosides)

FOOD POISONING

Clinical spectrum of food poisoning
1 *Staphylococcus aureus*
   a) Short incubation period 1–6 hours (pre-formed toxin)
   b) Source — uncooked food (dairy foods, sliced meats, salads)
   c) Vomiting prominent, no fever
2 *Bacillus cereus*
   a) Incubation period 1–6 hours (pre-formed toxin)
   b) Source — fried rice
   c) Vomiting, pain, diarrhoea
3 *Clostridium botulinum*
   a) Incubation period 24 hours (pre-formed toxin)
   b) Source — canned food
   c) Vomiting followed by paralysis; constipation; cranial nerve palsies; apnoea
   Clostridium perfringens (formerly *welchii*)   A
   a) Incubation period 12–24 hrs (pre-formed toxin)
   b) Source — poorly cooked meat dishes
   c) Abdominal pain, diarrhoea
4 *Salmonella spp.* (esp. *typhimurium* and *enteritidis*); also *Campylobacter*
   a) Incubation period 12–48 hours (toxin and infection)
   b) Source — contaminated meat/chicken/eggs/milk powder
   c) Fever, pain, diarrhoea; may last several days
   cf. **Typhoid**
   a) Incubation period 1–3 weeks
   b) Source — (human) faecal–oral transmission; polluted drinking water
   c) Headache, initial constipation, fever (cf. cholera) cough, orchitis, ototoxicity
5 *Vibrio parahaemolyticus*
   a) Incubation period 24 hours (toxin and infection)
   b) Source — seafood/shellfish (esp. shrimp)
   c) Vomiting, diarrhoea; may last up to 5 days
6 *Listeria monocytogenes* ('Vacherin cheese disease')
   a) Incubation period one week
   b) Source — undercooked hot dogs and chicken, soft cheese, coleslaw
   c) Predilection for pregnant women — → intrauterine fetal death
   d) Immunosuppressed or sporadic cases → meningitis, septicaemia
7 Eustrongylidiasis — from eating sushi

Common pathogens implicated in traveller's diarrhoea
1 Enterotoxigenic *E. coli*
2 *Salmonella* spp., *Shigella* spp., *Vibrio* spp., *Campylobacter*
3 *Giardia lamblia*
4 *Aeromonas hydrophila*
5 Norwalk virus; rotavirus (in children; see p. 124)

PRESENTATIONS OF INFECTIOUS DISEASE

'Spot' diagnosis of infectious diseases
1 Horder's spots — facial macules in psittacosis
2 Forschheimer's spots — soft palate lesions in rubella
3 Koplik's spots — bluish-grey buccal nodules in measles
4 Roth spots — pale-centred retinal infarcts in SBE due to either septic microemboli or vasculitis
5 Rose spots — truncal rash in 20% typhoid patients
6 Target lesions (erythema multiforme) — *M. pneumoniae*, herpes simplex (esp.)

Clinical features of toxic shock syndrome
1 Toxic (fever > 39°C)
2 Shock (systolic BP < 90 torr)
3 Rash
   a) Initially a diffuse 'sunburn-like' macular erythroderma
   b) About 10 days post-onset generalized desquamation supervenes, particularly affecting palms and soles
4 At least three of
   a) Vomiting or diarrhoea
   b) Mucosal (conjunctival/oropharyngeal/vaginal) hyperaemia
   c) Myalgias ± rhabdomyolysis (↑ CPK)
   d) Sterile pyuria and/or azotaemia
   e) Abnormal liver function tests
   f) Thrombocytopenia
   g) Confusion (in absence of shock or high fever)
5 Vaginal/endocervix cultures for *Staph. aureus* (phage gp 1) are positive in about 98% of untreated patients*
   Cultures of blood, throat and CSF are generally negative (very occasionally blood cultures may grow *S. aureus*)
   Staphylococcal exotoxin may be identified
6 Treatment consists of supportive measures (since symptoms are primarily toxin-mediated) ± flucloxacillin

UNUSUAL MICROORGANISMS

The rickettsioses: clinical syndromes
1 *R. rickettsi* — Rocky Mountain spotted fever
2 *R. tsutsugamushi* — scrub typhus
3 *R. prowazekii*
   a) Epidemic typhus (louseborne; human reservoir)
   b) Brill-Zinser disease (recrudesence of latent disease)
4 *R. typhi* — endemic typhus (fleaborne; rodent reservoir)

Lyme disease (*Borrelia burgdorferi*): features
1 Skin lesions (erythema chronicum migrans)
2 Neurological — meningism, cranial nerve palsies, peripheral neuropathy
3 Cardiac — AV block, myopericarditis
4 Arthritis — recurrent, asymmetric, often affects knee

---

*Not all cases occur in tampon users; e.g. nasal surgery may also predispose

Clinical spectrum of *Mycoplasma pneumoniae* infection
1 Community-acquired pneumonia, esp. in young patients
2 Cold agglutinin production ± haemolytic anaemia
3 Erythema multiforme, Stevens-Johnson syndrome
4 Non-specific musculoskeletal and/or gastrointestinal upset
5 Neurological effects — Guillain-Barré, cranial nerve palsies, polio-like syndrome, aseptic meningitis

Catscratch disease
1 Transmitted by cats; probably caused by bacterium
2 Presentation
  a) Red papule with regional adenopathy
  b) Adenopathy suppurative in 30%
3 Differential diagnosis — mycobacterial lymphadenitis
4 Diagnosis — biopsy with Warthin-Starry stain
5 Treatment — symptomatic

PARASITIC DISEASE

Malarial subtypes: the clinical distinction
1 *P. falciparum*
  a) Highest mortality; dense parasitaemia, frequent drug resistance
  b) → 'Cerebral malaria'
  c) → 'Blackwater fever'
    — Haemolysis/haemoglobinuria (blackwater)
    — Acute renal failure, DIC; hypoglycaemia
    — Pulmonary oedema
2 *P. vivax*
  a) Most difficult to eradicate (due to exoerythrocytic phase)
  b) 10% of cases present over a year after exposure
  c) Typically manifests with persistent splenomegaly and/or anaemia
  d) Prone to splenic rupture (may be spontaneous)
  e) Blood film shows Schüffner's dots within parasitized red cell
  f) Symptoms may recur every few months for up to 10 years
3 *P. ovale*
  a) Also exhibits exoerythrocytic phase and Schüffner's dots (hence primaquine required in treatment; see p. 184)
4 *P. malariae*
  a) Long incubation period; severe prodromal symptoms
  b) Red cell parasitization may persist for decades
  c) Late recrudescences may occur for up to 50 years; splenomegaly tends to persist
  d) Haematuria, nephrotic syndrome common

Classical presentations of parasitic disease
1 'Duodenal ulcer' type pain
  — *Strongyloides stercoralis*
  — Hookworm *(Ancylostoma/Necator)*
2 Intestinal obstruction
  — *Ascaris lumbricoides*
3 Rectal prolapse
  — *Trichostrongylus; Trichura* (whipworm)
4 Malabsorption
  — Giardiasis (a protozoön), capillariasis

5 Pruritus ani
  — *Enterobius* (pinworm, threadworm)
6 Haemoptysis
  — Paragonomiasis
7 'Anchovy sauce' expectoration
  — Amoebiasis (a protozoön) (hepatic)
8 'Grape skin' expectoration
  — Echinococcosis (hydatid disease)
9 Terminal haematuria
  — *Schistosoma haematobium*
10 Portal hypertension
  — *Schistosoma japonicum*
11 Pulmonary hypertension
  — *Schistosoma mansoni*
12 'Swimmer's itch'
  — Non-human schistosome cerceriae (cf. 'swimming pool granuloma'← *Mycobacterium marinum)*
13 Cholangitis, pancreatitis, cholangiocarcinoma:
  — *Clonorchis sinensis*
14 Lymphoedema, elephantiasis
  — Filariasis
15 Vitamin B$_{12}$ deficiency
  — *Diphyllobothrium latum*
16 Megaoesophagus/-colon, cardiomyopathy
  — Chagas' disease *(Trypanosoma cruzi)*

VIRAL DISEASES

Lymphotropic viruses
1 EBV
2 CMV
3 HHV-6: human herpesvirus 6; also known as human B-cell lymphotropic virus (HBLV)
4 Adenoviruses

Distinguishing features of mononucleosis-like syndromes
1 EBV
  a) Affects mainly adolescents (12–25 years)
  b) Pharyngitis/tonsillitis prominent; may be exudative
  c) Palatine petechiae characteristic, fever common
  d) Tender cervical lymphadenopathy usual, splenomegaly frequent
  e) Lymphocytosis in 90% of cases
    — Relative lymphocytosis >50%
    — Atypical lymphocytosis >10%
  f) Liver function tests abnormal in 90%; jaundice in 5–10%
  g) Ampicillin rash in 90% of exposed cases
2 CMV
  a) Affects mainly young adults (25–35 years)
  b) Pharyngitis absent; fever prominent
  c) Lymphadenopathy/splenomegaly unusual
  d) Hepatomegaly usual (granulomatous hepatitis on biopsy); liver function tests often abnormal (esp. alkaline phosphatase); jaundice rare
  e) Atypical lymphocytosis less common than with EBV
  f) May occur following transfusions
  g) Virus isolable from urine for long periods postinfection

h) Also isolable from secretions (e.g. saliva) or from buffy coat (i.e. leucocyte) blood fraction (best test)
i) Ampicillin rashes occur with same frequency as EBV
3 Toxoplasmosis (a protozoön)
   a) Affects all age groups
   b) Systemic symptoms unusual (most infections are subclinical)
   c) Pharyngitis absent
   d) Non-tender rubbery lymphadenopathy common, splenomegaly unusual; lymphadenopathy may persist for up to 12 months
   e) Liver dysfunction and atypical lymphocytosis usually absent
   f) Ampicillin rash not associated
   g) May respond to antibiotics (spiramycin; cotrimoxazole, pyrimethamine/sulphadimidine)
4 HHV-6 (human herpesvirus-6)
   a) Mononucleosis-like syndrome affects adults; children develop exanthem subitum (roseola infantum)
   b) Fever unusual; non-specific viral syndrome
   c) Non-tender cervical adenopathy
   d) Atypical lymphocytosis usual
5 Early HIV infection
   a) Affects mainly homosexuals (>i.v. drug abusers)
   b) Occurs within 2–6 weeeks of primary HIV infection
   c) Sudden onset (cf. EBV: insidious), short duration (about 2 weeks)
   d) Prominent *rash* (+ fever/pharyngitis/adenopathy/lethargy)
   e) Often associated with oral/genital/anal *ulcers* ?reflecting portal of virus entry; cough and/or watery diarrhoea also common
   f) *No* atypical lymphocytosis
   g) *No* hepatosplenomegaly or abnormal liver function tests
   h) Neurological abnormalities unusual (cf. later HIV syndromes)
   i) Patients usually well for 2–3 years subsequently

Parvovirus B19: the clinical spectrum
1 Erythema infectiosum ('fifth disease', 'slapped-cheek syndrome')
2 Aplastic crises (e.g. in sickle-cell disease) Anaemia in patients with malignancy (e.g. ALL)
3 Symmetric polyarthropathy in adults
4 Fetal abnormalities in utero

Human papillomavirus (HPV): clinical associations
1 Type 1 — plantar warts
2 Type 3 — flat warts
3 Type 5/8 — skin SCCs in transplant patients
4 Type 7 — common warts in food handlers
5 Types 6 and 11
   a) Condylomata acuminata (genital warts)
   b) Juvenile laryngeal papillomatosis
6 Type 13 — oral leukoplakia
7 Type 16 (and others, esp 18)
   a) SCC cervix
   b) SCC penis
   c) SCC vulva
8 Type 30 — SCC larynx

Complications of viral infections
1 Influenza A — staphylococcal/pneumococcal pneumonia
2 Measles
   a) Reactivation of pulmonary TB
   b) Bacterial pneumonia
   c) Encephalomyelitis, SSPE
3 Mumps
   a) Meningitis, deafness, thyroiditis, pancreatitis
   b) Paroxysmal cold haemoglobinuria
   c) Orchitis (common), sterility (rare)
4 Varicella-zoster
   a) Miliary calcification on CXR
   b) DIC
5 CMV
   a) Guillain-Barré syndrome
   b) Myopericarditis
   c) Necrotizing pneumonitis in transplant patients
   d) ? *P. carinii* pneumonia
   e) ? Kaposi's sarcoma
6 Coxsackie A
   a) Aseptic meningitis, paralysis
   b) Herpangina
   c) 'Hand, foot and mouth' disease
7 Coxsackie B
   a) Pleurodynia; myopericarditis
   b) Pancreatitis, orchitis
   c) ? Diabetes mellitus
8 JC virus (a papovavirus) — Progressive multifocal leucoencephalopathy
9 Parvovirus
   a) Fifth disease ('slapped cheek' syndrome)
   b) Aplastic crisis in sickle-cell disease
10 Jakob-Creutzfeldt
   a) Myoclonic jerks; dementia
   b) Transmissible by corneal transplantation

VIRAL HAEMORRHAGIC FEVERS

Classification of the viral haemorrhagic fevers
1 Togaviruses
   a) Alphaviruses (mosquito-borne)
      — Chikungunya fever (Asia)
      — O'nyong nyong (Africa)
   b) Flaviviruses (mosquito- and tick-borne)
      — Dengue fever (Asia, Africa, Pacific, Caribbean)
      — Yellow fever (Africa, S. America)
      — Kyasanur Forest disease (Asia)
      — Omsk haemorrhagic fever (Central Asia)
2 Bunyaviruses (mosquito- and tick-borne)
   a) Congo-Crimean fever (Africa, Asia)
   b) Rift Valley fever (Africa)
   c) Korean haemorrhagic fever (Hantaan virus: Asia)
3 Arenaviruses (rodent-borne)
   a) Lassa fever (Africa)
   b) Argentinian haemorrhagic fever (Junin virus)
   c) Bolivian haemorrhagic fever (Machupo virus)
4 Filoviruses (nosocomial transmission)
   a) Marburg virus ('green monkey') disease (Europe, Asia, Africa)
   b) Ebola virus disease (Africa)

The viral haemorrhagic fevers: differential diagnostic features

1 Marburg/Ebola viruses
  a) Filoviruses; African endemicity
  b) Nosocomial spread (transmissible by blood products)
  c) Tertiary cases rare
  d) Different incubation periods, similar clinical manifestations
  e) Presentation
    — Abrupt onset
    — Headache, conjunctivitis, back pain, arthralgias
    — Diarrhoea ± melaena
    — Pleurisy, psychosis, proteinuria
    — DIC; characteristic haemorrhagic rash
2 Lassa fever
  a) An arenavirus; African endemicity
  b) Similar syndromes seen with other arenaviruses, notably Junin (Argentinian) and Machupo (Bolivian) fevers
  c) Rodent-borne
  d) Transmission similar to Marburg/Ebola viruses
  e) Presentation
    — *Insidious* onset (many cases may be subclinical)
    — Pharyngitis, lymphadenopathy, nephrosis
    — Hypoxic death, esp. in pregnancy
  f) Management
    — Barrier nursing
    — Ribavirin
    — Junin type: 500 ml high-titre immune (convalescent) plasma
3 Dengue fever
  a) A flavivirus (four serotypes); South Pacific endemicity
  b) Rash, DIC tendency similar to above
  c) Most severe (→ shock) in infants and children, esp. if history of previous infection
4 Korean haemorrhagic fever with renal syndrome
  a) Caused by Hantaan virus (a bunyavirus); rodent-borne
  b) Same virus probably responsible for *nephropathica epidemica* in Scandinavia, while a closely-related bunyavirus may be the cause of Balkan nephropathy
  c) Presentation
    — Nephrosis, acute renal failure
    — *Mild* haemorrhagic signs in Korean variant
5 Congo-Crimean fever
  a) Tick-borne
  b) Similar syndrome seen in Kyasanur Forest disease (India)
  c) Presentation
    — *Severe* haemorrhagic sequelae
    — Chest pains, oropharyngitis
6 Yellow fever
  a) Mosquito-borne
  b) Similar syndrome seen in Rift Valley fever (also in Africa)
  c) Presentation
    — Arthritis
    — Retinal damage
    — Jaundice in convalescent phase

INVESTIGATING INFECTIOUS DISEASE

Diagnoses suggested by direct microscopy

1 Acid-fast bacteria to Ziehl-Neelsen staining
  a) *Mycobacteria* spp.
  Catalase-positive, niacin-negative, INH-resistant in vitro
  b) Atypical (non-tuberculous) mycobacteriosis
2 *Weakly* acid-fast organisms
  a) *Nocardia* (aerobic) spp.
  b) *Actinomyces* (anaerobic) spp.
3 Dark-field examination — *Treponema pallidum*
4 Silver methenamine stain — *P. carinii*
5 Indian ink stain (CSF) — *Cryptococcus neoformans*
6 Romanowsky-type stain
  Thick and thin films } —Plasmodia spp.
7 Gram-negative diplococci within leucocytes (endocervical/urethral swab) } —*Neisseria gonorrhoeae*
8 Inclusion bodies within urethral epithelial cells } — *Chlamydia trachomatis*
9 Pyogenic meningitis in adults
  a) Gram-positives in CSF — Pneumococcal meningitis
  b) Gram-negatives in CSF — Meningococcal meningitis } —Presumptive diagnoses

Diagnostic value of throat swabs

1 Gp A β-haemolytic strep (diagnosis excluded by negative swab)
2 Gonococcal pharyngitis
3 *Mycoplasma pneumoniae*
4 Diphtheria, pertussis
5 Some viral infections: polio, rubella

Diagnostic utility of bone marrow culture

1 Miliary tuberculosis
2 Brucellosis
3 Typhoid
4 Kala-azar

TUBERCULOSIS: INVESTIGATIONS

Diagnostic criteria in pulmonary tuberculosis

1 Suggestive
  a) Clinical context
  b) Radiographic appearance (NB: *activity* of TB *cannot* be assessed from CXR)
  c) Positive tuberculin test, esp. if previously negative
2 Presumptive
  a) Acid-fast bacilli in sputum/gastric washings
  b) Caseating granulomata on biopsy
3 Definitive: *Mycobacterium tuberculosis* isolated on culture

Diagnosis of tuberculous meningitis

1 Routine CSF examination
  a) ↑ Mononuclears
  b) ↑ Protein
  c) ↓ Glucose

2 Special CSF examination
   a) ↓ Chloride
   b) ↓ Serum/CSF bromide partition ratio
   c) Positive tryptophan assay
3 Diagnosis CSF examination — acid-fast bacilli on Ziehl-Neelsen staining, confirmed as tuberculous on culture (usually negative)
4 CXR, tuberculin test — useless

The false-negative tuberculin test: differential diagnosis

1 Extremes of age
2 Very recent infection (<2–10 weeks since inoculation)
3 Viraemia (e.g. measles, influenza)
   Following live vaccination (e.g. rubella)
4 Severe systemic disease
   a) Septicaemia (incl. miliary tuberculosis)
   b) Carcinomatosis and/or cytotoxic therapy
   c) Uraemia, malnutrition
   d) Tuberculous meningitis
5 Defective T-cell function
   a) Hodgkin's disease and/or thymic irradiation
   b) Sarcoidosis
   c) Wiskott-Aldrich, di George, SCID
   d) AIDS (NB: test hazardous to perform)
6 Drugs — steroids, other immunosuppressives
7 Technical problems
   a) Inadvertent subcutaneous injection
   b) Adsorption of antigen to syringe
   c) Substandard potency of preparation

SYPHILIS SEROLOGY

What sort of tests are available for diagnosing syphilis?

1 Darkfield examination (for direct spirochaetal identification)
2 Reaginic (flocculation) tests
   a) VDRL (best test; quantitative)
   b) WR (little used now)
   c) RPR (used in outlying areas)
3 Specific tests
   a) FTA-ABS
   b) TPI
   c) TPHA

Sensitivity of reaginic tests (e.g. VDRL) in established syphilis

1 Primary syphilis — positive in 80% (reliably negative within two years of successful treatment)
2 Secondary syphilis — positive in 99%
3 Late/latent syphilis — positive in 70% (may remain positive for long periods despite successful therapy of late syphilis)
4 Neurosyphilis — CSF positive in 50% (i.e. 50% false-negative rate; cf. CSF VDRL false-positives rare unless 'bloody tap' contaminates sample)

Causes of chronic reaginic false-positives

1 Autoimmune disease (e.g. SLE, Hashimoto's)

2 Sarcoidosis
3 Narcotic abuse
4 Lymphoma
5 Leprosy
6 Pregnancy

Choosing the most appropriate test in suspected syphilis

1 Primary (recent) exposure
   a) Darkfield examination of primary chancre
   b) FTA-ABS is the first test to become positive
2 Secondary syphilis
   a) Darkfield examination if skin/mucosal lesions present
   b) VDRL
3 Screening (pregnant women, prostitutes, contacts of cases)
   a) VDRL
   b) If positive, do FTA-ABS
4 Follow-up (of primary/secondary/late syphilis) after therapy
   a) VDRL at 3,6,12 months
   b) If titre unchanged after 12 months, re-treat
5 Exclusion of neurosyphilis — CSF FTA-ABS (negativity reliably excludes diagnosis)

Diagnostic significance of syphilis serology

1 Positive VDRL
  Positive FTA-ABS } —Syphilis (yaws, pinta, bejel)
2 Positive VDRL
  Negative FTA-ABS } —Biological false-positive
3 Negative VDRL
  Positive FTA-ABS } —Early, latent, late or treated syphilis
4 Positive FTA-ABS (IgM) — congenital syphilis (cf. IgG only: passive transfer of maternal antibody)

Positive dark-field examination: differential diagnosis

1 Primary syphilitic chancre
2 Secondary syphilis (mucosal lesions)
3 Congenital syphilis (mucosal lesions)
4 Non-pathogenic oral or rectal treponemes

Neurosyphilis: CSF monitors during treatment

1 Total protein
2 Mononuclear cell count
3 Quantitative VDRL titre if positive prior to treatment

FEVER OF UNKNOWN ORIGIN

Approach to the investigation of unexplained fever
(i.e. negative examination, CXR, MSU, and blood cultures)

1 Exclude drug allergy/surreptitious drug abuse/factitious fever
2 Bone marrow examination (lymphoma)
   Bone marrow culture (q.v.)
3 Thick and thin blood film (malarial parasitaemia)
4 CT/ultrasound if abscess suspected
5 Scintigraphy
   a) Gallium-67-scanning
   b) Indium-111-leucocyte (or -IgG) scanning
6 HIV serology

Fever of unknown origin: diagnoses localized by gallium scan
1 Abscess (e.g. subphrenic)
2 Lymphoma
3 Hepatoma
4 Sarcoidosis

Infections commonly causing profound peripheral eosinophilia
1 Trichinosis (diagnosis by serology or muscle biopsy)
2 Visceral larva migrans *(Toxocara canis)* esp. in children
3 Tropical pulmonary eosinophilia (filariasis)

OTHER INFECTIONS

Infectious mononucleosis: making sense of the serology
1 VCA (viral capsid antibody; IgG) — positivity indicates past or present infection
2 EA (antibody to EBV 'early antigen')
   a) Appears within 2–3 weeks of symptom onset
   b) 'D' (diffuse) component disappears within months; useful marker of current infection if positive
   c) 'R' (restricted) component may persist for years, esp. in relapsing disease
3 EBV specific IgM (i.e. to viral capsid antigen)
   a) Tends to parallel heterophile antibody rise (see below)
   b) Generally becomes negative within 3 months of symptom onset
   c) Extremely useful in heterophile-negative cases; the best test for confirming acute disease
4 EBNA (EB virus-associated nuclear antigen)
   a) Viral antigen detected by immunofluorescence
   b) Indicates infected cells harbouring viral genome
5 EBNA antibody (IgG)
   a) Appears late
   b) Indicates previous infection; persists lifelong
6 Heterophile antibody (IgM)
   a) i.e. Heterophile agglutinins for sheep erythrocytes
   b) Basis of Paul-Bunnell test (diagnostic); present in 90%
   c) Similar (Forssman-type) agglutinins seen in hepatitis, lymphomas, etc; absorbed out by guinea pig kidney (cf. positive Paul-Bunnell in EBV: antibodies preferentially absorbed out by ox erythrocytes)
   d) May be misleadingly negative for up to one month following symptom onset; tedious and expensive to perform

Weil-Felix reactions: diagnostic significance
1. Epidemic *(R. prowazekii)* typhus — OX-19 positive Brill-Zinsser disease (recurrent epidemic typhus) — all negative
2 Scrub *(R. tsutsugamushi)* typhus — OX-K positive
3 Rocky Mountain *(R. rickettsii)* spotted fever — OX-19 and OX-2 positive
4 Q *(Coxiella burneti)* fever — all negative

5 *Proteus* spp. infections
  Brucellosis, typhoid, leptospirosis } — false-positives

Laboratory characterization of genital ulcers
1 Positive dark-field examination — primary syphilis
2 *H. ducreyi* on microscopy — chancroid
3 Donovan bodies on microscopy — granuloma inguinale
4 *Chlamydia* on culture/serology — lymphogranuloma venereum
5 Herpes simplex on viral culture — genital herpes
6 Negative microbiology — consider Behçet's/Reiter's syndrome

Laboratory diagnosis of specific infections
1 Gonorrhoea
   a) Immediate plating and Gram-stain
   b) Urethral culture in chocolate (blood) agar
   c) Endocervical/anorectal/pharyngeal culture in Thayer-Martin (antibiotic-enriched) medium
2 Typhoid
   a) Blood cultures; stool and urine cultures
   b) Widal test — >4 × ↑ Ab titre to 'O' (cell wall) antigen
3 Cryptococcal meningitis
   a) Cryptococcal antigen in CSF (most sensitive test)
   b) CSF culture (most specific test)
   c) Indian ink stain (quickest test)
4 Q fever — complement fixation test (CFT)
   a) Acute disease → 4× ↑ phase II antibody titre
   b) Chronic disease → persistent ↑ phase I and II Ab titre
   c) Endocarditis → > 1 : 200 phase I Ab titre

MANAGING INFECTIOUS DISEASE

PRINCIPLES OF ANTIBIOTIC CHEMOTHERAPY

Mechanisms underlying antibiotic activity
1 Interference with bacterial cell wall synthesis
   a) β-lactams (penicillins, cephalosporins) — prevent peptidoglycan crosslinking
   b) Vancomycin — inhibits peptidoglycan formation
2 Interference with fungal cell wall synthesis — imidazoles (ketoconazole, miconazole, clotrimazole) — inhibit ergosterol synthesis, making cells 'leaky'
3 Interference with bacterial RNA/ribosome interaction (i.e. inhibition of protein synthesis)
   a) Aminoglycosides (prevent correct mRNA ribosomal attachment and translation)
   b) Tetracycline (prevents tRNA binding to 30S ribosomal subunit)
   c) Chloramphenicol (prevents mRNA binding to 50S ribosomal subunit by blocking peptidyl transferase reaction)
   d) Erythromycin (blocks ribosomal translocation)
4 Interference with folate metabolism
   a) Sulphonamides (PABA analogues)
   b) Trimethoprim (inhibits bacterial DHFR)
   c) 5FC (fungal antimetabolite)
5 Interference with bacterial DNA gyrase

(topoisomerase II)
a) Nalidixic acid
b) Ciprofloxacin
6 Other mechanisms
a) Metronidazole — inhibition of anaerobic electron transfer
b) Nitrofurantoin — interference with bacterial acetyl CoA
c) Rifampicin — inactivation of bacterial RNA polymerase
d) Acyclovir — inhibition of viral DNA polymerase (the drug is selectively activated by *viral* thymidine kinase)

Bioavailability of antibiotics at specific sites of infection
1 CSF
a) Chloramphenicol
b) Erythromycin; metronidazole
c) Penicillins (during meningitis *only*)
d) Isoniazid/rifampicin/pyrazinamide
2 Bile
a) Penicillins
b) Cephalosporins
c) Erythromycin
3 Urine
a) Penicillins, cephalosporins
b) Sulphonamides
c) Aminoglycosides
d) Nitrofurantoin, nalidixic acid
e) Ethambutol

Non-absorbable antibiotics
1 Nystatin
2 Neomycin
3 Colistin
4 Framycetin
5 Vancomycin

TREATMENT OF ANAEROBIC INFECTIONS

Antibiotics with anaerobic specificity
1 Metronidazole
  Imipenem-cilastatin } — Good activity against *Bacteroides fragilis*
  Clindamycin
  Chloramphenicol
2 Cefoxitin
  Latamoxef } — Moderate activity against *Bacteroides fragilis*
  Ticarcillin
3 Penicillin G
  Tetracycline } — Poor activity against *Bacteroides fragilis*
  Erythromycin

Metronidazole: exclusive indications for parenteral administration
1 Prior to urgent surgery if anaerobic sepsis suspected
2 Proven anaerobic infections resistant to oral or rectal therapy
3 Patients with vomiting, diarrhoea, and anaerobic sepsis
4 Major uncharacterized sepsis in patients with predispositions to anaerobic source

PROPHYLACTIC ANTIBIOTICS

Antibiotic prophylaxis regimens
1 Rheumatic fever (*maintenance* prophylaxis)
a) 1×10^6 U benzathine penicillin i.m. monthly, **or**
b) 250 mg penicillin V orally b.d. until adulthood; lifelong prophylaxis recommended if there is significant valve disease
2 Infective endocarditis (*intermittent* prophylaxis)
a) Dental work — amoxycillin 3 g orally 1 hour before- and 6 hours after
b) Genitourinary/colonic instrumentation: ampicillin 1 g i.v. and gentamicin 2 mg/kg i.v. 30 minutes before, then amoxycillin 1 g orally 6 hours later
c) Penicillin allergy: vancomycin 1 g i.v. infusion prior to procedure
3 Tuberculosis
a) Isoniazid 300 mg daily p.o. for 12 months, *plus*
b) Pyridoxine 25 mg daily p.o. for 12 months
4 Malaria*
a) Endemic resistance — pyrimethamine plus dapsone weekly until 6 weeks following return to non-endemic area
b) Non-resistant area — chloroquine
c) *Falciparum* endemic — mefloquine, *or* chloroquine + proguanil
5 *Pneumocystis carinii* (in marrow transplant recipients)
a) trimethoprim/sulphamethoxazole
b) inhaled pentamidine

MANAGING MYCOBACTERIAL DISEASE

Relative indications for BCG vaccination
1 Medical or laboratory workers exposed to tubercle bacilli
2 Neonates exposed to active TB
3 Tuberculin-negative children and adolescents in endemic areas

Principal indications for tuberculin skin testing
1 To assess need for isoniazid prophylaxis in non-BCG-treated contacts (esp. children) of active tuberculosis cases
2 To assess need for BCG immunization in children
3 To assess TB prevalence in different communities
4 To investigate individuals suspected of having active TB

Indications for prophylactic isoniazid
1 A tuberculin-positive individual younger than 50 (esp. a child)
a) Is a member of a household in which a recent diagnosis of TB has been made
b) Has a chest X-ray suggesting TB
2 A tuberculin-positive individual
a) Is about to commence immunosuppressive treatment
b) Has
   — Hodgkin's disease, leukaemia (e.g. CLL, hairy cell)
   — Silicosis, sarcoidosis, alcoholism

---

*Recommendations change often
†*Very limited* role in this context

— Poorly controlled insulin-dependent diabetes
c) Has had a gastrectomy
3 Documented recent tuberculin conversion in absence of history of BCG vaccination

Chemotherapy of established tuberculosis
1 Standard (pre-sensitivity) regimen for pulmonary TB
  a) 6 months isoniazid and rifampicin (strongly bactericidal), plus
  b) 2 months pyrazinamide (weakly bactericidal), plus
  c) 2 months of either ethambutol (bacteriostatic) or streptomycin (weakly bactericidal)
  NB: if cavities present on initial CXR, continue isoniazid and rifampicin for 9 months
2 Sputum cultures still positive after 4 months of above regimen?
  a) Reculture and check for acquired resistance
  b) If no resistance demonstrable, recommence therapy and maintain for 9 months duration
  c) If resistance demonstrated, substitute second-line drug(s)
3 Pulmonary TB in pregnancy or during lactation
  a) Isoniazid (plus pyridoxine supplements) for 9 months
  b) Ethambutol may be added for the first 2 months if resistance suspected
  c) Rifampicin probably safe in second and third trimesters
  d) Avoid streptomycin at all stages
4 Pulmonary TB in child <16 years old
  a) Isoniazid and rifampicin for 9 months
  b) *Not* mandatory to add a third drug unless resistance suspected
5 Immunosuppressed patients
  a) Isoniazid and rifampicin for 12 months
  b) Ethambutol and pyrazinamide for 2 months
6 Renal TB — avoid streptomycin and ethambutol in renal impairment

Indications for corticosteroids in tuberculosis
(NB: Steroid administration is absolutely contraindicated *unless* the patient is receiving maximal anti-tuberculous chemotherapy)
1 Absolute indication — acute hypoadrenalism due to tuberculous ablation of the adrenal glands
2 Controversial indications
  a) Spinal or ureteric stenosis
  b) Pericarditis
  c) Acute miliary dissemination with septic shock
  d) Refractory large pleural effusion(s)
  e) Tuberculous meningitis

Toxicity of antituberculous chemotherapy
1 Isoniazid
  a) Hepatitis
  b) SLE
  c) Pyridoxine deficiency (rare)
    — Pellagra-like rash
    — Neuropathy; optic neuritis (↓ green vision)
    — Sideroblastosis
    Commoner in
    — High dosage schedule (>15 mg/kg/day)
    — Slow acetylation status

— Alcoholism
— Pregnancy
  d) *Potentiation* of phenytoin, warfarin
2 Rifampicin
  Daily administration
  a) *Antagonism* of oral contraceptives, warfarin, steroids, digoxin, and short-acting sulphonylureas
  b) Asymptomatic elevation of transaminases
  Intermittent administration
  a) Flu-like illness — occurs in Caucasians who have been receiving treatment less than 3 times per week for 3–6 months; 20% mortality
  b) Clinical hepatitis*
  c) Haemolysis, thrombocytopenia; azotaemia; DVT
3 Streptomycin
  a) Hypersensitivity reactions
    — Rash, malaise
    — PUO; eosinophilia
  b) Vestibular damage (esp. if renal impairment)
  c) Teratogenicity
4 Ethambutol — optic neuritis, esp. in renal impairment
5 Pyrazinamide — hepatotoxic in⁻ 10%
6 Cycloserine — fits, psychoses, pyridoxine deficiency

Ethionamide	— hepatotoxicity
Prothionamide	— neuropathy
	— nausea; psychoses

Features of isoniazid-associated hepatotoxicity
1 Occurs in about 1%; usually within 3 months; occasionally fatal
2 *Not* dose-related; *not* consistently related to acetylator phenotype, though an association with rapid acetylation has been reported.
3 Risk factors
  a) Male sex
  b) Age >35 years (8-fold increase if >65 years)
  c) Alcoholism
  d) Other hepatotoxic drugs
    — Rifampicin
    — Pyrazinamide
    — Ethionamide
4 Clinically indistinguishable from viral hepatitis
5 Liver function tests should *only* be routinely performed in
  a) The latter 'at-risk' group
  b) Symptomatic patients
6 Consideration should be given to cessation of therapy if the transaminase level exceeds 3 times the upper limit of normal

Problems in managing the alcoholic with tuberculosis
1 Poor compliance necessitating supervised (intermittent) treatment schedule, thereby predisposing to rifampicin toxicity
2 Increased risk of hepatotoxicity
3 Increased risk of toxic amblyopia
4 Increased risk of pyridoxine deficiency
5 Neuropathy/optic neuritis, rash, and sideroblastosis may arise due to other (non-iatrogenic) alcohol-related causes

*Also colours urine orange

Therapy of non-tuberculous mycobacteria

1 *Mycobacterium avium-intracellulare*
   a) Indolent disease — standard anti-TB regimens (for up to two years)
   b) Aggressive local disease — surgery (lobectomy)
   c) Aggressive widespread disease — five- or six-drug combinations, possibly including ethionamide, prothionamide or cycloserine for two years
2 *Mycobacterium marinum*
   a) Expectant
   b) Excision of involved skin
   c) Rifampicin, ethambutol, doxycycline
3 *Mycobacterium scrofulaceum* — lymphadenectomy
4 *Mycobacterium fortuitum-chelonei*
   a) Excision of soft-tissue abscesses
   b) Doxycycline; amikacin, sulphonamides, erythromycin
5 *Mycobacterium kansasii*
   a) Isoniazid ⎫
   b) Rifampicin ⎬ — For 2 years
   c) Ethambutol ⎭
6 *Mycobacterium xenopi* — standard anti-TB therapy

Leprosy: therapeutic options

1 Acedapsone/dapsone
2 Clofazimine
3 Rifampicin
4 Ethionamide/prothionamide
5 Thalidomide (for reactions following antibiotics in males)

Diseases which may respond to dapsone

1 Leprosy
2 Dermatitis herpetiformis
3 Pyoderma gangrenosum
4 Relapsing polychondritis

ANTIBIOTIC PRESCRIBING STRATEGIES

Antibiotic therapy of venereal disease

1 Genital gonorrhoea — tetracycline 500 mg q.i.d. for 5 days (or single-dose ciprofloxacin)
2 Gonococcal pharyngitis — trimethoprim/sulphamethoxazole for 5 days (usually unresponsive to amoxycillin or spectinomycin)
3 Gonococcal proctitis — spectinomycin 4 g i.m. (unresponsive to tetracycline in males and, usually, to amoxycillin)
   Gonococcal proctitis with positive VDRL — procaine penicillin (see below)
4 Syphilis — procaine penicillin 600 000 U i.m. daily
   a) Primary/secondary — for 10 days ⎫
   b) Latent/gummatous — for 15 days ⎬ —Resistant to spectinomycin
   c) Neurological/aortitic — for 20 days ⎭
5 Chlamydial urethritis — tetracycline 500 mg q.i.d. for 14 days (resistant to spectinomycin)

Treatment strategies in malaria

1 *P. falciparum* (sensitive) — chloroquine (base)

600 mg stat orally, then 300 mg 6 hours later, then 300 mg daily for 2 days
2 *P. falciparum* (resistant, fulminant or cerebral)
   a) Exchange transfusion (5–10 units) if parasitaemia >10%
   b) IV quinine dihydrochloride 20 mg/kg (=15 mg/kg quinine base) over first 4 hours, then 10 mg/kg q 8 hours; run 5% dextrose infusion throughout to obviate risk of hypoglycaemia; or
      — Amodiaquine 600 mg/day ± tetracycline; or
      — Mefloquine 20 mg/kg for two doses
      — No steroids
3 *P. vivax/ovale* — due to involvement of exoerythrocytic (cryptobiotic) phase, add primaquine (base) 7.5 mg orally b.d. for 2 weeks to the chloroquine-based regimen
4 *P. malariae* — relapse *not* prevented by primaquine; relapses may occur decades later, and each must be fully retreated with chloroquine
5 Malaria prophylaxis in pregnancy — chloroquine

Antibiotic chemotherapy of infection in the AIDS patient

1 *P. carinii* — cotrimoxazole; pentamidine
2 *C. albicans* (mucosal)
   a) Topical clotrimazole
   b) Oral ketoconazole
   C. albicans (oesophageal, invasive or disseminated) — i.v. amphotericin B ± 5-FC
3 *T. gondii* — pyrimethamine/sulphadiazine
4 *C. neoformans* — amphotericin B/5-FC
5 *Salmonella/Shigella* spp. — i.v. ampicillin
6 Herpes simplex, varicella-zoster — acyclovir
   CMV — ganciclovir

OPTIMIZING ANTIBIOTIC THERAPY

Drug of choice: erythromycin

1 Legionnaires' disease
2 *Mycoplasma* pneumonia
3 *Campylobacter* enterocolitis (if treatment indicated)
4 *C. diphtheriae* carrier state

Drug of choice: tetracycline

1 Chlamydial disease (NSU, trachoma, psittacosis, LGV)
2 Brucellosis
3 Whipple's disease; bacterial overgrowth; *Yersinia* enteritis; cholera; tropical sprue
4 Rickettsioses
5 Acne vulgaris/rosacea

Drug of choice: chloramphenicol

1 Pyogenic meningitis/encephalitis in childhood (3 months–5 years)
2 Cerebral abscess
3 Severe (para)typhoid fever
4 Acute epiglottitis
5 High oral bioavailability required (e.g. in refractory chest infections due to cystic fibrosis)

Drug of choice: co-trimoxazole (trimethoprim/sulphamethoxazole)

1 *Klebsiella* spp.

2 *Serratia/Enterobacter* spp.
3 *Pneumocystis carinii*
4 Nocardiosis

Drug of choice: vancomycin
1 Pseudomembranous colitis
2 Methicillin-resistant *Staph. aureus*
3 Bacterial endocarditis
   a) Penicillin allergy
   b) Prosthetic valve involvement
4 Shunt infections in haemodialysis patients
   (vancomycin *not* dialysable)

Drug of choice: metronidazole (or tinidazole)
1 Giardiasis
2 Trichomoniasis, *Gardnerella* vaginitis
3 Amoebic dysentery
4 Anaerobic infections
5 Abscesses (incl. hepatic, cerebral)

NB: Many liver abscesses are due to **microaerophilic** strep. — *St. milleri* — and may therefore be resistant

CEPHALOSPORINS

A general guide to the cephalosporins
1 First generation
   a) Cephalothin
   b) Cephazolin
   c) Cephalexin (oral formulation)
   —Good activity against Gram-positives
   —Little activity against Gram-negatives
2 Second generation
   a) Cefoxitin
   b) Cephamandole
   c) Cefuroxime
   —Medium activity against Gram-positive (except *S. aureus*)
   —Improved activity against β-lactamases
   —Medium activity against Gram-negatives (except *Ps. aeruginosa*, coliforms)
3 Third generation
   a) Cefotaxime
   b) Latamoxef
   —Minor activity against Gram-positives (not *St. faecalis*)
   —Variable activity against β-lactamases
   —Good activity against Gram-negatives, esp. *Ps. aeruginosa*

Problems associated with cephalosporin therapy
1 Expense
2 Poor penetration of sputum and CSF
3 Development of Gram-negative resistance
4 Significant incidence of cross-sensitivity in penicillin allergy
5 Potentiation of aminoglycoside nephrotoxicity by cephaloridine and cephalothin
6 Risk of coagulopathy (responsive to vitamin K) with latamoxef use

PENICILLINS

Microorganisms highly sensitive to penicillin G
1 Non-enterococcal streptococci (*viridans, pyogenes,* most pneumococci)

2 *Clostridia* spp. (**except** *C. difficile*)
3 *Actinomyces* spp., *Corynebacteria* spp., *Listeria monocytogenes*
4 *Neisseria meningitidis*
5 *Treponema pallidum*
6 DF-2 (dysgonic fermenter 2); *Pasteurella multocida* (dog bite)

Presumptive antibiotic therapy in penicillin allergy
1 Pyogenic meningitis / Aspiration pneumonia / Typhoid — chloramphenicol
2 Lobar pneumonia / Rheumatic fever prophylaxis — erythromycin
3 Acute bronchitis / Sinusitis, otitis — cotrimoxazole
4 Osteomyelitis — clindamycin
5 Gonorrhoea, syphilis — erythromycin
6 Bacterial endocarditis
   a) Prophylaxis — vancomycin
   b) Staphylococcal or non-enterococcal streptococcal — vancomycin, or oral ciprofloxacin + rifampicin
   c) Enterococcal
      — Penicillin desensitization → ampicillin/aminoglycoside, or
      — Vancomycin (depending on *in vitro* studies: MIC, MBC, synergy) ± aminoglycoside

Pneumococcal infections: approximate duration of therapy
1 Otitis media — 5 days
2 Pneumonia — 10 days
3 Meningitis — 2 weeks
4 Septic arthritis — 4 weeks
5 Empyema — 6 weeks

ANTIBIOTIC SENSITIVITY AND RESISTANCE

Patterns of antibiotic resistance
1 *Klebsiella* spp. — penicillins (incl. ampicillin, ticarcillin)
2 *Haemophilus influenzae* — penicillin G, cephalosporins; up to 5% of strains may now be resistant to ampicillin also.
3 Streptococci / Anaerobes — aminoglycosides
   (*Enterococcal* streptococci are only 'sensitive' to aminoglycosides when used in conjunction with a penicillin)

Patterns of bacterial susceptibility to antibiotics
1 *Pseudomonas aeruginosa*
   a) Aminoglycosides
   b) Ticarcillin — esp. in combination
   c) Azlocillin, piperacillin, mezlocillin
   d) Other β-lactams: ceftazidime, aztreonam, imipenem ± cilastatin
   e) 4-quinolones — norfloxacin, ciprofloxacin
2 *Staph aureus*
   a) (Flu)cloxacillin; methicillin (*in vitro* only); nafcillin
   b) Vancomycin, fusidic acid, rifampicin — useful in *multiresistant* strains
   c) Clindamycin, erythromycin
   d) Amoxicillin plus clavulanic acid — 2nd-line drugs

3 *Haemophilus influenzae*
  a) Chloramphenicol
  b) Ampicillin

Established synergy of antibiotic combinations
1 *Pseudomonas* infections — β-lactam plus an aminoglycoside (e.g. ticarcillin/tobramycin)
2 *Strep faecalis* endocarditis — ampicillin/gentamicin
3 Cryptococcal meningitis — amphotericin B/5-FC

Antibiotics rapidly engendering bacterial resistance if used alone
1 Rifampicin, streptomycin, pyrazinamide (T8)
2 Fusidic acid, rifampicin, erythromycin (*S. aureus*)
3 Nalidixic acid
4 5-FC
5 Cefoxitin (appears to induce β-lactamase); similarly, other 2nd- and 3rd-generation cephalosporins

Drug therapy of miscellaneous infections and infestations
1 Giardiasis: metronidazole 2 g once daily for 3 days or tinidazole 2 g stat (single dose)
2 Hepatic amoebiasis — metronidazole 400 mg t.d.s. for 5 days (alternative: chloroquine)
  Caecal amoebiasis — metronidazole 800 mg t.d.s. for 5 days (alternative: emetine)
3 Toxoplasmosis — pyrimethamine/sulphadiazine; spiramycin
4 Scabies, lice — topical gammabenzene hexachloride 1%
5 Hookworm, whipworm,
  echinococcus   —Mebendazole
  Strongyloides, Toxocara   —Thiabendazole
  Ascaris, pinworm   —Pyrantel pamoate
  Schistosoma japonicum   —Praziquantel
6 Onchocerciasis ('river blindness') — ivermectin

ANTIBIOTIC TOXICITY

Potential morbidity of antibiotic use
1 Nitrofurantoin
  a) Neuropathy (esp. with renal impairment)
  b) Pulmonary fibrosis
  c) Haemolytic anaemia; megaloblastosis
  d) Cholestasis → chronic active hepatitis
2 Chloramphenicol
  a) Idiosyncratic aplastic anaemia
  b) Dose-related myelosuppression
  c) Neuropathy, optic atrophy
  d) Depression of antibody synthesis
3 Erythromycin
  a) Abdominal pain (gastritis)
  b) Phlebitis (with i.v. use)
4 Ticarcillin
  a) Fluid (sodium) overload; hypokalaemia
  b) Impaired platelet aggregation
  c) Leucopenia, thrombocytopenia
  d) Inactivation of gentamicin/tobramycin if admixed
5 Metronidazole
  a) Dysgeusia
  b) Disulfiram-type reactions

  c) Painful neuropathy
6 Amphotericin B
  a) Fever, rigors; vomiting
  b) Hypokalaemia
  c) Myelosuppression

Tetracyclines: toxic manifestations
1 Common — diarrhoea, oesophagitis, moniliasis
2 Benign intracranial hypertension
3 Photosensitization (demeclocycline), vertigo (minocycline)
4 Worsening of renal failure
5 Hepatotoxicity, esp.
  a) Intravenous use
  b) In pregnant women
  c) With pre-existing renal impairment
6 Teeth staining when administered to children aged <8 years or to pregnant women; ingestion during the third trimester may result in staining of the child's secondary (permanent) dentition

Aminoglycoside toxicity: variations between drugs
1 Deafness (cochlear VIII toxicity) — esp. amikacin (a kanamycin derivative), neomycin
2 Ataxia (vestibular VIII toxicity) — esp. streptomycin, gentamicin (also tobramycin, netilmicin)
3 Nephrotoxicity
  a) Esp. gentamicin
  b) Worsened by concurrent frusemide or cephalothin
  c) Less nephrotoxicity from netilmicin

Disadvantages of aminoglycosides
1 Narrow therapeutic range (must monitor levels to avoid toxicity)
2 Ineffective against anaerobes
3 Failure to penetrate CSF, bile, abscesses

IATROGENIC INFECTIONS

Infections occurring in prosthetic appliances
1 Prosthetic valves, arterial grafts
  a) *S. albus*
  b) *S. aureus*
  c) *St. viridans*
  d) Gram-negative bacilli
2 Prosthetic joints
  a) *S. albus*
  b) *S. aureus*
  c) Gram-negative bacilli
3 CSF shunts
  a) *S. albus* (75%)
  b) *S. aureus*
  c) Gram-negative bacilli
4 Intraocular lens implant
  a) *S. albus*
  b) *S aureus*

Microorganisms transmissible by blood transfusion
1 Hepatitis B virus; delta agent (hepatitis D virus)
2 Non-A, non-B hepatitis
3 HIV

4 CMV
5 Syphilis
6 Malaria
7 *Trypanosoma cruzi* (Chagas' disease)
8 Rare
   a) Brucellosis
   b) EBV
   c) Hepatitis A

Approach to the febrile neutropenic patient
1 Culture blood, urine, and other relevant sites
2 Commence aminoglycoside + antipseudomonal
   β-lactam
3 Add amphotericin B if:
   a) Fever and neutropenia persist > 1 week
   b) Fever persists > 3 days and condition
      deteriorating
   c) Fever persists despite resolution of neutropenia

ANTIFUNGAL DRUGS

Principles of antifungal chemotherapy
1 Any severe or disseminated fungal infection, e.g.
   invasive aspergillosis, candiduria (in the absence of
   an indwelling catheter), rhinocerebral
   mucormycosis — intravenous amphotericin B ±
   oral 5-FC
2 Candiduria with indwelling catheter in situ — oral
   5-FC ± amphotericin B bladder washouts
3 Refractory superficial candidal infections —
   intravenous miconazole
4 Chronic mucocutaneous candidiasis
   a) (Oral) ketoconazole — for induction
   b) Transfer factor — for maintenance
5 Trivial infections
   a) Oropharyngeal candidiasis — amphotericin
      lozenges ± nystatin drops or topical clotrimazole
   b) Tinea capitis — oral griseofulvin
   c) Tinea corporis — topical clotrimazole/tolnaftate
6 Cryptococcal meningitis
   a) IV (intravenous or intraventricular) amphotericin
      B, plus
   b) Oral (or intravenous) 5-FC

Toxicity of ketoconazole
1 Nausea
2 Hepatotoxicity
3 Inhibition of steroid hormone synthesis
   a) Impotence (antiandrogenic action useful in Ca
      prostate)
   b) Dysfunctional uterine bleeding
   c) Hypoadrenalism (useful in Cushing's syndrome)

Drug interactions with ketoconazole
1 Absorption of ketoconazole inhibited by cimetidine
   (and other drugs causing achlorhydria)
2 Disulfiram-like effect with alcohol
3 Rifampicin antagonism (hepatic metabolism
   induced by ketoconazole)
4 Induction of ketoconazole metabolism by rifampicin
   (and isoniazid)
5 Potentiation of cyclosporin A toxicity in renal
   transplantation

ANTIVIRAL CHEMOTHERAPY

Antibiotic regimens for viral infections
1 Herpes simplex
   a) Keratitis — 3% acyclovir ointment
   b) Labialis — 5% acyclovir cream
   c) Genital (acute attack) — 1 g/day acyclovir p.o.
   d) Genital (prophylaxis) — 500 mg/day acyclovir
      p.o.
   e) Disseminated — acyclovir by intravenous
      infusion
2 Varicella-zoster
   a) Mild shingles — acyclovir 500 mg/day p.o. for
      one week
   b) Severe shingles — acyclovir: up to 500 mg t.d.s.
      i.v.
   c) Ophthalmic — 3% ointment plus oral acyclovir
   NB: Acyclovir therapy does *not* affect subsequent
   incidence or severity of postherpetic neuralgia
3 HIV — zidovudine (AZT) 250 mg q 4 h orally
4 Influenza A (prophylaxis or therapy) — amantadine
   or rimantidine, 200 mg/day for one week
5 Influenza B, RSV — ribavirin aerosol
6 Lassa fever — ribavirin orally
7 HPV (in juvenile laryngeal papillomatosis) —
   interferon i.v.
8 Rhinovirus (in the common cold) — interferon
   intranasally
9 CMV in the immunosuppressed patient —
   ganciclovir

VACCINES

Active immunization: mechanisms of vaccine action
1 Toxoids — tetanus, diphtheria, botulinum
2 Recombinant vaccines
   a) Hepatitis B
   b) Cholera
3 Pooled surface proteins — pneumococcus, *H.
   influenzae* #B
4 Attenuated (live) organisms (contraindicated in
   immunosuppressed patients)
   a) Polio, measles, rubella, mumps
   b) BCG, yellow fever, rabies; varicella-zoster
5 Killed organisms (ineffective in immunosuppressed
   patients)
   a) Influenza A; hepatitis A
   b) Typhoid, pertussis

Indications for pneumococcal vaccine
1 Patients aged 2–70
   a) Hyposplenism — post-splenectomy or sickle-cell
      anaemia
   b) Chronic renal failure
2 Patients aged 55–70
   a) Diabetes mellitus
   b) Chronic liver disease
   c) Cardiac and/or pulmonary disease
   d) CSF leaks

Indications for passive immunization
1 Pooled gammaglobulin
   a) Hepatitis A

— Family contacts
— Institutional outbreaks
— Exposed travellers in tropical and/or developing countries (every 4 months)
b) Measles — immunosuppressed contacts of acute cases exposed less than 6 days previously

2 Hyperimmune globulin
a) Hepatitis B
— Percutaneous or mucosal exposure to positive sera
— Sexual contacts of acute cases (optional)
— Newborns of HBsAg+ mothers (at birth, 3 and 6 months)
b) Rh isoimmunization
— Rh(D)-negative mother on delivery of Rh+ infant
— Rh(D)-negative mother after aborted pregnancy with Rh+ father
— Rh(D)-negative mother following inadvertent transfusion of Rh+ blood
c) Varicella-zoster
— Immunesuppressed contacts of acute case
— Newborn contacts of acute case
d) Rabies — subjects exposed to rabid animals
e) Tetanus
— Prophylaxis following significant exposure of unimmunized subject
— Therapeutically — immediately on diagnosis of disease

UNDERSTANDING INFECTIOUS DISEASE

A simplified classification of microorganisms
1 Viruses
a) RNA
— Myxoviruses (e.g. influenza)
— Paramyxoviruses (e.g. measles, mumps, RSV)
— Picornaviruses (e.g. enteroviruses — ECHO, polio, and Coxsackie — or hepatitis A)
— Reoviruses (e.g. rotavirus)
— Rhabdoviruses (e.g. rabies)
— Arenaviruses (e.g. Lassa fever)
— Togaviruses (e.g. rubella, dengue)
— Retroviruses (e.g. HIV, HTLV)
b) DNA
— Herpesviruses (HSV, V-Z, CMV, EBV)
— Adenoviruses
— Parvoviruses
— Papovaviruses (e.g. HPV, JC virus)
— Hepadnaviruses (hepatitis B)
2 Bacteria
a) Cell-wall-deficient — Mycoplasmas
b) Obligate intracellular — Chlamydiae, Rickettsiae
c) Helically coiled — spirochaetes (e.g. Treponema, Leptospira, Borrelia)
d) 'Higher' bacteria
— Mycobacteria spp.
— Corynebacteria spp.
— Actinomyces, Nocardia
e) Eubacteria (the rest)
3 Fungi

a) Yeasts (grow as hyphae, increase by budding), e.g.
— Candida albicans
— Cryptococcus neoformans
b) Moulds (grow as mycelia, increase by branching), e.g.
— Aspergillus fumigatus
— Dermatophytes (e.g. tinea)
c) Dimorphic, e.g. Histoplasma capsulatum
4 Protozoan parasites
a) Plasmodium spp.
b) Toxoplasma gondii
c) Entamoeba histolytica
d) Giardia lamblia
e) Pneumocystis carinii*
f) Trichomonas vaginalis
5 Multicellular parasites (worms)
a) Schistosoma spp.
b) Strongyloides stercoralis
c) Echinococcus granulosus
d) Toxocara canis
e) Filariasis

Gram-staining: clinically relevant organisms
1 Gram-positive cocci
a) Staphylococcus spp.
b) Streptococcus spp.
2 Gram-negative cocci — Neisseria spp. (gonococcus, meningococcus)
3 Gram-positive bacilli
a) Clostridium spp.
b) Bacillus spp.
c) Corynebacterium diphtheriae
d) Actinomyces israeli
e) Gardnerella vaginalis
f) Listeria monocytogenes
4 Gram-negative bacilli
a) Enterobacteriaceae (E. coli, Proteus, Klebsiella, Salmonella/Shigella spp.)
b) Pseudomonas aeruginosa
c) Haemophilus influenzae
d) Campylobacter jejuni/coli
e) Brucella abortus
5 Acid-fast bacilli
a) Mycobacteria spp.
b) Nocardia asteroides (weakly acid-fast)

EPIDEMIOLOGY OF INFECTIOUS DISEASE

Periodicity of infectious disease
1 Summer/autumn
a) Legionnaires' disease
b) Leptospirosis
c) Polio; enteroviruses
d) Arboviruses (e.g. Ross River virus)
2 Autumn/winter
a) Hepatitis A
b) Coxsackie B
3 Winter/spring

*Recent evidence suggests that Pneumocystis may be a fungus; see ref. 7.3

a) Mumps
b) Infectious mononucleosis
c) Lymphocytic choriomeningitis
d) Rotavirus/Norwalk (parvovirus)

Vectors of infectious disease
1 Malaria — (female) *Anopheles* mosquito
2 Yellow fever — *Aëdes* mosquito
3 Leishmaniasis — *Phlebotomus* sandfly
4 Trypanosoma cruzi — *Reduviid* arthropod
5 Trypanosoma gambiense — *Tsetse* fly

Incubation periods of various infective agents
1 Less than 1 week (rapid-onset)
a) Cholera
b) Scarlet fever
c) Diphtheria
d) Gonorrhoea
e) Meningococcus
f) Herpes simplex
g) Bacillary dysentery
h) *Haemophilus influenzae*
i) Yellow fever
j) Anthrax
2 More than 3 weeks (delayed-onset)
a) Hepatitis A/B
b) Epstein-Barr virus
c) Syphilis
d) Filariasis
e) Leprosy
f) Rabies
g) Leishmaniasis
h) Trypanosomiasis
i) Schistosomiasis
j) Amoebiasis (often)

Infectious disease: periods of infectivity
1 Hepatitis A — prior to icteric phase
2 Measles — from prodrome until 4 days after onset of rash
3 Mumps — three days pre-parotitis until one week after
4 Rubella ⎫ One week prior to onset of rash
  Chicken pox ⎬ until one week after
5 Scarlet fever ⎫ Onset until three weeks after
  Diphtheria ⎬ (shortened by antibiotic therapy)

Nosocomial sources of infection
1 Air conditioners — aspergilli, staphylococci
2 Humidifiers
a) *Acinetobacter* spp.
b) *Pseudomonas* spp.
3 Water reservoirs — *Legionella pneumophila*, *Pseudomonas* spp.
4 Foods (e.g. salads) — Gram-negatives, staphylococci, streptococci
5 Endogenous flora — *Enterobacteriaceae*, staphylococci
6 Reactivation — TB, herpesviruses, mycoses
7 Parenteral nutrition — candidiasis, staphylococci
8 Blood transfusions
a) Hepatitis B, CMV, non-A non-B
b) Malaria, Chagas' disease (developing countries)

9 Hydrotherapy pools — *Ps. aeruginosa* folliculitis
10 Other patients and staff
—Herpesviruses (esp. zoster)
—*Listeria* spp.
—*Cl. difficile*

Pathogen or contaminant? A guide to normal bacterial flora
1 Mouth
a) Anaerobes
b) *St. viridans*
c) Pneumococcus
d) *Haemophilus influenzae*
2 Skin
a) *Propionibacterium acnes*
b) *Staphylococcus* spp.
3 Colon
a) Anaerobes
b) Enterobacteriaceae, esp. *E. coli*
4 Vagina
a) Lactobacilli
b) Anaerobes
c) Gp B streptococci

Infections which commonly persist in the host
1 Viral
a) EBV
b) Varicella-zoster
c) Herpes simplex
d) CMV
2 Toxoplasmosis
3 Malaria (esp. *P. malariae*)
4 *Strongyloides stercoralis*

Dental caries: the most prevalent infectious disease of humans
1 *St. mutans* is clearly the most cariogenic bacterium found in plaque (an accretion on tooth enamel in which acid accumulates)
2 Dietary sucrose reduces plaque pH, thus inducing demineralization of hydroxyapatite enamel
3 Immunization against *St. mutans* reduces plaque load and caries by stimulating production of secretory IgA (and systemic IgG) antibodies
4 Fluoride also reduces caries

MECHANISMS OF INFECTIOUS DISEASE

Microorganisms which form spores
1 Fungi
2 *Clostridium* spp. (e.g. botulism)
3 *Bacillus* spp. (e.g. anthrax)

Diseases mediated by exotoxins
1 Clostridial disease
a) Tetanus (*Cl. tetani*)
b) Botulism (*Cl. botulinum*)
c) Gas gangrene (*Cl. perfringens*)
d) Antibiotic-associated colitis (*Cl. difficile*)
2 Diphtheria
3 Cholera

4 Staphylococcal food poisoning; toxic shock syndrome
5 Enterotoxigenic *E. coli* diarrhoea

Microbiological determinants of the 'gay bowel' syndrome
1 Pruritus ani
   a) *Enterobius vermicularis* (pinworm)
   b) *Pthirus pubis* (pubic lice)
   c) *Sarcoptes scabiei* (scabies)
2 Perianal lesions
   a) Condylomata acuminata (HPV 6, 11)
   b) Condylomata lata (secondary syphilis)
   c) Primary syphilitic chancre (simulates fissure)
   d) Granuloma inguinale (*H. ducreyi*: donovanosis)
   e) Herpetic vesicles
3 Proctitis
   a) *C. trachomatis* (non-LGV serotypes)
   b) *N. gonorrhoea*
   c) *T. pallidum*
   d) Herpes simplex
4 Proctocolitis
   a) *C. trachomatis* (LGV serotypes)
   b) *Shigella flexneri*
   c) *Campylobacter* spp.
   d) *Entamoeba histolytica* (NB: may be non-pathogenic commensal)
5 Enteritis — *Giardia lamblia*
6 HIV-associated gastrointestinal infections
   a) Cryptosporidiosis (small intestine)
   b) Candidiasis (oesophageal)
   c) *M. avium-intracellulare* (may mimic Whipple's disease)
   d) *Isospora belli*

Predispositions to mucormycosis (invasive zygomycosis)
1 Diabetes (→ rhinocerebral)
2 Malnutrition (→ gastrointestinal)
3 Burns (→ cutaneous)
4 Leukaemia (→ pulmonary)
5 Immunosuppression (→ disseminated)

DISEASE SUBTYPES

Clinical manifestations of *Haemophilus influenza* (HI) infection
1 Capsulated HI responsible for
   a) Acute epiglottitis ⎫
   b) Meningitis ⎬ —in children
   c) Septic arthritis ⎭
2 Non-capsulated HI
   a) Otitis media ⎫
   b Conjunctivitis ⎬ —in children
   c) Exacerbation of chronic bronchitis — in adults

Varieties and features of chlamydial infection
1 Non-specific urethritis (NSU)
   a) Caused by *C. trachomatis* serotypes D-K
   b) Commonest sexually transmitted disease
   c) Presentations
      — Seropurulent urethral discharge

      — Persistent symptoms after gonorrhoea therapy
      — Failure of presumptive β-lactam therapy
      — Reiter's syndrome; Fitz-Hugh Curtis syndrome
      — Pelvic inflammatory disease, infertility
   d) Diagnosis — chlamydial isolation
2 Lymphogranuloma venereum (LGV)
   a) Caused by *C. trachomatis* serotypes L1-3
   b) Systemic venereal disease endemic in tropics
   c) Commonest in males (5: 1), esp. homosexuals
   d) Presentations
      — Painful inguinal adenopathy (may suppurate)
      — 'Groove sign' (node mass indented by inguinal ligament)
      — Ulcerative proctitis; rectal stricture
      — Rectovaginal or rectovesical fistula
      — Genital elephantiasis (esp. in women)
   e) Diagnosis — serology
3 Trachoma inclusion conjunctivitis (TRIC)
   a) Caused by *C. trachomatis* serotypes A-C (hyperendemic type)
   b) Estimated to affect 500 million people
   c) Commonest avoidable cause of blindness (corneal scarring)
   d) Diagnosis: chlamydial isolation
4 Psittacosis
   a) Caused by *C. psittaci*
   b) Occupational hazard of bird-fanciers
   c) Presentations
      — Atypical pneumonia
      — Myocarditis, endocarditis (rarely)
   d) Diagnosis — serology
5 Epidemic pneumonia (TWAR)
   a) Caused by *C. pneumoniae* (named TWAR after first two isolates, TW-183 and AR-39); morphologically resembles *C. psittaci*
   b) Responsible for 30% of epidemic pneumonia and 5% of sporadic pneumonia in Finland
   c) Presentations
      — Prolonged, often relapsing illness
      — Prominent pharyngitis, laryngitis
      — Atypical pneumonia mimics *Mycoplasma*/psittacosis
   d) Resistant to erythromycin (cf. other atypical pneumonias), responds to tetracycline
   e) Diagnosis — serology (distinguishable from *C. psittaci*)

STREPTOCOCCI

Principal pathogenicity of streptococci
There are three main clinical groups of streptococci
1 *St. pyogenes*
   a) Acute invasive suppurative effects
      — Impetigo
      — Cellulitis
      — Pharyngitis
   b) Other acute sequelae
      — Scarlet fever
      — Erysipelas
   c) Late non-suppurative sequelae
      — Rheumatic fever
      — Postinfective nephritis

2 *St. pneumoniae* (pneumococci)
   a) Pneumonia, esp. community-acquired lobar
   b) Meningitis
   c) Otitis media
3 *St. 'viridans'* — a broad term, including:
   a) *St. sanguis* — infective endocarditis (commonest causative streptococcus)
   b) *St. faecalis* (enterococci)
      — Urinary tract infection
      — Infective endocarditis (notoriously penicillin-resistant)
   c) *St. bovis* (enterococci) — infective endocarditis (exquisitely penicillin-sensitive)
   d) *St. milleri* — liver and/or brain abscess
   e) *St. mutans* — dental plaque/caries

Characterization of streptococci

1 Diagnostically relevant Lancefield antigen groups
   a) Gp A — *St. pyogenes*
   b) Gp D — enterococci
2 Diagnostically relevant *in vitro* haemolysis
   a) α-Haemolytic*
      — *St. viridans*
      — Pneumococci
   b) β-Haemolytic[†] — *St. pyogenes*

---

* α-Haemolytic organisms convert unlysed red cell haemoglobin in 5% blood agar to greenish (hence, 'viridans') compounds.
[†] β-Haemolytic organisms lyse red cells in 5% blood agar

Pyogenic streptococci

1 *St. pyogenes* (i.e. Gp.A β-haemolytic strep)
2 Pneumococci (Gram-positive diplococci on microscopy)
3 *St. milleri*

NB: *St. pyogenes* and pneumococci **rarely** cause streptococcal endocarditis

Streptococcal infections: clinical correlations

1 Untreated gpA streptococcal pharyngitis predisposes to development of rheumatic fever (cf. primary skin infections)
2 Both pharyngeal *and* cutaneous gpA streptococcal infections predispose to development of post-strep. glomerulonephritis
3 Prompt antibiotic therapy does *not* appear to prevent the development of post-strep. glomerulonephritis (cf. rheumatic fever)
4 Latent periods between initial infection and development of complications average four weeks for rheumatic fever, two weeks for glomerulonephritis following impetigo, and one week for synpharyngitic nephritis
5 ASO titres tend to be strongly positive in strep. pharyngitis but only weakly so in skin sepsis
6 Elevated or changing ASO titres may also be observed in association with erythema nodosum or Henoch-Schönlein purpura

Reviewing the Literature: Infectious Diseases

7.1 Wiesel J, Rose D N, Silver Al et al 1985 Lumbar puncture in asymptomatic late syphilis: an analysis of the benefits and risks. Archives of Internal Medicine 145: 465–469

Presumptive treatment with parenteral penicillin was more cost-effective and less morbid than routine lumbar puncture in patients with neurological or psychiatric syndrome

7.2 Levine M M, Herrington D, Losonsky G et al 1988 Safety, immunogenicity and efficacy of recombinant live oral cholera vaccines CVD 103 and CVD 103-HgR. Lancet ii: 467–470

Genetically engineered vaccine developed by deleting genes encoding the toxic subunit of cholera toxin from a pathogenic strain

7.3 Edman J C, Kovacs J A, Masur H et al 1988 Ribosomal RNA sequence shows *Pneumocystis carinii* to be a member of the Fungi. Nature 334: 519–521

Although morphological and ultrastructural criteria have led to *Pneumocystis* being traditionally characterized as a protozoon, phylogenetic analysis of the ribosomal RNA sequence suggests that the organism may in fact be a fungus

7.4 Erice A et al 1989 Progressive disease due to ganciclovir-resistant cytomegalovirus in immunocompromised patients. New England Journal of Medicine 320: 289–293

Erlich K S et al 1989 Acyclovir-resistant herpes simplex virus infections in patients with the acquired immunodeficiency syndrome. New England Journal of Medicine 320: 293–296

Chatis P A et al 1989 Successful treatment with foscarnet of an acyclovir-resistant mucocutaneous infection with herpes simplex virus in a patient with acquired immunodeficiency syndrome. New England Journal of Medicine 320: 297–299

Three reports illustrating that acquired resistance to antiviral chemotherapy has now become a reality, e.g. via development of mutant viral genomes associated with deficient thymidine kinases. New drugs which are not dependent upon viral thymidine kinase such as foscarnet (a pyrophosphate analogue which inhibits viral DNA polymerase) or (S)-HPMPA (S-9-3-hydroxy-2-phosphonylmethoxypropyladenine) may be useful in this setting

7.5 Saikku P et al 1988 Serological evidence of an association of a novel *Chlamydia*, TWAR, with chronic coronary heart disease and acute myocardial infarction. Lancet ii: 983–986

Finnish study of 70 patients with ischaemic heart disease demonstrating a strong serologic association with TWAR chlamydia

7.6 Allason-Jones E, Mindel A, Sargeaunt P, Williams P 1986 *Entamoeba histolytica* as a commensal intestinal parasite in homosexual men. New England Journal of Medicine 315: 354–356

20% of 354 randomly selected homosexuals attending a VD clinic had amoebae in their stools, all of which proved to be non-pathogenic zymodemes. No correlation was found with gastrointestinal symptoms. The authors conclude that it is useless to treat asymptomatic gay cyst passers

Chuck S L, Sande M A 1989 Infections with *Cryptococcus neoformans* in the acquired immunodeficiency syndrome. New England Journal of Medicine 321: 794–799

Retrospective study of 106 AIDS patients, concluding that addition of 5FC to amphotericin conferred no benefit in terms of either survival or infective relapse (only toxicity), but that long-term prophylaxis with ketoconazole or amphotericin was associated with improved survival

7.7 Taylor D N, Echeverria P, Blasser M J et al 1985 Polymicrobial aetiology of travellers' diarrhoea. Lancet i: 381–383

Of 30 episodes of travellers' diarrhoea, one-third of cases yielded 2–4 potential pathogens. Enterotoxigenic *E. coli* was found in 37% of cases, but other organisms included *C.jejuni*, *Aeromonas*, *V. parahaemolyticus*, Norwalk and rotaviruses. Fifteen symptomless infections were also documented.

7.8 Douglas R M, Moore B W, Miles H B et al 1986 Prophylactic efficacy of intranasal α-2-interferon against rhinovirus infections in the family setting. New England Journal of Medicine 314: 65–70

Double-blind Australian study of 120 patients demonstrating 76% shorter duration of symptoms from rhinovirus infection. A cure for the common cold at last?

7.9 Whitley R J, Alford C A, Hirsch M S et al 1986 Vidarabine versus acyclovir therapy in herpes simplex encephalitis. New England Journal of Medicine 314: 144–149

Prospective study of 69 patients with biopsy-proven herpes simplex encephalitis confirming that acyclovir is indeed the drug of choice in this disorder, with significant reductions in morbidity and mortality

7.10 Esmann V et al 1987 Prednisolone does not prevent postherpetic neuralgia. Lancet ii: 126–129

Danish randomized double-blind trial of 78 patients showing that about a quarter of zoster patients get postherpetic neuralgia irrespective of whether they receive steroids

CHAPTER 8

Metabolism, nutrition and genetics

Physical examination protocol 8.1 You are asked to assess the nutritional status of a patient with diarrhoea

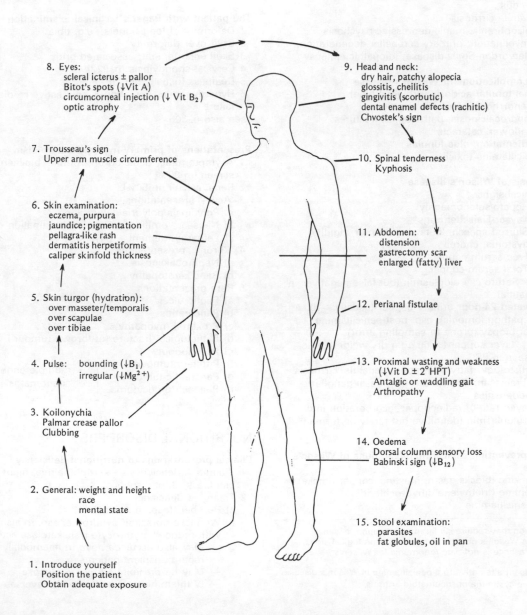

8. Eyes:
   scleral icterus ± pallor
   Bitot's spots ($\downarrow$Vit A)
   circumcorneal injection ($\downarrow$ Vit B_2)
   optic atrophy

7. Trousseau's sign
   Upper arm muscle circumference

6. Skin examination:
   eczema, purpura
   jaundice; pigmentation
   pellagra-like rash
   dermatitis herpetiformis
   caliper skinfold thickness

5. Skin turgor (hydration):
   over masseter/temporalis
   over scapulae
   over tibiae

4. Pulse: bounding ($\downarrow B_1$)
            irregular ($\downarrow Mg^{2+}$)

3. Koilonychia
   Palmar crease pallor
   Clubbing

2. General: weight and height
            race
            mental state

1. Introduce yourself
   Position the patient
   Obtain adequate exposure

9. Head and neck:
   dry hair, patchy alopecia
   glossitis, cheilitis
   gingivitis (scorbutic)
   dental enamel defects (rachitic)
   Chvostek's sign

10. Spinal tenderness
    Kyphosis

11. Abdomen:
    distension
    gastrectomy scar
    enlarged (fatty) liver

12. Perianal fistulae

13. Proximal wasting and weakness
    ($\downarrow$Vit D ± 2°HPT)
    Antalgic or waddling gait
    Arthropathy

14. Oedema
    Dorsal column sensory loss
    Babinski sign ($\downarrow B_{12}$)

15. Stool examination:
    parasites
    fat globules, oil in pan

CLINICAL ASPECTS OF METABOLIC DISORDERS

COMMONEST METABOLIC SHORT CASES

1 Paget's disease
2 Marfan's syndrome

WILSON'S DISEASE

Potential misdiagnoses in Wilson's disease

1 Coombs-negative haemolytic anaemia due to unexplained hypersplenism
2 Idiopathic ('lupoid', HBsAg-negative) chronic active hepatitis
3 'Juvenile cirrhosis'
4 Schizophrenia, manic-depressive psychosis
5 Demyelination; primary cerebellar degeneration; Hallervorden-Spatz disease; idiopathic epilepsy

Other complications of Wilson's disease

1 Renal tubular acidosis (proximal type)
2 Amenorrhoea, recurrent abortions
3 Chondrocalcinosis; pathological fractures
4 'Sunflower' cataracts
5 Pigmentation, blue lunules
6 Penicillamine toxicity

Diagnosis of Wilson's disease

1 Clinical signs
   a) Hepato/splenomegaly
   b) Kayser-Fleischer rings*
   c) Slurred speech, 'batswing' tremor, rigidity, dystonia, chorea
2 ↑ *Free* serum copper
   ↓ *Total* serum copper
   ↓ ↓ Serum caeruloplasmin (but false-negatives in hepatitis)
3 Elevated 24-hour urinary copper (usually >100 μg; not pathognomonic), esp. post-penicillamine
4 Liver biopsy (prone to sampling error)
   a) ↑ Liver copper (> 60 μg/g dry weight); also seen in PBC
   b) Histology: fatty infiltration, hepatitis, cirrhosis
5 CT brainscan: cortical atrophy, basal ganglia hypodensities
6 Delayed rate of radiocopper incorporation into caeruloplasmin (definitive but rarely performed)

Drugs preventing clinical manifestations of Wilson's disease

1 Oral zinc (blocks gastrointestinal copper uptake)
2 Trientine (triethylene dihydrochloride)†
3 D-penicillamine

---

*Exclusion may require slit-lamp examination; absence excludes Wilson's disease as cause of neurological signs, while presence is not pathognomonic for Wilson's

†Used as an alternative to D-penicillamine in Wilson's disease, but not in cystinuria or rheumatoid arthritis

SKELETAL DISORDERS

Diagnostic criteria for Marfan's syndrome

1 Major criteria
   a) Mitral valve prolapse with regurgitation
   b) Dilated aortic root with regurgitation
   c) Dissecting ascending aortic aneurysm
   d) Lens dislocation with iridodonesis (shaky iris)
2 Minor criteria
   a) Isolated mitral valve prolapse
   b) Severe myopia (>4 dioptres)
   c) High arched palate
   d) Scoliosis, 'funnel' chest, asthenic build
   e) Spontaneous pneumothorax
   f) Arachnodactyly; flat feet
   g) Joint hypermobility (esp. ankle)
   h) Positive family history

The patient with Paget's*: clinical examination

1 Deformity of long bone(s), e.g. tibia
2 Bruit over deformity
3 Skull enlargement; associated bruit
4 Cervical spondylosis (p. 222)
5 Deafness (usually nerve)
6 Hyperdynamic circulation ± congestive cardiac failure

*see also p. 305

Presentations of primary hyperparathyroidism

1 Asymptomatic; detected on 'routine' biochemical screen (in 30%)
2 Renal calculi (in 50%)
3 'Acute' presentations
   a) Polydipsia/polyuria/dehydration
   b) Nausea, vomiting, anorexia, constipation
   c) Lethargy, dementia, psychosis
4 'Chronic' presentations
   a) Nephrocalcinosis
   b) Band keratopathy
5 Rare presentations
   a) **P**eptic ulcer
   b) **P**ancreatitis
   c) **P**roximal myopathy
   d) **P**athological fracture (of 'brown tumour')
   e) **P**seudogout
   f) **P**ituitary tumours
   g) **P**ancreatic tumours } —multiple endocrine
   h) **P**haeochromocytoma } adenomatosis

NUTRITIONAL DISORDERS

Clinical presentations of nutritional deficiency

1 Vitamin A deficiency — xerophthalmia, night blindness, Bitot's spots
2 Thiamine deficiency
   a) Beri-beri (esp. in Asians)
   b) Wernicke-Korsakoff syndrome, esp. in alcoholics with reduced erythrocyte transketolase activity
   — May also occur *de novo* in haemodialysis or renal transplant patients
   — May be precipitated by i.v. glucose
   — IV thiamine treatment usually reverses

coma and ocular palsies, but nystagmus or
ataxia often persist
— May be mimicked by niacin deficiency
3 Pellagra (niacin deficiency)
   a) Dermatitis
   b) Diarrhoea
   c) Dementia
4 Strachan's syndrome (? vitamin B-complex
   deficiency)
   a) Orogenital dermatitis
   b) Amblyopia
   c) Painful peripheral neuropathy
5 Scurvy (ascorbic acid deficiency)
   a) Weakness, fatigue, arthralgias
   b) Ulcers, poor wound healing
   c) Gingivitis, purpura
   d) Subperiosteal haemorrhages (may be palpable)
6 Osteomalacia/rickets (vitamin D deficiency)
   a) Tetany (in children)
   b) Bone disease
   c) Proximal myopathy
7 Vitamin E deficiency (e.g. in cystic fibrosis, ileal
   resection, hereditary abetalipoproteinaemia)
   a) Peripheral neuropathy
   b) Spinocerebellar degeneration
   c) Haemolysis
8 Zinc deficiency — occurs in genetic form, short
   bowel syndrome, alcoholism, or TPN
   a) Acrodermatitis enteropathica
   b) Poor wound healing
   c) Alopecia
   d) Photophobia
9 Selenium deficiency: commoner in China (Keshan's
   disease: childhood cardiomyopathy) but ?may
   occur in TPN

Differential diagnosis of a pellagra-like rash
1 Pellagra (dietary niacin deficiency) — esp. with
   high-maize (leucine-rich, tryptophan-poor) diet:
   leucine inhibits conversion of tryptophan to niacin
2 Hartnup disease (inherited aminoaciduria) —
   tryptophan malabsorption → nicotinamide
   deficiency
3 Carcinoid syndrome — excess 5-hydroxytryptamine
   synthesis → tryptophan depletion
4 Isoniazid toxicity — prevents pyridoxine activation,
   depleting niacin precursors

Sorting out vitamin B_6 metabolism
1 'Niacin' = nicotinic acid = pyridine 2-carboxylic
   acid
2 Nicotinic acid is a precursor of nicotinamide which
   is in turn a precursor of NAD (nicotinamide
   adenine dinucleotide) and NADP (NAD phosphate),
   both of which participate in cellular
   oxidation/reduction reactions
3 'Pyridoxine' (vitamin B_6) = one of three pyridine
   (niacin precursor) moieties in the diet; it is
   converted to the active coenzyme, pyridoxal
   phosphate
4 Pyridoxal phosphate is involved in intermediary
   amino acid metabolism, and also binds to muscle
   glycogen phosphorylase

HYPOTHERMIA

Predispositions to hypothermia
1 Any severe illness, esp. if elderly or otherwise
   debilitated
2 Poverty, poor housing, esp. in elderly
3 Exposure
4 Drug overdose, esp.
   a) Alcohol
   b) Phenothiazines
5 Hypothyroidism
6 Erythroderma

Metabolic complications of hypothermia
1 Acidosis, hyperkalaemia
2 Tissue hypoxia; hypovolaemia; hypoglycaemia
3 Erosive gastritis, pancreatitis, pneumonia
4 ECG abnormalities — 'J' waves, ventricular
   dysrhythmias
5 Myocardial infarction if externally rewarmed
   without i.v. fluid replacement
6 Rewarming may also lead to drug toxicity when
   normal metabolism restored

Metabolic considerations in near-drowned patients
1 Fresh-water (hypotonic, hypervolaemic) drowning
   — often leads to *mild* hypoxia only, due to
   surfactant inactivation and/or intravascular
   haemolysis
2 Salt-water (hypertonic) drowning — often leads
   rapidly to *severe* hypoxia, due to induction of
   pulmonary oedema
3 'Dry drowning' — death may occur due to reflex
   laryngospasm without aspiration
4 Post-resuscitative course may be complicated by
   a) Aspiration pneumonia
   b) Acute tubular necrosis
   c) Disseminated intravascular coagulation
5 Prognosis following resuscitation is indicated to
   some extent by the presence of hypothermia
   (improved prognosis) or neurological signs (poor
   prognosis)

HYPERTHERMIA

Differential diagnosis of hyperthermia
1 Fever (due to infection)
2 Heat stroke — exacerbated by anticholinergic
   therapy
3 Iatrogenic (general)
   a) Bleomycin, L-asparaginase, interferon
   b) MAOI or sympathomimetic overdose ± tricyclics
4 Malignant hyperthermia ⎫
5 Neuroleptic malignant ⎬ — see below
   syndrome   ⎭

Malignant hyperthermia or neuroleptic malignant syndrome?
1 Malignant hyperthermia (MH)
   a) Autosomal dominant aetiology
   b) Precipitated by many inhalational anaesthetics,
      e.g. halothane, suxamethonium (cf.

pseudocholinesterase deficiency: specific for
suxamethonium)
  c) *Peripheral* origin (postsynaptic muscle
  contraction)
  d) High fever develops *rapidly* (within minutes);
  may be fatal
  e) Frequently complicated by metabolic acidosis,
  hyperkalaemia
  f) Muscle necrosis may be accompanied by
  myoglobinuria with renal failure and
  hypercalcaemia
  g) Associated with central core disease and
  myotonic dystrophy
  h) Prophylaxis or therapy: dantrolene sodium
2 Neuroleptic malignant syndrome (NMS)
  a) Idiosyncratic aetiology (impossible to predict)
  b) Precipitated by phenothiazines/butyrophenones;
  also seen in L-DOPA 'drug holidays' in
  Parkinson's disease
  c) *Central* origin (inhibition of CNS dopaminergic
  transmission)
  d) Develops *insidiously* over 1–3 days;
  characterized by fluctuating consciousness,
  dystonias, autonomic instability
  e) 20% mortality due to aspiration pneumonitis,
  acute myoglobinuric renal failure, arrhythmias
  f) Neuromuscular blockers (e.g. pancuronium) may
  cause flaccid paralysis (cf. MH: no effect)
  g) Therapy — dantrolene or bromocriptine
  (recovery takes days)

AROMATIC ABNORMALITIES

Olfactory clues in diagnosis of metabolic disorders
1 Breath
  a) Rotten apples (salicylism)
  b) Bitter almonds (cyanide intoxication)
2 Vomitus: garlic (arsenic poisoning)
3 Skin
  a) Salty (cystic fibrosis)
  b) Caramel (maple syrup urine disease)
  c) Sweaty feet (isovaleric acidaemia)
4 Urine
  a) Stale fish (methylaminuria)
  b) Mouse-like (phenylketonuria)
5 Bizarre subjective sensations
  a) Parosmia (e.g. accompanying temporal lobe
  tumours)
  b) Olfactory hallucinations, e.g. 'burning monkeys'
  (in temporal lobe epilepsy)

Anosmia: differential diagnosis
1 Post-traumatic, e.g. skull fracture (commonest
  cause)
2 Frontal meningioma
  Olfactory groove meningioma (→ asymptomatic
  unilateral loss)
3 Inherited disease — Kallman's syndrome, Refsum's
  disease
4 Postcoryzal or chronic rhinitis; cadmium poisoning
5 Sjögren's syndrome, Paget's disease
6 CNS disease: Alzheimer's disease, Parkinson's
  disease

UNUSUAL DISORDERS

Diagnoses worth considering in obscure clinical presentations
1 Malignancy, esp. Ca lung/liver/kidney, lymphoma
2 Tuberculosis; syphilis; infective endocarditis
3 Sarcoidosis
4 Polyarteritis nodosa
5 Iatrogenic
6 Functional
  a) Alcoholism/narcotic addiction
  b) Depression
  c) Hysteria
  d) Self-inflicted disease

Fibrosing syndromes in clinical medicine
1 Retroperitoneal fibrosis
2 Constrictive pericarditis
3 Sclerosing cholangitis
4 Riedel's thyroiditis
5 Peyronie's disease
6 Fibrosing alveolitis
7 Systemic sclerosis (scleroderma)

Clinical varieties of histiocytosis
1 Benign sinus histiocytosis — presents as massive
  cervical lymphadenopathy
2 Malignant histiocytosis
  a) Gut tumours in coeliac disease ('true histiocytic'
  lymphomas)
  b) Histiocytic medullary reticulosis: relentless
  neoplasm of adults manifesting with extranodal
  (esp. bony) tumours, adenopathy, rash,
  cytopaenias, fever and weight loss
3 Histiocytosis X (probably benign)
  a) Letterer-Siwe disease — fatal soft-tissue disease
  of infants — manifests with
    — Hepatosplenomegaly/lymphadenopathy
    — Cytopenias (marrow infiltration by H-X cells)
    — Lung infiltrates, recurrent pneumothoraces
  b) Hand-Schüller-Christian disease — affects
  children and adolescents — manifests with skull
  lesions
    — Exophthalmos
    — Aural discharge
    — Diabetes insipidus (in 30%)
  c) Eosinophilic granuloma — slowly progressive
  disease of adults — manifests with
    — Multiple lytic bony deposits (esp. in skull)
    — Malaise, weight loss, fever
    — Lung fibrosis

CLINICAL PRESENTATIONS OF INHERITED DISEASE

Gaucher's (adult non-neuronopathic) disease: features
1 Occurs due to deficiency of β-glucosidase
2 Presents with
  a) Hypersplenism ± massive splenomegaly
  b) Bone pain due to
    — Infarcts/aseptic necrosis
    — Bone cysts (→distal femur)
    — Vertebral collapse
    — Pathological fracture

c) Pingueculae; pigmentation
d) Pneumonia
3 Normal life expectancy (i.e. in adult — type III — disease)
4 Best screening test is serum acid phosphatase (tartrate-resistant)
5 Definitive diagnosis is by demonstration of Gaucher cells in marrow, liver or node — PAS +ve cells with 'crumpled silk' cytoplasm (may also be seen in CGL, myeloma, ITP)

Clinical spectrum of mitochondrial disease
1 Progressive external ophthalmoplegia, incl. Kearns-Sayre ('oculocraniosomatic') syndrome — ophthalmoplegia + retinitis pigmentosa + complete heart block + increased CSF protein
2 Hypermetabolic proximal myopathy — e.g. Luft's: heat intolerance, fever, diaphoresis and weakness (may mimic thyrotoxicosis)
3 'Ragged red fibre' syndrome
   a) Myopathy resembles facioscapulohumeral dystrophy
   b) May be associated with myoclonic epilepsy, lactic acidosis
4 Cytochrome deficiencies — e.g. Menke's ('kinky hair') syndrome

NB: diseases due to abnormal mitochondrial DNA are inherited strictly via the *maternal genome*

Inborn abnormalities of connective tissue: features
1 Marfan's syndrome
   a) Autosomal dominant, variable penetrance
   b) Increasing frequency with paternal age
   c) 30% sporadic mutation rate
   d) Occurs due to ↓ type I collagen
   e) Signs
      — Armspan > height; scoliosis
      — Joint hypermobility
      — Arachnodactyly → 'wrist', 'thumb' signs
      — High palate, iridodonesis
      — Pectus deformity; MVP, AI
2 Osteogenesis imperfecta — occurs due to *qualitatively abnormal* type I collagen
3 Homocystinuria (autosomal recessive)
   Some phenotypic similarity to Marfan's but —
   a) Atherothrombotic tendency
   b) Subclinical osteoporosis
   c) Downward lens dislocation
   d) 30% incidence of mental retardation
   e) Responds to
      — Dietary methionine restriction
      — Cystine supplements
      — Pyridoxine (in 50%)
      — Betaine
4 Pseudoxanthoma elasticum (dominant or recessive)
   a) Flexural xanthoma-like lesions, lax skin
   b) Fundal angioid streaks
   c) Premature atherosclerosis (→hypothyroidism *inter alia*)
   d) Diagnostic calcium deposition on skin biopsy
   e) Occurs due to production of *abnormal elastin*
5 Ehlers-Danlos syndromes (dominant or recessive)
   a) Characterized by
      — Joint hypermobility, recurrent dislocations
      — Purpura
      — 'Fish-mouth' scarring
      — Diverticulosis, pneumothoraces
   b) Type IV
      — GI bleeding, visceral perforation, aneurysm rupture
      — Occurs due to ↓ type III collagen
   c) Type VI
      — Retinal detachment, corneal perforation
      — Occurs due to ↓ lysyl hydroxylase
   d) Type VII
      — Velvety skin, short stature
      — Occurs due to ↓ procollagen protease
   e) Type VIII manifests as periodontitis
6 Disorders due to reduced lysyl oxidase activity
   a) Ehlers-Danlos Type V (X-linked)
   b) Cutis laxa (X-linked) → emphysema, pulmonary hypertension
   c) Menke's 'kinky hair' syndrome (defective copper absorption)

Laurence-Moon vs Bardet-Biedl syndrome: the clinical distinction
1 Features in common
   a) Mental retardation
   b) Hypogonadism
   c) Obesity
   d) Retinopathy
2 Additional features of Laurence-Moon syndrome
   a) Ataxia
   b) Spastic paraparesis
3 Additional features of Bardet-Biedl syndrome
   a) Polydactyly
   b) Renal abnormalities
      — Persistent fetal lobulation
      — Cystic dysplasia, clubbed calices
      — Nephrogenic diabetes insipidus
      — Aminoaciduria

INVESTIGATING METABOLIC DISORDERS

Causes of misleading results
1 (Pseudo)hyponatraemia
   a) High-grade paraproteinaemia
   b) Chylomicronaemia (diabetic ketoacidosis, hyperlipidaemia type I or type V)
   c) Intravenous therapy (incl. mannitol or parenteral fat emulsions)
2 Spurious hyperkalaemia
   a) (Leukaemic) white cell count > 200 000/ml
   b) Difficult venepuncture ⎫ Haemolysis
   c) Delay in processing ⎬ –in vitro
      specimen ⎭
3 Spurious hyperchloraemia — bromism
4 Spurious hyperglycaemia — venepuncture adjacent to dextrose infusion site
5 Spurious hypercalcaemia
   a) Prolonged venous stasis
   b) Rarely, binding of calcium by myelomatous paraprotein
      Spurious normocalcaemia — profound hypoalbuminaemia (e.g. in patients with carcinomatosis)

6 Elevated triglycerides
Elevated gastrin } —patient not fasted
Low growth hormone
7 Elevated CPK — recent intramuscular injection
8 Elevated acid phosphatase — recent rectal examination
9 Negative urinalysis for ketones — alcoholic ketoacidosis (leads to high β-hydroxybutyrate but normal acetone)

ELECTROLYTE DISORDERS AND THE ANION GAP

The high-anion-gap metabolic acidosis: common precipitants
1 Uraemia
2 Ketoacidosis (diabetic or alcoholic)
3 Lactic acidosis (± dehydration, alcohol intoxication)
4 Overdose
  a) Aspirin
  b) Methanol, ethylene glycol
  c) Paraldehyde

Lactic acidosis: antecedents and diagnosis
1 Type A — may be precipitated by *any* cause of severe tissue hypoxia
2 Type B
  a) 'Idiopathic' onset in elderly debilitated patients
  b) Alcohol abuse and/or liver disease
  c) Uraemia
  d) Some leukaemias, myeloproliferative disorders
  e) Diabetes mellitus ± metformin ± ketoacidosis
3 Clinical — hyperventilation without dehydration (cf. hyperosmolar coma: vice versa)
4 Definitive diagnosis depends on exclusion of other causes of high-anion-gap acidosis, and/or demonstration of elevated plasma lactate

Examples of mixed metabolic acidosis
1 Normal- and high-anion gap acidoses
  a) Renal tubular acidosis leading to nephrocalcinosis
  b) Diabetic with hyporeninaemic hypoaldosteronism developing ketoacidosis
2 Mixed normal-anion gap acidoses
  a) Acetazolamide therapy in patients with pre-existing renal tubular acidosis
3 Mixed high-anion gap acidoses
  a) Alcoholic ketoacidosis complicated by lactic acidosis
  b) Methanol intoxication and lactic acidosis

Differential diagnosis of a low anion gap
(may mask biochemical recognition of metabolic acidosis)
1 Hypoalbuminaemia
2 Paraproteinaemia
3 Electrolyte imbalance
  a) Hypercalcaemia
  b) Hypermagnesaemia
  c) Lithium intoxication

Hyperchloraemic (normal anion gap) acidosis: pathogeneses
(anion gap = $Na^+ - Cl^- - HCO_3^-$; normal range = 8–12 mEq/L)
1 Renal tubular acidosis
2 Gastrointestinal
  a) Diarrhoea, esp. in neonates
  b) Pancreatic/biliary fistula
  c) Ureteroenterostomy ± obstructed ileal bladder/vesicocolic fistula
3 Iatrogenic
  a) Acetazolamide
  b) Cholestyramine
  c) Parenteral nutrition with fructose, sorbitol

Normal anion gap acidosis with hyperkalaemia*: causes
(*type 4 renal tubular acidosis)
1 Treated diabetic ketoacidosis
2 Obstructive uropathy
3 Early uraemic acidosis, esp. if due to medullary disease
4 Mineralocorticoid deficiency or insensitivity

Some causes of hypouricaemia
1 Proximal renal tubular disease (e.g. Wilson's disease)
2 SIADH (e.g. acute intermittent porphyria, Guillain-Barré)
3 Chronic liver disease
4 Carcinomatosis
5 Hereditary xanthinuria (xanthine oxidase deficiency)
6 Drug-induced — allopurinol, high-dose aspirin, NSAIDs, sulphinpyrazone, diflunisal, probenecid

Indications for serum magnesium estimation
1 Severe or intractable diarrhoea and/or malabsorption, e.g.
  a) Short bowel syndrome
  b) Inflammatory bowel disease
2 Life-threatening alcohol withdrawal
3 Refractory cardiac arrhythmias (esp. ventricular) Unexplained digoxin toxicity
4 Apathetic thyrotoxicosis
5 Hypocalcaemia and/or tetany unresponsive to calcium supplements
6 Neuromuscular symptoms following *cis*-platinum and/or mannitol infusion

Clinically important causes of hypophosphataemia
1 Insulin treatment of diabetic ketoacidosis
2 Alcoholic withdrawal supported with dextrose infusions
3 Proximal renal tubular dysfunction
4 Following starvation or severe burns
5 Iatrogenic — hyperalimentation, phosphate-binding antacids, haemodialysis, paracetamol overdose
6 Osteomalacia (unless associated with renal failure)

Manifestations of hypophosphataemia
1 Tissue hypoxia (due to reduced erythrocyte 2,3DPG) leading to ataxia, confusion, convulsions; esp. in ketoacidosis

2 Leucocyte dysfunction
   → sepsis
   Platelet dysfunction → } Due to ↓ intracellular ATP
   bleeding
   Haemolytic anaemia
3 Rhabdomyolysis (esp. in alcoholics) ±
   cardiomyopathy, renal failure, delayed
   hypercalcaemia

HYPERCALCAEMIA

Common causes of hypercalcaemia
1 Hyperparathyroidism
2 Malignancy

Steroid-suppressible hypercalcaemia: differential diagnosis
1 Sarcoidosis
2 Vitamin D intoxication
3 Multiple myeloma

Differential diagnosis of hypercalcaemia with detectable iPTH
1 Hyperparathyroidism
   a) Primary
   b) Tertiary
   c) Secondary, *if* there has been overzealous
      prescription of phosphate binders
2 Immobilization (urinary cAMP normal)
3 Malignancy (urinary cAMP commonly elevated
   without ↑ iPTH)
4 Phaeochromocytoma
   a) Part of MEA type II (Sipple's syndrome)
   b) Catecholamine-stimulated PTH release

Steps in the diagnosis of primary hyperparathyroidism:
1 ↑ Ca^{2+}; ± ↓ PO_4^{2-} (normalization may presage
   renal failure)
2 Phosphaturia (> hypercalciuria); mild ↑ alk. phos.
3 Hyperchloraemic acidosis with alkaline urine
4 ↑ iPTH
   a) Normal levels do not exclude the diagnosis,
      though undetectable levels do
   b) The carboxy-terminal fragment is generally
      assayed, though the amino-terminal fragment
      confers activity
5 Elevated nephrogenous cAMP (non-suppressible
   with oral calcium tolerance test)
6 Glandular hyperplasia/adenoma demonstrated at
   neck exploration; resection followed by
   normalization of serum calcium

Hypercalcaemia: selected clinical aspects
1 Dehydration may arise due to any combination of
   a) Vomiting
   b) Reduced fluid intake (anorexia, obtundation)
   c) Nephrogenic diabetes insipidus
   Azotaemia may supervene due to
   a) Prerenal failure (i.e. secondary to dehydration)
   b) Renal vasoconstriction, ↓ glomerular
      permeability (acute)
   c) Tubular vacuolization and/or nephrocalcinosis
      (chronic)

2 Immobilization hypercalcaemia (and hypercalciuria)
   occurs more frequently in patients with Paget's
   disease. Corticosteroids and phosphate (oral, i.v.)
   therapy are contraindicated in the treatment of
   immobilization hypercalcaemia
3 Gut hyperabsorption contributes to the
   hypercalcaemia of
   a) Sarcoidosis
   b) 'Milk-alkali' syndrome
   c) Primary hyperparathyroidism
4 Rhabdomyolysis may lead to initial hypocalcaemia
   with azotaemia followed by hypercalcaemia during
   the early phase of renal recovery
5 Familial hypocalciuric ('benign familial')
   hypercalcaemia classically presents as a failed neck
   exploration for hyperparathyroidism; it is the
   commonest cause of hypercalcaemia in patients
   aged less than 10 years

VITAMIN D

Abnormal patterns of vitamin D metabolism in disease
1 Vitamin D intoxication
   a) ↑ 25-Hydroxycholecalciferol ($25-D_3$)
   b) Normal $1,25-D_3$
2 Sarcoidosis
   a) Normal $25-D_3$
   b) ↑ $1,25-D_3$ (even in *anephric* patients)
3 Chronic renal failure
   a) Normal $25-D_3$
   b) ↓ $1,25-D_3$
   c) ↑ $24,25-D_3$
4 Rickets
   a) Normal $1,25-D_3$ (vitamin D-resistant rickets)
   b) ↓ $1,25-D_3$ (type I vitamin D-dependent rickets)
   c) ↑ $1,25-D_3$ (type II vitamin D-dependent rickets)

Differential diagnosis of abnormal vitamin D metabolism
1 ↑ $1,25-D_3$
   a) Primary hyperparathyroidism
   b) Pregnancy
   c) Sarcoidosis
2 ↓ $1,25-D_3$
   a) Malignancy-induced hypercalcaemia
   b) Postmenopausal osteoporosis
   c) Chronic renal failure
3 ↑ $25-D_3$—vitamin D intoxication
   ↓ $25-D_3$
   a) Osteomalacia
   b) Hypomagnesaemia
   c) Chronic liver disease (e.g. PBC)
   d) Chronic peritoneal dialysis
   e) Nephrotic syndrome
   f) Phenytoin use

DIAGNOSTIC ASPECTS OF METABOLIC BONE DISEASE

Diagnostic significance of elevated urinary hydroxyproline*

---

*Indicates collagen breakdown; correlates with serum alkaline
phosphatase

1 Paget's disease (often $>50 \times \uparrow$)
2 Hereditary
  hyperphosphatasia } (often $>50 \times \uparrow$)
3 Hyperparathyroidism
4 Osteomalacia (*except* renal tubular type)
5 Thyrotoxicosis

Diagnostic features of pseudohypoparathyroidism

1 Hypocalcaemia, hypocalciuria, hyperphosphaturia (cf. 'pseudopseudo-' variant)
2 No enamel hypoplasia or candidiasis (cf. 'idiopathic' variety)
3 No associated autoimmune diathesis
  Positive (maternal) family history (inheritance is X-dominant)
4 Short fourth and fifth metacarpals (cf. Turner's syndrome — short fourth metacarpal; Down's syndrome — short, curved middle phalanx of fifth finger)
5 Mental retardation (variable), dwarfism, obesity, subcutaneous calcification — all more consistently present in pseudo-pseudohypoparathyroidism
6 Normal or elevated serum iPTH
  Subnormal increment of urinary phosphate and nephrogenous cAMP following PTH infusion } — cf. idiopathic hypoparathyroidism
  Responsive to pharmacological doses of calcitriol

Diagnostic considerations in osteomalacia

1 The main source of vitamin D for most people is sunlight; however, elderly people with little sun exposure may develop osteomalacia following dietary malabsorption induced (say) by gastrectomy
2 Proximal myopathy may be a prominent presenting symptom; it is thought to arise in part due to hypophosphataemia and in part due to vitamin D deficiency *per se*
3 In addition to the characteristic radiographic features (q.v.), the diagnosis is suggested by the biochemical triad of hypocalcaemia, hypophosphataemia, and elevated serum alkaline phosphatase
4 Definitive diagnosis is made by bone biopsy

RADIOGRAPHIC FEATURES OF METABOLIC DISORDERS

Radiological stigmata of hyperparathyroidism

1 Generalized osteopenia
2 Subperiosteal resorption of radial aspects of middle phalanges of second and third fingers (highly specific)
  Resorption of distal phalangeal tufts (and/or distal clavicles)
3 Bone cysts, 'brown tumours' → phalanges, metacarpals, long bones
4 'Fleabitten' mandible
  'Salt-and-pepper' skull

5 Loss of (dental) lamina dura
  Clavicular erosions
6 Nephrocalcinosis, renal calculi
  Chondrocalcinosis
  Vascular calcification (in secondary hyperparathyroidism)

Classical spinal X-rays in metabolic bone disease

1 'Rugger-jersey' spine
  a) Renal osteodystrophy
  b) Osteopetrosis ('bone-within-bone')
2 'Ivory vertebrae'
  a) Paget's disease
  b) Hodgkin's disease
3 'Codfish' vertebrae
  a) Osteoporosis
  b) Osteomalacia
  c) Sickle-cell disease

Classical skull X-rays in metabolic bone disease

1 Osteoporosis circumscripta: Paget's disease
2 'Raindrops' — myeloma (numerous lytic lesions without surrounding osteoblastic reaction)
3 'Salt-and-pepper' skull — hyperparathyroidism
4 Wormian bones — osteogenesis imperfecta
5 'Hair-on-end' appearance — inherited anaemias
6 'Punched-out' skull lesions — histiocytosis X
7 Enlarged frontal sinuses — acromegaly (cf. *absent* frontal sinuses: Kartagener's syndrome)
8 Hyperostosis frontalis interna — normal variant (esp. in women)

Other radiographic anomalies in bone disease

1 Rickets — widened epiphyseal plate with indistinct borders; splaying of bone ends (esp. wrists, knees); deformities — tibial bowing, frontal bossing
2 Osteomalacia
  Pseudo-('Milkman's') fractures, Looser's zones:
  — Pubic rami
  — Proximal femurs
  — Lateral scapulae
  — Ribs
3 Scurvy
  a) Sclerotic bone edge ('dense white line') at epiphysis
  b) No widening of epiphyseal plate (cf. rickets)
  c) Periosteal elevation due to haemorrhage — seen after treatment
4 Heavy metal poisoning — dense 'white line' at metaphysis (cf. scurvy)
5 Osteoid osteoma — densely sclerotic lesion comprising radiolucent zone around a central nidus; presents as aspirin-sensitive bone pain in a young patient
6 Osteopetrosis — 'Erlenmeyer flask' deformity of metaphyses

Possible indications for isotope bone scanning

1 Suspected metastatic bone disease
2 Suspected (X-ray negative) fracture, esp.
  a) Stress
  b) Sternum
  c) Scaphoid

3 Suspected aseptic necrosis (efficacy limited by non-specificity)
4 Suspected sacroiliitis with non-diagnostic X-ray findings (value in this context is controversial)
5 Suspected periprosthetic infection (gallium scanning)
6 Paget's disease

INVESTIGATION OF GENETIC DISEASE

Screening tests available for inborn errors of metabolism
1 Benedict's test (copper reduction) — galactosaemia
2 DNP (dinitrophenylhydrazine) test — maple syrup urine disease
3 Nitroprusside test — homocystinuria
4 Alkaline silver reduction — alkaptonuria (ochronosis)
5 Urinary colorimetry — orotic aciduria

Presymptomatic disease identifiable by genetic linkage analysis
1 Huntington's chorea
2 Myotonic dystrophy
3 Duchenne muscular dystrophy
4 Neurofibromatosis (incl. acoustic variant)
5 Cystic fibrosis
6 α/β-thalassaemias
7 Adult polycystic kidney disease (one type)
8 Multiple polyposis
9 Multiple endocrine adenomatosis type IIa

Diagnosis of familial Mediterranean fever (recurrent polyserositis)
1 Clinical
   a) Ethnic origin
   b) Previous attacks ± failed exploratory laparotomy
   c) Positive family history
   d) Rapid defervescence
2 Mild leucocytosis
   ↑ ESR, ↑ fibrinogen } —During attacks
3 Proteinuria (in amyloidosis)
4 ↑ Plasma dopamine β-hydroxylase (normalizes with colchicine; *best test*)
5 Negative microbiology (incl. joint fluid)
   Normal amylase
   Negative ANA and rheumatoid factor
6 Therapeutic response to prophylactic colchicine

MANAGING METABOLIC DISEASE

Therapeutic priorities in metabolic derangements
1 Lactic acidosis
   a) Removal of underlying cause (e.g. alcohol)
   b) IV bicarbonate ± dichloroacetate
2 Alcoholic ketoacidosis
   a) Intravenous glucose, *plus*
   b) Intravenous thiamine
3 Diabetic ketoacidosis
   a) Insulin
   b) Fluid and electrolyte balance
4 Hyperosmolar (non-ketotic diabetic) coma

   a) IV fluid replacement (use hypotonic saline unless hypotensive)
   b) Insulin (usually *not* necessary in *long-term* therapy; cf. DKA)
5 Hypoglycaemic coma
   a) Prevention
   b) Immediate therapeutic trial of i.v. dextrose (±naloxone) in any undiagnosed unconscious patient*
6 Myxoedema coma
   a) *Active exclusion* of associated hypothermia/-glycaemia/-natraemia/-adrenalism
   b) Low-dose increments of i.v. thyroid hormone with presumptive i.v. hydrocortisone supplementation

MANAGEMENT OF ELECTROLYTE ABNORMALITIES

Hypokalaemia: when is prophylactic supplementation indicated?
1 Patients clinically hypovolaemic due to gastrointestinal losses who are commencing resuscitation with i.v. fluids
2 Patients undergoing insulin and fluid replacement for diabetic ketoacidosis unless hyperkalaemic **and**
   a) ECG changes of hyperkalaemia or
   b) Biochemical evidence of prerenal failure or
   c) Known coexisting hyporeninaemic hypoaldosteronism
3 Patients with anticipated large renal losses, e.g.
   a) Postobstructive diuresis
   b) Sjögren's syndrome postpartum
   c) Wilson's disease with renal tubular dysfunction and cirrhosis
4 Patients commencing therapy with
   a) Loop diuretics
   b) Ticarcillin
   c) Amphotericin B
5 Patients stabilized on digoxin and commencing therapy with
   a) Thiazides
   b) Corticosteroids

An approach to acute hyperkalaemia
1 Exclude diabetic ketoacidosis as a cause, since the hyperkalaemia of insulin deficiency may be associated with total body potassium deficit (and hence require potassium *supplements* with insulin)
2 Check result on fresh specimen to exclude haemolysis artefact
3 Identify and remove precipitating cause if possible
4 Administer 50 ml 50% dextrose i.v. followed by soluble insulin (8–12 units)
5 Administer 50 ml 8.4% sodium bicarbonate i.v.
6 Administer 20 ml 10% calcium gluconate i.v. if ECG changes present
7 Prescribe 15 g cation-exchange resin orally sixth-hourly, and 30 g per rectum 12-hourly
8 Dialysis (esp. peritoneal) may be indicated

---

*If associated Wernicke-Korsakoff syndrome suspected, be sure to give i.v. thiamine at the same time

Approach to management of severe hyponatraemia
($Na^+ < 110$ mmol/L)

1 Asymptomatic patient on diuretics, normotensive, low plasma sodium found on routine testing
   a) Discontinue diuretic
   b) Restrict water intake
   c) Encourage dietary salt intake until Na^+ normal
2 Minimally symptomatic patient, hypotensive, no CNS signs
   a) Restrict water intake
   b) IV normal saline to re-expand plasma volume
3 Symptomatic patient, CNS signs present (e.g. postop)
   a) Slow hypertonic (3%) saline infusion — calibrate rate to increase plasma Na^+ by a maximum of 1 mmol/h until Na^+ >125 mmol/l (more rapid infusion may precipitate *central pontine myelinolysis*); then,
   b) Restrict water intake

Hazards of bicarbonate administration in metabolic acidosis

1 High sodium/osmotic load
2 Aggravation of tissue hypoxia ($\uparrow$ Hb affinity for oxygen)
3 Paradoxical fall in CSF pH, leading to hypoventilation

MEDICAL TECHNOLOGY

Potential indications for hyperbaric oxygen therapy

1 Gas gangrene
   Other infections
   a) Anaerobic sepsis with tissue necrosis
   b) Mucormycosis, actinomycosis
   c) Refractory chronic osteomyelitis
2 Carbon monoxide poisoning (controversial)
   Other poisonous inhalations
   a) Hydrogen cyanide (adjunctive only)
   b) Hydrogen sulphide
   c) Smoke inhalation
3 Decompression sickness ('the bends')
4 Air embolism
5 Wound healing
   a) Radiation necrosis
   b) Severe thermal burns
   c) Ischaemic crush injury

Iatrogenic consequences of synthetic implantable devices

1 Infection, e.g.
   a) Prosthetic hip
   b) Cardiac valve replacement
   c) CSF shunts
   d) Soft contact lenses; lens implants
   e) Long-term vascular access catheters
   f) Indwelling urinary catheters
2 Thromboembolism, e.g.
   a) Vascular grafts
   b) Valve replacements
3 Specific valve problems
   a) Valve failure (acute incompetence)
   b) Valve thrombosis (acute stenosis)

   c) Haemolysis
4 Specific IUD problems
   a) Pelvic inflammatory disease, infertility
   b) Ectopic pregnancy; septic abortion
   c) Uterine perforation, peritonitis
   d) *Actinomyces*/fungal infections (with plastic IUDs)

NUTRITIONAL SUPPLEMENTATION

Indications for high-dose vitamin supplements

1 Vitamins A,D,E,K
   a) Hereditary abetalipoproteinaemia
   b) Biliary atresia
   c) Cystic fibrosis
2 Vitamin B_6
   a) Homocystinuria
   b) Idiopathic refractory sideroblastic anaemia
   c) Renal oxalate stones
   d) Unexplained infantile convulsions
3 Vitamin B_{12}
   a) Transcobalamin II deficiency
   b) Juvenile pernicious anaemia
   c) Homocystinuria
4 Folate—congenital megaloblastosis
5 Vitamin K — coagulopathy due to liver disease (esp. postpartum)

Toxicity of vitamin overdosage

1 Vitamin A
   a) Skin dryness, fissuring, hair loss
   b) Bone pain, hypercalcaemia
   c) Raised intracranial pressure ('pseudotumour')
   d) Hepatic fibrosis
2 Vitamin B_3 (niacin)
   a) Pruritus, hair loss
   b) Peptic ulcer
   c) Abnormal liver function tests
3 Vitamin B_6 (pyridoxine)
   a) Sensory neuropathy
   b) Antagonism of L-DOPA
4 Vitamin C—renal oxalate stones
5 Vitamin D
   a) Hypercalcaemia
   b) Hypertension
6 Vitamin E—warfarin potentiation (impairment of vitamin K absorption)
7 Vitamin K—haemolysis

Drug-induced vitamin deficiencies

1 Pyridoxine (B_6)
   a) Isoniazid (in slow acetylators)
   b) Cycloserine
   c) D-penicillamine
   d) Hydralazine; chloramphenicol; L-DOPA
   e) ?Oral contraceptives
2 Folate
   a) Cholestyramine
   b) Phenytoin
   c) 'Antifolates': methotrexate, pyrimethamine, trimethoprim, triamterene, pentamidine
   d) Sulphasalazine, oral contraceptives (may 'unmask' pre-existing borderline deficiency)

3 B_{12}
   a) Chloramphenicol
   b) Longterm PAS, metformin, oral neomycin
4 B_1 (thiamine): nitrofurantoin
   B_2 (riboflavin): thalidomide
5 Vitamin D
   a) *Long-term* phenytoin/phenobarbitone (?due to hepatic induction → inactivation of 1,25DHCC)
   b) Cadmium poisoning ('ouch-ouch' disease — Itai-Itai — osteomalacia in Japan)
6 Vitamin K
   a) Warfarin
   b) Aspirin
   c) Latamoxef
   d) 'Megadose' vitamin E

Disorders which may respond to pyridoxine
1 Homocystinuria
2 Primary hyperoxaluria
3 Idiopathic refractory sideroblastic anaemia
4 Alcoholics developing neuropathy while taking isoniazid
5 Depression in women taking contraceptive pill
   Vomiting in pregnant women
   Convulsions of obscure cause in neonates

Indications for hyperalimentation (parenteral nutrition)
1 Short bowel syndrome
2 Crohn's disease with severe malabsorption
3 Prolonged ileus
4 Pancreatic/intestinal fistula
5 Hypermetabolism (e.g. severe sepsis or burns)
6 Hyperemesis gravidarum (or other cause of temporary feeding difficulty)

Metabolic complications of total parenteral nutrition
1 Hyperglycaemia (may be aggravated by occult chromium deficiency) if insufficient insulin added to infusion
   Hypoglycaemia (most commonly due to kinking of dextrose infusion containing insulin which continues to act)
   Hyperosmolar coma (may be precipitated by sepsis)
2 Hypercalcaemia (e.g. due to hypervitaminosis A or D)
   Osteomalacia (in long-term TPN)
3 Hyperchloraemic acidosis (preventable with acetate supplement)
   Lactic acidosis (→ fructose infusions in neonates)
4 Hypophosphataemia (esp. during dextrose infusions)
   Pseudohyponatraemia (during infusion of fat emulsions)
   Hypokalaemia, hypomagnesaemia, copper/zinc deficiency
5 Exfoliative dermatitis — hypervitaminosis A, fatty acid deficiency, zinc deficiency
6 Liver disease
   a) Fatty infiltration
   b) Lymphocytic infiltration (± transaminitis)
   c) Jaundice (± cholestasis, sepsis)
   d) Hyperammonaemia (± encephalopathy)

MANAGEMENT OF METABOLIC BONE DISEASE

Hyperparathyroidism: indications for surgical management
1 Renal calculi
   Progressive renal impairment due to nephrocalcinosis
2 Recurrent peptic ulceration (exclude associated gastrinoma)
3 Progressive reduction in height (vertebral osteopenia)
   Recurrent pancreatitis
   Recent onset of psychiatric symptoms
4 Severe or progressive radiological abnormalities (e.g. osteitis fibrosa cystica associated with 2°/3° hyperparathyroidism in chronic renal failure)
5 High serum calcium (e.g. > 3.0 mmol/l) in a patient living in a remote location

NB: Provided that experienced surgeons are available, it is probably wisest to proceed to operation if there is any doubt concerning the presence of symptoms

Potential therapeutic modalities in postmenopausal osteoporosis
1 Hormone replacement therapy
   a) Oestrogens
   b) Progestogens
2 Exercise
3 Calcium supplements
4 Subcutaneous or intranasal calcitonin
5 Controversial—vitamin D supplements, sodium fluoride

UNDERSTANDING METABOLIC DISEASE

Racial predispositions to disease
1 Ashkenazy Jews
   a) Gaucher's
   b) Tay-Sachs
   c) Riley-Day
   d) Niemann-Pick
   e) Bassen-Kornzweig
   f) Bloom's
   Non-Ashkenazy (Sephardic) Jews — familial Mediterranean fever (recurrent polyserositis)
2 African negro, Mediterranean littoral
   a) Sickle-cell anaemia
   b) Thalassaemias
   c) Hb C
3 Lebanese
   a) Hypercholesterolaemia
   b) Behçet's
4 Chinese
   a) α-Thalassaemia
   b) Alactasia
5 Northern European caucasians
   a) Idiopathic haemochromatosis
   b) Phenylketonuria
   c) Acute intermittent porphyria
   Swedes
   a) Cystic fibrosis

b) Giant-cell arteritis
c) α-1-Antitrypsin deficiency
d) LCAT deficiency
Finns
a) Imerslund's disease
b) *Diphyllobothrium latum* infestations
c) Mulibrey nanism (→ pericarditis)
d) Congenital nephrosis
6 Eskimos (esp. Yupik)
a) Congenital adrenal hyperplasia
b) Pseudocholinesterase deficiency
c) Rapid acetylation status (in up to 100%)
7 Other races
Thais — Hb H disease (Hb Constant Spring →
2–5%)
Pima Indians/Micronesians/Yemenite Jews — type
II (non-insulin-dependent) diabetes mellitus
South Africans — variegate porphyria
Scottish — peptic ulceration (acid hypersecretion)
Quebecois — tyrosinaemia (→ cirrhosis, renal
tubular acidosis)

INHERITED DISEASE

Factors maintaining the heterozygote frequency of genetic disease
1 Duchenne muscular dystrophy *et al* — new
mutations
2 Haemoglobinopathies (e.g. sickle-cell anaemia) —
resistance to malaria
3 Lipid storage diseases
Peptic ulcer diathesis   } resistance to TB
4 Congenital adrenal hyperplasia — resistance to *H. influenzae* #B
5 Idiopathic haemochromatosis — resistance to
iron-deficiency anaemia (in women)
6 Type I (insulin-dependent) diabetes mellitus —
reduced incidence of miscarriage (? due to HLA
association)
Type II (non-insulin-dependent) diabetes mellitus
protects against starvation

Autosomal dominant inheritance of suspected single-gene defects
1 Familial hypercholesterolaemia
2 Multiple polyposis
3 Neurofibromatosis
4 Tuberose sclerosis
5 Myotonic dystrophy
6 Huntington's chorea
7 Marfan's syndrome
8 Acute intermittent porphyria
9 Adult polycystic kidney disease

Autosomal recessive inheritance of suspected single-gene defects
1 Cystic fibrosis
2 β-Thalassemia
3 Sickle-cell anaemia
4 Phenylketonuria
5 Galactosaemia

6 Tay-Sachs disease
7 Infantile polycystic kidney disease

X-linked recessive inheritance of suspected single-gene defects
1 Haemophilias A and B
2 Duchenne muscular dystrophy
3 Alport's syndrome
4 Lesch-Nyhan syndrome
5 Nephrogenic diabetes insipidus
6 Testicular feminization syndrome
7 G6PD deficiency

GENETIC COUNSELLING

Referral for genetic counselling: potential indications
1 Suspected chromosomal abnormality
2 Diagnosed congenital and/or heritable abnormality
3 Abnormal mental or physical development
4 Abnormal sexual development
5 Unexplained infertility
6 Repeated abortions

Risk assessment in genetic counselling (general)
1 Risk of spontaneous abortion in established
pregnancy—10–15%
2 Risk of married couple's infertility—10%
3 Risk of baby being born with physical or mental
defect—2%
4 Risk of perinatal death or stillbirth—1%
5 Risk of death in infancy—0.5%

GENETIC DIAGNOSIS

Methods of localizing abnormal genes to specific chromosomes
1 Gene linkage (i.e. of a disease phenotype with a
mapped gene), e.g.
a) 21-hydroxylase deficiency with HLA gene cluster
b) Myotonic dystrophy with secretor (Se) gene
2 Linkage disequilibrium (i.e. between a suspected
gene mutation and a mapped restriction fragment
length polymorphism), e.g.
a) Huntington's chorea
b) Duchenne muscular dystrophy
c) Cystic fibrosis
d) Neurofibromatosis; tuberose sclerosis
e) Adult polycystic kidney disease (one type)
f) Haemophilias, α-Thalassaemias
3 Mutation-specific gene probes, e.g.
a) Sickle-cell anaemia
b) α$_1$-Antitrypsin deficiency
c) β-Thalassaemias
d) Phenylketonuria

Dermatoglyphic stigmata of Down's syndrome
1 Distal axial triradius (demonstrable in 85%)
2 Simian crease (single transverse palmar flexion
crease)—50%
3 Supernumerary ulnar loops

Reviewing the Literature: Metabolism, nutrition and genetics

8.1 Stunkard A J, Sorensen T I A, Harris C et al 1986 An adoption study of human obesity. New England Journal of Medicine 314: 193–198

Danish study of 540 adoptees revealed a strong link between degree of body fat in probands and biological (not adoptive) parents, suggesting a predominantly genetic — rather than environmental — mode of inheritance for this trait

Peterson H R et al 1988 Body fat and the activity of the autonomic nervous system. New England Journal of Medicine 318: 1077–1083

Study of 56 male patients which demonstrated a significant correlation between body fat and activity of the sympathetic and parasympathetic nervous system

8.2 Worthley L I G, Thomas P D 1986 Treatment of hyponatraemic seizures with intravenous 29.2% saline. British Medical Journal 292: 168–170

Report of 5 severely hyponatraemic fitting patients treated by rapid i.v. infusion of hypertonic saline, all of whom did well

8.3 Straus S E et al 1988 Acyclovir treatment of the chronic fatigue syndrome: lack of efficacy in a placebo-controlled trial. New England Journal of Medicine 319: 1692–1698

No effect of acyclovir in 27 patients with chronic fatigue syndrome ('epidemic myalgia', 'myalgic encephalomyelitis', 'Royal Free disease'), tending to make possibility of an occult systemic viral aetiology (esp. EBV) less likely

8.4 Baggio G et al 1986 Apolipoprotein C-II deficiency syndrome: clinical features, lipoprotein characterisation, lipase activity, and correction of hypertriglyceridaemia after apo C-II administration. Journal of Clinical Investigation 77: 520—527

Patients with apo C-II deficiency were characterized by recurrent pancreatitis, xanthomas, hepatomegaly and type I hyperlipidaemia; symptoms resolved with infusion of normal plasma or synthesized apo C-II

8.5 Whang R et al 1985 Frequency of hypomagnesaemia in hospitalized patients receiving digitals. Archives of Internal Medicine 145: 655—656

In this study, hypomagnesaemia was found to be twice as common as hypokalaemia, both of which were associated with diuretic use. Furthermore, refractory hypokalaemia was found to respond to magnesium supplementation in patients who were also hypomagnesaemic

8.6 Stewart A F et al 1986 Hypocalcaemia associated with calcium-soap formation in a patient with a pancreatic fistula. New England Journal of Medicine 315: 496–498

Case report strongly suggesting that the well-recognized hypocalcaemia of acute pancreatitis is indeed mediated by intrapancreatic saponification

8.7 Corlew D S et al 1985 Observations on the course of untreated primary hyperparathyroidism. Surgery 98: 1064–1070

Study of 47 patients in which over a third of the patients died or experienced complications of hyperparathyroidism, leading the authors to conclude that surgery is indicated even for asymptomatic primary hyperparathyroidism

Wilson R J et al 1988 Mild asymptomatic primary hyperparathyroidism is not a risk factor for vertebral fractures. Annals of Internal Medicine 109: 959–962

Study of 174 patients concluding that surgery is not indicated in mild symptomatic hyperparathyroidism; it suggests that the increased rates of vertebral fractures seen in other series are due to inappropriate controls and/or selection bias

8.8 Silverberg S J et al 1989 Abnormalities in parathyroid hormone secretion and 1,25-dihydroxyvitamin D_3 formation in women with osteoporosis. New England Journal of Medicine 320: 277–281

Case-control study of 18 women suggesting that older women need more PTH stimulation than younger women to maintain vitamin D homeostasis, and that osteoporotic women were characterized by a failure to increase PTH secretion sufficiently (i.e. as well as the recognized reduction in vitamin D responsiveness seen in ageing)

8.9 Klibanski A, Greenspan S L 1986 Increase in bone mass after treatment of hyperprolactinaemic amenorrhoea. New England Journal of Medicine 315: 542–546

Improvement (but not normalization) of bone density was seen in 32 anovulatory women following correction of hyperprolactinaemia

8.10 Riis B, Thomsen K, Christiansen C 1987 Does calcium supplementation prevent postmenopausal bone loss? New England Journal of Medicine 316: 173–177

A double-blind controlled Danish trial showing a minor improvement in cortical (but not trabecular) bone following calcium supplementation. Calcium therapy was clearly inferior to oestrogen replacement

Dalsky G P et al 1988 Weight-bearing exercise training and lumbar bone mineral content in postmenopausal women. Annals of Internal Medicine 108: 824–828

Training resulted in a 5% increase in bone mineral content; following 12 months without training, this improvement disappeared

CHAPTER 9

Neurology

Physical examination protocol 9.1 You are asked to examine the cranial nerves

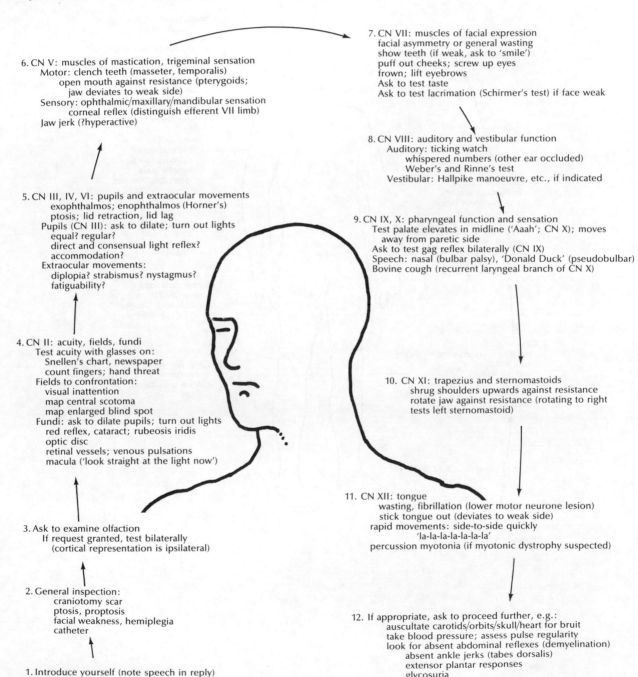

7. CN VII: muscles of facial expression
   facial asymmetry or general wasting
   show teeth (if weak, ask to 'smile')
   puff out cheeks; screw up eyes
   frown; lift eyebrows
   Ask to test taste
   Ask to test lacrimation (Schirmer's test) if face weak

6. CN V: muscles of mastication, trigeminal sensation
   Motor: clench teeth (masseter, temporalis)
   open mouth against resistance (pterygoids;
   jaw deviates to weak side)
   Sensory: ophthalmic/maxillary/mandibular sensation
   corneal reflex (distinguish efferent VII limb)
   Jaw jerk (?hyperactive)

8. CN VIII: auditory and vestibular function
   Auditory: ticking watch
   whispered numbers (other ear occluded)
   Weber's and Rinne's test
   Vestibular: Hallpike manoeuvre, etc., if indicated

5. CN III, IV, VI: pupils and extraocular movements
   exophthalmos; enophthalmos (Horner's)
   ptosis; lid retraction, lid lag
   Pupils (CN III): ask to dilate; turn out lights
   equal? regular?
   direct and consensual light reflex?
   accommodation?
   Extraocular movements:
   diplopia? strabismus? nystagmus?
   fatiguability?

9. CN IX, X: pharyngeal function and sensation
   Test palate elevates in midline ('Aaah'; CN X); moves
   away from paretic side
   Ask to test gag reflex bilaterally (CN IX)
   Speech: nasal (bulbar palsy), 'Donald Duck' (pseudobulbar)
   Bovine cough (recurrent laryngeal branch of CN X)

4. CN II: acuity, fields, fundi
   Test acuity with glasses on:
   Snellen's chart, newspaper
   count fingers; hand threat
   Fields to confrontation:
   visual inattention
   map central scotoma
   map enlarged blind spot
   Fundi: ask to dilate pupils; turn out lights
   red reflex, cataract; rubeosis iridis
   optic disc
   retinal vessels; venous pulsations
   macula ('look straight at the light now')

10. CN XI: trapezius and sternomastoids
    shrug shoulders upwards against resistance
    rotate jaw against resistance (rotating to right
    tests left sternomastoid)

3. Ask to examine olfaction
   If request granted, test bilaterally
   (cortical representation is ipsilateral)

11. CN XII: tongue
    wasting, fibrillation (lower motor neurone lesion)
    stick tongue out (deviates to weak side)
    rapid movements: side-to-side quickly
    'la-la-la-la-la-la-la'
    percussion myotonia (if myotonic dystrophy suspected)

2. General inspection:
   craniotomy scar
   ptosis, proptosis
   facial weakness, hemiplegia
   catheter

12. If appropriate, ask to proceed further, e.g.:
    auscultate carotids/orbits/skull/heart for bruit
    take blood pressure; assess pulse regularity
    look for absent abdominal reflexes (demyelination)
    absent ankle jerks (tabes dorsalis)
    extensor plantar responses
    glycosuria

1. Introduce yourself (note speech in reply)
   Position yourself opposite patient

Physical examination protocol 9.2 You are asked to assess a patient who has had difficulty walking

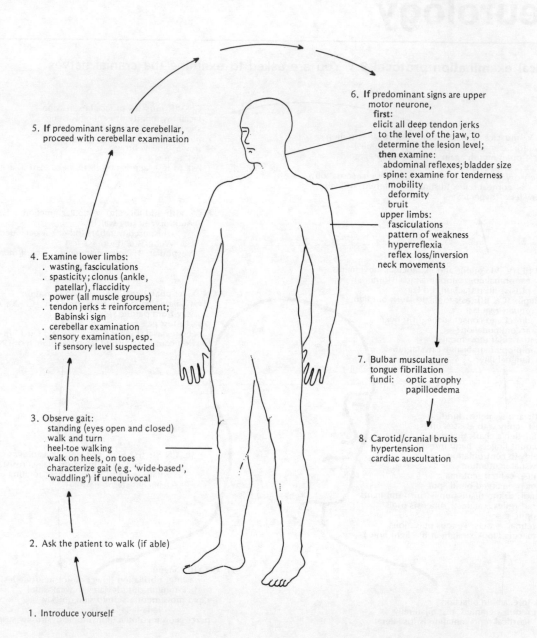

5. **If** predominant signs are cerebellar, proceed with cerebellar examination

6. **If** predominant signs are upper motor neurone,
   first:
   elicit all deep tendon jerks to the level of the jaw, to determine the lesion level;
   then examine:
   abdominal reflexes; bladder size
   spine: examine for tenderness
   mobility
   deformity
   bruit
   upper limbs:
   fasciculations
   pattern of weakness
   hyperreflexia
   reflex loss/inversion
   neck movements

4. Examine lower limbs:
   . wasting, fasciculations
   . spasticity; clonus (ankle, patellar), flaccidity
   . power (all muscle groups)
   . tendon jerks ± reinforcement; Babinski sign
   . cerebellar examination
   . sensory examination, esp. if sensory level suspected

7. Bulbar musculature
   tongue fibrillation
   fundi: optic atrophy
   papilloedema

3. Observe gait:
   standing (eyes open and closed)
   walk and turn
   heel-toe walking
   walk on heels, on toes
   characterize gait (e.g. 'wide-based', 'waddling') **if** unequivocal

8. Carotid/cranial bruits
   hypertension
   cardiac auscultation

2. Ask the patient to walk (if able)

1. Introduce yourself

Physical examination protocol 9.3 You are asked to examine a patient who has noticed wasting of the hand muscles

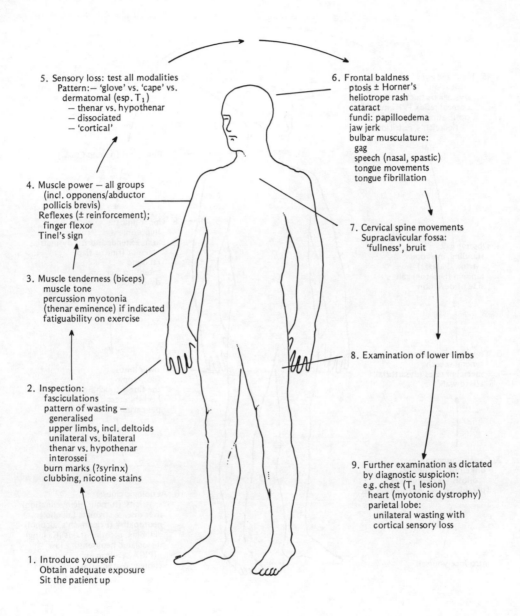

5. Sensory loss: test all modalities
   Pattern:– 'glove' vs. 'cape' vs.
   dermatomal (esp. T_1)
   — thenar vs. hypothenar
   — dissociated
   — 'cortical'

4. Muscle power — all groups
   (incl. opponens/abductor
   pollicis brevis)
   Reflexes (± reinforcement);
   finger flexor
   Tinel's sign

3. Muscle tenderness (biceps)
   muscle tone
   percussion myotonia
   (thenar eminence) if indicated
   fatiguability on exercise

2. Inspection:
   fasciculations
   pattern of wasting –
   generalised
   upper limbs, incl. deltoids
   unilateral vs. bilateral
   thenar vs. hypothenar
   interossei
   burn marks (?syrinx)
   clubbing, nicotine stains

1. Introduce yourself
   Obtain adequate exposure
   Sit the patient up

6. Frontal baldness
   ptosis ± Horner's
   heliotrope rash
   cataract
   fundi: papilloedema
   jaw jerk
   bulbar musculature:
      gag
      speech (nasal, spastic)
      tongue movements
      tongue fibrillation

7. Cervical spine movements
   Supraclavicular fossa:
      'fullness', bruit

8. Examination of lower limbs

9. Further examination as dictated
   by diagnostic suspicion:
   e.g. chest (T_1 lesion)
      heart (myotonic dystrophy)
      parietal lobe:
         unilateral wasting with
         cortical sensory loss

Physical examination protocol 9.4 You are asked to examine the patient's cerebellar function

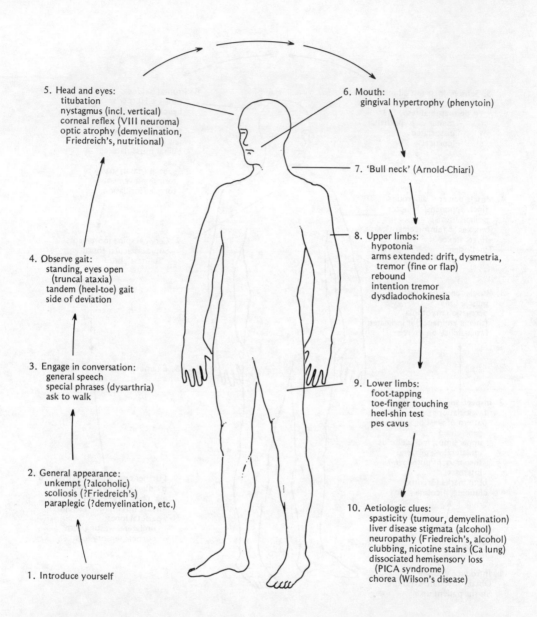

5. Head and eyes:
   titubation
   nystagmus (incl. vertical)
   corneal reflex (VIII neuroma)
   optic atrophy (demyelination,
   Friedreich's, nutritional)

6. Mouth:
   gingival hypertrophy (phenytoin)

7. 'Bull neck' (Arnold-Chiari)

4. Observe gait:
   standing, eyes open
   (truncal ataxia)
   tandem (heel-toe) gait
   side of deviation

8. Upper limbs:
   hypotonia
   arms extended: drift, dysmetria,
   tremor (fine or flap)
   rebound
   intention tremor
   dysdiadochokinesia

3. Engage in conversation:
   general speech
   special phrases (dysarthria)
   ask to walk

9. Lower limbs:
   foot-tapping
   toe-finger touching
   heel-shin test
   pes cavus

2. General appearance:
   unkempt (?alcoholic)
   scoliosis (?Friedreich's)
   paraplegic (?demyelination, etc.)

1. Introduce yourself

10. Aetiologic clues:
    spasticity (tumour, demyelination)
    liver disease stigmata (alcohol)
    neuropathy (Friedreich's, alcohol)
    clubbing, nicotine stains (Ca lung)
    dissociated hemisensory loss
    (PICA syndrome)
    chorea (Wilson's disease)

Physical examination protocol 9.5 You are asked to examine a patient for signs of parkinsonism

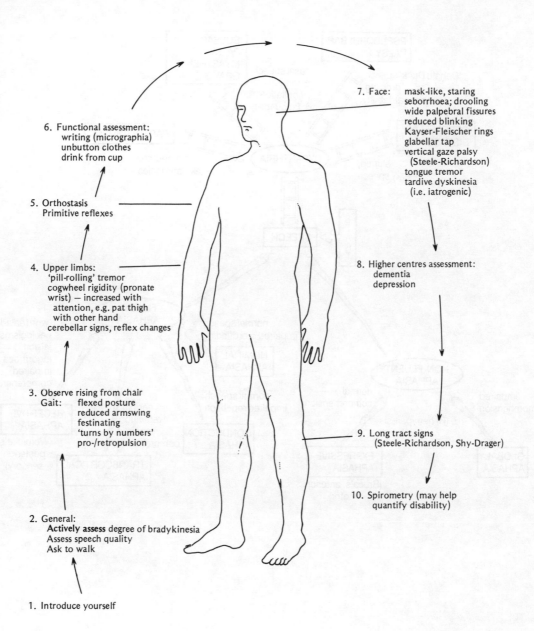

7. Face: mask-like, staring
            seborrhoea; drooling
            wide palpebral fissures
            reduced blinking
            Kayser-Fleischer rings
            glabellar tap
            vertical gaze palsy
             (Steele-Richardson)
            tongue tremor
            tardive dyskinesia
             (i.e. iatrogenic)

6. Functional assessment:
   writing (micrographia)
   unbutton clothes
   drink from cup

5. Orthostasis
   Primitive reflexes

8. Higher centres assessment:
   dementia
   depression

4. Upper limbs:
   'pill-rolling' tremor
   cogwheel rigidity (pronate
   wrist) — increased with
   attention, e.g. pat thigh
   with other hand
   cerebellar signs, reflex changes

3. Observe rising from chair
Gait: flexed posture
         reduced armswing
         festinating
         'turns by numbers'
         pro-/retropulsion

9. Long tract signs
   (Steele-Richardson, Shy-Drager)

10. Spirometry (may help
    quantify disability)

2. General:
   Actively assess degree of bradykinesia
   Assess speech quality
   Ask to walk

1. Introduce yourself

Diagnostic pathway 9.1 This patient has a speech defect. What do you make of it?

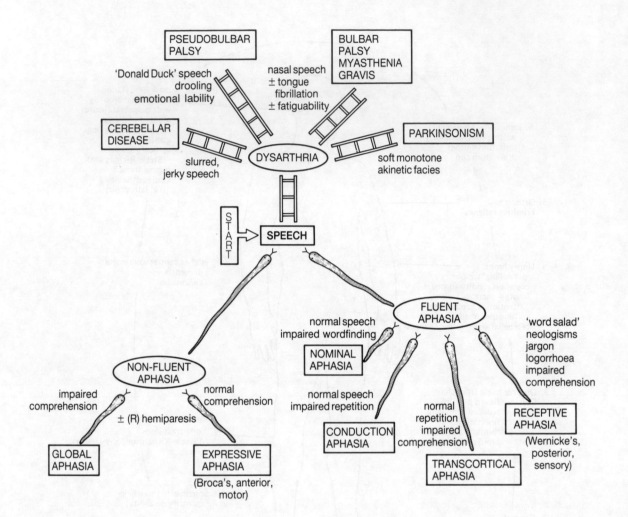

Diagnostic pathway 9.2 This patient is troubled by ptosis. Can you shed any light on the pathophysiology?

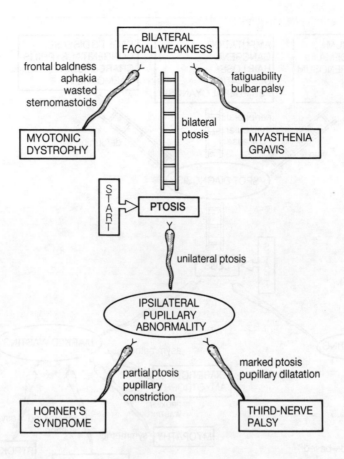

Diagnostic pathway 9.3 The patient is concerned about his legs. What do you think is the problem?

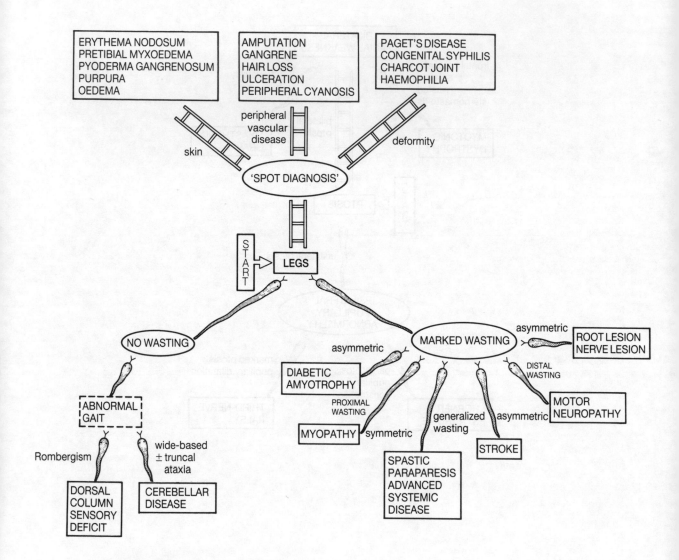

CLINICAL ASPECTS OF NEUROLOGICAL DISEASE

COMMONEST NEUROLOGICAL SHORT CASES
1 Spastic paraparesis
2 Peripheral neuropathy
3 Ocular palsy

Clinical assessment of muscle weakness (MRC criteria)
1 Grade 1 — flicker of voluntary muscle activity (paralysis = O)
2 Grade 2 — able to move with gravity eliminated
3 Grade 3 — able to move against gravity
4 Grade 4 — able to move against resistance
5 Grade 5 — normal power

Multiple CNS deficits: causes
1 Multiple sclerosis
  Multifocal leucoencephalopathy
2 Multiple infarcts
3 Multiple metastases
  Meningeal carcinomatosis
4 Meningovascular syphilis
5 Vasculitis (e.g. PAN)

Multiple cranial nerve palsies: causes
1 Malignancy
  a) Brainstem tumour (incl. nasopharyngeal carcinoma)
  b) Meningeal carcinomatosis
  c) Perineural tumour infiltration
2 Infection
  a) Basal meningitis (pneumococcal, cryptococcal, tuberculous)
  b) Meningovascular syphilis
3 Sarcoidosis
4 Vasculitis
5 Paget's disease

Signs suggesting brainstem pathology
1 Conjugate gaze palsy/internuclear ophthalmoplegia
2 Vertical nystagmus
3 Opisthotonos and/or cerebellar signs
4 Crossed (cranial nerves vs long tract) signs
5 Deviation of eyes and head towards paralysed side (cf. cortical)
6 Bilateral extensive deficit

Signs suggesting extracapsular (cortical) disease
1 Localized deficit
2 Dysphasia (cf. capsular lesion → pure dysarthria)
3 Hemianopia
4 Decreased proprioception/two-point discrimination
5 Apraxia
6 Obtundation

Clinical distinction between meningitis and encephalitis
1 Meningitis
  a) Conscious state unimpaired
  b) Meningism (including headache) — marked, early-onset
  c) Prominent fever
  d) ± Cranial nerve lesions (lower motor neurone)
2 Encephalitis
  a) Early impairment of consciousness (drowsiness, coma)
  b) Focal neurological signs (upper motor neurone)
  c) Convulsions
  d) Associated features, e.g. hydrophobia (rabies), temporal lobe epilepsy (HSV)

Assessment of neurological function in the unconscious patient
1 Pupils
  a) Midbrain lesions
    — Light reflex may be lost
    — Hippus (fluctuation in pupil size)
    — Ciliospinal reflex (dilatation on pinching ipsilateral neck skin)
  b) Pontine lesions
    — Pinpoint pupils
  c) Lateral medullary lesions
    — Horner's syndrome
  d) Diffuse cerebral damage
    — Fixed dilated pupils (not diagnostic)
  e) Metabolic depression (e.g. overdose)
    — Loss of all brainstem reflexes except pupillary light reflex
2 Conjugate gaze deviation (p. 220)
3 Caloric and oculocephalic testing (p. 222)
4 Reflexes
  a) Corneal (depressed in bilateral cerebral damage)
  b) Jaw jerk (hyperactive in bilateral UMN lesions)
  c) Gag reflex
5 Spontaneous respiratory movements

CEREBROVASCULAR DISEASE: BACKGROUND

Symptoms suggesting carotid insufficiency
1 Amaurosis fugax
2 Dysphasia
3 Unilateral limb weakness/paraesthesiae without other (brainstem) features

Clinical significance of transient ischaemic attacks
1 30% of patients will have only one episode
2 30% will continue to have TIA's alone
3 30% will have a completed stroke within 3 years
4 30% of the latter will do so within 3 months of presentation
5 30% of asymptomatic carotid bruits will go on to TIA and/or CVA
6 30% of patients with carotid-type TIAs will be found to have relatively normal arteriography

Carotid-type TIAs: factors predictive of angiographic disease
1 Ipsilateral retinal emboli
2 Reduced superficial temporal and/or carotid artery pulse

3 Presence of forehead/scleral collaterals
4 Ipsilateral central retinal artery pressure (diastolic) < 20 mmHg
5 Ipsilateral carotid bruit, esp. if diastolic extension present; severe stenosis may cause a high-pitched, low-intensity bruit

Neurological syndromes directly due to hypertension
1 Lacunar infarcts
2 Intracranial haemorrhage
3 Hypertensive encephalopathy

Common sites of intracranial haemorrhage
1 Putamen
2 Thalamus
3 Pons
4 Cerebellum

PRESENTATIONS OF CEREBROVASCULAR DISEASE

Features suggestive of intracerebral haemorrhage
1 Gradual onset, smooth progression
2 Obtunded sensorium
3 Vomiting (95%), headache (50%)
4 Hypertension ± fundal stigmata/cardiomegaly
5 Diagnostic confirmation by CT

Signs suggestive of basal pontine haemorrhage
1 Rapid onset of decerebrate rigidity progressing to coma
2 Ophthalmoplegia with (classically) small reactive pupils
3 Abnormal oculocephalic and oculovestibular reflexes
4 Cheyne-Stokes/ataxic respiration
5 Sweating

Signs and symptoms of cerebellar haemorrhage
1 Subacute onset of occipital headache, vertigo and vomiting
2 Skew deviation of the eyes; ocular bobbing (nystagmus unusual)
3 Paresis of gaze to affected side
4 Hemiparesis unusual (cf. putaminal/thalamic type)
5 Good recovery after prompt surgical evacuation

Clinical patterns of lacunar infarction
1 Pure motor hemiplegia
   a) Pontine
   b) Posterior limb of internal capsule
      — Associated with dysarthria
      — Typically affects upper limb more than lower
2 Dysarthria-clumsy hand syndrome
   a) Caused by pontine infarction
   b) Associated with homolateral facial weakness
3 Pure hemisensory loss
   — Due to thalamic infarction (posterolateral nucleus)
4 Ipsilateral ataxia/crossed hemiparesis
   — Due to midbrain infarction
5 Dementia/incontinence/affective lability
   — Due to bipyramidal (pseudobulbar) palsy (DD$_x$ = normal pressure hydrocephalus)

Reasons for clinical deterioration in a patient with an apparently completed stroke
1 Infarct extension
2 Haemorrhage into infarct
3 Further emboli
4 Worsening cerebral oedema/vasospasm
5 Misdiagnosis (e.g. tumour/vasculitis)

Presentations of arteriovenous malformations
1 Epilepsy (45%)
2 Haemorrhage (40%; may mimic aseptic meningitis)
3 Headache (often migrainous: 15%)
4 Pseudotumour (neurological deficit due to vascular 'steal')
5 Apparent 'spontaneous' stroke:
   a) Age under 20
   b) During third trimester

Diagnostic considerations in the young patient with 'stroke'
1 Disseminated sclerosis
2 Cardiac disease
   a) Arrhythmias (esp. atrial fibrillation)
   b) Valvular disease (esp. mitral valve stenosis/prolapse)
   c) Infective endocarditis
3 Vascular disease
   a) Vasculitis (e.g. SLE)
   b) Severe hypertension
   c) Hypercoagulable state
4 Arteriovenous malformation/aneurysm
5 Intracranial tumour
6 Encephalitis (e.g. HSV type 1); neurosyphilis
7 Postictal
8 'Classical' migraine
9 Hyperventilation (may simulate TIA)
10 Hysteria

Clinical features of lateral medullary (PICA*) syndrome
1 Abrupt onset of vertigo and hiccupping
2 Bilateral nystagmus
   a) Maximal to side of lesion
   b) Often varies with posture
3 Contralateral body anaesthesia for pain and temperature
4 Ipsilateral
   a) Facial anaesthesia for pain and temperature
   b) Palatal paresis
   c) Taste loss
   d) Horner's syndrome
   e) Ataxia

LOCALIZING PATTERNS IN CEREBRAL DISEASE

Clinical manifestations of frontal lobe lesions
1 Anosmia — homolateral

---

*Posterior inferior cerebellar artery

Ataxia   — Brun's
Aphasia   — Broca's
Apathy
Amnesia
Atrophy (optic)
2 Mass effects (papilloedema, field defects, Foster-Kennedy syndrome)
3 Incontinence
4 Spastic paraparesis or contralateral UMN signs
5 Primitive reflexes (palmar-mental/grasp/snout/pout/suck)

Clinical manifestations of temporal lobe lesions
1 Superior quadrantanopia
2 Fluent aphasia (lesion in Wernicke's area)
3 Uncinate fits, depersonalization, micro-/macropsia,
4 Bilateral disease (rare)
  a) Deafness
  b) Severe amnesia
  c) Kluver-Bucy syndrome

Clinical manifestations of parietal lobe lesions
1 Non-dominant lobe lesions
  a) Dressing apraxia
  b) Constructional apraxia (draw clockface, house, five-pointed star)
  c) Anosognosia
2 Dominant lobe lesions:
  a) Ideomotor apraxia ('brush teeth, use saw, drink from cup, undo safety pin')
  b) Receptive dysphasia (in inferior lesions)
  c) Gerstmann's
    — Alexia
    — Acalculia
    — Finger agnosia
    — Left-right confusion
  d) Agraphia (in posterior lesions)
3 Anterior lobe lesions
  a) Astereognosis/graphaesthesia
  b) Sensory inattention
  c) ↓ Proprioception/two-point discrimination
  d) Focal sensory deficits
4 Posterior lobe lesions
  a) Visual inattention, sensory inattention
  b) Homonymous (albeit incongruous) hemianopia/inferior quadrantanopia
  c) ↓ Opticokinetic nystagmus
5 Wasting (→ 'parietal lobe weakness')

Clinical manifestations of occipital lobe lesions
1 'Cortical' blindness **or** altitudinal hemianopia **or** congruous crossed hemianopia
2 Smooth pursuit defects, impaired opticokinetic nystagmus
3 Visual agnosia; visual hallucinations
4 Achromatopsia; prosopagnosia; topographical amnesia

EXAMINING THE EYES

Clinical criteria for characterizing blindness
1 Complete blindness — absent pupillary reactions and opticokinetic nystagmus

2 Hysterical blindness — normal pupillary reactions and optikokinetic nystagmus
3 Cortical blindness — normal pupillary reactions (to light) but absent opticokinetic nystagmus
4 Anton's syndrome — cortical blindness denied by patient (? due to destruction of visual association areas) ± hallucinations and memory loss

Causes of painful visual loss
1 Optic neuritis
2 Acute glaucoma
3 Giant cell arteritis ⎫
4 Central retinal artery (CRA) occlusion ⎬ → amaurosis fugax
5 Migraine

Classical patterns of visual field defect
1 Central field defects
  a) Central scotoma — *macular* pathology, e.g. demyelination (often associated with, but not caused by, optic neuritis)
  b) Central arcuate scotoma — early glaucoma
  c) Pericentral scotoma (normal acuity)
    — Retinitis pigmentosa
    — Chloroquine retinopathy
  d) Centrocaecal scotoma (extends to involve blind spot) — toxic optic neuropathies, e.g. methanol, 'nutritional'
  e) Congruous homonymous scotoma — localized lesions of occipital cortex
2 Hemianopias
  a) Bitemporal hemianopia — central chiasmal lesion, esp. pituitary tumour (see below)
  b) Incongruous homonymous hemianopia — optic tract lesion (rare)
  c) Congruous homonymous hemianopia — lesion of occipital lobe optic radiation
  d) Homonymous hemianopia with macular sparing — lesion of occipital cortex (usually vascular aetiology)
  e) Bilateral homonymous hemianopia due to bilateral posterior cerebral artery occlusion — small island of central vision
3 Quadrantanopias (usually due to tumours)
  a) Superior — lesion of temporal lobe optic radiation
  b) Inferior — lesion of parietal lobe optic radiation
4 Field defects in one eye only
  a) Retinal detachment
  b) Branch retinal vein occlusion
  c) Ischaemic optic neuropathy (→ inferior defect)
  d) Vasculitis
5 Concentric visual field constriction
  a) Hysteria ('tubular' vision)
  b) Advanced glaucoma or papilloedema
  c) 'Panretinal' laser photocoagulation (→ peripheral field loss with normal acuity; cf. diabetic maculopathy → reduced acuity with peripheral sparing)
6 Other patterns of field defect
  a) Enlarged blind spot — early papilloedema
  b) Visual inattention — lesion of posterior parietal lobe

Chiasmal lesions: clinical signs aiding localization

1 Posterior chiasm lesions
   a) Due to suprasellar or third ventricle tumours
   b) Typically involve macular fibres only
   c) Manifest with central scotoma only
2 Anterosuperior chiasm lesions
   a) Due to meningiomas (sphenoid ridge, frontal lobe) or aneurysms (anterior cerebral, anterior communicating)
   b) Manifest with inferior temporal quadrant loss
3 Anteroinferior chiasm lesions
   a) Due to pituitary tumour, meningitis
   b) Typically involve maculopapillary bundle as well as compressing chiasm
   c) Manifest with bitemporal hemianopia *plus* central scotoma
4 Posteroinferior chiasm lesions
   a) Due to pituitary tumours
   b) Manifest initially with bitemporal superior quadrantanopia
   c) May progress to
   — Optic atrophy
   — Inferior temporal field loss
   — Nasal field loss (optic tract involvement)

'Examine the eyes': important extra details

1 Position the patient in front of you (e.g. in chair, side of bed) if practicable
2 Specific features to note on inspection
   a) Proptosis (view orbits from all angles); ± pulsating
   b) Enophthalmos (esp. if pupil constricted), dry skin
   c) Ptosis (unilateral or bilateral)
   d) Rubeosis iridis; arcus senilis; band keratopathy
   e) Glasses (e.g. thick lenses, for aphakic patients)
3 Visual acuity
   a) Test with patient's glasses on (newsprint, eye chart)
   b) Unilateral blindness? exclude glass eye
4 Visual fields
   a) Test for visual inattention
   b) Map blind spot (and central scotoma, if present)
5 Fundoscopy
   a) Look for red reflex
   b) Characterize opacities (e.g. cataract)
   c) Indicate that you would like to dilate the pupils
   d) Comment on retinal vessels, venous pulsations, disc
   e) Inspect macula last ('look straight at the light now')
6 Extraocular movements
   a) Ask re diplopia in any direction, and cover eyes sequentially when double image maximal (peripheral image is from the diseased eye)
   b) Is nystagmus present? look for optic atrophy, dysarthria, bulbar palsy, cerebellar signs, etc.
   c) Is there fatiguability?
7 Pupils
   a) Check for regularity and circularity
   b) Turn off lights if possible to examine reactivity
   c) Test both the direct and consensual response to light in each eye
   d) Horner's syndrome? check for ipsilateral facial anhidrosis (signifies lesion proximal to carotid bifurcation, e.g. in brachial plexus)
8 Palpate globes and temporal arteries for tenderness
9 Auscultate orbits (and skull if indicated)
10 Auscultate carotids if CVA suspected

THE ABNORMAL FUNDUS

Papilloedema: fundoscopic criteria
1 Loss of physiological cup
2 Elevation of disc head (quantifiable in dioptres)
3 Blurring of disc margins
4 Distended non-pulsatile veins
5 Subhyaloid haemorrhages at disc margins

Differential diagnosis of optic disc swelling
1 Pseudopapilloedema — benign congenital anomalies, e.g.
   a) Drüsen of the disc (may → field defect)
   b) Hypermetropia
2 Papilloedema
   a) Disc swelling: usually bilateral (cf. papillitis)
   b) Visual field testing: enlarged blind spot
   c) Visual acuity: normal (unless longstanding disease)
3 Papillitis
   a) Disc swelling — unilateral (may → optic atrophy)
   b) Visual field testing — → central scotoma (use red pin) due to *macular* involvement
   c) Associated subjective loss of brightness and colour
   d) Pain on eye movement, tenderness on globe palpation
   e) Marcus-Gunn phenomenon (p. 219)
   f) Visual acuity — early, marked reduction
(cf. Retrobular neuritis: similar to papillitis, but
   a) *No* visible disc swelling; may be temporal disc pallor
   b) Commoner presentation of demyelination)
4 Posterior uveitis:
   a) Disc swelling — may be unilateral or bilateral
   b) Visual field testing — usually normal
   c) Visual acuity — only reduced if macular oedema present
   d) Cellular infiltrate visible in vitreous
5 Ischaemic optic neuropathy
   a) Disc swelling — pale, asymmetric
   b) Visual field testing — inferior altitudinal defect
   c) Hypertensive/arteriosclerotic vascular changes; otherwise clinically resembles papillitis

Disorders causing retinal arteriolar constriction
1 Malignant hypertension
2 Central retinal artery occlusion
3 Retinitis pigmentosa
4 Cinchonism

Disorders causing dilated retinal veins
1 Polycythaemia, hyperviscosity
2 Central retinal vein (CRV) thrombosis
3 Increased intracranial pressure
4 CO_2 retention
5 Carotico-cavernous fistula

Causes of angioid streaks
(breaks in Bruch's membrane)
1 Paget's disease
2 Acromegaly
3 Pseudoxanthoma elasticum
4 Ehlers-Danlos syndrome
5 Hereditary hyperphosphatasia
6 Sickle-cell anaemia

RETINOPATHY

Retinal haemorrhages: their morphological significance
1 'Dot' haemorrhages
  a) Microaneurysms in the posterior pole of the retina
  b) The hallmark of diabetic retinopathy
2 'Blot' haemorrhages
  a) Small haemorrhages deep in the posterior retinal pole
  b) Vertical course of nerve fibres restricts spread here
  c) Also characteristic of diabetic retinopathy
3 'Flame' haemorrhages
  a) Rupture of superficial retinal capillary plexus
  b) Track horizontally along superficial nerve fibre layer
  c) Characteristic of grade III/IV hypertensive retinopathy
4 Preretinal ('subhyaloid') haemorrhages
  a) Fluid level visible between retina and vitreous
  b) Caused by new vessel rupture (e.g. proliferative diabetic retinopathy), or rapid increase in intracranial pressure (e.g. in subarachnoid or intracerebral haemorrhage)
5 Subretinal haemorrhages
  a) Greenish/brown appearance
  b) Indicate choroidal pathology
6 Full-thickness haemorrhages
  a) Widespread, dark, irregular appearance
  b) Indicate retinal ischaemia; predispose to new vessels

Retinopathy: hypertensive or diabetic?
1 Hypertensive
  a) AV (arteriovenous) nipping*
  b) Flame haemorrhages } —only occasionally seen in diabetic retinopathy
  c) Papilloedema
2 Diabetic
  a) Microaneurysms
  b) Dot and blot haemorrhages
  c) New vessel formation

CLINICAL SIGNS IN THE ANTERIOR EYE

Causes of a small pupil
1 Horner's syndrome
2 Neurosyphilis (Argyll-Robertson pupils)
3 Myotonic dystrophy
4 Pontine lesions
5 Acute iritis
6 Opiates; organophosphate poisoning

---

*not useful in assessing severity of hypertension

Causes of a large pupil
1 Third nerve palsy (if due to compressive lesion)
2 Holmes-Adie syndrome
3 Midbrain lesions
4 Congenital syphilis
5 Trauma (local)
6 Anticholinergics, benzodiazepines, cocaine, mydriatics

Pupillary responses to mydriatics
1 Hyperactive (excessive mydriasis)
  a) Holmes-Adie syndrome ('tonic' pupil; see below)
2 Hypoactive (sluggish response)
  a) Myotonic dystrophy ('contratonic' pupil)
  b) Argyll-Robertson pupil
3 Autonomic neuropathy
  a) *Hyperactive* response to topical adrenaline 1:1000 (similarly, hyperactive constriction to 2.5% topical methacholine), indicating denervation hypersensitivity
  b) *Hypoactive* response to topical cocaine (2.5%) or hydroxyamphetamine, indicating depletion of endogenous noradrenaline

Causes of Horner's syndrome
1 Pancoast tumour
2 Sympathectomy
3 Syringomyelia
4 Lateral medullary syndrome
5 Shy-Drager syndrome (may be alternating)

Double-barrelled eponymous pupillary anomalies
1 Holmes-Adie syndrome
  a) 'Tonic pupil'; usually unilateral; commoner in women
  b) Pupil reacts abnormally slowly to light (and accommodation), but exhibits denervation hypersensitivity to mydriatics
  c) Associated with hyporeflexia and peripheral anhidrosis
2 Argyll-Robertson pupils
  a) Small irregular pupils, frequently unequal
  b) React to accommodation but not to light
  c) Hallmark of neurosyphilis; rarely seen in diabetes
3 Marcus-Gunn phenomenon
  a) Pupil constricts weakly to direct illumination, strongly to consensual illumination ('swinging light' test)
  b) Indicates relative afferent pupillary defect
  c) Hallmark of optic neuritis (and hence, in practice, of multiple sclerosis)

Characteristic cataracts
1 'Snowflake' — insulin-dependent diabetes (now rare)
2 'Sunflower' — Wilson's disease (do not impair vision)
3 'Stellate' (punctate, radially distributed) — hypoparathyroidism
4 'Scintillatory' (polychromatophilic, dustlike) — myotonic dystrophy
5 Subcapsular posterior
  a) Steroid-induced (dose- and duration-dependent)
  b) Chronic uveitis (± steroid eyedrops)
  c) Irradiation

OCULAR PALSIES

Clinical characterization of ptosis
1 Bilateral — muscle disease (myasthenia gravis, myotonic dystrophy)
2 Partial unilateral
  a) Horner's syndrome ('everything is smaller'; ptosis, miosis, enophthalmos)
  b) Partial third nerve palsy
  c) Congenital ptosis (commonest cause in healthy people)
3 Complete unilateral — third nerve palsy

Diplopia: signs favouring myopathic aetiology
1 Bilateral ptosis or exophthalmos
2 Bifacial weakness (incl. orbicularis oculi)
3 Normal pupils
  Worsening of diplopia } In myasthenia gravis
  with fatigue

Syndromes with impaired vertical gaze
1 Parinaud's
2 Richardson-Steele
3 Graves' disease
4 Thalamic haemorrhage

Painful ophthalmoplegic syndromes
1 Third nerve palsy
  a) Posterior communicating artery aneurysm Intracavernous internal carotid artery aneurysm
  b) Diabetes mellitus; vasculitis
  c) Migraine (esp. in children)
2 Sixth nerve palsy
  a) Tolosa-Hunt syndrome
  b) Gradenigo's syndrome
  c) Nasopharyngeal carcinoma
  d) Infraclinoid (extradural) internal carotid artery aneurysm
3 Total ophthalmoplegia (± proptosis) — superior orbital fissure syndrome

Varieties of nystagmus and their clinical significance
1 Physiological (opticokinetic) nystagmus
  a) Reflex elicited by objects moving through fixed line of sight (e.g. looking out a train window)
  b) Mediated by angular and supramarginal gyri in posterior parietal lobe (i.e. independent of vestibular nuclei)
  c) Reduced (impaired) when looking at striped drum rotating towards side of destructive cerebral lesion
  d) Provides evidence of sightedness in infants, retarded or aphasic patients, hysterics and malingerers
2 Rotary nystagmus
  a) Usually due to labyrinthine lesions; hence, often accompanied by vertigo, deafness and/or tinnitus
  b) Horizontal direction defined by fast (saccadic) phase
  c) Severity maximal when eyes deviated in direction of fast phase
  d) Saccadic correction is made by the paramedian pontine reticular formation (PPRF) on the 'fast' side

In benign positional nystagmus (due to utricle pathology)
  a) Fast phase towards dependent ear (e.g. clockwise rotation if left ear maintained in dependent position)
  b) Nystagmus characterized by latency (10–20 s period prior to onset after repositioning) and adaptation (lessening of nystagmus following repeated repositioning)
3 Pendular nystagmus (i.e. no 'fast' phase)
  a) Arises due to difficulty fixating and/or maintaining gaze
  b) Seen in congenital or familial nystagmus (even if eyes midposition)
    — Acquired amblyopia
    — Myopathies, esp. myasthenia gravis
    — Pontine/cerebellar lesions affecting the PPRF
4 Vertical nystagmus
  a) Indicates brainstem/cerebellar, rather than vestibular, pathology
  b) In diffuse cerebellar lesions, nystagmus may occur on fixation in any direction
  c) Upbeat nystagmus (fast phase up) — due to lesions of pontine tegmentum or floor of fourth ventricle
  d) Downbeat nystagmus — cerebellar atrophy, or lesion at foramen magnum (may be surgically remediable)
5 Ataxic nystagmus
  a) i.e. Internuclear ophthalmoplegia — brainstem lesion
  b) Bilateral horizontal nystagmus of abducting eye with paralysis of adducting eye
  c) (Almost) pathognomonic of multiple sclerosis
6 Ocular bobbing
  a) Indicates caudal pontine lesion
  b) Rapid downward movement of eyes followed by slow return

Lateralization of pathological eye signs
1 Nystagmus
  a) Maximal on looking away from side of vestibular lesion
  b) Maximal on looking towards side of cerebellar lesion
2 Conjugate deviation:
  a) Eyes turned towards side of CVA (i.e. away from hemiplegic arm or leg) in a hemispheric stroke
  b) Eyes turned away from side of irritative cortical (i.e. hemispheric) epileptogenic focus during seizure
  c) Eyes turned away from side of lateral pontine lesion (i.e. towards hemiplegic arm or leg) in brainstem disease
  d) Eyes turned towards the ear irrigated with ice-cold water during caloric testing of patients with intact brainstem and labyrinth
3 Homonymous hemianopia — hemianopic field defect on the side opposite the cortical lesion (i.e. on the same side as the hemiplegic arm or leg) in hemispheric pathology
4 Diplopia — when looking in direction of maximal diplopia, the more peripheral image disappears when the abnormal eye is covered

THE FACE IN NEUROLOGICAL DISEASE

Differential diagnosis of facial pain in trigeminal distribution

1 Trigeminal neuralgia
   a) Tends to occur in patients > 50 years
   b) Pain → maxillary and mandibular branches of CN V
2 Paratrigeminal neuralgia (Raeder's syndrome)
   a) May be caused by malignancy at skull base
   b) Pain → ophthalmic branch of CN V; → orbital pain, Horner's
3 Postherpetic neuralgia
   a) Tends to occur in elderly patients
   b) Pain →ophthalmic branch of CN V
4 Intracavernous internal carotid artery aneurysm
   a) May cause ophthalmoplegia, esp. CN III
   b) Pain and sensory loss → ophthalmic (± maxillary) CN V
5 Superior orbital fissure syndrome
   a) Often caused by tumour invasion
   b) Pain → ophthalmic CN V (± ophthalmoplegia, proptosis)
6 Gradenigo's syndrome
   a) Due to petrous temporal lesions, e.g. chronic otitis media
   b) Pain → CN V distribution; associated CN VI palsy; now rare

Non-trigeminal patterns of facial pain

1 Ramsay-Hunt syndrome (geniculate neuralgia)
   a) Varicella-zoster of the geniculate ganglion of CN VII
   b) Preauricular pain, facial paralysis, vesicles in ear and/or ipsilateral fauces, ± involvement of CN VIII ('otic zoster')
2 Costen's syndrome
   a) Affects patients with jaw malocclusion
   b) Pain → temporomandibular region
3 Tolosa-Hunt syndrome
   a) Usually occurs due to granulomatous angiitis or tumours
   b) Painful ophthalmoplegia (palsies of CN III, IV and/or VI)
4 Glossopharyngeal neuralgia
   a) Similar pain to trigeminal neuralgia; affects elderly
   b) Pain → CN IX, provoked by speaking or swallowing; rare
5 Jaw claudication
   a) Usually due to giant-cell arteritis (elderly patients)
   b) Pain → jaw and/or tongue when eating or speaking

Clinical characterization of facial weakness

1 Unilateral upper motor neurone weakness (e.g. CVA)
   a) Upper face *spared* (bilateral innervation of frontalis and orbicularis oculi)
   b) No lower facial sagging (tone preserved)
   c) Facial paresis may disappear during emotion (mediated via extrapyramidal fibres)
   d) Often associated with ipsilateral hemiplegia

2 Unilateral lower motor neurone weakness (e.g. Bell's palsy)
   a) Upper face weak (loss of forehead wrinkling)
   b) Lower facial sagging (± mild dysarthria)
   c) Inability to voluntarily close eye (eye rolls up: Bell's sign) due to paralysis of orbicularis oculi →ectropion, conjunctivitis
   d) Progressively more proximal lesions
      — Loss of taste over ipsilateral anterior two-thirds tongue ± sensory loss in external auditory meatus (chorda tympani involvement)
      — Hyperacusis (involvement of nerve to stapedius)
      — Reduced lacrimation (greater petrosal nerve involvement) or aberrant lacrimation during nerve recovery (e.g. 'crocodile tears' precipitated by eating)
   e) Involvement of neighbouring cranial nerves
      CN VI (e.g. brainstem lesion)
      CN VIII (e.g. in Ramsay-Hunt syndrome)
      CN V, VIII (e.g. cerebellopontine angle tumour; CN VII palsy more often due to surgery than compression)
3 Myopathy (e.g. myotonic dystrophy)
   a) Symmetric facial wasting → long, haggard appearance
   b) Ptosis (may be asymmetric; *absent* in CN VII lesions)
   c) Ophthalmoplegia (common in myasthenia gravis, rare in myasthenic syndrome or polymyositis); usually asymmetric; pupils normal (cf. CN III palsy)
   d) 'Transverse smile' (myotonic dystrophy)
   e) 'Myasthenic snarl' (myasthenia gravis)
   f) Periorbital oedema/heliotrope rash (polymyositis)
   g) Fatiguability

Facial presentations of systemic disease

1 Trigeminal neuralgia in a young patient
   a) Multiple sclerosis
   b) Cerebellopontine angle tumour
2 Bilateral lower motor neurone facial palsy
   a) Guillain-Barré syndrome
   b) Mikulicz syndrome — bilateral parotid infiltration, e.g. due to sarcoidosis/tuberculosis/actinomycosis
3 Facial neuromyopathy
   a) Myotonic dystrophy
   b) Facioscapulohumeral dystrophy
   c) Myasthenia gravis

DISORDERS AFFECTING THE LOWER CRANIAL NERVES

Characterizing and lateralizing hearing loss

1 Weber's test
   a) Lateralizes to deaf side in conduction deafness (e.g. otosclerosis)
   b) Lateralizes to normal side in nerve deafness (e.g. acoustic neuroma)
2 Rinne's test
   a) Bone > air conduction on affected side in conduction deafness

b) Air > bone conduction on both sides in nerve deafness

Clinical evaluation of vestibular function
1 Caloric testing
  a) Tests integrity of one labyrinth at a time by slowly irrigating ear with hot (44°C) or cold (30°C) water
  b) Patient lies flat with head elevated 30–45° to make horizontal semicircular canal vertical
  c) Nystagmus induced may exhibit two possible abnormalities
    — Canal paresis, i.e. weaker nystagmus on affected side
    — Directional preponderance, i.e. longer duration of nystagmus on stimulation of one labyrinth
  d) Principal diagnostic use
    — Menière's disease
    — Acoustic neuroma
    — Unconscious patients: demonstration of brainstem integrity, CN III or VI palsies
2 Oculocephalic testing
  a) Tests integrity of both labyrinths together by holding eyelids open and sharply rotating head to one side
  b) 'Doll's-eye' movements are those in which the eyes initially lag behind head, but come to occupy original resting position
  c) Doll's-eye movements indicate loss of hemispheric suppression, i.e. unconsciousness, but with preservation of brainstem function

Distinction of acoustic neuroma from Menière's disease
1 Discrete symptomatic episodes unusual
2 Vertigo uncommon; rarely occurs in isolation
3 May be associated with postauricular/suboccipital pain, facial spasms or paraesthesiae, or dysphonia/dysphagia
4 Physical signs may include limb ataxia, cranial nerve palsies (esp. V) or hemianaesthesia/-paresis
5 Impaired oculovestibular (caloric) response
  High frequency deafness with recruitment on audiometry
6 Radiology
  a) MRI — modality of choice for cerebellopontine angle tumours
  b) CT (± air contrast for small tumours)
  c) SXR may reveal widening of internal auditory meatus or erosion of petrous temporal bone, but is no longer routinely indicated

SPINAL CORD DISEASE: GENERAL

Clues to localizing a spinal cord lesion
1 Radicular pain (indicating myotome) and weakness
2 Pattern of reflex changes
3 Sensory level (indicating dermatome)
4 Spinal tenderness to percussion (esp. acute epidural abscess/malignancy)
5 Vertebral bruit (indicating tumour/AVM)

Clinical sequelae of spinal cord lesions
1 Hypotension; poikilothermia
2 Paralytic ileus; sphincter dysfunction
  Chronic UTI → amyloidosis
3 Pressure sores; contractures
4 Immobilization →
  a) Hypercalcaemia
  b) Renal calculi
  c) Osteoporosis
  d) Venous thrombosis
5 Excessive sweating below lesion level

NEUROLOGY OF THE UPPER SPINE

Cranial nerve signs of high cervical cord disease
1 Ipsilateral hemifacial dissociated sensory loss (pain, temperature)
2 Horner's syndrome
3 Rarely — nystagmus, optic neuritis/atrophy

Signs of craniocervical junction anomaly (e.g. Arnold-Chiari)
1 Occipital pain; facial sensory loss; ± Pagetoid appearance
2 Cerebellar signs (due to foraminal tonsillar herniation)
3 Downbeat nystagmus
4 Finger de-afferentation (esp. proprioception) → pseudotremor
5 Bulbar palsy, spastic quadriparesis (may simulate MND)

Physical findings in cervical spondylosis
1 Limitation of neck movements
2 Absent tendon jerk(s) at level of lesion (root compression)
3 Increased tendon jerks below lesion (cord compression)
4 Inversion of reflexes
5 Dermatomal sensory loss in upper limbs
6 Dorsal column sensory loss in upper and lower limbs
7 Rombergism
8 Spastic paraparesis

Thoracic outlet syndrome: clinical features
1 Physical examination
  a) Supraclavicular 'fullness'/tenderness/bruit
  b) Dilated venous collaterals
  c) Arm pallor/cyanosis/oedema
  d) Arm claudication
  e) Wasted interossei
  f) Sensory loss in C8–T1 distribution
  g) Arm abduction (to 90°) and external rotation leads to
    — Reproduction of symptoms
    — ↓ Systolic BP in arm by > 15 mmHg
    — Loss or reduction of radial pulse
2 Investigation
  a) Plain X-ray of thoracic outlet, cervical spine and apical lordotic chest views
  b) Cervical myelography
  c) Angiography (bilateral) *if* cervical rib present

C4 root lesions: clinical findings
1 Ipsilateral hemidiaphragmatic paralysis
2 C4 sensory loss (abutting T2 dermatome) at shoulder

C5 root lesions
1 Total loss of shoulder abduction
2 Axillary nerve involvement
  a) Weak elbow flexion
  b) Reduced biceps jerk
  c) Larger sensory loss than circumflex nerve palsy
3 Supraspinatus wasting ± scapula winging

THE MOTOR SYSTEM

Distinguishing upper and lower motor neurone lesions
1 Upper motor neurone lesions
  a) Increased tone ± clonus
  b) Increased tendon reflexes
  c) Absent abdominal reflexes
  d) Extensor plantar response(s)
  e) 'Pyramidal' pattern of weakness (see below)
2 Lower motor neurone lesions
  a) Prominent wasting
  b) Fasciculation (in anterior horn cell disorders)
  c) Reduced tone
  d) Reflexes may be reduced or absent

Patterns of weakness in upper motor neurone lesions
1 Elbow and wrist extension
2 Finger extension and abduction — Upper limb extensors
3 Hip and knee flexion
4 Ankle dorsiflexion and eversion — Lower limb flexors
5 Fine movements of fingers and feet (esp. in capsular lesions)

Absent abdominal reflexes: differential diagnosis
1 Upper motor neurone lesions, esp.
  a) Multiple sclerosis
  b) General paresis of the insane (neurosyphilis)
  c) Spinal cord lesions above T7
2 Old age
  Gross obesity
  Multiparity

NB: superficial abdominal reflexes are usually *preserved* in motor neurone disease

Signs suggesting upper motor neurone lesions
1 Babinski sign — dorsiflexion of great toe and fanning of other digits on stroking lateral sole of foot
2 Oppenheim's sign — dorsiflexion of great toe on applying firm pressure while sliding thumb and forefinger down anterior tibia
3 Hoffman's sign — adduction and flexion of all digits after passively flexing and releasing distal phalanx of middle finger
4 Finger-flexor — adduction and flexion of all digits induced by tapping the palmar surface of relaxed fingers with tendon hammer

NB: exaggerated finger flexion is indicative of hypertonia rather than an upper motor neurone lesion *per se*

Fasciculations: differential diagnosis
1 Motor neurone disease
2 Acute phase of poliomyelitis
3 Thyrotoxicosis
  Severe hyponatraemia
4 Localized
  a) Neuralgic amyotrophy
  b) Cervical spondylosis
  c) Syringomyelia
5 Drugs
  a) Clofibrate
  b) Salbutamol
  c) Lithium

THE SENSORY SYSTEM

Characteristic patterns of sensory loss
1 Symmetric 'glove-and-stocking' sensory loss to all modalities — *peripheral neuropathy*
2 Dermatomal sensory loss — nerve root lesion
3 Ipsilateral loss of pain and temperature; Contralateral loss of proprioception/two-point discrimination — *Brown-Séquard syndrome*
4 Bilateral loss of pain and temperature
  Normal proprioception/two-point discrimination —'Dissociated' sensory loss
  a) *Syringomyelia*
  b) *Anterior spinal artery thrombosis*
5 Loss of proprioception/two-point discrimination/vibration
  Loss of deep pain (e.g. in testes, Achilles' tendon)
  Patchy loss of pinprick sensation (e.g. along side of nose) — *tabes dorsalis*

Symptoms of dorsal column pathology
1 Difficulty with fine movements ('clumsy')
2 Limb 'tightness' (as though bandaged)
3 'Cotton-wool' sensation over skin

Causes of reduced dorsal column function
1 Subacute combined degeneration
2 Cervical spondylosis
3 Friedreich's ataxia
4 Tabes dorsalis
  (cf. syringomyelia, anterior spinal artery thrombosis: normal dorsal column function is usual)

TESTING NERVE ROOT INTEGRITY

Clinical assessment of nerve root integrity: reflex levels
1 Biceps/supinator jerk present — C6 intact

2 Triceps jerk present — C7 intact
3 Finger flexor elicitable — C8 intact
4 Abdominal reflexes present — T7–12 intact
5 Cremasteric reflex present — L1/2 intact
6 Knee jerk present — L3/4 intact
7 Ankle jerk/plantars present — S1 intact
8 Anal reflex present — S3/4 intact

Quick testing of nerve root integrity in the upper limb
1 C5: shoulder abduction (deltoid) — 'make wings; keep them up, don't let me push them down'
2 C5/6: elbow flexion (biceps) — 'pull me towards you'
3 C7: elbow extension (triceps) — 'now push me away'
4 C8: finger flexion (long and short finger flexors) — 'squeeze my fingers, try to break them'
5 T1: finger abduction/adduction (intrinsics) — 'spread your fingers apart, don't let me push them in'

Quick testing of nerve root integrity in the lower limb
1 L1/2: hip flexion (iliopsoas) — 'push up against my hand; keep it up'
2 L2/3: hip adduction (adductors) — 'pull your knees together against my hands'
3 L3/4: knee extension (quadriceps) — 'try to straighten your knee; kick out against my hand'
4 L4: ankle dorsiflexion (tibialis anterior) — 'curl your ankle up, don't let me straighten it'
5 L5: great toe plantarflexion (extensor hallucis longus) — 'push your big toe down into my hand'
6 S1: ankle plantarflexion (gastrocnemius) — 'try to straighten out your foot; don't let me bend it back'

NEUROLOGY OF THE UPPER LIMB

Clinical spectrum of radial nerve palsy
1 High axillary injury ('crutch palsy')
  a) All supplied muscles paralysed
  b) Paralysis includes triceps
    — Loss of elbow extension
    — Absent triceps jerk
  c) Sensory deficit may extend to posterolateral upper arm and dorsal forearm/hand
2 Humeral midshaft injury ('Saturday night palsy')
  a) Wrist- and finger-drop
  b) Triceps spared — normal elbow extension and triceps jerk
  c) Paralysis → brachioradialis/supinator/forearm extensors
  d) Sensory deficit limited to dorsum of hand
4 Posterior interosseous nerve injury (distal to supinator)
  a) Loss of thumb/index extension
  b) Loss of thumb abduction
  c) Brachioradialis/supinator/forearm extensors spared
  d) No sensory deficit

Small hand muscles affected by median nerve lesion
'LOAF'
1 **L**ateral two lumbricals
2 **O**pponens pollicis
3 **A**bductor pollicis brevis (best test of median nerve integrity)
4 **F**lexor pollicis brevis

Wasting of the small muscles of both hands
1 Disuse
  a) Old age
  b) Rheumatoid arthritis
2 Spinal cord disease
  a) Syringomyelia
  b) Motor neurone disease
3 Spinal cord compression
  a) Cervical spondylosis
  b) C8/T1 tumour
4 Bilateral nerve root compression
  a) Cervical spondylosis
  b) Thoracic outlet syndrome
5 Peripheral neuropathy
  a) Charcot-Marie-Tooth disease
  b) Lead poisoning, acute intermittent porphyria

NB: myotonic dystrophy causes prominent forearm wasting but characteristically spares the small hand muscles

Wasting of the small muscles of one hand
1 Ulnar nerve lesion
2 T1 nerve root lesion (e.g. bronchogenic carcinoma)

Differentiation of T1 root lesion from ulnar nerve palsy
NB: ulnar nerve lesion at *wrist* (rare) also produces no sensory loss
1 No sensory deficit in the hand
2 Dermatomal sensory loss in medial arm
3 Weakness of opponens pollicis/abductor pollicis brevis (supplied by median nerve; i.e. T1 root lesion affects *all* intrinsics)

NEUROLOGICAL SIGNS IN THE LOWER LIMB

Absent ankle jerks with extensor plantar responses
1 Subacute combined degeneration
2 Friedreich's ataxia
3 Taboparesis
4 Rare causes
  a) Meningeal carcinomatosis
  b) Coexisting lumbar and cervical spondylosis
  c) Motor neurone disease
  d) Diabetic amyotrophy
  e) Conus medullaris lesion
  f) Spinal shock

Clinical assessment of paraparesis
1 Cauda equina compression
  a) Early onset of lumbosacral pain, precipitated by walking
  b) Flaccid paralysis — wasted calves/absent ankle jerks
  c) Sphincter involvement/perianal anaesthesia occur late
2 Conus medullaris lesion
  a) Pain occurs late

b) Spastic paraparesis — wasted quadriceps/upgoing toes

c) Sphincter dysfunction occurs early

3 Parasagittal meningioma
a) Spastic paraparesis, extensor plantar response(s)
b) Distal weakness often prominent
c) Papilloedema

Clinical assessment of footdrop
1 Lateral popliteal nerve palsy
a) Equinovarus deformity due to impaired eversion
b) Variable sensory loss (usually none)
c) Great toe — sensation/dorsiflexion usually normal

2 L5 root lesion
a) Eversion unimpaired (cf. S1 root lesion)
b) Dermatomal sensory loss (dorsum of foot)
c) Great toe — sensation/dorsiflexion usually impaired

3 Charcot-Marie-Tooth disease
a) Equinovarus deformity with pes cavus
b) 'Inverted champagne bottle' appearance of limbs
c) Mild glove-and-stocking sensory loss
d) Bilateral signs; possible hand involvement

Diagnostic significance of abnormal posture
1 Rombergism (loss of balance with eyes closed) — proprioceptive deficit
2 Truncal ataxia (same with eyes open or closed) — cerebellar (flocculonodular lobe) disease
3 Simian posture — parkinsonism

Diagnostic significance of abnormal gait
1 Wide-based ('drunken') gait — cerebellar (vermis) disease; same with eyes open or closed
2 Stamping ('footslapping') gait; may also be wide-based
a) Sensory (esp. dorsal column) ataxia; worse with eyes closed
b) Typically associated with rombergism, e.g. in tabes dorsalis
3 High-stepping ('equine') gait — footdrop, e.g. Charcot-Marie-Tooth disease
4 Circumducting ('sticky') gait — hemiplegia
5 Scissors ('walking through mud') gait — spastic paraparesis
6 Waddling ('duck-like') gait — myopathy
7 Festinating gait (± propulsion, retropulsion, turns-by-numbers) — parkinsonism
8 Marche à petits pas ('sputtering'/apraxic gait) — 'magnetic foot'
a) Pseudobulbar palsy
b) Alzheimer's disease
c) Normal pressure hydrocephalus

NB: in practice it is best to delay classifying the gait (if possible) until *after* the other signs have established the diagnosis!

PATTERNS OF PERIPHERAL NEUROPATHY

Important causes of hypertrophic (palpable) neuropathies
1 Charcot-Marie-Tooth disease

2 Acromegaly
3 Lepromatous leprosy
4 Amyloidosis

Predominantly motor neuropathies
1 Charcot-Marie-Tooth
2 Guillain-Barré syndrome
3 Acute intermittent (or variegate) porphyria
4 Diphtheria
5 Lead poisoning
6 Herpes zoster (common but usually subclinical)

Predominantly sensory neuropathies
1 Diabetes
2 Paraneoplastic
3 Nutritional (incl. B_{12}/folate deficiency, alcohol)
4 Uraemia
5 Amyloid

Frequently painful neuropathies
1 Diabetic amyotrophy
2 Nutritional — alcoholic neuropathy, beri-beri, Strachan's syndrome
3 Toxic — metronidazole, thallium poisoning
4 AIDS-related neuropathy

Cranial nerve involvement in peripheral neuropathy
1 Diphtheria (CN IX)
2 Guillain-Barré (CN VI, VII); Miller-Fisher variant (III, IV)
3 Sarcoidosis (CN VII)
4 Diabetes (CN III)

Drugs commonly associated with peripheral neuropathy
1 Vincristine, vindesine
2 Nitrofurantoin
3 Metronidazole
4 Perhexiline maleate
5 Gold
6 Isoniazid (B_6 deficiency), ethambutol Phenytoin (folate deficiency)

Guillain-Barré syndrome: diagnostic criteria
1 Major criteria
a) Progressive lower motor neurone weakness of > one limb
b) Maximal deficit induced within four weeks of onset
c) No other cause of neuropathy demonstrable
2 Minor criteria
a) Lack of fever
b) Symmetrical weakness with only mild sensory signs
c) ↑ CSF protein with normal cell count one week after onset
d) Segmental demyelination pattern of nerve conduction
e) Antiperipheral nerve myelin antibodies detectable acutely
f) Successful trial of plasmapheresis within first week

AUTONOMIC NEUROPATHY

Principal causes of autonomic neuropathy
1 Diabetes mellitus
2 Uraemia
3 Amyloidosis
4 Guillain-Barré syndrome
5 Liver disease ± alcoholism
6 Idiopathic (acquired): Shy-Drager syndrome
7 Idiopathic (congenital): Riley-Day syndrome

Presentations of autonomic neuropathy
1 Supine hypertension   } DD$_x$ — antihypertensive
  Postural hypotension } therapy
2 Fixed resting tachycardia (indicating vagal paresis) or postural tachycardia
3 Facial ('differential') gustatory sweating (anhidrosis elsewhere)
  Pupils — anisocoria, Horner's
4 Nocturnal hyperdefaecation
  Faecal incontinence
  Chronic intestinal pseudo-obstruction (→ constipation, or diarrhoea due to bacterial overgrowth)
5 Epigastric pain (gastroparesis, oesophageal reflux)
6 Reduced pain sensation
  a) 'Silent' myocardial infarction
  b) Absence of 'deep' pain (e.g. on compressing Achilles' tendon or testicle)
  c) Coexisting loss of peripheral pain and temperature sensation (small-fibre neuropathy)
7 Impotence (rarely if ever presents in isolation)
8 Urinary retention with overflow incontinence (urgency)
9 Hypoglycaemic unawareness (e.g. in treated diabetics)

Assessment of autonomic neuropathy
1 Measurement of variation in heart rate/blood pressure, ECG R-R intervals, and plasma noradrenaline/renin activity
  a) Posturing using tilt-table
  b) Valsalva manoeuvre (4-phase response)
  c) Isometric handgrip
  d) Mental arithmetic (serial 7, s)
  e) Hands in iced water (for 90 s)
  f) Hyperventilation (for 30 s)
  g) Carotid sinus massage
  h) Response to amyl nitrite/atropine/isoprenaline/noradrenaline
2 Pupillary responses
  a) Intraocular adrenaline 1: 1000 → no dilatation normally, but *dilates* in autonomic neuropathy (denervation hypersensitivity)
  b) Intraocular cocaine 2.5% → dilatation normally, but *not* in autonomic neuropathy
  c) Intraocular methacholine 2.5% → no constriction normally, but *constricts* in autonomic neuropathy (parasympathetic denervation)
3 Sweat tests
  a) Heat patient to cause 1°C rise in oral temperature
  b) Response to i.m.i. pilocarpine or intradermal methacholine
4 Bladder urodynamics (cystometry)

INVESTIGATING NEUROLOGICAL DISEASE

INVESTIGATING THE CENTRAL NERVOUS SYSTEM

Diagnosis of brain death
1 Sufficient cause (exclude hypothermia/sedative overdose)
2 No response to noxious stimuli except spinal reflexes
3 Fixed pupils
4 Loss of oculovestibular and oculocephalic reflexes
5 Absent gag/corneal/cough reflexes
6 No spontaneous respiratory movements after ventilator disconnected and patient observed for five minutes with oxygen supplied via tracheal catheter.

Aseptic meningitis: diagnostic considerations
1 Partly-treated pyogenic meningitis
2 Tuberculous meningitis
  Cryptococcal meningitis } — i.e. may not be
  Neurosyphilis } identified on ordinary
  Leptospirosis } microscopy/culture
  Brucellosis
3 Viral (e.g. HSV#2, polio)
  HIV
4 Non-infectious causes
  a) Vasculitis (esp. SLE)
  b) Meningeal carcinomatosis ('carcinomatous meningitis')
  c) Sarcoidosis
  d) Behçet's/Whipple's disease; Vogt-Koyanagi syndrome

Markedly elevated CSF protein: differential diagnosis
1 Pyogenic meningitis
2 Meningeal carcinomatosis
3 Guillain-Barré syndrome
4 Froin's syndrome (spinal block)
5 Rare: alcoholism, amyloidosis, diabetes, acoustic neuroma

Evoked responses: diagnostic utility
1 Visual evoked responses (VERs)
  a) Multiple sclerosis: may be useful
    — Prior to firm (clinical) diagnosis or
    — Monitoring disease progress
  b) Retinal disease
  c) Hemispheric disease (e.g. 'cortical' blindness vs hysteria)
2 Brainstem auditory evoked responses (BAERs)
  a) Suspected acoustic neuroma
  b) Comatose patient
  c) Hysterical deafness
  d) Multiple sclerosis
3 Somatosensory evoked responses (SSERs)
  a) Localization of peripheral nerve pathology vs spinal cord/root lesion
  b) Multiple sclerosis

ELECTROENCEPHALOGRAPHY (EEG)

Normal EEG patterns
1 Awake (eyes closed) — alpha waves (8–12 cps); detected over parieto-occipital region
2 Non-REM sleep — delta waves (0–3 cps)
3 REM sleep — beta waves (> 13 cps); detected over frontal region
4 Hyperventilation — theta waves (4–7 cps)

Capabilities of the EEG
1 May confirm epileptic activity
2 May demonstrate functional disturbance due to metabolic disorder (e.g. liver failure)
3 May suggest focal pathology
4 May provide an explanation for sleep disturbances and/or drop attacks
5 May help distinguish petit mal from temporal lobe epilepsy

Limitations of the EEG
1 Cannot exclude epilepsy
2 Cannot be used to assess adequacy of antiepileptic treatment
3 Cannot exclude focal pathology
4 Cannot suggest structural nature of focal pathology

Principal indications for EEG
1 Diagnosis and management of epilepsy
2 Diagnosis of brain death
3 Initial investigation of presenile dementia
4 Evaluation of birth asphyxia
5 Any unexplained organic brain syndrome

Suggestive diagnostic EEG patterns
1 Hepatic encephalopathy — triphasic waves (*not* seen in Wernicke's or DT's) and/or slow (delta) waves
2 Barbiturate overdose — excess fast-wave activity
3 'Alpha coma' — follows infarction of midbrain tegmentum
4 Absence (petit mal) seizures — characteristic 3 cps spike-and-wave pattern
5 HSV encephalitis ⎫
  SSPE   ⎬ Slow background repetitive sharp waves
  Jakob-Creutzfeldt ⎭

The unconscious patient: utility of the EEG
1 Helps distinguish diffuse encephalopathy (e.g. myxoedema → diffuse slowing; dialysis dementia → paroxysmal spike-and-wave pattern) **from**
2 Space-occupying lesions (e.g. frontal lobe tumour → focal slowing) **or**
3 Other focal pathology (e.g. HSV encephalitis → temporal lobe slowing) **or**
4 Depressive pseudodementia (normal EEG)

INVESTIGATING CAROTID DISEASE

Techniques available for assessing carotid disease
1 Direct tests
  a) Angiography (incl. digital subtraction angiography)
  b) 'Duplex scan' — B-mode (real-time) ultrasound + multigated pulsed-Doppler ultrasound
2 Indirect tests
  a) Ophthalmodynamometry
  b) Oculoplethysmography
  c) Periorbital directional Doppler ultrasonography
  d) Radionuclide angiography

Which investigation to choose in carotid disease?
1 Angiograpy
  a) Advantages
    — Reveals location *and* severity of disease
    — Still the 'gold standard' for preop. diagnosis
  b) Disadvantages
    — Invasive; may precipitate stroke
    — May fail to reveal intramural pathology
2 'Duplex scan'
  a) Advantages
    — Non-invasive; useful in monitoring known disease
    — May detect plaque haemorrhage or ulceration
    — *Normal* study may obviate need for angiography
  b) Disadvantages — abnormal study may still require angiography prior to surgery
3 Indirect tests (ophthalmic artery flow/pressure studies)
  a) Advantages — non-invasive
  b) Disadvantages
    — Only reliably detect *unilateral* disease
    — Only reliably detect *advanced* (>75% stenosis) disease
    — Only reliably detect *occlusive* disease (misses ulcerated plaques)

Indications for angiography in cerebrovascular disease
1 Operable patient *plus*
2 Symptoms suggesting carotid pathology, *or*
3 Subclavian steal syndrome

INVESTIGATING THE PERIPHERAL NERVOUS SYSTEM

Investigation of peripheral neuropathy
1 Qualitative tests
  a) Nerve conduction studies
  b) Nerve biopsy
2 Aetiological tests
  a) Blood film, MCV
  b) B_{12}, folate
  c) GGT/urate (ethanol)
  d) Fasting blood sugar level, HbA_{1c}, GTT
  e) Lead, mercury levels
  f) Urinary porphobilinogen/ALA
  g) CSF protein and cell count
  h) Carcinoma search (e.g. CXR) only if clinically indicated

Nerve conduction studies: diagnostic significance
1 General
  a) Myopathy
    — Normal nerve conduction velocity
    — Reduced amplitude and duration of motor units

b) Neuropathy
  — Reduced nerve conduction velocity
  — Reduced number of motor units
2 Neuropathy — *segmental demyelination* (e.g. Guillain-Barré)
  a) Marked slowing of conduction velocity
  b) Amplitude may be normal
  c) Clinical correlations
    — Early loss of reflexes and vibration sense
    — Mononeuritis multiplex
    — Rapid recovery (often)
3 Neuropathy — *axonal degeneration* (e.g. nutritional deficiency)
  a) Marked reduction of motor unit amplitude
  b) Mild slowing of conduction velocity
  c) Clinical correlations
    — Early onset of wasting
    — Incomplete recovery (usually)
4 Upper motor neurone lesion
  a) Normal evoked muscle potentials
  b) Low firing rate; slow in reaching full interference pattern
  c) Unexpected 'H' reflexes

Indications for nerve biopsy
1 Definitive distinction between *axonal degeneration* and *segmental demyelination* (thereby allowing prognostic clarification)
2 Definitive diagnosis of neuropathies due to
  a) Polyarteritis/vasculitis
  b) Amyloidosis
  c) Sarcoidosis
  d) Leprosy
  e) Déjerine-Sottas disease

DIAGNOSTIC ASPECTS OF MUSCLE DISEASE

Muscle biopsy: diagnostic value
1 Polymyositis
2 Polyarteritis
3 Myotonic dystrophy
4 Trichinosis, toxoplasmosis
5 Metabolic muscle disease (e.g. glycogen storage) Special myopathies (e.g. mitochondrial)

Pathological patterns in electromyography (EMG)
1 Polymyositis — may cause fibrillation (brief low-amplitude action potentials due to denervation hypersensitivity), indicating pathology at the motor end-plate (i.e. in addition to the known muscle fibre pathology)
2 Myotonia — 'dive-bomber' EMG (high-frequency discharge of action potential)
3 Myasthenia gravis — decremental response to repetitive ('tetanic') stimulation; increased 'jitter'
4 Myasthenic (Eaton-Lambert) syndrome — incremental response to repetitive stimulation ('post-tetanic facilitation')

Myotonic dystrophy: recognition and diagnosis
1 Percussion myotonia best demonstrated in thenar eminence, forearm, quadriceps

2 Pattern of weakness/wasting
  a) Myopathic facies
    — Ptosis
    — Hanging jaw
    — Temporalis wasting
  b) Weakness of neck flexion, wasting of sternomastoids
  c) Distal limb weakness with wasted brachioradialis
  d) Monotonous voice; oesophageal dilatation
3 Frontal baldness
  Craniofacial abnormalities (incl. hyperostosis frontalis interna)
4 Cataracts; aphakia (iatrogenic)
5 End-organ resistance to insulin (impaired glucose tolerance) and gonadotrophins (↑ FSH/LH, hypogonadism)
6 Cardiac conduction defects (e.g. primary heart block, atrial arrhythmias); cardiomyopathy
7 Hypoventilation
  Postanaesthetic respiratory failure
8 Hypogammaglobulinaemia
9 Hypersomnolence; subnormal intellect
10 Management includes
  a) Family screening using FSH levels and/or EMG
  b) Drugs: quinine, phenytoin, procainamide

NEURORADIOLOGY

Intracranial calcification on skull X-ray
1 Oligodendroglioma, meningioma
  a) 20% calcify ('ball of calcium')
  b) May be associated with overlying bony hyperostosis
2 Craniopharyngioma, esp. in children
  a) 75% calcify
  b) May be intra- or suprasellar
3 Pineal gland
  a) Calcified in 60% adults, 10% children
  b) Midline shift may indicate intracranial mass lesion
4 Tuberous sclerosis — multiple discrete lesions → temporal lobes
5 Sturge-Weber syndrome
  a) Subcortical 'tramline' calcification → parieto-occipital
  b) ± Ipsilateral facial haemangioma, contralateral hemiparesis
6 Infection
  a) Toxoplasmosis
  b) CMV; TB
7 Vascular
  a) Aneurysm ('ring' calcification)
  b) Angioma (spotty flecks of calcification)
  c) Atheroma (curvilinear)
  d) Chronic subdurals (outlined by calcification; rare)
8 Basal ganglia calcification — esp. in hypoparathyroidism

Characteristic CT scan appearances
1 Normal pressure hydrocephalus: large ventricles with minimal cortical atrophy
2 Benign intracranial hypertension: small ventricles

3 Intracerebral abscess: enhancing ring ± satellite oedema

False-negative CT brainscans
1 Non-enhancing lesions < 1 cm diameter
2 Diffuse lesions (e.g. microgliomatosis)
3 Bilateral subdurals isodense with brain
4 Lesions near skull base or anterior optic pathways

Indications for CT brainscan in the 'stroke' patient
1 Young patient
2 Diagnostic uncertainty (e.g. ?tumour, ?subdural)
3 Atypical clinical course, esp. unexpectedly rapid deterioration
4 Suspected cerebellar (i.e. surgically evacuable) haemorrhage
5 Subarachnoid haemorrhage (CT is now investigation of choice)
6 Recent history of anticoagulant therapy

Other indications for CT brainscan
1 Head injury with disturbance of consciousness
2 Head injury with focal signs
3 Late-(adult)-onset epilepsy, esp. with focal signs
4 Presenile dementia

MAGNETIC RESONANCE IMAGING (MRI)

Advantages of magnetic resonance imaging over CT
1 *No* ionizing radiation with MRI; consists of radiofrequency radiation emitted within magnetic field → resonance of magnetic elements (e.g. H_2) in body
2 MRI can provide imaging sections in *any* anatomic plane
3 Compact bone does not produce any signal with MRI, hence no artefacts, e.g. in posterior cranial fossa (cf. CT)

Specific scenarios where MRI is superior to CT
1 Posterior fossa lesions, esp. tumours
2 Cerebellopontine angle pathology, e.g. acoustic neuroma
3 Craniocervical junction pathology, e.g. Arnold-Chiari
4 Demyelinating plaques, esp. if gadolinium contrast used
5 Spinal pathology: cord/vertebral tumours, disc disease
6 Hydrocephalus
7 Contrast allergy

Contraindications to MRI
1 Cerebral aneurysm clips in situ
2 Permanent pacemaker
3 Pregnancy

Conditions in which CT may be superior to MRI
1 Acute skull trauma
2 Acute stroke, e.g. subarachnoid haemorrhage
3 Cerebral aneurysm or arteriovenous malformation

MANAGING NEUROLOGICAL DISEASE

CEREBROVASCULAR DISEASE

Management considerations in cerebrovascular disease
1 A carotid bruit with stenosis is highly predictive for the development of ischaemic heart/peripheral vascular disease
2 In symptomatic patients, the more severe the stenosis, the higher the risk of stroke, *but*
3 Many severe (even occlusive) stenoses are asymptomatic; if so, the risk of stroke is < 2%
4 Atheromatous carotid lesions may regress
5 Absence of a bruit is not a contraindication to angiographic assessment (severe stenoses may be inaudible)
6 Hypertension is the single biggest risk factor for a cerebrovascular event; in patients with TIAs, reducing diastolic BP by 5–10 mmHg may reduce stroke risk by up to 40–50%

Important therapeutic negatives in cerebrovascular disease
1 Prophylactic endarterectomy is *not* indicated for asymptomatic carotid bruits
2 High-dose steroids are of *no* benefit in cerebral infarction
3 Extracranial-intracranial bypass grafting appears to be of *no* benefit to symptomatic patients with internal carotid/middle cerebral artery disease

Rationâle for aspirin prophylaxis in cardiovascular disease
1 Reduces morbidity and mortality of carotid-type TIAs in males
2 Reduces reinfarction (20%) and mortality (10%) following myocardial infarction
3 Reduces 'event rates' in unstable angina
4 Enhances coronary artery bypass graft patency
5 Helps prevent venous thrombosis after hip surgery in males
6 May retard progression of peripheral vascular disease

Indications for anticoagulation
1 TIAs associated with cardiac disease (e.g. mitral stenosis and/or atrial fibrillation; postinfarct)
2 Carotid-type TIAs
   a) In a potentially operable patient prior to angiography
   b) In a female patient unsuitable for surgery
      — Unfit
      — Normal angiogram
   c) In a male patient unsuitable for surgery *and* unresponsive to aspirin prophylaxis
3 Vertebrobasilar insufficiency in a female patient *or* in a male patient despite aspirin prophylaxis (Rare exception: subclavian steal syndrome may be surgically treated)
4 Relative need for anticoagulation is increased with
   a) Recent onset (<6/12) of TIAs

b) Increasing frequency of attacks
c) Longer duration of attacks
d) Accumulating (residual) neurological deficit with repeated attacks

SURGERY IN CEREBROVASCULAR DISEASE

Carotid endarterectomy: when should it be considered?
1 Logistic prerequisites
   a) Fit patient with symptomatic carotid disease
   b) Experienced vascular surgical team available
2 Principal indication — >70% stenosis (residual lumen < 2 mm) accompanied by appropriate symptoms
3 Less definite indications
   a) Ulcerated (potentially embologenic) carotid lesion
   b) Clots (luminal filling defects) ± tight stenosis
   c) Acute phase occlusion with mild/fluctuating deficit

Common scenarios for inappropriate carotid endarterectomy
1 Stenosis too mild
2 Symptoms related to contralateral cerebral hemisphere
3 Established total carotid occlusion
4 Patient unfit for general anaesthesia

SPASTICITY

Antispasticity drugs: therapeutic considerations
1 General — drug therapy tends to be more effective in spasticity of spinal rather than intracranial origin
2 Diazepam
   a) CNS GABA agonist
   b) Dosage limited by sedation
3 Baclofen
   a) CNS GABA agonist
   b) May reduce seizure threshold
4 Dantrolene
   a) Peripheral effect on skeletal muscles; inhibits calcium release from sarcoplasmic reticulum
   b) May exacerbate weakness (therefore less popular)
   c) Occasionally associated with hepatotoxicity

Surgical measures in spasticity management
1 Neurolysis — phenol/absolute alcohol injection into nerve or dorsal nerve root
2 Tenotomy — e.g. hamstring, adductor, heelcord
3 Myotomy — e.g. iliopsoas
4 Neurectomy — e.g. obturator; pudendal (for detrusor instability)
5 Myelotomy
6 Cordectomy — a drastic measure for intractable symptoms, e.g. uncontrollable flexor/adductor spasms

ANTICONVULSANT THERAPY

Choosing an anticonvulsant for epileptic disorders
1 Tonic-clonic ('grand mal') seizures alone

   a) Drug of choice — phenytoin (NB: may worsen absence seizures)
   b) Other drugs
      — Carbamazepine (esp. if focal seizures)
      — Phenobarbitone/primidone
2 Complex partial ('temporal lobe') ± tonic-clonic seizures
   a) Drug of choice — carbamazepine
   b) Other drugs — phenytoin, sodium valproate
3 Status epilepticus
   a) Drug of choice — diazepam (slow i.v.i. or infusion)
   b) Other drugs
      — Clonazepam/lorazepam
      — Thiopentone, chlormethiazole (in intensive care)
      — Phenytoin infusion (ECG and plasma monitoring required)

Epileptic disorders best treated by sodium valproate
1 Absence ('petit mal') seizures (other drugs: ethosuximide*
2 Tonic-clonic seizures associated with absence seizures (other drugs: phenytoin, phenobarbitone)
3 Myoclonic epilepsy (other drugs: clonazepam, nitrazepam)
4 Febrile convulsion prophylaxis (other drugs: phenobarbitone)
5 Minor motor seizures (infantile spasms)

MECHANISMS OF ANTICONVULSANT ACTION

Anticonvulsants acting as GABA agonists
(i.e. act by enhancing GABA-mediated CNS inhibition)
1 Valproate
2 Benzodiazepines
3 Barbiturates
4 Baclofen

Anticonvulsants acting as membrane stabilizers
1 Phenytoin — increases membrane binding of calcium
2 Carbamazepine — structurally related to tricyclics (*not* to benzodiazepines)

Pharmacokinetics of anticonvulsant therapy
1 Phenytoin
   a) $t^{\frac{1}{2}} \approx 24$ hours
   b) Time to plateau ≈ 5 days
   c) Once-daily dosage schedule is satisfactory
   d) Children may require up to double the usual adult maintenance dose due to enhanced liver metabolism
   e) Exhibits saturation kinetics (similar to aspirin, alcohol)
2 Phenobarbitone
   a) $t^{\frac{1}{2}} \approx 100$ hours
   b) Time to plateau ≈ 2–3 weeks
   c) Once-daily dosage schedule is satisfactory

*Worsens tonic-clonic seizures

3 Carbamazepine
   a) $t^{\frac{1}{2}}$ 12 hours
   b) Time to plateau $\approx$ 3 days (but may take longer since *initial* $t^{\frac{1}{2}} \approx$ 36 hours; shortens due to autoinduction)
   c) Administered three times daily
4 Sodium valproate
   a) Plasma $t^{\frac{1}{2}} \approx$ hours, but this bears no relation to therapeutic effect (which presumably relates better to intracellular levels)
   b) Administered twice- or thrice-daily

PROBLEMS WITH ANTICONVULSANT THERAPY

Specific indications for monitoring anticonvulsant plasma levels
1 Phenytoin therapy, esp. if
   a) Poor seizure control
   b) Suspected toxicity
   c) New drug added (e.g. valproate)
2 Carbamazepine therapy in initial stages (subsequent plasma levels tend to be proportional to dose)
3 Renal or liver disease
4 Mentally retarded patients (if difficult to assess toxicity)
5 Suspected non-compliance

Side-effects of phenytoin
1 Acute toxicity with i.v. use
   a) Hypotension
   b) Arrhythmias
   c) CNS depression
2 Acute toxicity with oral use
   a) Dose-dependent; correlates with toxic serum drug levels
   b) Nystagmus → ataxia → drowsiness
3 Chronic toxicity with routine oral use
   a) Dose-dependent, but may occur at therapeutic drug levels
   b) Vitamin D deficiency — osteomalacia, hypocalcaemia
4 Idiosyncratic
   a) Not necessarily dose-related
   b) Nausea, vomiting, diarrhoea
   c) Skin rash
   d) SLE; pseudolymphoma
5 Epilepsy-related
   a) May cause *worsening* of absence seizures
   b) High-dose therapy may be associated with increased frequency of tonic-clonic seizures

Side-effects of other anticonvulsants
1 Sodium valproate
   a) Tremor (dose-dependent)
   b) Hair thinning (reversible), hair curling
   c) Increased appetite, weight gain; ankle oedema
   d) Drowsiness (but less than most other anticonvulsants)
   e) Stupor, encephalopathy ± hyperammonaemia/hyperglycinaemia
   f) Reye's-like hepatotoxicity (idiosyncratic); affects

1/10 000, esp. age <3 years; often preceded by increased seizure frequency; potentially fatal
2 Carbamazepine
   a) Drowsiness (esp. if co-prescribed with phenytoin)
   b) SIADH with fluid retention (may precipitate CCF in elderly)
   c) Anticholinergic effects (carbamazepine structurally resembles tricyclics)
   d) Leucopenia, agranulocytosis (rare)
3 Phenobarbitone and congeners (e.g. primidone)
   a) Drowsiness/confusion, esp. in elderly
   b) Hyperactivity in children
   c) Megaloblastosis

Anticonvulsant interactions of clinical significance
1 *Phenytoin, phenobarbitone* and (especially) *carbamazepine* all **induce** hepatic metabolism; hence,
   a) After commencing monotherapy with such drugs, dosage may need to be increased due to autoinduction of drug metabolism
   b) Adding any of these agents to treatment of a patient already stabilized on monotherapy (e.g. valproate) may lead to a paradoxical worsening of epileptic control initially due to enhanced drug metabolism
   c) These drugs may also antagonize other medications, including oral contraceptives, steroids, quinidine, warfarin, and theophylline; conversely, toxicity of the latter drugs may be precipitated by (say) carbamazepine withdrawal
2 *Sodium valproate* may **inhibit** hepatic metabolism, hence adding valproate tends to precipitate toxicity of other anticonvulsants such as phenobarbitone (which may in turn reduce the effect of valproate) or clonazepam
3 Other inhibitors of hepatic metabolism (e.g. isoniazid) may also precipitate phenytoin toxicity (in the case of isoniazid, this is particularly true for slow acetylators)
4 *Valproate* may also precipitate *phenytoin toxicity* even in the absence of raised serum phenytoin levels, due to **plasma protein displacement** (i.e. increased free — but not total — phenytoin)

Considerations in managing the pregnant epileptic
1 Seizure control may deteriorate due to reduction in plasma drug concentration. If dosage increased, toxicity may supervene in the puerperium unless drug levels are closely monitored
2 Antagonism of vitamin K-dependent coagulation factors by anticonvulsants, esp. barbiturates, may predispose to fetal or neonatal haemorrhage (cf. haemorrhagic disease of the newborn: no bleeding until at least 24 hours postpartum)
3 Phenytoin and phenobarbitone/primidone therapy is associated with reduced folate levels
4 A small but significant increased incidence of congenital malformations is seen in the offspring of epileptics, incl.
   a) Epileptic mothers *not* being treated with anticonvulsants
   b) Epileptic fathers (i.e. married to non-epileptic mothers)

PARKINSON'S DISEASE

Therapeutic options in Parkinson's disease
1 Mild disease (symptoms without disability):
  a) Anticholinergics (e.g. benzhexol, orphenadrine)
    — Best avoided in elderly patients (→ confusion)
    — Most effective in controlling salivation
    — Also useful in treating bradykinesia and/or rigidity; less useful in treating tremor
    — Confer additive benefit to levodopa
  b) Amantadine
    — Weak non-specific dopamine receptor agonist
    — Useful for mild bradykinesia; tremor may worsen
    — Minimal toxicity: oedema, livedo reticularis
    — Amphetamine-like effect → insomnia; high dosage → confusion
    — Tolerance may be a problem
  c) Deprenyl
    — MAO inhibitor proven to defer disability
2 Moderately disabling disease — levodopa
  a) Taken up by dopaminergic neurones and converted to dopamine by decarboxylation
  b) Usually combined with peripheral (extracerebral) decarboxylase inhibitor, e.g. carbidopa, benserazide
  c) Mainstay of therapy for bradykinesia, rigidity
  d) Antagonized by phenothiazines (e.g. prescribed for levodopa-induced nausea) or pyridoxine
3 Advanced or refractory disability
  a) Bromocriptine
    — Specific dopamine receptor agonist
    — Prime indication: late failure of levodopa
    — Longer duration of action than levodopa
    — Expensive and relatively toxic ('first-dose' reactions, psychosis)
  b) Stereotactic surgery
    — Rarely used
    — Sole indication: incapacitating tremor (esp. if unilateral) refractory to levodopa
4 Adjunctive measures
  a) Physiotherapy
  b) Laxative (esp. if on anticholinergics)
  c) Tricyclic antidepressants
  d) β-blockers (for tremor)
  e) Benzodiazepines (for myalgias)

PROBLEMS IN MANAGING PARKINSON'S DISEASE

Primary levodopa resistance in parkinsonism: things to exclude
1 Non-compliance (± dementia, depression)
2 Coadministration of phenothiazines or pyridoxine
3 Misdiagnosis
  a) Richardson-Steele syndrome (progressive supranuclear palsy)
  b) Multiple system atrophy
    — Olivopontocerebellar atrophy
    — Striatonigral degeneration
    — Shy-Drager syndrome (progressive autonomic failure)

Limitations of levodopa therapy
1 Episodic exacerbations of bradykinesia ('on-off' effect)
2 End-of dose deterioration ('wearing-off' effect)
3 Dose-limiting effects
  a) Confusion; nightmares
  b) Depression, paranoid ideation
4 Dose-dependent toxicity
  a) Vomiting (CNS effect and delayed gastric emptying)
  b) Hypotension, orthostasis
  c) Dyskinesias, blepharospasm, akathisia
5 Minimal effect in treating tremor (cf. rigidity, bradykinesia)

The 'on-off' effect: therapeutic approaches
1 Add deprenyl to levodopa
2 Substitute bromocriptine for levodopa
3 Levodopa 'drug holiday'
4 Experimental — transplantation of fetal substantia nigra

IATROGENIC NEUROLOGICAL DISEASE

Neurological sequelae of oral contraceptives
1 Migraine
2 Cerebral thrombosis/infarction
3 Hypertensive intracerebral haemorrhage
4 Subarachnoid haemorrhage
5 Dural sinus thrombosis
6 Chorea (Sydenham's); benign intracranial hypertension

Benign intracranial hypertension: iatrogenic causes
1 Tetracycline
2 Oral contraceptives, corticosteroids
3 Vitamin A
4 Nitrofurantoin; nalidixic acid; perhexiline

Varieties of drug-induced eye disease
1 Corneal microdeposits
  a) Amiodarone (usually asymptomatic)
  b) Chloroquine (reversible)
2 Cataracts
  a) Steroids (incl. eyedrops)
  b) Phenothiazines (usually asymptomatic)
3 Optic neuritis
  a) Ethambutol
  b) Chloramphenicol
4 Retinopathy
  a) Chloroquine ('bull's-eye' macula)
  b) Thioridazine (retinitis pigmentosa-like)
5 Stevens-Johnson syndrome — e.g. sulphonamides

UNDERSTANDING NEUROLOGICAL DISEASE

Neurotransmitters in CNS disease
1 Excitatory
  a) Glutamate
  b) N-methyl-D Aspartate (NMDA)

2 Inhibitory
  a) Glycine (but *enhances* NMDA excitation)
  b) GABA (decarboxylation product of glutamate)

NB: these are *amine* neurotransmitters; *peptide* neurotransmitters do not lend themselves to such simple categorization

Parkinson's disease vs Huntington's chorea: what's different
1 Predominant site of neuronal loss in Parkinson's — pigmented nuclei: substantia nigra, locus caeruleus
  Predominant site of neuronal loss in Huntington's — caudate nucleus (± frontal lobes, putamen)
2 Neurotransmitter loss in Parkinson's — dopamine
  Neurotransmitter loss in Huntington's — acetylcholine (and GABA)
3 Pathophysiology of Parkinson's — relative excess of acetylcholine → parkinsonism
  Pathophysiology of Huntington's — relative excess of dopamine → chorea (cf. *tardive dyskinesia:* thought to arise due to acquisition of striatal supersensitivity to dopamine)
4 Dopamine receptor agonists (e.g. levodopa) in Parkinson's → improvement of parkinsonism
  Dopamine receptor agonists in Huntington's → exacerbation of chorea
5 Dopamine receptor antagonists (e.g. phenothiazines) in Parkinson's → exacerbation of parkinsonism
  Dopamine receptor antagonists in Huntington's → improvement of chorea

Movement disorders: predominant sites of pathology
1 Kernicterus — caudate and lenticular nuclei
2 Haliervorden-Spatz disease — substantia nigra (zona reticulata)
3 Hemiballismus — subthalamus (contralateral)
4 Wilson's disease — putamen
  Kayser-Fleischer rings — Descemet's membrane (absence of these on slit-lamp examination reliably excludes Wilson's disease as a cause of neurological — cf. hepatic — dysfunction)

Classical localization of selected intracranial pathologies
1 Herpes simplex encephalitis — temporal lobes
2 Wernicke's encephalopathy — mamillary bodies, mamillothalamic tracts
3 Pick's disease — anterior frontal and temporal lobes
4 Sturge-Weber syndrome
  a) Forehead haemangioma → occipital lobe involvement
  b) Facial haemangioma → frontoparietal involvement
5 Tuberous sclerosis — temporal lobe calcification

Predispositions to chronic subdural haematomata
1 Epilepsy
2 Alcoholism
3 Haemodialysis
4 Anticoagulant therapy
5 Poor socioeconomic status

Features of chronic subdurals
1 Headache occurs in 75%
2 History of head trauma in 50% (only)
3 Fluctuating level of consciousness in less than 25%

Predispositions to cerebral aneurysms
1 Aortic coarctation
2 Polycystic disease
3 Renal artery stenosis due to fibromuscular dysplasia
4 Essential hypertension
5 Ehlers-Danlos syndrome type IV
6 PAN/Wegener's/SBE

Sequelae of subarachnoid haemorrhage
1 Cerebral vasospasm
2 Rebleeding (40% within 12 months); 20% have multiple aneurysms
3 Excessive catecholamine release (acute phase)
  a) Hypertension
  b) ECG abnormalities (e.g. T-wave inversion)
  c) Glycosuria
4 Normal pressure hydrocephalus (long-term)

NEUROSYPHILIS
Clinical varieties of neurosyphilis
1 Meningovascular syphilis
  a) Non-specific mental changes
  b) Cranial nerve palsies
  c) Argyll-Robertson pupils, papilloedema
  d) Cerebral infarction
  e) Limb paresis
2 Tabes dorsalis:
  a) Symptoms — lightning pains, gastric crises, impotence
  b) Argyll-Robertson pupils, optic atrophy
  c) Pseudo-ptosis (overactive frontalis)
  d) Reduced vibration/proprioception/deep pain
  e) Patchy loss of temperature/pinprick sensation — nose, tibia
  f) Charcot joints, trophic foot ulcers
  g) Rombergism, stamping gait (sensory ataxia)
  h) Hypotonia, hyporeflexia; flexor plantar responses
3 General paresis of the insane
  a) Dementia, incontinence, fits
  b) Argyll-Robertson pupils
  c) Dysarthria
  d) Tongue ('trombone') tremor
  e) Upper motor neurone signs, incl. extensor plantar responses

NEUROLOGY AND THE AIDS PATIENT
Neurological indications for HIV serology
1 Unexplained mental deterioration
  a) Encephalitis
  b) Encephalopathy
  c) Dementia
2 Myelopathy (aseptic meningitis, transverse myelitis)
3 Inflammatory neuropathy

Neurological manifestations of AIDS
1 AIDS-dementia complex
  a) Affects > 50% of AIDS patients with advanced disease
  b) Causes ataxia, incontinence, mutism, paraplegia
  c) Subacute encephalitis may be due to HIV itself (or CMV)
2 Opportunistic CNS infection — e.g. toxoplasmosis, cryptococcosis, JC virus
3 Vacuolar myelopathy — bilateral leg weakness, incontinence
4 Atypical aseptic meningitis — may be recurrent, involve cranial nerves and/or long tracts
5 Inflammatory demyelinating polyneuropathy — may mimic GBS; mononeuritis multiplex — may precede AIDS diagnosis
6 CNS lymphoma (EBV-induced)
7 Zidovudine neurotoxicity (rare)
  a) Idiosyncratic confusion, seizures
  b) Dose-related ataxia/nystagmus
  c) Symptom precipitation if drug abruptly withdrawn

MULTIPLE SCLEROSIS

Diagnosis of multiple sclerosis
1 Clinical: at least two remitting episodes of at least two focal lesions
2 Supporting investigations
  a) Delayed evoked responses, esp. VERs
  b) Oligoclonal bands on CSF EPG (90% sensitive; also seen in sarcoid, syphilis, SLE, etc.)
  c) Demyelinating plaques visible on magnetic resonance imaging with gadolinium contrast (best single test); positive in 95%

Predictors of poor prognosis in multiple sclerosis
1 Advanced age at onset
2 Incomplete recovery (esp. persistent weakness) from initial attack
3 Presentation with acute brainstem syndrome (simulating stroke)
4 Early onset of cerebellar ataxia
5 Early loss of mental acuity (may be associated with euphoria)

Common presentations of multiple sclerosis
1 CN II involvement — optic neuritis
2 Brainstem involvement
  a) Diplopia (CN VI or internuclear palsy)
  b) Nystagmus, vertigo
3 Spinal cord involvement — asymmetrical leg weakness and/or numbness

Uncommon presentations of multiple sclerosis
1 Facial presentations
  a) Trigeminal neuralgia
  b) Facial palsy (*upper* motor neurone type)
  c) Facial myokymia (continuous rippling of one side)
2 'Useless hand' with proprioceptive loss and no other signs (differential diagnosis includes hysteria)
3 Lhermitte's sign ('electric' pains on flexing neck)

4 Uhthoff's phenomenon (worsening of weakness or vision with heat, e.g. hot bath or exercise)

Presentations suggesting alternative aetiological diagnoses
1 Peripheral neuropathy
2 *Persistent* loss of skin sensation
3 Epilepsy

Multiple sclerosis vs Friedreich's ataxia
1 Similarities
  a) Optic atrophy
  b) Nystagmus
  c) Cerebellar signs
  d) Extensor plantar responses
2 Factors favouring Freidreich's
  a) Family history
  b) Absent ankle jerks
  c) Pes cavus/scoliosis
  d) Cardiomegaly
3 Factors favouring multiple sclerosis
  a) History of Lhermitte's or Uhthoff's phenomena
  b) Trigeminal neuralgia (esp. bilateral)
  c) Absent abdominal reflexes
  d) Bladder enlargement
  e) Brisk ankle jerks

SPINAL DISEASE

Transverse myelitis: features
1 Presentation
  a) Pain (often interscapular), typically localizing to segment of final sensory level.
  b) Lower limb paraesthesiae, ascending weakness
  c) Sphincter dysfunction
2 Established clinical deficit
  a) Flaccid paralysis
  b) Complete sensory loss (typically to thorax)
3 Investigations
  a) Usually no aetiology can be found
  b) Myelogram usually normal
  c) CSF may reveal non-specific pleocytosis, ↑ protein
  d) VERs usually normal
4 Features associated with poor prognosis
  a) Fulminant onset
  b) Pain
  c) Spinal shock

Common vertebral levels of various pathologies
1 Cervical cord
  a) Syphilitic myelitis
  b) Syringomyelia
2 Thoracic cord
  a) Subacute combined degeneration
  b) Anterior spinal artery thrombosis (~ T4)
  c) Pott's disease
3 Thoracolumbar
  a) Ependymoma; metastatic tumours
  b) Transverse myelitis
4 Lumbosacral: tabes dorsalis

Neurological deficits in cervical spondylosis
1 Lateral disc protrusion — root compression
2 Foraminal osteophytes — root compression
3 Osteophytes — vertebral artery insufficiency
4 Posterior disc protrusion — cord compression
5 Posterior disc protrusion — vascular myelopathy

Predispositions to kyphoscoliosis and/or pes cavus
1 Friedreich's ataxia
  Hereditary spastic paraplegia
2 Charcot-Marie-Tooth disease
3 Polio
4 Neurofibromatosis
5 Syringomyelia

Associations of neurofibromatosis
1 Café-au-lait spots (>5, >1.5 cm diameter)
  Axillary freckling
  Melanoma
2 Optic glioma, cerebral glioma
  Acoustic neuroma(ta), meningioma
  Ependymoma, malignant schwannoma
  Syringomyelia
3 Berry aneurysms
  Aortic coarctation
  Renal artery stenosis; phaeochromocytoma
  Mesenteric ischaemia
4 Limb deformities (tibial bowing, pes cavus)
  Vertebral scalloping
5 Pulmonary fibrosis
  Diabetes insipidus
  Hypospadias
  Intellectual impairment

CEREBELLAR DISEASE

Patterns of cerebellar disease
1 Vermis involvement
  a) Often due to alcoholism
  b) Spinocerebellar tract connexions involved
  c) Signs
    — Wide-based gait (deviates to affected side)
    — Impaired tandem gait
    — Slurred speech
2 Flocculonodular lobe involvement
  a) May be due to PICA syndrome/medulloblastoma
  b) Vestibular connexions involved
  c) Signs
    — Truncal ataxia (unable to sit/stand without
      support)
    — Nystagmus (may be vertical)
    — Titubation
3 Posterior lobe involvement
  a) Many causes
  b) Cortical connexions involved
  c) Signs
    — Hypotonia
    — Limb ataxia ('drift')
    — Dysmetria ('past-pointing')
    — Dysdiadochokinesis
    — Intention tremor

MYASTHENIA GRAVIS

Examining the patient with myasthenia gravis: special manoeuvres
1 Sustained lateral/upward gaze
  a) →Ptosis
  b) →Diplopia $\Big\}$ ± Diurnal variation
  c) →Ophthalmoplegia
2 Count to 50 → slurring of speech
3 Drink a large glass of water → regurgitation,
  dysphagia
4 Abduct one shoulder repeatedly, then compare
  power of other
5 Elevate limb for long period, assess power; then
  note any improvement with rest (cf. psychogenic
  fatigue: rest doesn't help)

Investigating the patient with suspected myasthenia gravis
1 Edrophonium ('Tensilon') test
  a) Pretreat with atropine to prevent bradycardia,
    nausea
  b) Give 1 mg test dose prior to 5 mg test proper
  c) False-negatives occur in up to 10% (e.g. due to
    severe wasting)
2 EMG
  a) Post-tetanic inhibition (decremental response to
    repetitive stimulation)
  b) Increased 'jitter'
3 AChRAb:
  a) 90% sensitivity (70% in ocular myasthenia)
  b) False-positives occur in
    — First-degree relatives
    — Myasthenics in remission
    — RA patients on D-penicillamine

Approach to management
1 Anticholinesterase therapy (losing popularity)
  a) Commence with pyridostigmine 30 mg qid
  b) Beware of cholinergic crisis when increasing
    dosage
  c) May test integrity of bulbar/respiratory muscle
    power by injecting edrophonium 2 mg i.v.i
2 Corticosteroid therapy
  a) 1 mg/kg alternate days
  b) Indications
    — Seriously ill before thymectomy
    — Insufficiently improved after thymectomy
    — Ocular myasthenia
    — Now often used as initial therapy
  c) Initial deterioration common (? due to
    anticholinesterase potentiation), therefore
    commence steroids as inpatient.
3 Azathioprine
  a) Improvement apparent at 6–12 weeks
  b) Improvement maximal at 6–12 months
  c) Better results if
    — Patient > 40 years
    — Male sex
    — Long-standing disease (> 10 years)
    — Absent HLA-B_8DRw$_3$
    — High AChRAb levels
4 Thymectomy
  a) 80% of patients without thymoma improve

b) Improvement may be delayed up to five years
c) *Less* effective if thymoma present (but all the more necessary)
d) Thymoma may be managed with trans-sternal thymectomy and/or thymic irradiation
5 Plasma exchange — may be indicated as a holding measure in myasthenic crisis or prior to thymectomy
6 Unexpected deterioration? exclude:
a) Thyrotoxicosis
b) Pregnancy
c) Sepsis
d) Drugs
— Quin(id)ine, procainamide; phenytoin
— Propranolol; lignocaine
— Aminoglycosides
— CNS depressants
— D-penicillamine
— Hypokalaemia (e.g. due to diuretics)

CLASSIFICATION OF NEUROMUSCULAR DISEASE: THERAPEUTIC SIGNIFICANCE

Myasthenia gravis
1 Ocular
a) Lowest AChRAb levels (25% are normal)
b) Unresponsive to thymectomy; responsive to corticosteroids
2 Thymoma
a) Highest AChRAb levels
b) Positive antistriated muscle antibodies commonly (epiphenomenal; non-pathogenic antibodies which cross-react with thymic myoid cells)
3 'Thymitis' (age <40 years)
a) Female > male
b) HLA-B$_8$DRw$_3$ commonly

c) Associated with other autoimmune disease
d) Negative antistriated muscle antibodies
e) Best response to thymectomy (80%)
4 'Thymitis' (age >40 years)
a) Male > female
b) HLA-A$_3$-B$_7$DRw$_2$ commonly
c) Low levels of AChRAb
d) Best response to corticosteroids
5 Do not confuse with non-autoimmune 'congenital myasthenia'
a) Associated with consanguinity
b) Absent AChRAb
c) No response to thymectomy/plasmapheresis

Periodic paralysis
1 Hypokalaemic
a) May be
— Familial, or
— Associated with thyrotoxicosis (esp. in oriental males), or
— Associated with primary aldosteronism
b) Paralysis precipitated by
— Carbohydrate meal ($\uparrow$ insulin $\rightarrow$ $\downarrow$ K$^+$)
— Rest after exertion (duration: hours – days)
c) Prophylaxis with
— Potassium supplements
— Acetazolamide
— Spironolactone
2 Normokalaemic
a) Paramyotonia (von Eulenberg's disease)
b) Weakness and/or myotonia inducible by cold
c) Treat with tocainide
3 Hyperkalaemic (Gamstorp's disease)
a) Often familial
b) Typically affects eye muscles (duration ~ 30 minutes)
c) Precipitated by cold weather
d) Acute attack responds to intravenous calcium gluconate

Reviewing the Literature: Neurology

9.1 De la Monte S M et al 1985 Risk factors for the development and rupture of intracranial berry aneurysms. American Journal of Medicine 78: 957–964

Strongest predictor of aneurysm *development* was hypertension. Strongest predictors of aneurysm *rupture* were: presence of multiple aneurysms, size of aneurysm(s), alcohol or aspirin use

Wiebers DO et al 1987 The significance of unruptured intracranial saccular aneurysms. Journal of Neurosurgery 66: 23–29

Study of 78 patients showing that no aneurysm < 10 mm diameter ruptured, but that 15/51 > 10 mm diameter did rupture

9.2 Plato CC et al 1986 Amyotrophic lateral sclerosis and parkinsonism and dementia on Guam: a 25-year

prospective case-control study. American Journal of Epidemiology 124: 643–656

Study documenting increased risk of motor neurone disease in spouses (but not offspring) of patients, suggesting that environmental factors may be important in aetiology of these disorders

Bhagavati S et al 1988 Detection of human HTLV #1 DNA and antigen in spinal fluid and blood of patients with chronic progressive myelopathy. New England Journal of Medicine 318: 1141–1147

Ten out of 13 patients with chronic progressive myelopathy had serum antibodies to HTLV#1, while 11/11 had HTLV#1 DNA detectable in peripheral blood monocytes

9.3 Norris J W, Hachinki V C 1986 High-dose steroid treatment in cerebral infarction. British Medical Journal 292: 21–23

Canadian double-blind randomized trial of 113 patients showed no significant benefits of steroid therapy in terms of mortality or quality of survival

Poungvarin N et al 1987 Effects of dexamethasone in primary supratentorial intracerebral haemorrhage. New England Journal of Medicine 316: 1229–1233

Double-blind randomized trial of 93 patients did not improve short-term survival, but rather led to a higher incidence of complications

9.4 Lebel M H et al 1988 Dexamethasone therapy for bacterial meningitis. New England Journal of Medicine 319: 964–971

Double-blind placebo-controlled trial of 200 children examining effect of adding dexamethasone to conventional antibiotic therapy of bacterial meningitis. Steroid-treated patients had more rapid defervescence, more rapid CSF normalization, and lower incidence of hearing loss and learning deficits

9.5 Antiplatelet Trialists' Collaboration 1988 Secondary prevention of vascular disease by prolonged antiplatelet treatment. British Medical Journal 296: 320–331

Aspirin 300 mg/day was effective in secondary prevention of stroke and myocardial infarction; it reduced non-fatal stroke/MI by 30%, and reduced fatal stroke/MI by 15%. The authors add the caveat that one should theoretically not commence aspirin in stroke patients until a CT brainscan (performed 2 weeks after onset of symptoms) has excluded intracranial haemorrhage

9.6 Winslow C M et al 1988 The appropriateness of carotid endarterectomy. New England Journal of Medicine 318: 721–727

This study concluded that carotid endarterectomy is 'substantially overused', and that up to 2/3 of such operations may be unnecessary. Moreover, the authors emphasize that there is no hard evidence that carotid endarterectomy reduces the risk of stroke in any patient subset

9.7 EC/IC Bypass Study Group 1985 Failure of extracranial-intracranial arterial bypass to reduce the risk of ischaemic stroke: results of an international randomized trial. New England Journal of Medicine 313: 1191–1200

Controlled prospective trial of 1377 'at-risk' patients failed to identify any subgroup benefiting from surgery; perioperative morbidity actually worsened the outcomes of surgically treated patients

9.8 Mayeux R et al 1985 Reappraisal of temporary levodopa withdrawal ('drug holiday') in Parkinson's disease. New England Journal of Medicine 313: 724–728

Retrospective study suggesting lack of benefit of levodopa drug holidays

Goetz C G et al 1989 Multicenter study of autologous adrenal medullary transplantation to the corpus striatum in patients with advanced Parkinson's disease. New England Journal of Medicine 320: 337–341

Follow-up study to the controversial Madrazo et al publication (which had documented the efficacy of adrenal medullary transplantation to the right caudate nucleus), suggesting that autologous adrenal transplantation significantly ameliorated the 'on-off' phenomenon but that antiparkinsonian medications needed to be maintained in full dosage

Tetrud J W, Langsont J W 1989 The effect of deprenyl (Seleciline) on the natural history of Parkinson's disease. Science 244: 519–521

Parkinson Study Group 1989 Effect of deprenyl on the progression of disability in early Parkinson's disease. New England Journal of Medicine 321: 1364–1371

Two randomised studies showing beneficial effects of the monoamine oxidase B inhibitor, deprenyl, in prolonging the onset of disability (defined as the necessity of prescribing levodopa) from Parkinson's disease

9.9 Snead O C, Hosey L C 1985 Exacerbation of seizures in children by carbamazepine. New England Journal of Medicine 313: 916–921

Fifteen patients with complex partial seizures deteriorated on receiving carbamazepine; EEG deterioration also noted

9.10 Schroth G et al 1987 Early diagnosis of herpes simplex encephalitis by magnetic resonance imaging. Neurology 37: 179–183

Preferential limbic system involvement by HSV may be demonstrated by MRI well prior to CT, thus allowing early prescription of acyclovir

CHAPTER 10

Pharmacology and toxicology

Physical examination protocol 10.1 You are asked to examine a patient known to be a drug addict

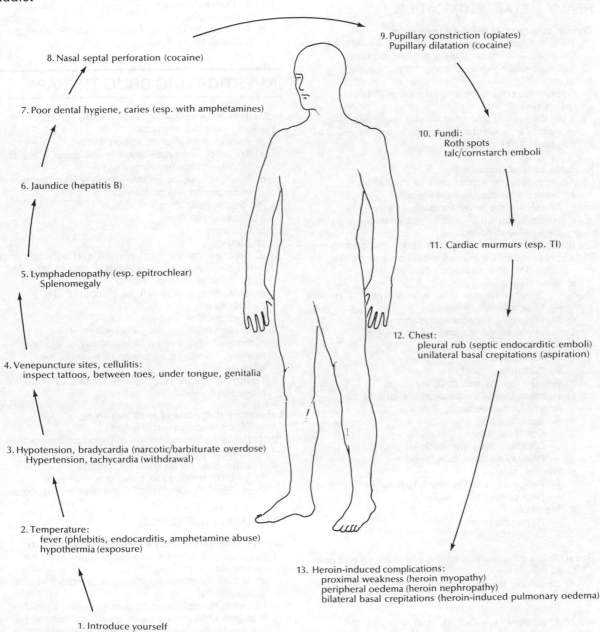

8. Nasal septal perforation (cocaine)

7. Poor dental hygiene, caries (esp. with amphetamines)

6. Jaundice (hepatitis B)

5. Lymphadenopathy (esp. epitrochlear)
   Splenomegaly

4. Venepuncture sites, cellulitis:
   inspect tattoos, between toes, under tongue, genitalia

3. Hypotension, bradycardia (narcotic/barbiturate overdose)
   Hypertension, tachycardia (withdrawal)

2. Temperature:
   fever (phlebitis, endocarditis, amphetamine abuse)
   hypothermia (exposure)

1. Introduce yourself
   Position the patient
   Obtain adequate exposure

9. Pupillary constriction (opiates)
   Pupillary dilatation (cocaine)

10. Fundi:
    Roth spots
    talc/cornstarch emboli

11. Cardiac murmurs (esp. TI)

12. Chest:
    pleural rub (septic endocarditic emboli)
    unilateral basal crepitations (aspiration)

13. Heroin-induced complications:
    proximal weakness (heroin myopathy)
    peripheral oedema (heroin nephropathy)
    bilateral basal crepitations (heroin-induced pulmonary oedema)

CLINICAL ASPECTS OF PHARMACOLOGY AND TOXICOLOGY

COMMONEST TOXICOLOGICAL SHORT CASES
1 Heavy metal poisoning
2 Drug eruption

HEAVY METAL INTOXICATION

Clinical stigmata of mercury poisoning
1 Tremor ('hatter's shakes') → tongue, eyelids, legs
2 Erethism — irritability, easy embarrassment
3 Salivation, gingivitis, pharyngeal pain, bloody diarrhoea
4 Nephrosis, renal tubular dysfunction (often reversible)
5 'Pink disease' (acrodynia) — skin hypersensitivity in infants exposed to *topical* mercury-containing solutions (10% mortality)

Features of lead poisoning
1 Acute poisoning (commoner in children)
  a) Musculoskeletal — arthralgias
  b) Renal — tubular dysfunction
  c) Haematological — haemolytic anaemia ± basophilic stippling
  d) Gastrointestinal — colicky abdominal pain precipitated by alcohol ingestion and relieved by palpation or intravenous calcium
  e) Neurological
    — Encephalopathy (ataxia, vomiting, fits, stupor)
    — Headache
  f) Metabolic — hepatocellular injury
2 Chronic poisoning (commoner in adults)
  a) Musculoskeletal
    — Arthropathy
    — 'Saturnine' gout
  b) Renal — gouty nephropathy
  c) Haematological — basophilic stippling ± haemolytic anaemia
  d) Gastrointestinal
    — Constipation
    — Gingival 'blue line' (adults)
    — Premature tooth loss (children)
  e) Neurological
    — Peripheral neuropathy (predominantly motor)
    — Neuropsychiatric sequelae
  f) Metabolic
    — Hyperuricaemia
    — Subfertility

Reversibility of complications in heavy metal poisoning
1 Lead poisoning
  a) Chelation therapy (p. 242) is effective in reversing the gastrointestinal and haematological effects
  b) Treatment is *not* effective in reversing the neurological, renal or metabolic sequelae
2 Wilson's disease (copper overload)
  a) Penicillamine therapy is effective in reversing the renal tubular dysfunction

  b) Penicillamine is *not* effective in reversing end-stage hepatic or neurological disease; liver disease may require transplantation
3 Haemochromatosis (iron overload)
  a) Phlebotomy may *prevent* all sequelae, incl. cardiac disease
  b) Phlebotomy *prolongs life* in symptomatic patients with established disease
  c) Phlebotomy is *not* effective in *reversing* established
    — Hypogonadotropic hypogonadism
    — Diabetes mellitus
    — Arthropathy
  d) Phlebotomy does *not* reduce *hepatoma risk* in established *cirrhosis*

INVESTIGATING DRUG THERAPY

Indications for monitoring plasma drug levels
1 Life-threatening overdose
  a) Paracetamol (if urine screen +ve)
  b) Tricyclics, salicylate (peak levels occur late due to delayed gastric emptying)
  c) Methanol, salicylate (very high levels dictate early use of haemodialysis)
2 Routine regular dose calibration
  a) Aminoglycosides
  b) Lithium
  c) Digoxin
  d) Anticonvulsants — phenytoin, carbamazepine
3 Initial calculation of maintenance dosage (esp. in cardiac, renal or liver failure)
  a) Quinidine, procainamide, disopyramide, lignocaine
  b) Theophylline
4 High probability of drug interaction — e.g. commencing quinidine in maintenance digoxin therapy, or adding valproate to maintenance phenytoin
5 Treatment failure (esp. in context of suspected non-compliance)

Laboratory diagnosis of lead poisoning
1 ↑ Blood lead (esp. in children)
2 ↑ Urinary coproporphyrin III (good screening test)
3 ↑ Urine and serum ALA
4 ↑ Urine lead (± EDTA-mobilization)
5 ↑ Serum iron and red cell protoporphyrin (non-specific indicators of ineffective erythropoiesis)

PHARMACOGENETICS

Genetic polymorphisms determining drug toxicity
1 Pseudocholinesterase deficiency (autosomal recessive)
  a) Manifests as suxamethonium (succinylcholine) sensitivity
  b) Leads to prolonged apnoea postanaesthesia
2 Malignant hyperthermia (autosomal dominant) — hypercatabolic response to various anaesthetic agents, esp. halothane and suxamethonium; also tricyclics, MAOIs, nitrous oxide
3 Favism (G6PD deficiency — X-linked dominant)

a) Manifests as haemolysis
b) May be precipitated by many drugs, incl. primaquine, sulphonamides, nitrofurantoin
4 Acute intermittent porphyria (autosomal dominant)
a) Manifests as abdominal pain (acute), neuropathy (chronic)
b) Precipitated by many drugs, esp. barbiturates, alcohol
5 Steroid-induced glaucoma (autosomal recessive)
a) Precipitated by topical (or long-term systemic) steroids
b) Occurs in about 5% of the population
6 Slow acetylation (autosomal recessive) — generally manifests as drug toxicity
Rapid acetylation (autosomal recessive) — generally manisfests as drug insensitivity
7 Sulphonylurea flushing (autosomal dominant)
a) Precipitated by chlorpropamide or tolbutamide
b) Occurs in about 30% of Caucasians
8 Warfarin resistance (autosomal dominant)—rare

METABOLIC POLYMORPHISMS

Rationale for determining the acetylation phenotype
(50% of the population are slow acetylators)
1 Isoniazid
a) Slow acetylators
  — ↑ Peripheral neuropathy (B_6-responsive)
  — ↑ Iatrogenic SLE
  — ↑ Phenytoin/carbamazepine toxicity
  — ↑ Rifampicin-induced hepatotoxicity
b) Rapid acetylators
  — Failure of once-weekly TB therapy
  — ↑ Isoniazid-induced hepatitis
2 Sulphasalazine — slow acetylators
a) ↑ Toxicity from sulphapyridine moiety, esp. headaches, leucopenia
b) ↑ Haemolysis in G6PD-deficient patients
3 Hydralazine
a) Slow acetylators — ↑ iatrogenic SLE, esp. in females
b) Rapid acetylators — failure of antihypertensive therapy
4 Procainamide — slow acetylators: ↑ iatrogenic SLE
5 Dapsone
a) Slow acetylators — ↑ haemolysis in G6PD-deficient patients
b) Rapid acetylators — failure of therapy for dermatitis herpetiformis

Diseases associated with slow acetylation phenotype
1 Gilbert's syndrome
2 Sjögren's syndrome
3 Arylamine-induced bladder cancer

Clinical associations of 'poor' debrisoquine oxidation phenotype (50% of the population are poor metabolizers of debrisoquine, i.e. have homozygous monoxygenase deficiency)
1 Excessive hypotension with
a) Debrisoquine
b) Propranolol, metoprolol, timolol
2 Methaemoglobinaemia with phenacetin

3 Lactic acidosis with phenformin
4 Neuropathy/hepatotoxicity with perhexiline
5 Agranulocytosis with captopril
6 Confusion with nortriptyline (plus other anticholinergic effects)

MANAGING DRUG THERAPY

APPROACH TO THE POISONED PATIENT

Treatment options in life-threatening overdosage
1 Forced alkaline diuresis (urine pH → 7.5–8.5)
a) (Pheno)barbitone
b) Salicylate
2 Forced acid diuresis (urine pH → 5.5–6.5)
a) Quin(id)ine
b) Amphetamine, phencyclidine
3 Peritoneal dialysis — formerly used in management of lithium or ethylene glycol poisoning, but less popular now
4 Haemodialysis
a) Lithium (if plasma level > 5 mmol/l)
b) CCl_4 (within 48 h of ingestion)
5 Charcoal haemoperfusion
a) Theophylline (if > 60 mg/l)
b) Barbiturates, methaqualone
c) Paraquat

Clinical use of oral activated charcoal ('gastrointestinal dialysis')
1 Technically simpler than haemoperfusion or dialysis
2 Suitable for use in district hospitals or remote locations
3 Most effective for weakly acidic drugs with small volume of distribution, e.g. phenobarbitone, salicylate

Paracetamol overdose: principles of management
1 Gastric lavage ± charcoal adsorption, if
a) Ingestion of at least 10 g paracetamol within last 4 hours, or
b) Time and/or quantity of ingested dose unknown
2 Specific therapy (if overdose taken within last 16 hours)
a) Best guide — plasma paracetamol level > 4 h postingestion
b) If above reference level for toxicity, infuse N-acetylcysteine according to nomogram (e.g. 150 mg/kg over 15 min, then 50 mg/kg over 4 h, then 100 mg/kg over 16 h)
c) Specific therapy indicated if overdose taken within 24 hours of presentation; may require continuation until 72 hours postingestion
3 If N-acetylcysteine unavailable, use oral methionine (both are glutathione precursors)
4 Prothrombin time and transaminases should be monitored closely (may become elevated within 12 hours of overdose)
5 In patients at risk of hepatic necrosis (esp. if massive overdose and/or late presentation), give 5% dextrose infusion to obviate risk of hypoglycaemia

Specific antidotes
1 Carbon monoxide
   a) 100% oxygen
   b) Hyperbaric (2 atm./200 kPa) if unconsciousness supervenes
2 Cyanide
   a) Dicobalt EDTA IV, or
   b) Sodium nitrite then sodium thiosulphate i.v., or
   c) Amyl nitrite inhaled every five minutes, or
   d) Hydroxocobalamin i.v. in mild cases, e.g. due to use of sodium nitroprusside; plus
   e) 100% oxygen ± sodium bicarbonate i.v.
3 Ethylene glycol or methanol
   a) Gastric lavage, plus
   b) 50 g ethanol i.v. loading dose, plus
   c) IV 4-methylpyrazole, or
   d) 5% ethanol infusion + forced alkaline diuresis + early dialysis
4 Organophosphate insecticides (cholinesterase inhibitors)
   a) IV atropine every 10 minutes (to keep heart rate > 60)
   b) Pralidoxime (PAM) slow IVI hourly
5 Tricyclics/anticholinergics
   a) IV neostigmine over 60 seconds using ECG monitor
6 Lead
   a) Calcium disodium EDTA slow i.v. b.d. ± dimercaprol
   b) Intramuscular administration is less hazardous in children suspected of developing encephalopathy
   c) Oral or intragastric administration is absolutely contraindicated
7 Iron (presents with GI bleeding or hepatic necrosis)
   a) Desferrioxamine (DFO) ± charcoal adsorption
      — By gastric lavage
      — Then leave in stomach
      — Then deep intramuscular loading dose
      — Then *slow* infusion
   (NB: DFO should *not* be used in patients receiving vitamin C due to attendant risk of cardiac damage)
8 Mercury, arsenic, gold — dimercaprol (BAL) by deep intramuscular injection
9 Zinc (→ 'metal-fume fever')
   a) D-Penicillamine p.o. (also effective in lead, mercury, arsenic, gold, or copper poisoning)
   b) Dimercaprol (BAL)
10 Thallium (used in rodenticides) — Prussian (Berlin) blue via nasogastric tube (also effective in iron, cyanide poisoning)
11 Bromism
   a) Saline infusion (also helpful in poisoning with lithium)
   NB: gastric lavage contraindicated following ingestion of paraffin, kerosene, or petrol (due to risk of aspiration pneumonitis)

SALICYLISM

Salicylate overdose: therapeutic options
1 Mild poisoning (salicylate level <500 mg/l) — fluid and electrolyte balance alone

2 Moderate (level <500 mg/l plus acidosis, or <750 mg/l alone)
   a) Forced alkaline diuresis, or
   b) Oral activated charcoal
3 Severe (<750 mg/l plus renal impairment, or <900 mg/l alone)
   a) Charcoal haemoperfusion, or
   b) Haemodialysis

Metabolic complications of salicylate overdosage
1 Fever, sweating (due to uncoupling of oxidative phosphorylation)
2 Confusion (neuroglycopenia, esp. in adults)
3 Epigastric discomfort, vomiting (delayed gastric emptying)
4 Tachypnoea (primary respiratory alkalosis occurs in adults due to direct stimulation of the respiratory centre)
5 Primary metabolic acidosis (in infants; multifactorial pathogenesis incl. lactic acidosis)
6 Prerenal failure (dehydration, renal vasoconstriction)
7 Hypo- or hyperglycaemia; hypo- or hypernatraemia
8 Pulmonary oedema and/or hypokalaemia (esp. if forced alkaline diuresis)
9 Gastrointestinal bleeding (unusual despite gastric irritation, platelet dysfunction and/or hypoprothrombinaemia)

CLINICAL PHARMACOKINETICS

Drugs exhibiting saturation kinetics
1 Phenytoin
2 Salicylate
3 Alcohol

Approximate incidences of some adverse drug reactions
1 Retroperitoneal fibrosis due to methysergide — 1 in 250
2 Pseudomembranous colitis due to clindamycin — 1 in 5000
3 Aplastic anaemia due to chloramphenicol — 1 in 6000
   Aplastic anaemia due to phenylbutazone — 1 in 10 000
4 Thrombotic complication due to oral contraceptive — 1 in 10 000
5 Hepatitis due to halothane — 1 in 10 000
6 Vaginal carcinoma due to maternal stilboestrol — 1 in 10 000

Important clinical contexts for drug interaction
1 Where dose and response are critically balanced
   a) Anticoagulants
   b) Oral hypoglycaemics
2 Where major toxicity may supervene
   a) Cytotoxics
   b) Digoxin
   c) Theophylline

d) Aminoglycosides
e) Lithium
3 Where loss of effect may be catastrophic
a) Antiarrhythmics (e.g. quinidine)
b) Anticonvulsants (e.g. valproate)
c) Corticosteroids (e.g. in temporal arteritis)
d) Oral contraceptives
4 Where indications for interacting drugs may be similar
a) Digoxin and loop diuretics ($\downarrow$ K$^+\rightarrow\uparrow$ digoxin toxicity)
b) Digoxin and quinidine, amiodarone ($\uparrow$ plasma digoxin)
c) Captopril and potassium-sparing diuretics ($\uparrow\uparrow$ K$^+$)
d) Beta-blockers and acetazolamide (acidosis may $\rightarrow$ CCF)
e) Beta-blockers and clonidine ($\uparrow$ risk of clonidine 'rebound')
f) Cimetidine and antacids ($\downarrow$ cimetidine absorption)
g) Azathioprine/6MP and allopurinol (four-fold cytotoxic potentiation)
— Ketoconazole and cyclosporin A ($\rightarrow$ cyclosporin nephrotoxicity)
— Tranylcypromine and clomipramine ($\rightarrow$ hypertensive crisis)

Pharmacokinetic considerations in elderly patients
1 Reduced renal clearance — e.g. digoxin, lithium, cimetidine, chlorpropamide
2 Reduced hepatic metabolism — e.g. tricyclics, chlormethiazole, propranolol
3 Reduced volume of distribution (for water-soluble drugs) — e.g. ethanol, digoxin, cimetidine
4 Reduce sensitivity — e.g. some antihypertensives
5 Increased sensitivity — e.g. benzodiazepines, warfarin, some diuretics

UNDERSTANDING DRUG THERAPY

CLINICAL PHARMACOLOGY

Pharmacokinetics: principles underlying clinical practice
1 For a given dosage, the plasma level of any drug is inversely proportional to its volume of distribution (V_D)
2 The loading dose of any drug is directly proportional to its V_D
The maintenance dose of any drug is directly proportional to its clearance
3 Drugs with low V_D (i.e. high concentration in plasma relative to tissues) tend to be heavily protein-bound
The lower the V_D of a given drug, the more readily it is removed by dialysis
4 The steady-state plasma level of any drug is achieved following regular administration for a period approximating 3–5 half-lives of the drug

5 Biliary excretion tends to be of minor pharmacokinetic significance; enterohepatic recirculation will occur until hepatic metabolism produces polar drug metabolites able to be renally excreted

Clinical significance of plasma protein binding
1 Drug interactions due to displacement from plasma protein binding sites tend to be transient and of minor clinical significance
2 Changes in protein binding may greatly affect assayed *total* plasma concentrations of drug
3 If assay for *free* drug not available, salivary concentration of phenytoin, isoniazid or theophylline may be used as a guide
4 Protein-bound drug molecules do not undergo glomerular filtration
Ionized drug molecules may undergo active tubular secretion irrespective of plasma protein binding status
Non-ionized (non-polar, liposoluble) drugs undergo passive renal tubular reabsorption and, thence, hepatic metabolism
5 Acidic drugs tend to be highly protein-bound

Examples of significant alterations in plasma protein binding
1 Precipitation of kernicterus by sulphonamides displacing bilirubin
2 Precipitation of mucositis by aspirin displacing methotrexate (and hence increasing free methotrexate levels)
3 Precipitation of hypoglycaemia by phenylbutazone displacing tolbutamide
4 Precipitation of haemorrhage by clofibrate displacing warfarin
5 Precipitation of phenytoin toxicity by uraemia, hepatic failure, or concomitant valproate administration
6 Antagonism of lignocaine/propranolol/disopyramide effect due to major increases in α-1 acid glycoprotein (an acute phase reactant elevated in burns, trauma, surgery, etc.)

CHARACTERISTICS OF DRUG STRUCTURE AND FUNCTION

Polar vs non-polar drugs: the clinical distinction
1 Polar (ionized, water-soluble) drugs typically exhibit
a) Heavy plasma protein-binding
b) Low V_D
c) Long plasma t$^{\frac{1}{2}}$
d) Low CNS penetration and toxicity
e) Acidic pK$_a$
f) Predominant renal excretion (via active tubular secretion without glomerular filtration) of unchanged drug
g) Examples — warfarin, frusemide
2 Non-polar (un-ionized, lipophilic) drugs typically exhibit
a) Little plasma protein binding
b) Large V_D

c) Short plasma t$^{\frac{1}{2}}$
d) High CNS penetrance and toxicity
e) Basic pK$_a$
f) Predominant hepatic metabolism (via glomerular filtration and passive renal tubular reabsorption)
g) Examples — propranolol, nortriptyline

Drugs excreted unchanged by the kidney
1 β-blockers — atenolol
2 Antibiotics — penicillins, cephalosporins, aminoglycosides, tetracycline
3 Diuretics — frusemide, chlorothiazide
4 Cardiac drugs — digoxin, procainamide
5 CNS drugs — lithium
6 Oral hypoglycaemics — chlorpropamide, metformin
7 Analgesics — aspirin (in overdosage only)
8 Other — cimetidine, ranitidine

Acidic vs. basic drugs
1 Acidic
   a) 'ates' — salicylate, clofibrate, valproate, barbiturate
   b) 'ins' — warfarin, phenytoin, penicillins, cephalosporins (exception: *prazosin* is basic)
   c) 'ids' — NSAIDs, probenecid
   d) Other — frusemide, thiazides, chlorpropamide, sulphonamides
2 Basic
   a) 'ines'
      — Chlorpromazine, imipramine, nortriptyline
      — Morphine, propoxyphene
      — Quinidine, cimetidine, triamterene (exceptions: *theophylline*, *thyroxine* are acidic)
   b) 'ols' — propranolol, ethambutol, dipyridamole
   c) Other
      — Verapamil
      — Trimethoprim, diazepam
      — Procainamide, disopyramide, amiloride

Drugs yielding active metabolites responsible for efficacy
1 Aspirin; phenacetin (→ paracetamol); phenylbutazone; sulindac
2 Carbamazepine; diazepam
3 Verapamil; enalapril; lignocaine; procainamide
4 Carbimazole (→ methimazole)
5 Amitriptyline; imipramine; chloral hydrate; L-DOPA
6 Cyclophosphamide; azathioprine (→ 6MP); prednisone (→ prednisolone)

Drugs yielding active metabolites responsible for toxicity
1 Isoniazid (→ acetylhydrazine, esp. in fast acetylators)
2 Methanol (→ formaldehyde)
3 Phenacetin (→ paracetamol); allopurinol (→ oxypurinol)
4 Clofibrate, procainamide
5 Cyclophosphamide (acrolein metabolites → bladder toxicity)
6 Alcohol (→ acetaldehyde)

MECHANISMS OF DRUG ACTION

Enzymes inhibited by drug therapy
1 Xanthine oxidase — allopurinol
2 Na$^+$/K$^+$-ATPase (cardiac) — digoxin
  Na$^+$/K$^+$-ATPase (loop of Henle) — frusemide
3 H$^+$/K$^+$-ATPase (gastric) — omeprazole
4 Angiotensin-converting enzyme (ACE) — captopril, enalapril
5 Prostaglandin synthetase — aspirin
6 Monoamine oxidase — phenelzine
7 Carbonic anhydrase — acetazolamide
8 DOPA decarboxylase — carbidopa
9 DNA topoisomerase II (bacterial) — nalidixic acid
  DNA topoisomerase II (human) — VP-16 (etoposide)
10 Acetylcholinesterase — neostigmine

Receptors involved in drug action
1 Endorphin receptors
   a) Agonist — morphine
   b) Antagonist — naloxone
2 Aldosterone receptors — antagonist: spironolactone
3 Histamine receptors
   a) H$_1$ antagonist — chlorpheniramine, promethazine, terfenadine
   b) H$_2$ antagonist — cimetidine, ranitidine, famotidine
4 Dopamine (CNS) receptors
   a) Agonist — bromocriptine
   b) Antagonist — chlorpromazine
5 α$_1$-adrenergic (postsynaptic) receptors — antagonist: prazosin
6 α$_2$-adrenergic (brainstem) receptors — agonist: clonidine
7 β$_1$-adrenergic receptors
   a) Agonist — dopamine
   b) Antagonist — metoprolol, atenolol
8 β$_2$-adrenergic receptors — agonist: salbutamol

DRUG METABOLISM BY HEPATIC MICROSOMAL ENZYMES

Drugs commonly inhibiting cytochrome P$_{450}$
1 Acute alcoholic binge
2 Antibiotics
   a) Isoniazid
   b) Erythromycin
   c) Sulphonamides
   d) Metronidazole
   e) Chloramphenicol
3 Anticonvulsants — valproate
4 Other drugs
   a) Cimetidine
   b) Allopurinol
   c) Chlorpromazine, imipramine
   d) Propranolol, metoprolol
   e) Dextropropoxyphene
   f) Disulfiram

Drugs commonly inducing cytochrome P$_{450}$
1 Chronic alcohol ingestion or cigarette smoking

2 Antibiotics — rifampicin
3 Anticonvulsants
  a) Phenytoin
  b) Carbamazepine
  c) Phenobarbitone, primidone
4 Other
  a) Aminoglutethimide
  b) Spironolactone
  c) Griseofulvin

Drugs undergoing major hepatic metabolism
1 β-blockers — propranolol, labetalol, metoprolol, oxprenolol
  β_2-agonists — salbutamol, terbutaline
2 Antibiotics — rifampicin, erythromycin
3 Diuretics — spironolactone
4 Cardiac drugs — glyceryl trinitrate, verapamil, nifedipine, lignocaine, prazosin, digitoxin
5 CNS drugs — chlormethiazole, tricyclics, phenothiazines, benzodiazepines, barbiturates, L-DOPA
6 Oral hypoglycaemics — glibenclamide, tolbutamide
7 Analgesics — paracetamol, pethidine, pentazocine, propoxyphene, aspirin

PROSTAGLANDINS

Physiological actions of prostaglandins
1 PGI_2 (prostacyclin), PGE_1 — → ↑ intracellular cAMP →
  a) Prevents calcium influx
  b) Relaxes vascular smooth muscle (i.e. vasodilates)
  c) ↓ Platelet aggregation
2 PGE_2
  a) Mediates oedema in inflammation
  b) Induces vasoconstriction
  c) ↑ Platelet aggregation
  d) Mediates diuretic effect of frusemide by inhibiting ADH in renal tubules
  e) Induces bronchodilatation
3 $PGF_{2\alpha}$
  a) Abortifacient
  b) Induces bronchoconstriction
4 TXA_2 (thromboxane A_2)
  a) Induces vasoconstriction (incl. pulmonary arterial)
  b) ↑ Platelet aggregation
  c) Implicated in
    — Primary pulmonary hypertension
    — Respiratory distress syndrome
    — Renal vasoconstriction with proteinuria

Drugs interacting with prostaglandins
1 Cyclo-oxygenase inhibitors
  a) Include aspirin and other NSAIDs
  b) Do *not* inhibit lipo-oxygenase; hence arachidonate metabolism is redirected away from prostaglandin synthesis and towards leukotriene synthesis (incl. the bronchoconstrictor SRS-A)
  c) The latter mechanism may underlie aspirin-induced asthma

2 Phospholipase A_2 inhibitors
  a) Include high-dose steroids, mepacrine, hydroxychloroquine
  b) Block both prostaglandin and leukotriene synthesis
3 Selective TXA_2 synthetase inhibitors — e.g. dazoxiben; remain in development

DRUGS AND THE REPRODUCTIVE SYSTEM

Drugs contraindicated in pregnant women
1 Alcohol, nicotine, narcotics
2 Antithyroid drugs (esp. [131]I); sulphonylureas
3 Drugs predisposing to kernicterus
  a) Sulphonamides
  b) Aspirin
  c) Vitamin K
4 Vasoactive drugs
  a) Ergotamine, propranolol (placental insufficiency)
  b) Guanethidine (mecomium ileus)
5 Antibiotics
  a) Tetracyclines (dental staining, enamel hypoplasia)
  b) Chloramphenicol ('grey syndrome': cardiovascular collapse in newborns)
  c) Aminoglycosides (esp. streptomycin) — deafness Vancomycin
  d) Sulphonamides (fetal abnormalities in first trimester; kernicterus in late pregnancy)

Recognized teratogens
1 Warfarin ('koala bear' facies)
2 Phenytoin (digital hypoplasia)
  Valproate (spina bifida)
  Phenobarbitone (cleft palate)
3 Lithium (congenital heart disease; cretinism)
4 Thalidomide (phocomelia)
5 Ergometrine (poland anomaly)
6 Cytotoxics (esp. methotrexate, alkylators)
7 Steroid hormones (DES → vaginal carcinoma in adolescent female progeny; androgens → cardiac/oesophageal defects; low-dose prednisone probably safe)
8 Alcohol (acetaldehyde metabolite → 'fetal alcohol syndrome')
9 Isotretinoin (13-cis-retinoic acid), etretinate High-dose vitamin D or vitamin A
10 Radioisotopes, esp. [131]I
  Live vaccines

Drugs contraindicated in breast-feeding mothers
1 Antibiotics — chloramphenicol, clindamycin, tetracycline
2 Vitamins — etretinate, high-dose vitamin A or D
3 Analgesics/anti-inflammatories — aspirin, indomethacin, gold salts, penicillamine
4 Other
  a) Lithium, doxepin
  b) Amiodarone
  c) Atropine
  d) Ergotamine

Relatively safe drugs in pregnancy
1 Digoxin
2 Heparin (does *not* cross placenta)*
3 Insulin, thyroxine
4 Antibiotics
   a) Penicillins
   b) Cephalosporins
   c) Erythromycin

---

*Heparin does not appear to be teratogenic, but has been associated with increased incidence of antepartum haemorrhage, prematurity and stillbirth, and may contribute to both maternal and fetal bone demineralization

   d) Ethambutol; INH (*plus* pyridoxine)
   e) Nystatin
5 Salbutamol (by inhaler)
6 Antihypertensives
   a) Methyldopa
   b) Hydralazine

Influences on drug metabolism in pregnancy
1 ↑ Glomerular filtration rate (→ ↑ clearance of digoxin, lithium)
2 ↑ Hepatic microsomal (P_{450}) enzyme activity → ↑ anticonvulsant metabolism
3 ↑ Volume of distribution (e.g. for cloxacillin)
4 ↓ Plasma protein binding (e.g. aspirin, phenytoin)
5 ↓ Gastric emptying

Reviewing the Literature: Pharmacology & Toxicology

10.1 Kumana C R et al 1985 Herbal tea-induced hepatic veno-occlusive disease: quantification of toxic alkaloid exposure in adults. Gut 26: 101–104

Association of pyrrolizidine alkaloid (e.g. in comfrey) ingestion with veno-occlusive disease of the liver

10.2 Griffiths R R et al 1986 Human coffee drinking: reinforcing and physical dependence-producing effects of caffeine. Journal of Pharmacology and Experimental Therapeutics 239: 416–425

Regular coffee drinkers exhibited pronounced withdrawal symptoms within 19 hours of coffee cessation. Symptoms became maximal over the next 48 hours, and consisted predominantly of headache and malaise; the authors conclude that caffeine is a typical drug of addiction

10.3 Wilcox A et al 1988 Caffeinated beverages and decreased fertility. Lancet ii: 1453–1455

Study of 104 healthy women desiring pregnancy, suggesting that those drinking more than 2 cups of coffee per day had only 25% of the chance of falling pregnant each month compared with non-caffeine drinkers

10.4 Langford H G et al 1987 Is thiazide-induced uric acid elevation harmful? Analysis of data from the Hypertension Detection and Follow-up program. Archives of Internal Medicine 147: 645–649

Study of 3693 thiazide-treated patients over 5 years revealed only 15 episodes of gout and no renal deterioration, suggesting that 'adjuvant' allopurinol (with the attendant expense and toxicity) is not indicated in patients being treated with thiazides

10.5 Zucker M L et al 1986 Low- versus high-dose aspirin: effects on platelet function in hyperlipidaemic and normal subjects. Archives of Internal Medicine 146: 921–925

Low-dose aspirin (0.45 mg/kg body weight) inhibited thromboxane A2 synthesis and platelet aggregation almost as well as high-dose (3.5 mg/kg body weight), and was just as effective in hyperlipidaemic patients. The

authors recommend that 75 mg aspirin/day is ample to achieve an antiaggregatory effect on platelets

10.6 Hormons J T et al 1986 Neurologic sequelae of chronic solvent vapor abuse. Neurology 36: 698–702

Report of 20 toluene-sniffers who exhibited chronic neurological deficits, principally cognitive impairment (70%), cerebellar dysfunction (45%), dementia (35%) and spasticity (30%); CT scanning revealed cerebral, cerebellar and even brainstem atrophy

10.7 Piper J M et al 1988 Heavy phenacetin use and bladder cancer in women aged 20 to 49 years. New England Journal of Medicine 313: 292–295

Case-control study of paracetamol/phenacetin abuse, confirming this medication as an independent risk factor for development of bladder TCC

10.8 Lange R A et al 1989 Cocaine-induced coronary-artery vasoconstriction. New England Journal of Medicine 321: 1557–1562

Even small doses of intranasal cocaine caused 20% reduction in coronary blood flow and 10% reduction in left coronary artery diameter due to a-adrenergic stimulation; these effects could be far greater in so-called 'recreational' drug use

10.9 Kornhauser D M et al 1989 Probenecid and zidovudine metabolism. Lancet ii: 473–475

Probenecid (an inhibitor of glucuronidation) increased AZT plasma concentrations and reduced the required dosing interval, thus permitting more economical use of the drug

10.10 First M R et al 1989 Concomitant administration of cyclosporin and ketoconazole in renal transplant recipients. Lancet ii: 1198–1200

Adding ketoconazole permitted a 75–80% reduction in cyclosporin dosage. The combination therefore may be used to reduce expenditure on cyclosporin, or else may lead to an increase in inadvertent cyclosporin toxicity

CHAPTER 11
Psychiatry

Physical examination protocol 11.1 You are told to begin by asking the patient a few questions

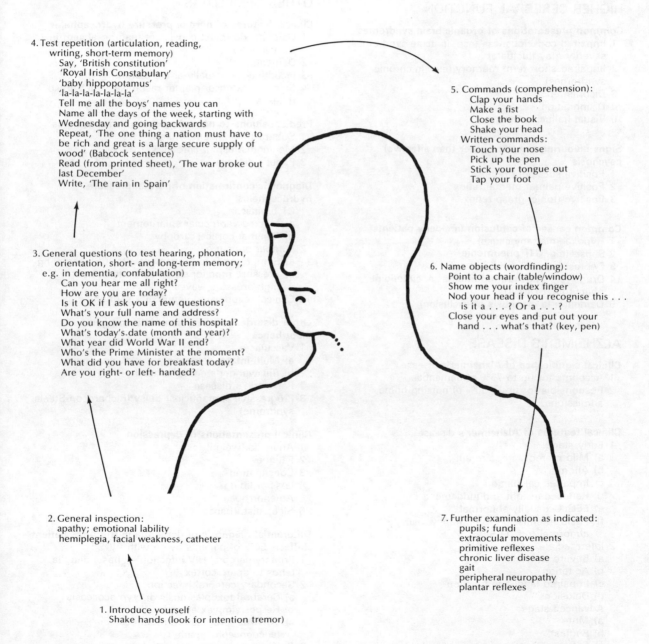

4. Test repetition (articulation, reading, writing, short-term memory)
   Say, 'British constitution'
   'Royal Irish Constabulary'
   'baby hippopotamus'
   'la-la-la-la-la-la-la'
   Tell me all the boys' names you can
   Name all the days of the week, starting with Wednesday and going backwards
   Repeat, 'The one thing a nation must have to be rich and great is a large secure supply of wood' (Babcock sentence)
   Read (from printed sheet), 'The war broke out last December'
   Write, 'The rain in Spain'

5. Commands (comprehension):
   Clap your hands
   Make a fist
   Close the book
   Shake your head
   Written commands:
   Touch your nose
   Pick up the pen
   Stick your tongue out
   Tap your foot

3. General questions (to test hearing, phonation, orientation, short- and long-term memory; e.g. in dementia, confabulation)
   Can you hear me all right?
   How are you are today?
   Is it OK if I ask you a few questions?
   What's your full name and address?
   Do you know the name of this hospital?
   What's today's.date (month and year)?
   What year did World War II end?
   Who's the Prime Minister at the moment?
   What did you have for breakfast today?
   Are you right- or left- handed?

6. Name objects (wordfinding):
   Point to a chair (table/window)
   Show me your index finger
   Nod your head if you recognise this . . . is it a . . . ? Or a . . . ?
   Close your eyes and put out your hand . . . what's that? (key, pen)

2. General inspection:
   apathy; emotional lability
   hemiplegia, facial weakness, catheter

7. Further examination as indicated:
   pupils; fundi
   extraocular movements
   primitive reflexes
   chronic liver disease
   gait
   peripheral neuropathy
   plantar reflexes

1. Introduce yourself
   Shake hands (look for intention tremor)

CLINICAL ASPECTS OF PSYCHIATRIC DISORDERS

COMMONEST PSYCHIATRIC SHORT CASES

1 Wernicke-Korsakoff syndrome
2 Tardive dyskinesia

HIGHER CEREBRAL FUNCTION

Common presentations of organic brain syndromes

1 Impaired consciousness (esp. in acute syndromes; severity may fluctuate)
2 Impaired short-term memory (esp. in chronic syndromes)
3 Disorientation
4 Disinhibition
5 Visual hallucinations

Signs favouring organic (rather than affective) psychosis

1 Positive suck/pout reflex
2 Positive palmar-mental reflex
3 Positive (tonic) grasp reflex

Common causes of confusion in elderly patients

1 Hypoxaemia (any cause)
2 Sepsis (e.g. UTI, pneumonia)
3 Depression
4 Drugs (e.g. digoxin, indomethacin, cimetidine, phenytoin, L-DOPA)
5 Dementia (a diagnosis of exclusion)

ALZHEIMER'S DISEASE

Clinical significance of Alzheimer's disease

1 Accounts for up to 75% of dementias
2 Responsible for up to 50% of nursing home admissions

Clinical features of Alzheimer's disease

1 Early stage:
   a) Mild memory impairment
   b) Anomia
   c) Impaired calculation
   d) Reduced insight and judgement
   e) EEG — usually abnormal
   f) Positron emission tomography: usually abnormal (ref. 11.6)
2 Intermediate stage:
   a) Severe amnesia
   b) Agitation
   c) Impaired language function
   d) Delusions
3 Advanced stage:
   a) Mute
   b) Bedfast
   c) Extrapyramidal deficit
   d) CT — cerebral atrophy
   e) EEG — frank slowing

Features suggesting dementias other than Alzheimer's

1 Convulsions
2 Gait disturbance

Important disorders to exclude prior to diagnosing Alzheimer's

1 Depression
2 Drug toxicity (alcohol, sedatives, L-DOPA, antihypertensives)

OTHER DEMENTIAS

Clinical features of normal pressure hydrocephalus

1 Gait apraxia (most consistent feature; absent in Alzheimer's)
2 Dementia
3 Incontinence (usually a late feature)
4 Signs — extensor plantar responses, suck/grasp reflexes

Predispositions to normal pressure hydrocephalus

1 Subarachnoid haemorrhage
2 Meningitis, esp. if chronic
3 Paget's disease

Diagnostic confirmation of normal pressure hydrocephalus

1 CT brainscan
   a) Marked ventricular enlargement
   b) Minimal cortical atrophy
2 Lumbar puncture
   a) Symptomatic improvement after CSF sampling
   b) Pressure monitoring reveals intermittent high-pressure waves
3 Clinical response to ventricular shunting

Other disorders causing dementia and gait disturbance

1 Vascular
   a) Multi-infarct dementia/pseudobulbar palsy
   b) Binswanger's encephalopathy
2 Parkinson's disease
3 Progressive supranuclear palsy (Richardson-Steele syndrome)

Clinical presentations of depression

1 Anorexia, weight loss
2 Fatigue
3 Constipation
4 Loss of libido
5 Amenorrhoea
6 Sleep disturbance

Differential diagnosis of dementia in the AIDS patient

(affects 50% of patients dying with AIDS)
1 Primary cerebral HIV infection — basal ganglia; tends to spare cortex
2 Secondary cerebral infection
   a) Cerebral toxoplasmosis or cryptococcosis
   b) Herpes simplex encephalitis
   c) JC virus (progressive multifocal leucoencephalopathy)
3 Cerebral neoplasm
   a) Cerebral lymphoma
   b) Cerebral Kaposi's

ALCOHOLISM

Confusion in the alcoholic patient: differential diagnosis
1 Acute intoxication
2 Delirium tremens (48–72 h post-withdrawal)
3 Hypoglycaemia (6–36 h post-binge)
4 Head injury — subdural haematoma
5 Post-ictal
6 Wernicke-Korsakoff syndrome
7 Ketoacidosis or lactic acidosis
8 Hepatic encephalopathy
9 Sepsis (e.g. *Klebsiella* pneumonia, aspiration pneumonia)
10 Unusual neurological syndromes
   a) Central pontine myelinolysis
   b) Marchiafava-Bignami disease (callosal demyelination; rarely diagnosed pre-mortem)

Neuropsychiatric manifestations of alcoholism
1 Epilepsy — may complicate
   a) Acute alcohol intoxication
   b) Chronic heavy alcohol ingestion
   c) Alcohol withdrawal
   d) Subdural haematoma
2 Withdrawal-related
   a) Tremulousness
   b) Agitation
   c) Delirium tremens
3 Toxic neuronal degeneration
   a) Cerebral atrophy ± dementia
   b) Cerebral atrophy
   c) Cerebral pontine myelinolysis (typically precipitated by use of hypertonic saline or lactulose)
   d) Callosal demyelination (Marchiafava-Bignami)
4 Nutrition-related (hypovitaminaemic)
   a) Wernicke's encephalopathy
   b) Korsakoff's psychosis ⎬ —thiamine-responsive ↓ transketolase
   c) Pellagra
   d) Neuropathy (typically painful)
   e) 'Tobacco-alcohol' amblyopia

The confused alcoholic: features suggesting DTs > encephalopathy
1 Severe agitation
2 Gross tremulousness without asterixis
3 Marked autonomic overactivity (sweats, fever, miosis, ↑ HR/BP)
4 Visual hallucinations
5 EEG — no triphasic waves
6 Improvement with sedation (NB: this is **not** a diagnostic test)

ANXIETY STATES

Differential diagnosis of recurrent acute anxiety attacks
1 Anxiety neurosis
2 Agoraphobia
3 Hyperventilation syndrome
4 Thyrotoxicosis
5 Phaeochromocytoma
6 Drug withdrawal (incl. alcohol)

Presentations of functional anxiety states
1 Panic attacks
  Sweating, palpitations ⎬ —May simulate phaeochromocytoma/ insulinoma
  Headaches
2 Presyncopal episodes
  Visual disturbance ⎬ —May simulate epilepsy or TIAs
  Paraesthesiae, tetany
3 Fatigue
  Breathlessness, ⎬ —May simulate thyrotoxicosis; pulmonary emboli; mitral valve prolapse
  tremulousness
  Atypical chest pain
4 Poor concentration
  Nightmares, headaches ⎬ —May simulate intracranial tumour; sleep apnoea; hepatic failure
  Sleep disturbance
5 Feelings of unreality
  Fear of madness ⎬ —May simulate schizophrenia; hysteria; aerophagy; agoraphobia
  Difficulty swallowing

Diagnosis of hyperventilation syndrome
1 High index of suspicion
2 Relief of symptoms following use of rebreathing bag
3 Reproduction of symptoms by forced voluntary overbreathing (the definitive test)
NB: measuring the P_aCO_2 during an attack is *not* a reliable test

'Funny turns': features favouring epilepsy
1 Clouding of consciousness
2 Prodromal irritability; premonitory stereotyped 'aura'
3 *Witnessed* absence or transiently impaired consciousness
  Regular, stereotyped tonic-clonic activity
  Tongue-bite, cyanosis or incontinence
4 Post-ictal paresis and/or confusion but *no* retrograde amnesia (cf. hysterical fugue)
5 Abnormal EEG during attack

HYSTERIA

Clinical spectrum of somatoform disorders
1 Hysteria
2 Psychogenic pain
3 Hypochondriasis
4 Münchausen's syndrome
5 Dermatitis artefacta
6 Compensation neurosis

Manifestations of hysteria
1 Conversion or dissociative symptoms, e.g.
   a) Paralysis
   b) Pseudoseizures
   c) Sensory disturbance
   d) Abnormal gait
2 Symptoms associated with
   a) *Belle indifference*
   b) Secondary gain
3 Briquet's (familial) syndrome — multiple recurrent somatic complaints
4 Ganser syndrome
   a) Amnesia, pseudodementia

b) Fugue state, hallucinations
c) Absurd answers, abrupt termination
5 Multiple personality
6 Mass hysteria

ANOREXIA NERVOSA

Physical findings in the patient with anorexia nervosa
1 Vital signs
   a) Bradycardia
   b) Hypotension
   c) Hypothermia
2 Musculoskeletal
   a) Marked weight loss
   b) Myopathy (nutritional)
   c) Weakness (hypokalaemic)
3 Cardiovascular
   a) Pallor (normochromic anaemia)
   b) Peripheral cyanosis
   c) Arrhythmias
4 Skin
   a) Carotenaemia
   b) Excessive lanugo hair
   c) Oedema (secondary hyperaldosteronism)
5 Gastrointestinal
   a) Parotidomegaly
   b) Rectal prolapse
6 Hypothermia

NB: Secondary sexual development is *normal* in anorexia nervosa

Investigating anorexia nervosa: potential abnormalities
1 Elevated BUN
2 Abnormal LFTs
3 'Sick euthyroid' (p. 88)
4 Elevated growth hormone, reduced somatomedin C
5 Multifollicular cystic ovaries on pelvic ultrasound

Complications of anorexia nervosa other than amenorrhoea
1 Dental caries
2 Gastric dilatation or atrophy
3 Constipation, cathartic colon
4 Renal calculi
5 Osteoporosis

INVESTIGATING PSYCHIATRIC DISORDERS

INVESTIGATION OF DEMENTIA

Investigation of the patient with presenile dementia
1 CT brainscan
2 Thyroid function tests/TSH   } Potentially reversible causes
3 Vitamin B_{12} assay
4 VDRL
5 HIV serology (in 'high-risk' patients)

Prerequisites for CT scanning in dementia
1 Presenile onset
2 Less than 2 years duration
3 Mild to moderate in severity
4 Patient fit for neurosurgery if indicated

Reversible pathologies excluded by CT scanning
1 Space-occupying intracerebral lesion (tumour, abscess)
2 Subdural haematoma
3 Normal pressure hydrocephalus
(NB: *unilateral* cerebral abnormalities generally do *not* affect conscious state)

THE ABNORMAL BRAIN BIOPSY

Definitive histological confirmation of Alzheimer's disease
1 Cerebral amyloid (type A4) angiopathy, *plus*
2 Neuritic amyloid plaques   } —correlate quantitatively with dementia severity
3 Neurofibrillary tangles

Dementia: neurofibrillary tangles in autopsied brain?
1 Alzheimer's disease
2 Post-encephalitic parkinsonism
3 Dementia pugilistica ('punch-drunk' syndrome)
4 Creutzfeldt-Jakob syndrome
5 SSPE

MANAGING PSYCHIATRIC DISEASE

IATROGENIC ORGANIC BRAIN SYNDROMES

Drugs commonly causing confusion in the elderly
1 Digoxin (may also → fatigue, euphoria)
2 Propranolol (also → nightmares, insomnia); methyldopa
3 Indomethacin (also → vertigo, headache)
4 Cimetidine (esp. in renal or hepatic insufficiency)
5 Amantadine, L-DOPA (esp. if used with anticholinergics)
6 Sedative-hypnotics, tricyclics, phenothiazines; alcohol

Psychiatric side-effects of steroid therapy
1 Commoner in
   a) High-dose treatment
   b) Prolonged duration of treatment
   c) Patient with psychiatric history
2 Commonest symptom — euphoria (cf. primary Cushing's disease: depression commoner)
3 Frank psychosis supervenes in about 5%

Clinical spectrum of lithium toxicity (plasma level > 1.5 mmol/l)*
1 CNS toxicity — lethargy → drowsiness → seizures → coma

*Lower plasma levels may result in toxicity, esp. in sodium-depleted patients (e.g. those on diuretics) or those with dehydration due to vomiting, diarrhoea or polyuria

2 Gastrointestinal toxicity — nausea, vomiting, diarrhoea
3 Cerebellar toxicity — tremulousness; dysarthria; ataxia
4 Renal toxicity — polyuria, polydipsia (nephrogenic diabetes insipidus; occurs in 30% but usually subclinical)
   May progress to frank renal failure if unrecognized
5 Thyroid toxicity — goitre, hypothyroidism
6 Cardiovascular
   a) ECG → T-wave flattening/inversion
   b) Cardiovascular collapse in massive overdose

TETRACYCLIC ANTIDEPRESSANTS

Clinical pharmacology of mianserin
1 Tetracyclic structure bears *no* similarity to tricyclics
2 Fewer arrhythmogenic and anticholinergic side-effects
3 Safer in overdose, hence possibly an advantage in treating potentially suicidal patients
4 Side-effects include neutropenia, agranulocytosis and aplastic anaemia
5 Doubts exist regarding the drug's therapeutic efficacy

NEUROLEPTIC SIDE-EFFECTS

Distinguishing features of drug-induced movement disorders
1 Neuroleptic-induced pseudo-Parkinsonism
   a) Usually appears after several months therapy
   b) Tends to occur more frequently with high dosage and in *elderly* patients
   c) May remit with continued treatment, respond to conventional anti-Parkinsonian therapy, or persist despite total drug withdrawal
   d) Is frequently indistinguishable from primary Parkinson's disease on clinical grounds alone
   e) Occurs in 20–30% of treated patients
   f) Treat with anticholinergics
2 Neuroleptic-induced acute dystonic reactions
   a) Usually appears within 24 hours of (often initial) dosage; may be induced by metoclopramide (rarely causes parkinsonism or tardive dyskinesia)
   b) Occurs more frequently in *men* than women, *young* than old
   c) Occurs within 48 hours of drug administration; duration variable
   d) May be preceded by akathisia, grimacing, hyperreflexia
   e) May manifest as oculogyric crisis, opisthotonus, trismus/torticollis
   f) Consistently responsive to intravenous administration of benztropine, diphenhydramine
   g) Occurs in approximately 2% of treated patients
3 Neuroleptic-induced tardive dyskinesia
   a) Insidious onset; may be 'unmasked' after dose reduction or discontinuation; affects 29–30% after 4 years' therapy, but has been reported after only 3 months

   b) Occurs in *women* more than men, *elderly* more than young
   c) Probably reflects dopamine receptor hypersensitivity
   d) No subjective patient distress
   e) Disappears during sleep; frequently worsened by withdrawal of neuroleptic
   f) 40% eventually remit following treatment cessation, while 60% persist or worsen
   g) Treat with tetrabenazine (depleted dopamine; also used in Huntington's chorea); *not* consistently effective
   h) Continued treatment with offending drug does not increase severity of the dyskinesia, but does reduce likelihood of eventual remission, i.e. disorder is not progressive

Differential diagnosis of tardive dyskinesia
1 Huntington's disease (patients may be receiving phenothiazines for associated psychiatric disorders, but may develop extrapyramidal symptoms *de novo*
2 Wilson's disease (as for Huntington's)
3 Gilles de la Tourette's syndrome (facial grimacing and verbal profanities in children) — important to diagnose, since eminently treatable with haloperidol

Features of tardive dyskinesia
1 Orofacial dyskinesia: hyperkinesis of cheeks/tongue/mouth
   a) 'Fly-catcher's tongue'
   b) 'Bon-bon' sign
   c) Rumination, pouting
2 Glottal dyskinesia — grunting
3 Blepharospasm; increased blink frequency
4 Torticollis
5 Upper limbs
   a) 'Piano-playing' fingers
   b) Choreiform or ballistic movements
   c) Shoulder shrugging
6 Lower limbs
   a) Foot-tapping
   b) Great toe dorsiflexion

ELECTROCONVULSIVE THERAPY (ECT)

Indications for ECT
1 Severe depression in patients resistant to tri-/tetracyclics
2 Severe depression complicated by dehydration or weight loss
3 Depression associated with suicidal ideation or delusions
4 Drug-resistant mania
5 Puerperal psychosis (treatment of choice)

Contraindications to ECT
1 Increased intracranial pressure
2 Known cerebral aneurysm
3 Past history of
   a) Cerebrovascular disease
   b) Myocardial infarction
   c) Aortic aneurysm
4 Unfit for general anaesthesia

PSYCHOSURGERY

Potential indications for psychosurgery
1 Cingulotomy — refractory incapacitating obsessional neurosis
2 Ventromedial frontal lobe surgery
   a) No longer used for schizophrenia
   b) Occasionally still used for severe depression refractory to tricyclics and ECT
3 Temporal lobectomy
   Callosal sectioning, } — Drug-resistant epilepsy
   commissurotomy

UNDERSTANDING PSYCHIATRIC DISEASE

Spectrum of self-inflicted diseases
1 Münchausen syndrome
2 Diuretic and/or laxative abuse (leading to symptomatic hypokalaemia ± nephropathy, *inter alia*)
3 Factitious fever
4 Factitious hypoglycaemia
5 Thyrotoxicosis factitia
6 Dermatitis artefacta

Clinical features associated with cannabis use
1 Anxiety, panic
   Paranoia; visual hallucinations
   Predisposition to schizophrenia in chronic users
2 Tachycardia
   Supine hypertension with postural hypotension
3 Bronchitis, emphysema

4 'Amotivational syndrome'
5 Symptomatic relief from nausea, glaucoma, spasticity

NEUROTRANSMITTER ABNORMALITIES

Recognized neurotransmitter abnormalities in schizophrenia
1 ↓ Somatostatin
2 ↓ CCK } —in the hippocampus

Recognized neurotransmitter abnormalities in Huntington's chorea
1 ↑ Somatostatin (preservation of *aspiny* neurones in caudate)
2 ↑ Dopamine
3 ↓ GABA
   ↓ Substance P
   ↓ Metenkephalin } —depletion of striatal *spiny* neurones
4 ↓ Acetylcholine

Recognized neurotransmitter abnormalities in Alzheimer's disease
1 ↓ Acetylcholine (neuronal degeneration in nucleus basalis)
2 ↓ Somatostatin (cortical degeneration of aspiny neurones)
3 ↓ Noradrenaline (neuronal degeneration in locus caeruleus)
4 ↓ Dopamine (neuronal degeneration in ventral tegmentum)
5 ↓ Serotonin (degeneration of raphé nucleus)

Reviewing the Literature: Psychiatry

11.1 Andreasson S et al 1987 Cannabis and schizophrenia: a longitudinal study of Swedish conscripts. Lancet ii: 1483–1485

Cohort of 45 000 showed relative six-fold risk of schizophrenia for people who had used cannabis on more than 50 occasions; this association was independent of social and psychological background

11.2 Kelsoe J R et al 1989 Re-evaluation of the linkage relationship between chromosome 11p loci and the gene for bipolar affective disorder in the Old Order Amish. Nature 342: 238–244

Retraction of a previous study claiming genetic linkage between the manic depressive phenotype and a locus on chromosome 11; the conclusions of the previous study are now regarded as spurious

11.3 Detera-Wadleigh S D et al 1989 Exclusion of linkage to 5q11–13 in families with schizophrenia and other psychiatric disorders. Nature 340: 391–393

Study suggesting that most cases of schizophrenia do not in fact involve the putative dominant gene located on chromosome 5 as reported in 1988. Oh well, maybe next year. . .

11.4 Klerman G L 1988 Overview of the Cross-National Collaborative Panic Study. Archives of General Psychiatry 45: 407–412

Documents the apparently successful treatment of agoraphobia, situational anxiety and panic attacks with high-dose alprazolam, a new benzodiazepine

11.5 Martyn C N et al 1989 Geographical relation between Alzheimer's disease and aluminium in drinking water. Lancet i: 59–62

Interesting but inconclusive study suggesting a 1.5-fold increase in Alzheimer's associated with polluted drinking water.

11.6 Duara R et al 1986 Positron emission tomography in Alzheimer's disease. Neurology 36: 879–887
PET scanning was shown to localize and quantify regional cerebral dysfunction (reduced glucose metabolism) in 21 Alzheimer's disease patients, making this modality a potential clinical tool here

11.7 Renvoize E B et al 1986 Identical twins discordant for presenile dementia of the Alzheimer type. British Journal of Psychiatry 149: 509–512

Case report of a patient remaining unaffected by

Alzheimer's 20 years after onset in identical twin, suggesting that at least some cases of Alzheimer's disease have exogenous cause

11.8   Mazziotta J C et al 1987 Reduced cerebral glucose metabolism in asymptomatic subjects at risk for Huntington 's chorea. New England Journal of Medicine 316: 357–362

Reduced striatal glucose metabolism (measured using PET scanning) predated occurrence of Huntington's disease

11.9   Phillips D P, King E W 1988 Death takes a holiday: mortality surrounding major social occasions. Lancet ii: 728–732

Study suggesting that patients can voluntarily 'postpone' death until after a major anticipated occasion has come to pass, suggesting in turn that the 'will to live' is a reality

11.10   Hale A S 1989 et al Tyramine conjugation test for prediction of treatment response in depressed patients. Lancet i: 234–236

30 depressed patients were found to excrete an oral tyramine load in inverse relationship to their responsiveness to tricyclic antidepressants, suggesting a role for abnormal tyramine metabolism in endogenous (but not reactive) depression and in therapeutic response

CHAPTER 12

Renal medicine

Physical examination protocol 12.1 You are asked to examine a patient for signs of renal disease

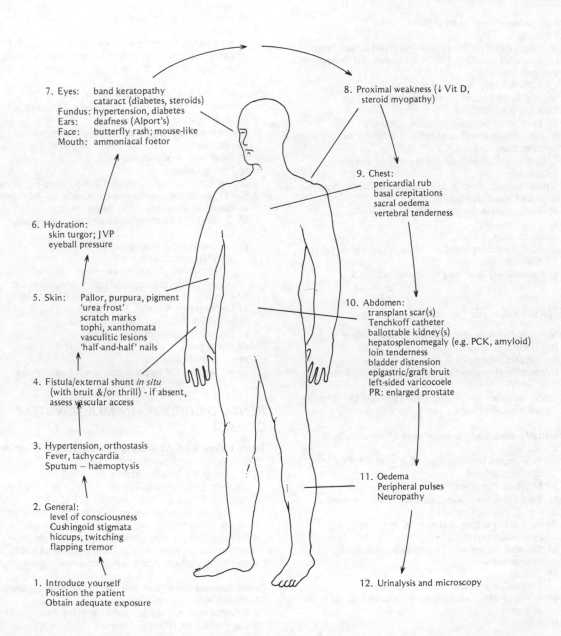

7. Eyes: band keratopathy
   cataract (diabetes, steroids)
   Fundus: hypertension, diabetes
   Ears: deafness (Alport's)
   Face: butterfly rash; mouse-like
   Mouth: ammoniacal foetor

8. Proximal weakness (↓ Vit D, steroid myopathy)

9. Chest:
   pericardial rub
   basal crepitations
   sacral oedema
   vertebral tenderness

6. Hydration:
   skin turgor; JVP
   eyeball pressure

5. Skin: Pallor, purpura, pigment
   'urea frost'
   scratch marks
   tophi, xanthomata
   vasculitic lesions
   'half-and-half' nails

10. Abdomen:
    transplant scar(s)
    Tenchkoff catheter
    ballottable kidney(s)
    hepatosplenomegaly (e.g. PCK, amyloid)
    loin tenderness
    bladder distension
    epigastric/graft bruit
    left-sided varicocoele
    PR: enlarged prostate

4. Fistula/external shunt *in situ*
   (with bruit &/or thrill) - if absent,
   assess vascular access

3. Hypertension, orthostasis
   Fever, tachycardia
   Sputum — haemoptysis

2. General:
   level of consciousness
   Cushingoid stigmata
   hiccups, twitching
   flapping tremor

11. Oedema
    Peripheral pulses
    Neuropathy

1. Introduce yourself
   Position the patient
   Obtain adequate exposure

12. Urinalysis and microscopy

CLINICAL ASPECTS OF RENAL DISEASE

COMMONEST RENAL SHORT CASES
1 Polycystic kidneys
2 Renal transplant (± cushingoid)

The abdominal mass: why do you think it's a kidney?
1 Able to get above it
2 Moves only slightly with respiration
3 Bimanually ballottable
4 Resonant on percussing above

Clinical assessment of hydration status
1 Vital signs
  a) Heart rate   ⎫ — marked orthostatic
  b) Blood pressure ⎬   response if dehydrated
2 Weight loss
  a) <3% (mildly dehydrated)
  b) >10% (profoundly dehydrated)
3 Skin turgor/elasticity
  a) Test over tibiae, scapulae, sternum
  b) Reduction implies at least moderate dehydration
  Eyeball pressure
4 CNS signs — confusion may reflect severe dehydration
5 Urine output — < 30 ml/h suggests hypovolaemia
6 Signs of fluid overload
  a) Tachycardia, tachypnoea
  b) Elevated JVP
  c) S_3, gallop
  d) Aortic incompetent murmur (may occur when dialysis overdue)
  e) Pulmonary and/or peripheral oedema

RENAL FAILURE

Features indicating chronicity of renal failure
1 Band keratopathy
2 Peripheral neuropathy
3 Bilaterally shrunken kidneys on plain abdominal film or IVP
4 CXR: annular calcification of mitral/aortic valve(s)
5 Renal osteodystrophy on X-ray and biopsy

Potentially reversible precipitants of renal failure
1 Vascular
  a) Prolonged hypotension (e.g. dehydration, cardiac failure)
  b) Malignant hypertension
  c) Vasculitis (esp. Goodpasture's syndrome)
  d) Renal vein thrombosis
2 Recent obstruction (exclude with ultrasound)
  a) Prostatomegaly
  b) Bladder atony (e.g. in diabetic autonomic neuropathy)
  c) Calculi
  d) Idiopathic retroperitoneal fibrosis
  e) Tumour infiltration (e.g. Ca bladder → ureteric orifices)
3 Infection

a) Pyelonephritis (may be secondary to subacute obstruction)
b) Septicaemia → acute tubular necrosis
c) Acute glomerulonephritis (e.g. *S. albus*: 'shunt nephritis')
d) Genitourinary TB → upper tract obstruction
e) Amyloidosis due to chronic sepsis (e.g. UTI in paraplegic)
4 Metabolic derangement
  a) Acute hyperuricaemia (e.g. tumour lysis syndrome)
  b) Hypercalcaemia
  c) Chronic hypokalaemia (laxative abuse, Conn's syndrome)
  d) Heavy metal poisoning
5 Iatrogenic
  a) Radiographic contrast examination, esp. IVP
  b) Drug toxicity (e.g. NSAIDs, aminoglycosides, tetracyclines)

Clinical evolution of renal dysfunction
1 Reduced renal reserve — creatinine clearance 60–100 ml/min: asymptomatic
2 Renal insufficiency — creatinine clearance 30–60 ml/min
  a) Nocturia; leg cramps
  b) Hypertension
  c) Hyperuricaemia; elevated blood urea nitrogen
3 Renal failure — creatinine clearance 15–30 ml/min
  a) Nausea, anorexia, diarrhoea
  b) Oedema; infections; occult bleeding, mouth ulcers
  c) — Phosphate retention
    — Metabolic acidosis
    — Impaired glucose tolerance
    — Anaemia (exception: polycystic disease)
4 Uraemia — creatinine clearance <15 ml/min
  a) Lethargy, irritability (→ fits, coma)
  b) Pruritus, hiccups, flapping tremor
  c) Pericarditis; pulmonary oedema
  d) Bone pain
  e) — Hyperkalaemia
    — Reciprocal hypocalcaemia; ↑ alk. phos.

RENAL DISORDERS IN MULTISYSTEM DISEASE

Renal failure with haemoptysis: differential diagnosis
1 Goodpasture's syndrome
  Wegener's granulomatosis
  Henoch-Schönlein purpura
  PAN, SLE, cryoglobulinaemia
2 Renal vein thrombosis with pulmonary embolism
3 Acute renal failure with pulmonary oedema
4 Right-sided infective endocarditis with septic pulmonary emboli and immune-complex nephritis
5 Infection: tuberculosis, Legionnaires' disease

Renal disease with jaundice: differential diagnosis
1 Haemolytic-uraemic syndrome
2 Hepatorenal failure (hepatic nephropathy)
3 Leptospirosis (Weil's disease)

4 Hepatitis B with nephrotic syndrome
5 Alcoholic cirrhosis with IgA nephropathy *or* renal tubular acidosis
6 Polycystic disease with congenital hepatic fibrosis
7 Stauffer's syndrome — renal cell carcinoma with non-metastatic hepatic dysfunction (e.g. cholestasis)
8 Toxic — CCl_4, methoxyflurane

Hepatorenal failure: clinical features
1 Typically occurs in context of advanced liver failure
2 May be precipitated by diuretic use, paracentesis, shunt surgery or biliary contrast radiography
3 Characterized by
  a) Oliguria
  b) Normal urinary sediment
  c) Urinary sodium < 5 mmol/l
4 No improvement following intravenous volume repletion (cf. prerenal failure)
5 Renal function becomes normal if kidneys transplanted into host with normal liver function

Diagnostic significance of skin lesions in renal failure
1 Impetigo ⎫ —Suggestive of
  Erythema nodosum ⎬ post-streptococcal
  ⎭ glomerulonephritis
2 Purpura
  a) Amyloid ('pinch'; post-proctoscopic periorbital type)
  b) Vasculitis (palpable)
  c) Henoch-Schönlein (→ thigh, buttock)
  d) Cryoglobulinaemia (± ulceration, gangrene)
3 Inherited nephropathies
  a) Scrotal angiokeratomata (Fabry's disease)
  b) Carotenaemic pigmentation (Balkan nephropathy)
  c) Hypoplastic nails (nail-patella syndrome)
  d) Adenoma sebaceum, ash-leaf macules (tuberous sclerosis; associated angiomyolipomata may cause massive haematuria)

SYMPTOMS AND SIGNS OF RENAL DISEASE

Renal disease with small kidney(s) size
1 Chronic glomerulonephritis (symmetrically smooth)
2 Chronic pyelonephritis (asymmetrically scarred cortical scars opposite dilated calices, esp. at upper poles)
3 Medullary cystic disease
4 Postobstructive atrophy
5 Renovascular insufficiency
6 Late stage of many diseases causing large kidneys initially

Renal disease with bilateral renal enlargement
1 Polycystic disease
2 Medullary sponge kidneys
3 Obstructive uropathy (bilateral hydronephrosis)
4 Acute nephropathies
  a) Acute glomerulonephritis
  b) Acute interstitial nephritis
  c) Acute tubular necrosis
  d) Acute urate nephropathy

5 Other
  a) Amyloidosis
  b) Renal vein thrombosis (± nephrosis, amyloid)
  c) Insulin-dependent diabetes
  d) Acromegaly (renal function typically normal)
  e) Radiation nephritis

Common features of interstitial nephritis
1 Fever, arthralgias, rash
2 Renal failure with microhaematuria ± polyuria/pyuria
3 Eosinophilia (esp. if drug-induced), eosinophiluria >5%
4 Abnormal liver function tests
5 Radiographically enlarged kidneys

Differential diagnosis of loin pain
1 Calculus; sloughed papilla
2 Pyelonephritis; perinephric abscess
3 Acute glomerulonephritis (esp. proliferative)
4 Vesicoureteric reflux
5 Haemorrhage into cyst; infected cyst
6 Segmental infarction (sickle-cell disease, embolism)

Nocturia: diagnostic significance
1 Prostatism
2 Oedematous states
3 Salt-losing nephropathies, e.g.
  a) Analgesic nephropathy
  b) Medullary sponge kidneys
  c) Sickle cell disease
4 Polyuric states, e.g.
  a) Diabetes mellitus/insipidus
  b) Primary polydipsia
  c) Post-ATN
5 Bladder pathology
  a) Tumour, fibrosis, infection
  b) Loss of reflex inhibition (e.g. multiple sclerosis)
  c) Vesicoureteric reflux ('double micturition' in children)

INVESTIGATING RENAL DISEASE

URINARY ABNORMALITIES

Highly diagnostic features on urine microscopy
1 Red cell casts (acute glomerulonephritis)
2 Doubly-refractile oval fat bodies (nephrotic syndrome)

Urinary stigmata of glomerular disease
1 Red cell casts
2 Heavy proteinuria (>2 g/day)
3 Pleomorphic red cells on phase-contrast microscopy

Clinically important causes of 'sterile pyuria'
1 Inadequately treated urinary tract infection
2 Genitourinary TB, or other fastidious organism, e.g.
  a) *Strep. morbillorum/agalactiae/milleri*
  b) *Corynebacteria*, lactobacilli

3 Inflammatory non-infective disease
  a) Papillary necrosis (esp. analgesic nephropathy)
  b) Calculi (renal or bladder)
  c) Interstitial nephritis/polycystic disease (light pyuria)
4 Lower tract inflammation
  a) Prostatitis
  b) Chemical cystitis (e.g. due to cyclophosphamide)
5 The 'dysuria-pyuria' (or 'urethral') syndrome
  a) Pathogenic bacteriuria $<10^5$ organisms/ml
  b) Chlamydial or gonococcal urethritis
  c) Periurethral herpes simplex
6 'False pyuria' (i.e. nil on suprapubic tap) — primary vaginal infection with poor specimen collection; e.g. due to *Gardnerella vaginalis, C. albicans, Trichomonas*

Urinary tract infection: factors favouring pyelonephritis
1 Clinical — loin pain/tenderness, fever, tachycardia, rigors
2 Urine microscopy — white blood cell casts
3 Blood — peripheral leucocytosis ± positive blood cultures
4 IVP — poor excretion of contrast on affected side
5 Therapy — failure of appropriate single-dose antibiotics

Iatrogenic causes of reddish urine
1 Drug excretion products
  a) Rifampicin
  b) Metronidazole
  c) Sulphasalazine
  d) Doxorubicin
  e) Desferrioxamine
2 Drug toxicity
  a) Drugs inducing acute intermittent porphyria (e.g. barbiturates)
  b) Drugs inducing rhabdomyolysis (e.g. clofibrate, heroin)
  c) Drugs inducing frank haematuria (e.g. warfarin, urokinase)

Myoglobinuria: precipitants and laboratory features
1 Causes
  a) Muscle crush injury
  b) Hyperthermia (e.g. malignant) ± convulsions
  c) Polymyositis
  d) McArdle's syndrome
  e) Meyer-Betz (familial) disease
  f) Haff disease
  g) Drugs
    — Acute alcoholic binge
    — Heroin, 'angel dust' (phencyclidine, PCP)
    — Clofibrate
2 Features
  a) Acute oliguric renal failure
  b) Initial profound hypocalcaemia
  c) → 'Rebound' hypercalcaemia
  d) ↑ Serum potassium, phosphate, urate
  e) Red urine
  f) Ward urinalysis 'haem-positive'
  g) No red cells on microscopy
  h) Serum clear (since myoglobin does not bind haptoglobin and is therefore renally cleared almost immediately; cf. early stages of intravascular haemolysis)

Crystalluria: differential diagnosis
1 Cystinuria (autosomal recessive)
2 Xanthinuria (hereditary **or** allopurinol-induced)
3 Hyperoxaluria
  a) Autosomal recessive (pyridoxine-responsive)
  b) Ileal disease (calculous tendency partly due to associated hypocitruria)
  c) Toxic
    — Ethylene glycol ingestion
    — Methoxyflurane
4 Orotic aciduria
5 Uricosuria
6 Drug-induced — sulphadiazine, nitrofurantoin, 5FC, acyclovir; acetazolamide

Differential diagnosis of normocalcaemic hypercalciuria
1 Idiopathic
2 Medullary sponge kidneys
3 Immobilization (esp. in Paget's disease)
4 Sarcoidosis
5 Acromegaly; Cushing's syndrome
6 (Mild) primary hyperparathyroidism (may be definitively diagnosed by documenting elevated serum iPTH and/or urinary cAMP)
7 Renal tubular acidosis
8 Iatrogenic
  a) Corticosteroids
  b) Frusemide

Diagnostic significance of urinary chloride in metabolic alkalosis
1 All forms of metabolic alkalosis have low *serum* chloride
2 *Urinary* chloride may be normal in some cases of metabolic alkalosis, e.g. hyperaldosteronism
3 Urinary chloride is typically *absent* in metabolic alkaloses associated with *hypovolaemia,* e.g.
  a) Gastric losses (vomiting, suction)
  b) Following excessive use of diuretics
4 This occurs because the hypovolaemic stimulus for hypothalamic ADH secretion *overrides* the hypo-osmolar stimulus for ADH suppression, i.e. renal Na^+ (and Cl^-) are conserved
5 The latter phenomenon leads to a *paradoxical aciduria* which will persist until NaCl (volume replacement) and KCl (electrolyte replacement) replenishment is achieved, i.e., resolution of the alkalosis is *chloride-dependent*

PROTEINURIA

Clinical sequelae of heavy proteinuria
1 Oedema
2 Weakness (muscle catabolism ± diuretic-induced hypokalaemia)
3 Frothy urine
4 Postural hypotension
5 Thromboembolism (incl. renal vein thrombosis)
6 Hypercholesterolaemia (xanthomata, vascular disease)

Laboratory characterization of proteinuria
1 'Selective' (glomerular) proteinuria is characterized by urinary losses of albumin and/or transferrin.

2 Non-selective proteinuria leads to loss of IgG (inter alia), and *selectivity* may therefore be quantitated by the ratio albumin/IgG (urine)

3 Similarly, the 'tubular' nature of proteinuria may be quantitatively confirmed by calculating the urinary β-2 microglobulin/albumin ratio

4 Low IgG/transferrin (albumin) ratios tend to be predictive of steroid responsiveness in nephrotic syndrome (e.g. 'minimal lesion' with selective proteinuria)

Characteristics of benign orthostatic proteinuria
1 Non-selective
2 Benign sediment
3 <1 g/day
4 Typical diurnal fluctuation
5 No increase with time

NEPHROTIC SYNDROME

Clinicopathological concomitants of the nephrotic syndrome
1 Low albumin
2 Low transferrin $\rightarrow$ iron-resistant hypochromic anaemia
3 Low IgG (hypogammaglobulinaemia); elevated α-2 globulins
4 Low plasma volume
   High fibrinogen, V, VII, VIII, X $\left.\right\}$ $\rightarrow$hypercoagulable state (e.g. $\rightarrow$ renal vein thrombosis)
5 Low 25-hydroxyvitamin D (due to urinary losses) $\rightarrow$ secondary reduction in 1,25 dihydroxyvitamin D
6 Hypercholesterolaemia $\rightarrow$ accelerated atherosclerosis
7 GFR may be overestimated by creatinine clearance. Reduced GFR (reflecting hypovolaemia rather than renal damage) may be more accurately measured using ^{51}Cr-EDTA clearance

Prognostic variables in the nephrotic syndrome
1 Clinical features portending poor prognosis
   a) Oliguria; haematuria
   b) Hypertension
   c) Purpura
2 Results portending poor prognosis
   a) Non-selective proteinuria
   b) Hypocomplementaemia
3 Aetiologic significance of steroid-resistance in minimal change disease
   a) Hodgkin's disease
   b) Amyloid
   c) Focal sclerosis (i.e. biopsy sampling error)
4 Indications for alkylator therapy in minimal change disease
   a) At least two relapses following initial response to steroids

GLOMERULAR DISEASE

Routine investigation of idiopathic glomerular disease
1 Careful microscopic examination of freshly voided urine

2 Serum albumin and 24-hour urine protein
3 ASO titre
   HBsAg
   VDRL
   Thick/thin film (if history of malarial exposure)
   Urine screen for glycosuria or opiate derivatives
   CXR (sarcoid, malignancy)
4 Blood cultures
   a) Infective endocarditis
   b) 'Shunt' (*Staph. albus*) nephritis
   c) Pneumococcal peritonitis
   d) Brucellosis, leptospirosis
5 ANA, rheumatoid factor; C_3, C_4
   Cryoglobulins
   Anti-GBM Ab
6 EPG/IEPG/urinary BJP ($\pm$ bone marrow pending result)
   Rectal biopsy
7 Renal biopsy
   a) Light microscopy
   b) Immunofluorescence
   c) Congo red
   d) Electron microscopy

Spectrum of renal pathology in diabetes
1 Renal enlargement (in early insulin-dependent diabetes); osmotic polyuria
2 Diffuse glomerulosclerosis
   Nodular glomerulosclerosis (Kimmelstiel-Wilson lesion) — suggests insulin-dependent diabetes
3 Glycogen deposition in tubules (Armanni-Ebstein lesion)
4 Interstitial nephritis
   Pyelonephritis $\rightarrow$ papillary necrosis
   Recurrent urinary tract infections
5 Hyporeninaemic hypoaldosteronism ($\uparrow$ K^+, $\uparrow$ Cl^-)

Spectrum of renal pathology in systemic lupus erythematosus (WHO classification)
1 Normal light microscopic appearances; positive mesangial immunofluorescence
2 Mesangial changes only
3 Focal proliferative glomerulonephritis
4 Diffuse proliferative glomerulonephritis
5 Membranous glomerulonephritis
6 Advanced sclerosis (an important biopsy diagnosis, since the absence of an inflammatory component contraindicates treatment)

Electron microscopy of renal disease
1 Minimal lesion nephrosis — epithelial podocyte fusion
2 Fanconi syndrome
   Congenital nephrosis $\left.\right\}$ 'Swan-neck' deformity and dilatation of proximal tubule
3 Alport's syndrome — splitting of lamina densa and lamina propria of glomerular basement membrane (similar appearance in chronic rejection)
4 Medullary cystic disease — cystic dilatation at corticomedullary junction
5 Medullary sponge kidneys
   Infantile polycystic kidneys $\left.\right\}$ Dilatation of collecting ducts
   (cf. adult polycystic kidneys — abnormality involves entire nephron)

IMMUNOPATHOLOGY OF THE NEPHRON

Some causes of membranous nephropathy
1 Paraneoplastic
2 Autoimmune disease, esp. SLE
3 Sarcoidosis
4 Infections — hepatitis B, syphilis; *P. malariae**
5 Drugs
  a) Gold, penicillamine
  b) Captopril (high-dose only; now unusual)

Immunofluorescence of glomerular disease
1 Helpful in diagnosing early membranous nephropathy (diffuse IgG $\pm$ C_3)
2 Distinguishes minimal change disease (IF-) from mesangial nephropathy (+IgM, weak +C_3)
3 Focal sclerosis: +IgM, +C_3
4 Mesangiocapillary GN
  a) Bright C_3 staining
  b) Modest Ig/C_{1q} staining
5 SLE
  a) Heavy IgG, A, M deposits
  b) +C_{1q}, C_3
  c) +ANA →5–10%; pathognomonic
6 IgA nephropathy/HSP: mesangial IgA and C_3 $\pm$ IgM, G but without C_{1q} (cf. SLE)
7 Goodpasture's: *linear IgG* (kidney and lung); rarely, may occur in SLE or transplant rejection. Associated with anti-GBM circulating antibody
8 Postinfectious — 'lumpy-bumpy' electron-dense deposits with +C_3

Complement levels in glomerulonephritis
1 Reduced ($\downarrow$ C_3)
  a) Postinfectious (SBE, 'shunt', post-strep)
  b) SLE; cryoglobulinaemia
  c) Mesangiocapillary type I and (esp.) II
    — May even be hypocomplementaemic with quiescent nephritis; C_3-nephritic factor may be detectable in type II
2 Normal
  a) Minimal lesion
  b) IgA nephropathy
  c) Goodpasture's syndrome; rapidly progressive GN (RPGN)
  d) PAN, HSP, Wegener's
  e) Membranous

INVESTIGATING RENAL FAILURE

Diagnostic approach to unexplained acute renal failure
1 Clinical
  a) Hypovolaemia (favours pre-renal cause)
  b) Fluid overload (favours renal/post-renal cause)
2 Urine microscopy/urinalysis/MSU — helps exclude glomerulonephritis, UTI
3 Renal ultrasound — excludes postrenal obstruction
4 Blood cultures, coagulation screen — helps exclude septicaemia, DIC
5 Renal biopsy $\pm$ high-dose IVP — confirms or refutes diagnosis of glomerulonephritis

---

*Cure of malaria will *not* necessarily lead to resolution of the nephropathy

Disproportionate elevation of blood urea vs creatinine
1 Nephrotic syndrome
2 Dehydration (loss of water *and* sodium)
3 Gastrointestinal haemorrhage
4 Congestive cardiac failure
5 High protein intake
6 Drugs
  a) Tetracycline
  b) Corticosteroids
  c) Cyclosporin A

Acute renal failure: 'prerenal' or acute tubular necrosis?
1 Prerenal
  a) Urinary sodium < 10 mEq/l
  b) Urinary osmolality > 500 mosm/l
  c) Urine: plasma osmolality >1.1
  d) Urine: plasma creatinine concentration > 20
2 ATN
  a) Urinary sodium >20 mEq/l
  b) Urinary osmolality < 400 mosm/l
  c) Urine: plasma osmolality = 0.9–1.05
  d) Urine: plasma creatinine concentration < 15

RENAL BIOPSY

Indications for renal biopsy
1 Haematuria with proteinuria
2 Haematuria with negative cystoscopy and IVP
3 Proteinuria > 1 g/day, esp. with renal impairment
4 Nephrotic syndrome in adults
5 Acute renal failure (esp. oliguric nephritic type) following exclusion of pre- and postrenal causes
6 Chronic renal failure (*not* end-stage) with radiographically normal kidneys
7 Renal vasculitis (before and during therapy)
8 Malfunctioning transplant kidney

Renal biopsy: complications and contraindications
1 Complications
  a) Persistent gross haematuria
  b) Pain ('clot colic', perinephric haematoma)
  c) Hypotension (transient), brady-/tachycardia
  d) Intrarenal A-V fistula
  e) Urinoma, urinary fistula
  f) Hypertension (chronic)
2 Contraindications
  a) Inadequate facilities for immunofluorescence and/or electron microscopy
  b) Abnormal coagulation; reduced platelet number and/or function
  c) Bilaterally small kidneys on IVP
  d) Diastolic BP > 120 mmHg
  e) Solitary (functioning) kidney
  f) Diabetic glomerulosclerosis clinically suspected
  g) Established uraemia

TUBULAR DISORDERS

Indicators of proximal tubular dysfunction
1 Glycosuria (i.e. without hyperglycaemia)
2 Phosphaturia

3 Uricosuria
4 Aminoaciduria

Indicators of distal tubular dysfunction
1 Urinary concentration defect
  a) Screen — overnight urine <700 mosm/l is abnormal
  b) Water deprivation test: <900 mosm/l is abnormal
  c) DDAVP stimulation: <800 mosm/l is abnormal
2 Urinary acidification defect — ammonium chloride test — pH > 5.0 is abnormal

Pathological spectrum of renal tubular dysfunction
(X = X-linked, A = autosomal, R = recessive, D = dominant)
1 Defective tubular responsiveness to hormones
  a) Nephrogenic diabetes insipidus (XR; distal tubular dysfunction)
  b) Bartter's syndrome (AR, distal)
  c) Liddle's syndrome (AD, distal)
  d) Pseudohypoparathyroidism (XD, proximal)
  e) Hypophosphataemic rickets (XD, proximal)
2 Primary tubular transport defects (often associated with corresponding intestinal transport defects)
  a) 'Renal' glycosuria (AD, proximal)
  b) Hartnup disease (AR, proximal; loss of tryptophan, leads to niacin deficiency)
  c) Cystinuria (AR, proximal; may manifest as recurrent calculi due to cystine loss, although ornithine, arginine and lysine — 'COAL' — are also lost)
  d) Cystinosis (AR, proximal; leads to uraemia and death in childhood)
  e) Fanconi syndrome (AR, proximal; multiple defects → aminoaciduria, glycosuria, phosphaturia, natriuria, hypercalciuria, uricosuria, 'tubular' proteinuria)
  f) Renal tubular acidosis type I (AD, distal)
3 Secondary tubular transport defects
  a) Distal tubule defects
    — Liver disease
    — Medullary sponge kidneys
    — Infantile polycystic disease
    — Amphotericin B ⎫
    — Cyclosporin A ⎬ toxicity
    — Lithium ⎭
  b) Proximal tubule defects
    — Wilson's disease; heavy metal poisoning
    — Medullary cystic disease
    — Fanconi's syndrome; cystinosis
    — Acetazolamide use
  c) Distal and/or proximal defects
    — Myeloma
    — Sjögren's syndrome, other autoimmune disorders
    — Renal transplant rejection
    — Longstanding hypercalciuria/-aemia or hypokalaemia
    — Obstructive uropathy
    — Analgesic nephropathy, chronic pyelonephritis

Renal tubular acidosis: clinical presentations in adults
1 Weakness (hypokalaemia)
2 Bone pain (osteomalacia)
3 Constipation
4 Renal calculi
  a) Calcium phosphate ($\pm$ nephrocalcinosis)
  b) Struvite (due to associated hypocitruria)
5 Renal failure

When to suspect renal tubular acidosis
1 High urine pH (>6 despite acidaemia in *distal* RTA) and negative urine culture
2 Hyperchloraemic hypokalaemic acidosis ($\uparrow Cl^-$, $\downarrow K^+$, $\downarrow HCO_3^-$)
3 Normal anion gap (i.e. $Na^+ - Cl^- - HCO_3^- = 8-12$; cf. uraemia)
4 Hypouricaemia and hypophosphataemia (proximal RTA)
5 Hypercalciuria; low urinary specific gravity; polyuria; failure of urinary acidification following oral ammonium chloride 100 mg/kg (distal RTA) despite normalization of systemic acidaemia (cf. proximal — 'bicarbonate wasting' — type)
6 Hyperkalaemia and acid urine — hyporeninaemic hypoaldosteronism in elderly diabetics or obstructive uropathy (RTA type 4)

Possible constituents of 'tubular proteinuria'
1 Tamm-Horsfall protein ⎫
2 β-2 microglobulin ⎬ 'physiological'
3 IgA ⎭
4 Myoglobin
5 Lysozyme
6 Bence-Jones protein

How to distinguish urinary concentrating defects
1 Water deprivation ⎫
  Exogenous DDAVP ⎬ —>1000 mosm/l:normal
2 Water deprivation ⎫ —no increase
  Exogenous DDAVP ⎬ nephrogenic diabetes insipidus
3 Water deprivation → no increase ⎫ —pituitary diabetes
  Exogenous DDAVP → major increase ⎬ insipidus
4 Water deprivation ⎫ —submaximal increase:
  Exogenous DDAVP ⎬ long-standing primary polydipsia

DISORDERS OF WATER METABOLISM

Primary polydipsia: its clinical significance
1 80% of primary polydipsia patients are schizophrenic
2 The most common presentation of primary polydipsia is fitting
3 10% of primary polydipsia patients die within 2 years of presenting

Features of nephrogenic diabetes insipidus
1 The diagnosis may be effectively *excluded* if any voided urine specimen has an osmolality exceeding 600 mosm/l or specific gravity exceeding 1.015. Conversely, if an overnight voided specimen has an osmolality less than 350 mosm/l, a formal water-deprivation test *may* be indicated
2 Distinction from 'central' diabetes insipidus may be

made if concentration defect persists following bilateral intranasal instillation of 20 μg dDAVP

3 Primary polydipsia *tends* to be associated with a low plasma osmolality (~275 mosm/l) whereas diabetes insipidus tends to be associated with a higher reading (~295 mosm/l). In *long-standing* primary polydipsia, however, definitive distinction from nephrogenic diabetes insipidus may *not* be possible on the basis of osmolalities and water-deprivation tests alone

4 Nephrogenic diabetes insipidus may occur as a primary X-linked recessive (XR) disorder or, more commonly, as a secondary manifestation of other disorders including sickle-cell disease/trait, obstructive uropathy, chronic hypercalcaemia or hypokalaemia, or drugs (e.g. lithium, amphotericin B)

5 Potentially useful management options include
   a) Treatment of underlying cause
   b) Thiazides (or ethacrynic acid) ± dietary salt restriction

(NB: Chlorpropamide, which is of potential benefit in incomplete central diabetes insipidus, is ineffective in nephrogenic diabetes insipidus)

Drug-induced disturbances of water metabolism
1 SIADH
   a) Chlorpropamide
   b) Carbamazepine
   c) Amitriptyline
2 Nephrogenic diabetes insipidus
   a) Lithium
   b) Demeclocycline
   c) Amphotericin B

Diagnosis of inappropriate ADH secretion
1 Plasma osmolality <275 mosm/l
2 Urinary osmolality inappropriately high (see below)
3 Urinary sodium >20 mmol/l

Inappropriate ADH secretion: features
(plasma osmolality = BUN + glucose + 2 × Na$^+$)
1 Remains a diagnosis of exclusion in the absence of a reliable and freely available assay for plasma ADH
2 *Not* clinically characterized by significant oedema, weight gain or hypertension despite hypervolaemia; however, elderly patients may develop cardiac failure
3 Development of symptoms may be more dependent on *rate* of decline of serum sodium than on absolute level.
4 Associated hypouricaemia may be a pointer to the cause of hyponatraemia in the absence of osmolalities; similarly, creatinine/BUN, haematocrit, and serum albumin may be low
5 Urinary osmolalities need only be *inappropriately* elevated for the diagnosis to be entertained; e.g. a urinary osmolality of 250 mosm/l would be consistent with SIADH in association with an identical plasma value (provided that urinary sodium is also elevated; see above)
6 Some drugs (e.g. chlorpropamide) are thought to increase sensitivity to ADH as well as quantitatively augmenting secretion. The mechanism of

hyponatraemia in myxoedema, on the other hand, is felt to be an ADH-independent impairment of free water clearance
7 Note that hyponatraemia in Addison's disease is associated with hyperkalaemia
8 Therapeutic options include
   a) Treatment of underlying cause
   b) Water restriction ± frusemide ± dietary salt supplements
   c) Demeclocycline (or lithium)
   d) V$_2$-receptor (renal tubular ADH receptor) antagonists
   e) Hypertonic saline (a desperation measure)

RENAL RADIOLOGY

Intravenous pyelography: risk factors for precipitation of renal failure
1 Myeloma
2 Diabetes (controversial)
3 Old age (esp. if hypovolaemic, e.g. nephrotic) Infants (esp. if dehydrated, since unable to concentrate urine)

NB: This complication may be prevented by avoiding routine preparatory dehydration

Retrograde pyelography: causes of 'spidery infundibula'
1 Polycystic kidneys
2 Intrarenal space-occupying lesion (e.g. tumour)
3 Renal vein thrombosis

Pelviureteric junction translucency: differential diagnosis on IVP
1 Carcinoma (TCC)
2 Clot
3 Calculus (radiolucent; p. 267)
4 Crystals (p. 258)

Differential diagnosis of papillary necrosis
1 Analgesic abuse
2 Diabetes mellitus
3 Sickle-cell disease
4 Tuberculosis

Common congenital renal abnormalities seen on IVP
(All may predispose to infection, obstruction, and calculi)
1 Duplex collecting systems
   a) Commoner in females
   b) Upper pole ureter drains to lower bladder, and vice versa
   c) Lower pole ureter is prone to vesicoureteric reflux
2 Horseshoe kidney — fused lower poles
3 Pelvic (ectopic) kidney
   a) May interfere with parturition
   b) May simulate a pathological pelvic mass
4 Crossed renal ectopia
   a) Ectopic kidney lies directly below orthotopic partner
   b) Fusion may occur
   c) Collecting system of ectopic kidney crosses midline to enter bladder on correct side

Rationale of isotope renal scans
1 ^{131}Iodo-hippuran
   a) 80% excreted by renal tubular secretion
   b) Helps assess effective renal plasma flow and, thereby, functional status of renal homograft
   c) Renography may be useful in follow-up of (diagnosed) obstructive uropathy and/or assessment of pelviureteric junction obstruction
2 $^{99}Tc^m$-labelled contrast agents
   a) Helps assess renal perfusion
   b) Useful in confirming integrity of post-transplant vascular anastomosis (*dynamic* — vascular phase — studies)
   c) Demonstration of gross hypoperfusion in a non-functioning transplant favours rejection rather than tubular necrosis
   d) Dynamic studies may also be useful in assessment of suspected renovascular trauma
   e) *Static* (parenchymal phase) studies may be useful in the delineation of renal cortical function in the presence of severe renal failure (more sensitive than IVP), and also in the evaluation of suspected intrarenal trauma
3 Gallium-66 — helpful in excluding graft infection, usually in conjunction with ultrasound and/or transplant biopsy

---

MANAGING RENAL DISEASE

THERAPY OF RENAL FAILURE

Immediate management priorities in acute renal failure
1 To treat life-threatening hyperkalaemia and/or pulmonary oedema (e.g. by continuous arteriovenous haemofiltration)
2 To establish the nature, and hence the reversibility, of the renal lesion

Management considerations in end-stage chronic renal failure
1 Exclude reversible factors contributing to azotaemia
2 Treat hypertension
3 Reduce protein intake if symptomatically uraemic (also assists in controlling acidosis and hyperkalaemia)
4 Administer bicarbonate (unless sodium restricted), phosphate binders and/or vitamin D analogues as necessary
5 Modify drug intake for degree of azotaemia
6 Realistically assess age, general condition, mental capacity and overall prognosis prior to definitive intervention
7 Assess logistic suitability of patient for chronic ambulatory peritoneal dialysis (CAPD) or haemodialysis
   a) Will the patient cope?
   b) How adequate is vascular access?
   c) When would a fistula be created?
   d) How is the patient's cardiovascular stability?
8 Document HBsAg status
9 Determine age and number of siblings, and document degree of 'matching' between patient and siblings with respect to ABO (essential), HLA

(B and DR: 'cytotoxic' crossmatch), and MLC (helps distinguish relative suitablity of similar HLA-matches) compatibility
10 Ensure regular blood transfusion if transplantation feasible

Treating the complications of chronic renal failure
1 Anaemia
   a) Folate, multivitamins
   b) Ferrous sulphate
   c) Erythropoietin (ref. 12.1)
   d) Dialysis
2 Acidosis
   a) Sodium bicarbonate
   b) Dialysis
3 Hyperuricaemia — allopurinol
4 Renal bone disease
   a) Phosphate binders (aluminium hydroxide)
   b) Vitamin D analogues (dihydrotachysterol)
   c) Calcium supplements, high-calcium dialysate
   d) Parathyroidectomy

PRESCRIBING IN RENAL DISEASE

Drugs competing for renal excretion: clinical significance
1 Probenecid — reduces tubular secretion of penicillin (+ aspirin, indomethacin, AZT), thus potentiating therapeutic effect
2 Quinidine
   Verapamil } —decrease tubular secretion of digoxin, thus increasing risk of digoxin toxicity
   Spironolactone
3 Thiazides
   Frusemide } —increase lithium reabsorption, thus increasing risk of lithium toxicity
4 Aspirin — reduces tubular secretion of methotrexate, increasing incidence and severity of methotrexate toxicity

'Safe' drugs in chronic renal failure
1 Antihypertensives — β-blockers, hydralazine
2 Antiarrhythmics — disopyramide
3 Antibiotics — amoxicillin, co-trimoxazole, cephalexin, doxycycline
4 Analgesics — paracetamol (low-dose)
5 Gastrointestinal — cimetidine, metoclopramide, loperamide
6 Hypnotic — temazepam

Principles of corticosteroid use in renal disease
1 Renal biopsy should precede steroid administration in adults with renal disease
2 Steroids may lead to rapid resolution of
   a) Minimal lesion nephrosis (esp. in children)
   b) Acute interstitial nephritis
   c) Mesangial proliferative glomerulonephritis
   d) Idiopathic retroperitoneal fibrosis (exclude TB first)
3 Steroid therapy will frequently need to be combined with other therapeutic modalities to achieve optimal results in
   a) RPGN (including Goodpasture's)
   b) PAN
   c) Multiple relapses of minimal-lesion nephrosis

4 Steroids are occasionally of value in membranous glomerulonephritis if used early
5 Steroid therapy is rarely if ever efficacious in sclerodermatous nephropathy

DIURETICS

Mechanisms of diuretic action
1 Acetazolamide
  a) Carbonic anhydrase inhibitor
  b) ↓ Proximal tubular transport of NaCl/bicarbonate
  c) *Ineffective* if serum bicarbonate <20 mEq/l
  d) Toxicity
    — Metabolic acidosis (hypokalaemic with normal anion gap) due to 'bicarbonate wasting'
    — Nephrocalcinosis
  e) Indications
    — Short-term treatment of oedema, esp: oedema in pregnancy; oedema in premenstrual syndrome; oedema with metabolic alkalosis
    — Urate nephropathy
    — Salicylism (forced alkaline diuresis)
2 Mannitol — delivers osmotic load to proximal tubule
3 Frusemide
  a) Blocks chloride pump in thick ascending limb of loop of Henle
    → Blocks countercurrent multiplier system
    → Blocks water reabsorption from collecting system
  b) *Also* increases renal cortical perfusion
  c) Systemic venodilator
  d) Effective at low clearances
4 Thiazides
  a) Act on thin ascending limb (cortical diluting segment) of distal tubule → block active sodium reabsorption
  b) *Reduce* renal perfusion
  c) Also useful in proximal renal tubular acidosis
  d) *Not* effective at clearance < 20 ml/min
5 Potassium-sparing diuretics:
  a) Triamterene → ↓ permeability of distal tubule/collecting ducts
  b) Amiloride → ↓ sodium/H_2O reabsorption, ↓K^+ loss
  c) Principal indication — diuretic for digoxin-treated patients
  d) Spironolactone — inhibits aldosterone action on distal tubule and collecting ducts; antiandrogenic side-effects
  e) Principal indication — diuretic for cirrhotics with ascites

Opposing indications for frusemide and thiazides
1 SIADH — frusemide (plus sodium supplements)
  Nephrogenic diabetes insipidus — thiazides (plus sodium restriction)
2 Hypercalcaemia — frusemide
  Idiopathic hypercalciuria — thiazides

Clinically significant diuretic side-effects in elderly patients
1 Commoner with potassium-sparing diuretics
  a) Hyperkalaemia (esp. in renal impairment)
  b) Hyponatraemia (symptomatic in up to 20%)
  c) Precipitation of prerenal failure
2 Commoner with thiazides/frusemide
  a) Hypokalaemia (esp. significant in patients on digoxin)
  b) Precipitation of gout (esp. in females)
  c) Precipitation of clinical diabetes
  d) Precipitation of incontinence

DRUG TOXICITY IN RENAL DISEASE

Nephrotoxicity of non-steroidal anti-inflammatory drugs
1 Electrolyte disturbances
  a) Sodium retention (oedema)
  b) Hyponatraemia ± SIADH
  c) Hyperkalaemia, esp. in diabetics (↓ renin release)
2 Acute renal failure in volume-contracted patients (see below) due to antagonism of prostaglandin-mediated renal arteriolar vasodilatation: usually reversible
3 Acute tubular necrosis
4 Interstitial nephritis (drug hypersensitivity)
5 Papillary necrosis (due to medullary ischaemia)
6 Minimal change nephrosis (indomethacin, naproxen)
7 Antagonism of antihypertensive therapy (e.g. frusemide, ACE inhibitors) by indomethacin

Patient subsets at increased risk of NSAID nephrotoxicity
1 Elderly
2 Pre-existing renal impairment
3 Volume contraction
  a) Diuretics
  b) Cardiac failure
  c) Cirrhosis, nephrosis
  d) Hypertension
  e) Perioperative

Spectrum of antibiotic-induced nephrotoxicity
1 Anti-anabolic effect (→ ↑BUN): tetracyclines (exception: doxycycline)
2 Interstitial nephritis
  a) Penicillins (esp. methicillin)
  b) Cephalosporins, sulphonamides
  c) Rifampicin (esp. intermittent)
3 Hypokalaemic alkalosis: penicillins (esp. ticarcillin)
4 Proximal tubular necrosis: aminoglycosides (potentiated by frusemide, cephaloridine)
  Distal tubular necrosis — amphotericin B
5 Nephrogenic diabetes insipidus: demethylchlortetracycline (demeclocycline)
6 Crystalluria (→ collecting duct obstruction)
  a) Sulphadiazine (for nocardiosis)
  b) Nitrofurantoin
  c) 5FC
  d) Acyclovir

Accumulation of toxic drug metabolites in chronic renal failure?
1 Allopurinol
2 Digoxin
3 Methyldopa, metoprolol
4 Clofibrate
5 Opiates; propoxyphene

ALTERED DRUG REGIMENS IN RENAL DISEASE

Modification of drug therapy in renal failure
1 Avoid due to toxicity
   a) Potassium-sparing diuretics (esp. in elderly or diabetics) ACE inhibitors }— life-threatening hyperkalaemia
   b) Tetracyclines (except doxycycline) Cephaloridine, cephalothin }—worsen azotaemia
   c) Nitrofurantoin (→neuropathy; also ineffective)
   d) Chloramphenicol (active drug does *not* accumulate, but myelotoxic inactive metabolites do)
   e) Lithium carbonate (toxicity potentiated by diuretic therapy)
   f) Metformin (→lactic acidosis)
   g) Clofibrate (→myopathy)
   h) Methotrexate
2 Avoid due to ineffectiveness
   a) Thiazides
   b) Nalidixic acid, mandelamine
3 Major dose reduction required (either according to nomogram or serum level)
   a) Digoxin, procainamide
   b) Cimetidine; amantadine
   c) Vancomycin; aminoglycosides; amphotericin B
   d) Penicillin G, ampicillin, ticarcillin
   e) Sulphonamides, cephalosporins
   f) 5-FC (→crystalluria)
   g) Ethambutol (→ optic neuritis)
4 No dose reduction usually required
   a) Digitoxin; frusemide (beware ototoxicity)
   b) Prazosin, minoxidil, hydralazine
   c) Tolbutamide, glibenclamide
   d) Prednisone, azathioprine, heparin
   e) Doxycycline
   f) Flucloxacillin, erythromycin, fusidic acid
   g) Isoniazid, rifampicin
   h) Griseofulvin, miconazole, ketoconazole, clotrimazole
5 Dosage may (rarely) require increase — phenytoin (reduced plasma protein binding → ↑ free drug → ↑ liver metabolism; renal excretion of phenytoin is insignificant)

Drugs requiring repeat dosage following dialysis
1 After *either* peritoneal dialysis or haemodialysis
   a) Aminoglycosides
   b) Ticarcillin
   c) Cefuroxime, cephalothin
   d) Isoniazid, ethambutol

   e) 5FC
   f) Methyldopa
   g) Aspirin
2 After haemodialysis only
   a) Penicillins (except cloxacillin)
   b) Cephalosporins
   c) Metronidazole, trimethoprim
   d) Acyclovir
   e) Allopurinol
   f) Paracetamol
   g) Azathioprine, cyclophosphamide, prednisolone
   h) Captopril, metoprolol, minoxidil, nadolol

NB: cf. heavily protein-bound drugs — **not** dialysable

HAEMODIALYSIS

Indications for dialysis in renal failure
1 Symptomatic uraemia (despite optimal conservative management)
2 Fluid overload (diuretic-resistant)
3 Refractory hyperkalaemia (after diet, resins, bicarbonate)
4 Unacceptable decline in quality of life (esp. if due to development of longterm complication, e.g. neuropathy, pericarditis)

Biochemical consequences of a haemodialysis treatment
1 Reduction in
   a) Plasma creatinine/BUN
   b) Plasma potassium
   c) Plasma phosphate
   d) Plasma osmolality
2 Increase in
   a) Plasma bicarbonate/pH
   b) Plasma sodium
   c) Plasma calcium

Conditions with poor prognosis when treated by haemodialysis
1 Diabetes mellitus
2 Amyloidosis
3 Scleroderma
4 SLE
5 Hypertensive nephrosclerosis

Acute complications of haemodialysis
1 Hypotension
2 Arrhythmias (± digoxin toxicity)
3 Cramps; nausea; headaches; fever (e.g. due to *Staph.* bacteraemias)
4 Air embolism (due to i.v. bags with airways)
5 Exsanguination (due to external shunts)
6 Disequilibrium syndrome (headaches, hypertension, confusion, fitting; occurs during first few dialyses due to rapid reduction of extracellular osmolarity leading to cerebral oedema)

Chronic complications of haemodialysis
1 Accelerated atherosclerosis (60% die from myocardial or cerebral infarction)

2 Hepatitis B
3 Sexual dysfunction, infertility, depression
4 Wernicke's syndrome; central pontine myelinolysis
5 Vascular
   a) Fistula thrombosis or endarteritis
   b) Haemorrhagic events (subdural haematoma, pericarditis ± tamponade, stroke, GI bleeding)
6 Dialysis dementia (due to cerebral aluminium overload)
7 Arthropathy (amyloidosis)
8 Nephrogenic ascites (indicates dire prognosis unless transplanted or switched to CAPD)

ALTERNATIVES TO HAEMODIALYSIS

Relative indications for chronic ambulatory peritoneal dialysis (CAPD) in end-stage renal failure

1 Unsuitability for haemodialysis
   a) Extremes of age
   b) Cardiovascular instability
   c) Inadequate vascular access
   d) Heparin contraindicated (e.g. in pericarditis)
   e) Geographical remoteness
   f) Religious conviction (Jehovah's Witness)
2 Symptomatic progression while on haemodialysis
3 Diabetic retinopathy
4 Scleroderma

Problems encountered in CAPD patients

1 Peritonitis (esp. due to *S. albus*; Gram-negatives may indicate visceral perforation by catheter); loculated ascites
2 Catheter blockage
3 Hyperglycaemia, hypertriglyceridaemia → obesity, accelerated atheroma, worsening of diabetic control (necessitating intraperitoneal insulin)
4 Protein and amino acid depletion
5 Basal atelectasis, pleural effusions
6 Hernias
   Ileus (constipation)

NB: technique precluded by previous laparotomy (→ adhesions)

Advantages of CAPD over haemodialysis

1 Early benefits
   a) Better blood pressure control
   b) Higher Hb
   c) Less muscle wasting and weight loss
   d) Less acidosis
   d) No dialysis disequilibrium
2 Long-term benefits
   a) Loss of pigmentation
   b) Return of menstruation
   c) Improved calcium/phosphate balance

RENAL TRANSPLANTATION

Specific indications for transplantation

1 Severe renal osteodystrophy
2 Inability to cope with dialysis, esp. in young patient

Contraindications to transplantation

1 Lack of compatible kidney donor
2 Advanced age or debility
3 Chronic infection (TB, HBV, bronchiectasis, osteomyelitis)
4 Malignancy
5 Peptic ulceration
6 Primary disease known to recur in grafts (p. 267)

Significance of hypertension in the renal transplant patient

1 Fluid overload
2 Chronic rejection
3 Steroid-induced
4 Stenosis of donor renal artery
5 Renin production from remnant kidneys (rare)
6 Cyclosporin A toxicity (i.e. *independent* of nephrotoxicity)

Features of cyclosporin nephrotoxicity

1 Acute toxicity — ↓ GFR/renal blood flow
2 Chronic toxicity — interstitial fibrosis, tubular atrophy
3 Toxicity may be potentiated by other drugs, esp. ketoconazole

Graft complications related to surgery in renal transplantation

1 Ureteric obstruction
2 Lymphocoele
3 Renal vein thrombosis
4 Renal artery stenosis

Prolonged post-transplant oliguria; differential diagnosis

1 Acute rejection
2 Acute tubular necrosis
3 Arterial (anastomotic) stenosis or thrombosis
4 Ureteric obstruction (lymphocoele, haematoma, ischaemia)
5 Cyclosporin A nephrotoxicity
6 Sepsis (e.g. CMV, UTI)

Management of prolonged post-transplant oliguria if rejection suspected

1 Exclude vascular and ureteric obstruction
2 Transplant biopsy — is rejection confirmed?
3 If not, measure intrarenal pressure manometrically using 25 g-needle (abnormally elevated in rejection)
4 If diagnosis still in doubt, decrease cyclosporin A dose
5 If no improvement in serum creatinine within 48 hours of CSA reduction, proceed with therapeutic trial of steroids or azathioprine (i.e. as for confirmed graft rejection)

Features of cytomegalovirus graft infection

1 Manifests with post-transplant azotaemia and/or oliguria
2 Most severe infections occur in seronegative patients receiving grafts from seropositive donors (to the extent that this now constitutes a relative contraindication to matching)
3 Other mechanisms of infection include reactivation

in seropositive hosts (occurs in 90%; generally mild) and transmission by granulocyte transfusions. An association with the use of antilymphocyte (-thymocyte) globulin is also recognized
4 Biopsy reveals diffuse glomerular lesions with minimal interstitial inflammatory response (cf. rejection)
5 The helper/suppressor ratio in peripheral blood T-lymphocytes is generally lower in CMV graft infection than in rejection, but this is inconsistently affected by the immunosuppressive regimen

Clinical stigmata of graft rejection
1 Hyperacute
   a) May occur within minutes
   b) Irreversible; graft nephrectomy mandatory
2 Acute
   a) May occur at any time
   b) Graft swelling, tenderness, fever
   c) Oliguria, azotaemia
   d) ↓ Urinary sodium
   e) Active urine sediment
   f) May respond to immunosuppression
3 Chronic
   a) Occurs after months to years
   b) Inexorable, irreversible decline in GFR
   c) May manifest as interstitial nephritis or proliferative glomerulonephritis

Late problems following renal transplantation
1 Recurrent glomerulonephritis (contraindicates further attempts at transplantation; see below)
2 Reflux nephropathy
3 Avascular necrosis of bone (usually head of femur) Other steroid-related morbidity, e.g. cataracts
4 Infections
5 Malignancy (lymphoma, cerebral microglioma, SCC skin/cervix)

Renal biopsy patterns classically recurring in transplants
1 Dense deposit disease (mesangiocapillary glomerulonephritis type II)
2 Focal sclerosis and hyalinosis (e.g. due to reflux, heroin or analgesic abuse)
3 Oxalosis, cystinosis, amyloidosis
4 Severe diabetic glomerulosclerosis
5 Vasculitis
   a) Anti-GBM disease (Goodpasture's syndrome)
   b) PAN
   c) Cryoglobulinaemia
6 IgA nephropathy

Graft biopsy in transplant rejection: implications for therapy
1 Acute rejection refractory to steroids
   a) Biopsy → cellular infiltrate — increase the steroids
   b) Biopsy → intimal proliferation — cease steroids and organize graft nephrectomy
2 Chronic rejection provisionally diagnosed
   a) Biopsy → recurrence of original disease process

— abandon graft; further transplantation contraindicated
   b) Biopsy → confirmation of chronic rejection — prepare for dialysis, and for retransplantation if possible

RENAL CALCULI

Radiological appearances predicting stone composition
1 Opaque stones
   a) Calcium oxalate
   b) Calcium phosphate
   c) Struvite ('infection' stones, 'triple phosphate': magnesium ammonium phosphate, MAP), esp. if large staghorn morphology
2 Semi-opaque — cystine
3 Lucent
   a) Urate
   b) Xanthine   — rare
   c) Orotic acid
   d) 2,8 dihydroxyadenine

Determining the aetiology of renal calculi
1 Family history
   a) Cystinuria, xanthinuria, hyperoxaluria
   b) Gout
   c) Multiple endocrine adenomatosis (→1° HPT)
2 Medication history
   a) Megadose vitamin therapy
   b) Milk-alkali syndrome
   c) Acetazolamide (→ alkaline urine → urea-splitting oganisms)
   d) Probenecid
3 Strain urine for passed stone fragments
   a) Quantitative chemical analysis — calcium, magnesium, ammonium, phosphate, oxalate, carbonate, urate
   b) Qualitative chemical analysis — cystine
   c) Bacteriological analysis — esp. for Proteus spp.
4 Urine specimen analysis
   a) pH
   b) Microscopy
   c) Culture (esp. for urea-splitting organisms: Proteus mirabilis, Pseudomonas aeruginosa, Klebsiella spp.)
   d) Sodium nitroprusside test (for cystine)
   e) Crystal counts (cystine, struvite) in freshly voided sample
5 Quantitative 24-hour urine analysis
   a) Volume
   b) Oxalate
   c) Calcium, phosphate, urate
   d) Cystine (if qualitative tests positive)
   e) cAMP (if indicated)
6 Plasma biochemical analysis
   a) Calcium, bicarbonate
   b) Urate (abnormally low? exclude xanthinuria)
   c) Creatinine
   d) iPTH (if calcium elevated)
7 IVP
   a) Polycystic kidneys
   b) Medullary sponge kidneys
   c) Duplex collecting system

Children with renal stones: diagnoses to exclude

1 Cystinuria
2 Distal RTA (calcium phosphate stones)
3 Hereditary hyperoxaluria
4 Medullary sponge kidneys (calcium oxalate stones in adolescents)

Long-term management of recurrent renal calculi

1 High fluid intake (indicated for all stone types)
2 Calcium oxalate stones (50%)
   a) Thiazides } — 'Coe regimen'
   b) Allopurinol
   c) Low-oxalate diet
   d) Pyridoxine (*if* hereditary hyperoxaluria)
   e) Cholestyramine (*if* ileal disease present)
3 Calcium phosphate stones (25%)
   a) Thiazides ($\rightarrow \downarrow$ urinary calcium)
   b) Urinary acidification (oral citrate)
   c) Cellulose phosphate (binds calcium in gut)
   d) Low-calcium diet
4 Struvite (15%)
   a) Surgery
   b) Percutaneous shock wave lithotripsy
   c) Percutaneous nephrostomy with lavage chemolysis
   d) Antibiotics
   e) Urinary acidification (pH < 5.5)
   f) Acetohydroxamic acid (a urease inhibitor)
5 Urate stones (5–10%)
   a) Allopurinol
   b) Urinary alkalinization (pH > 6.5): bicarbonate/acetazolamide
   c) Low purine diet
6 Cystine stones (0.5–3%)
   a) Aggressive hydration (3–5 L/day)
   b) D-Penicillamine (beware of drug-induced nephrosis)
   c) Urinary alkalinization (pH > 7.5); less effective than for urate stones

IMMEDIATE THERAPY OF RENAL CALCULI

Extracorporeal shock wave lithotripsy: contraindications

1 Radiolucent stones (cf. gallstones)
2 Large (> 3 cm diameter) staghorn stones
3 Ureteric stones (lower two-thirds of ureter)

Prerequisites for Dormia basket removal of ureteric stones

1 Stone diameter < 5 mm, *and*
2 Stone situated < 5 cm from ureteric orifice, *and*
3 Stone impacted < 5 weeks duration

Potential indications for surgical management of renal stones

1 Complete outflow tract obstruction
2 Large staghorn calculus
3 Multiple stones
4 Failure to pass stone despite 5-week trial of conservative management

MASSIVE BLADDER HAEMORRHAGE

Precipitants of massive bladder haemorrhage

1 Trauma
2 Bladder tumours (esp. postradiotherapy)
3 Long-term cyclophosphamide therapy (haemorrhagic cystitis)
4 Amyloidosis

Management modalities in massive bladder haemorrhage

1 Intravesical vasopressin — works only for as long as infusion continued
2 Intravesical alum irrigation — precipitates mucosal protein; no toxicity (cf. formalin)
3 Helmstein balloon compression — may cause fibrosis (similar to formalin instillation)
4 Arterial embolization — effective measure in trauma cases
5 Supravesical urinary diversion — for intractable bleeding
6 Emergency cystectomy — for life-threatening haemorrhage resistant to above measures

UNDERSTANDING RENAL DISEASE

COMPLICATIONS OF RENAL DISEASE

Major pathogenetic mechanisms of anaemia in renal failure

1 Reduced erythropoietin secretion
2 Reduced utilization of iron stores (anaemia of chronic disease) due to ? 'uraemic toxins'
3 Reduced production of glutathione by pentose phosphate pathway leading to shortened erythrocyte survival (haemolysis)
4 Marrow fibrosis due to secondary hyperparathyroidism
5 Occult blood loss due to
   a) Impaired platelet function
   b) Heparinization during haemodialysis
   c) Loss of blood and folate during haemodialysis
   d) Surreptitious ongoing aspirin ingestion
6 Diagnostic phlebotomies

Mechanisms of impotence in chronic renal failure

1 Depression
2 Reduced serum testosterone
3 Hyperprolactinaemia
4 Autonomic neuropathy
5 Antihypertensive medications

Psychiatric aetiologies in chronic renal failure

1 Uraemia
2 Water intoxication
3 Rapid electrolyte shifts
4 Dialysis disequilibrium syndrome (?cerebral oedema)
5 Dialysis dementia (?aluminium-induced)

Manifestations of disturbed calcium homeostasis in renal disease

1 Proximal myopathy (vitamin D deficiency)

2 Hyperparathyroidism — bone pain and deformity
3 Osteopaenia
4 Osteomalacia — bone pain, deformity, pathological fracture
5 Avascular necrosis of the femoral head (in transplants)
6 Extraskeletal calcification
   a) Band keratopathy
   b) Pruritus
   c) Vascular calcification
   d) Periarticular soft tissues

RENAL OSTEODYSTROPHY

Pathogenesis of renal bone disease
1 Nephron loss → ↓ GFR → phosphate retention
2 Nephron loss → ↓ dihydroxylation (activation) of vitamin D(25-HCC); ↓ 1,25-DHCC → osteomalacia
3 Skeletal PTH resistance⎫
  Phosphate retention ⎬→ ↓ ionized serum calcium
  ↓ 1,25-DHCC   ⎭
4 ↓ Ca² → secondary hyperparathyroidism
  ↑ PTH → osteosclerosis and/or osteitis fibrosa cystica
5 Aluminium in dialysate (or in oral phosphate-binding drugs) may aggravate osteomalacic tendency; heparin → osteoporosis
6 Anorexia → dietary deficiencies

Radiographic features of renal osteodystrophy
1 90% of biopsy-proven cases will exhibit radiological abnormalities
2 50% have vascular calcification
3 50% have 'rugger-jersey' spine
4 25% have subperiosteal lesions

Factors predicting incidence and severity of osteomalacia
1 Duration of dialysis (cf. transplant: osteomalacia rare)
2 Bone aluminium content

Approach to management of renal osteodystrophy
1 GFR < 30 ml/min: prophylactic calcium supplements (5 g/day calcium carbonate = 2 g/day elemental calcium)
2 Development of significant hyperphosphataemia — add oral phosphate binders
3 Indications for oral 1,25-DHCC/dihydrotachysterol
   a) Development of hypocalcaemia
   b) Development of myopathy and/or bone pain
   c) Radiographic erosions or fractures
   d) Elevation of serum alkaline phosphatase
4 Tertiary (or severe secondary) hyperparathyroidism
   a) Regular calcitriol (1,25-DHCC) *infusions*
   b) Subtotal parathyroidectomy
5 Use aluminium-free dialysate when dialysing

INCONTINENCE

Urinary incontinence: important physical signs
1 Fever, cachexia; foul urine (UTI)
2 Suprapubic tenderness

Bladder enlargement to ⎫ retention with overflow
percussion   ⎭
3 Pelvic and rectal examination for masses, fistula, uterine prolapse
4 Associated faecal   ⎫
    incontinence   ⎪
  ↓ Anal sphincter tone   ⎬ cauda equina syndrome
  ↓ Bulbocavernosus reflex⎪
  Perianal anaesthesia   ⎪
5 Pyramidal signs ⎫
  Sensory level ⎬ cord compression
6 Peripheral neuropathy; optic atrophy
  Postural hypotension (autonomic neuropathy)
7 Gait apraxia (normal pressure hydrocephalus)
  Dementia; primitive reflexes
8 Urinalysis (glycosuria, haematuria, nitrites)

Medical management of urinary incontinence
1 Stress incontinence
   a) Phenylpropanolamine
   b) Systemic or topical oestrogens if postmenopausal
2 Urge incontinence (best response to treatment)
   a) Propantheline
   b) Emepronium bromide
3 Overflow incontinence — bethanechol (though may exacerbate symptoms in elderly)
4 Functional (e.g. dementia) — no specific drug therapy

Other measures in treating urinary incontinence
1 Pelvic floor exercises
  Bladder retraining
  Biofeedback
2 Pessary
  Penile clamp
  Intermittent catheterization
3 Surgical repair (for stress incontinence)
  Electrical sphincter stimulation
  Artificial sphincters

RENAL CYSTIC DISEASE

Clinical spectrum of renal cystic disease
1 Medullary sponge kidneys (sporadic inheritance)
   a) Manifests with stones or UTI in adults
   b) Normal life expectancy
2 Medullary cystic disease (adult type = autosomal dominant)
   a) Causes renal failure and osteodystrophy in childhood
   b) Associated with liver fibrosis and retinitis pigmentosa
3 Infantile polycystic disease (autosomal recessive)
   a) Causes renal failure in childhood
   b) Associated with liver fibrosis and portal hypertension
4 Adult polycystic disease (autosomal dominant)
   a) Causes renal failure in middle life
   b) Associated with cysts in liver, pancreas, spleen, lungs

Features of medullary sponge kidneys
1 Asymmetrically enlarged kidneys

2 Probably underdiagnosed (as idiopathic hypercalciuria) in calcium stone-formers; IVP → 'grapelike clusters'
3 Presents between 10 and 40 years of age (bimodal) 60% get calculi; usually oxalate, but *S. albus* infections may lead to struvite stones
4 30% get
   — Haematuria
   — UTI
   — Papillary necrosis/nephrocalcinosis
5 Does not usually lead to uraemia; may be totally asymptomatic
6 Instrumentation should be avoided if possible

Features of medullary cystic disease
1 Asymmetrically shrunken kidneys
2 Histology similar to chronic interstitial nephritis
3 Hypertension rare
4 Urinalysis typically normal
5 No calcification on IVP
6 Progresses inexorably to uraemia via proximal RTA and/or salt-losing nephropathy

ADULT POLYCYSTIC KIDNEY DISEASE

Polycystic kidney disease: features
1 Episodic loin pain (cyst haemorrhage/torsion, clot colic, calculi)
2 Haematuria ± nocturia, mild proteinuria
3 Hypertension
4 Urinary tract infections
5 Anaemia (normochromic **or** hypochromic) **or** polycythaemia

Associations of polycystic kidney disease
1 Cysts in liver (30%), spleen, pancreas
2 Saccular aneurysms, esp. cerebral (10%)
3 Colonic diverticulosis
4 Aortic root dilatation, aortic incompetence Mitral valve prolapse, mitral incompetence
5 Rare
   a) Myotonic dystrophy
   b) Hereditary spherocytosis
   c) Peutz-Jeghers syndrome

Principles of management in adult polycystic disease
1 Prompt effective treatment of hypertension and urinary tract infection
2 Non-nephrotoxic analgesics for recurrent flank pain
3 Transplant work-up (if and when azotaemia supervenes)
4 Genetic counselling (normal IVP — ± ultrasound — at age 20 makes future development of polycystic disease unlikely)
5 Rarely, cyst puncture or nephrectomy may be indicated

MISCELLANEOUS RENAL DISORDERS

Pathogenetic mechanisms implicated in 'heroin nephropathy'
1 Nephritis due to contaminants (e.g. lead), typically focal sclerosing

2 Immune-complex mediated nephritis due to heroin acting as a hapten
3 Postinfective
   a) Staphylococcal bacteraemias
   b) Hepatitis B
4 Myoglobinuric nephropathy due to associated rhabdomyolysis

Clinical spectrum of analgesic-related disease
1 General
   a) Psychiatric disorder; passive aggression; headaches
   b) Premature ageing; pigmentation
   c) Dementia
2 Anaemia
   a) Normochromic (often disproportionate to azotaemia)
   b) Hypochromic (occult gastric bleeding)
   c) Megaloblastic (postgastrectomy)
3 Peptic ulceration (gastric); vague gastrointestinal symptoms
4 Hypertension (± renovascular component) Ischaemic heart disease
5 Renal complications
   a) Sterile pyuria; haemoproteinuria
   b) Salt-losing nephropathy, nocturia
   c) Nephrogenic diabetes insipidus
   d) Renal tubular acidosis
   e) Renal colic
   f) Osteomalacia
   g) Ureteric strictures
   h) Frequent UTI (esp. *Proteus*)
   i) Chronic renal failure
6 Malignancy — transitional cell carcinoma of renal pelvis

Spectrum of heredofamilial renal disease
1 Alport's syndrome (AD)
   a) Females are mildly affected; no nerve deafness
   b) Associated with lens abnormalities, platelet dysfunction, hyperprolinaemia and/or cerebral malfunction
   c) Does *not* recur after transplantation
2 Fabry's disease (AR) — ↓ α-galactosidase A
   a) Affected females have isolated renal impairment
   b) Associated with lower body punctate macules ('bathing trunk' distribution of angiokeratomas), corneal dystrophy, ischaemic heart disease, acroparaesthesiae in affected males
3 Nail-patella syndrome (AD)
   a) Dystrophic nails, esp. thumb and index
   b) Absent patellae
   c) X-ray → absent iliac horns
   d) Frequently manifests as nephrosis; characteristic 'moth-eaten' appearance of glomerular basement membrane

Retroperitoneal fibrosis: associations and features
1 Aetiologic associations (usually idiopathic)
   a) Methysergide, dexamphetamine, ergotamine
   b) Carcinoma; Crohn's disease
   c) Connective tissue disorders, Raynaud's
   d) Middle-aged males; HLA-B27
2 Clinical associations
   a) Mediastinal fibrosis (→ aortic/caval involvement)

b) Sclerosing cholangitis
c) Fibrosing alveolitis
d) Riedel's thyroiditis
e) Peyronie's disease
f) Pseudotumour oculi
g) Coronary arterial fibrosis
h) Constrictive pericarditis
(NB: sclerosing peritonitis due to practolol or carcinoid syndrome is a distinct entity)
3 Pathological features

a) Periaortic inflammation with lymphocyte and plasma cell infiltration commencing in lower abdomen or mediastinum — ureters fibrosed (lumen *not* occluded)
4 Radiographic features — medial deviation of lower two-thirds of both ureters on IVP
5 Therapeutic features — may respond dramatically to corticosteroids, but genitourinary TB leading to ureteric strictures must be *actively* excluded beforehand

Reviewing the Literature: Renal Medicine

12.1 Winearls C G et al 1986 Effect of human erythropoietin derived from recombinant DNA on the anaemia of patients maintained by chronic haemodialysis. Lancet ii: 1175–1177

First study to demonstrate the efficacy of recombinant erythropoietin in raising haematocrits of azotaemic patients

12.2 de Bold A J et al 1981 A rapid and potent natriuretic response to intravenous injection of atrial myocardial extract in rats. Life Sciences 28: 89–94

Original characterization of atrial natriuretic peptide, abnormalities of which have since been implicated in the pathogenesis of hypertension, oedema and cardiac failure

12.3 Taguma Y et al 1985 Effect of captopril on heavy proteinuria in azotaemic diabetics. New England Journal of Medicine 313: 1617–1620

Report suggesting that captopril reduced proteinuria without increasing creatinine or serum potassium, esp. in diabetic patients with hypertension

Bjorck S et al 1986 Beneficial effects of angiotensin converting enzyme inhibition on renal function in patients with diabetic nephropathy. British Medical Journal 293: 471–474

Small study showing a reduction in proteinuria, and slowing of renal deterioration, in diabetic patients.

12.4 Hossack K F et al 1988 Echocardiographic findings in autosomal dominant polycystic kidney disease. New England Journal of Medicine 319: 907—912

Patients with adult polycystic kidney disease (and their relatives) had an unexpectedly high incidence of mitral valve prolapse, mitral incompetence, aortic incompetence, tricuspid incompetence, and tricuspid valve prolapse, suggesting that the pathophysiology of adult PCK is related to a defect of extracellular matrix production

12.5 Johnson J P et al 1985 Therapy of antiglomerular basement membrane antibody disease: analysis of prognostic significance of clinical, pathologic and therapeutic factors. Medicine (Baltimore) 64: 219–227

Although plasma exchange seemed more effective than pulse i.v. methylprednisolone, the only independent predictors of outcome were histology and renal function (poor outcome associated with crescentic glomerulonephritis and low GFR)

12.6 Gregory M C et al 1988 Renal deposition of CMV antigen in IgA nephropathy. Lancet i: 11–13

31 out of 31 patients with IgA nephropathy (Berger's disease) had positive CMV antigen detected in renal biopsy specimens, compared with only 2 out of 39 patients with other glomerulopathies

Waldo F B et al 1989 Non-specific mesangial staining with antibodies against cytomegalovirus in IgA nephropathy. Lancet i: 129–132

Study of 12 patients suggesting that previous observations of anti-CMV antibody binding to IgA nephropathy glomeruli may have been an artefact due to contaminating antibodies

Snydman D R et al 1987 Use of CMV immune globulin to prevent CMV disease in renal transplant recipients. New England Journal of Medicine 317: 1049–1054

CMV immune globulin appeared effective in preventing CMV disease, esp. in CMV-seronegative recipients of CMV-seropositive organ donors

Balfour H H et al 1989 A randomized, placebo-controlled trial of oral acyclovir for the prevention of cytomegalovirus disease in recipients of renal allografts. New England Journal of Medicine 320: 1381–1387

Prophylactic oral acyclovir was a great success in preventing symptomatic CMV infection in recipients of cadaver kidneys, but did not make any difference in terms of either graft or patient survival

12.7 Chang C R et al 1986 Comparison of therapy of renal calculi by open surgery, percutaneous nephrolithotomy, and extracorporeal shock wave lithotripsy. British Medical Journal 292: 879–882

Study of 1052 patients concluded that ESWL was the cheapest and quickest way of returning patients to normal life — even though the apparatus at the time cost around two million dollars.

Roos N P et al 1989 Mortality and reoperation after open and transurethral resection of the prostate for benign prostatic hyperplasia. New England Journal of Medicine 320: 1120–1124

Eight-year retrospective study of 55 000 prostate resection patients, suggesting a lower age-specific mortality in patients having undergone open (transrectal) prostatectomy when compared to good old-fashioned TURP.

12.8 Reeders S T et al 1986 Prenatal diagnosis of autosomal

dominant polycystic kidney disease with a DNA probe. Lancet ii: 6–8

First report of successful prenatal screening for one type of adult-onset polycystic disease using recombinant DNA technology

12.9   Ortho Multicenter Transplant Study Group 1985 A randomized clinical trial of OKT3 monoclonal antibody for acute rejection of cadaveric renal transplants. New England Journal of Medicine 313: 337–342

Prospective randomized trial of 123 patients; 94% of antibody-treated patients resolved their rejection episodes, compared with 75% of patients treated with conventional high-dose steroids alone. This difference was associated with improved 12-month survival (62% vs 45%)

12.10   Ponticelli C, Zucchelli P, Imbasciati E et al 1984

Controlled trial of methylprednisolone and chlorambucil in idiopathic membranous nephropathy. New England Journal of Medicine 310: 946–950

A randomized trial of 67 patients which compared the results of symptomatic management with those obtained with immunosuppression. Significantly improved remission rates and renal function were documented in patients undergoing active treatment, the period of follow-up being 7 years

Cattran D C et al 1989 A randomized controlled trial of prednisone in patients with idiopathic membranous nephropathy. New England Journal of Medicine 320: 210–215

Prospective randomized trial of 158 patients with idiopathic membranous nephropathy, suggesting that a 6-month course of alternate-day steroids (45 mg/m^2) conferred no benefit. Hence, optimal therapy in this disorder remains controversial

CHAPTER 13
Respiratory medicine

Physical examination protocol 13.1 You are asked to examine the respiratory system.

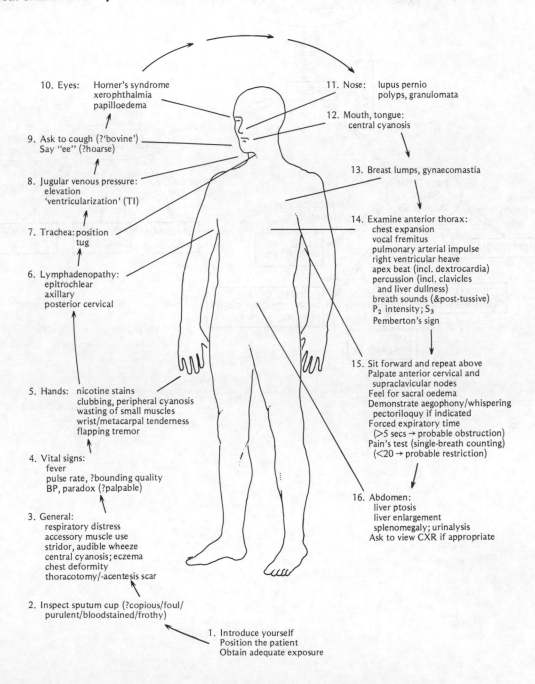

10. Eyes: Horner's syndrome
xerophthalmia
papilloedema

9. Ask to cough (?'bovine')
Say "ee" (?hoarse)

8. Jugular venous pressure:
elevation
'ventricularization' (TI)

7. Trachea: position
tug

6. Lymphadenopathy:
epitrochlear
axillary
posterior cervical

5. Hands: nicotine stains
clubbing, peripheral cyanosis
wasting of small muscles
wrist/metacarpal tenderness
flapping tremor

4. Vital signs:
fever
pulse rate, ?bounding quality
BP, paradox (?palpable)

3. General:
respiratory distress
accessory muscle use
stridor, audible wheeze
central cyanosis; eczema
chest deformity
thoracotomy/-acentesis scar

2. Inspect sputum cup (?copious/foul/
purulent/bloodstained/frothy)

1. Introduce yourself
Position the patient
Obtain adequate exposure

11. Nose: lupus pernio
polyps, granulomata

12. Mouth, tongue:
central cyanosis

13. Breast lumps, gynaecomastia

14. Examine anterior thorax:
chest expansion
vocal fremitus
pulmonary arterial impulse
right ventricular heave
apex beat (incl. dextrocardia)
percussion (incl. clavicles
and liver dullness)
breath sounds (&post-tussive)
P_2 intensity; S_3
Pemberton's sign

15. Sit forward and repeat above
Palpate anterior cervical and
supraclavicular nodes
Feel for sacral oedema
Demonstrate aegophony/whispering
pectoriloquy if indicated
Forced expiratory time
(>5 secs → probable obstruction)
Pain's test (single-breath counting)
(<20 → probable restriction)

16. Abdomen:
liver ptosis
liver enlargement
splenomegaly; urinalysis
Ask to view CXR if appropriate

Diagnostic pathway 13.1   This patient is breathless. Why do you think that might be?

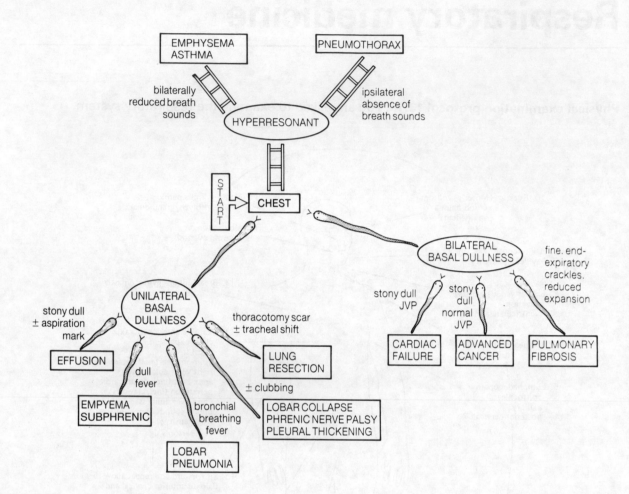

CLINICAL ASPECTS OF RESPIRATORY DISEASE

COMMONEST RESPIRATORY SHORT CASES

1 Pleural effusion
2 Chronic obstructive airways disease ($\pm$ cor pulmonale)

DYSPNOEA

Grading of exertional dyspnoea by clinical history
(Medical Research Council — MRC — criteria)
1 MRC I — troubled by dyspnoea when hurrying on level ground or walking up a slight hill
2 MRC II — troubled by dyspnoea when walking with people of one's own age on level ground
3 MRC III — troubled by dyspnoea (sufficient to necessitate stopping) when walking at one's own pace on level ground

Dyspnoea: typical rates of onset
1 Maximal within seconds
  a) Pneumothorax
  b) Pulmonary embolism
2 Maximal within hours
  a) Asthma
  b) Hypersensitivity pneumonitis
  c) Pneumonia
  d) Cardiac failure
  e) Haemorrhage
3 Maximal within days to months
  a) Progressive anaemia
  b) Progression of restrictive lung disease
  c) Exacerbation of obstructive airways disease
  d) Enlarging pleural effusion(s)
  e) Primary or secondary malignancy

'Blue bloater' or 'pink puffer'? Factors favouring dominant emphysema ($>$ chronic bronchitis)
1 Severe subjective dyspnoea
2 Scanty sputum, few infections
3 CXR — hypertransradiant lungs, 'thin' heart
4 $P_a\text{CO}_2 < 40$ mmHg
  $P_a\text{O}_2 > 60$ mmHg
5 Haematocrit not elevated
6 No signs of pulmonary hypertension or cor pulmonale

PRESENTATIONS OF RESPIRATORY DISEASE

Differential diagnosis of recurrent haemoptysis
1 Bronchiectasis; chronic bronchitis
2 Bronchial adenoma
3 Mitral stenosis; recurrent left ventricular failure
4 Recurrent pulmonary embolism with infarction
5 Telangiectasia (arteriovenous malformation)

Predispositions to recurrent lower respiratory tract infections
1 Hypogammaglobulinaemia

2 Ciliary dysfunction
  a) Cystic fibrosis
  b) Immotile cilia syndrome
  c) Pulmonary alveolar proteinosis
  d) Bronchiectasis
3 Autoimmune disease
  a) Sjögren's syndrome
  b) Relapsing polychondritis
4 Oesophageal disease
  a) Achalasia
  b) Scleroderma
  c) Riley-Day syndrome
  d) Pharyngeal pouch
5 Cardiovascular disease
  a) Atrial septal defect
  b) Mitral stenosis
  c) Pulmonary emboli

Diagnostic considerations in refractory pneumonia
1 Wrong antibiotics
2 Multiple or unusual organisms
3 Immunosuppressed patient (e.g. myeloma, AIDS, transplant)
4 Empyema/abscess formation
5 Recurrent aspiration (e.g. pharyngeal pouch)
6 Proximal endobronchial neoplasm
7 Misdiagnosis
  a) Lymphoma, alveolar cell carcinoma
  b) Pulmonary infarction
  c) Pulmonary haemorrhage
  d) Adult respiratory distress syndrome
  e) Hypersensitivity pneumonitis
  f) Pulmonary eosinophilia
  g) Pulmonary oedema
  h) Radiation pneumonitis
  i) Drug (incl. antibiotic) reaction

Differential diagnosis of unexplained pleuritic pain
1 Pleurodynia (Bornholm's disease, epidemic myalgia)
2 Pneumonia
3 Pneumothorax
4 Pulmonary infarction
5 Pericarditis
6 (Sub)phrenic abscess
7 Pancreatitis
8 Pathologic rib fracture

Some age-related causes of wheezing
1 Infant/young child — inhaled foreign body
2 Adolescent/young adult — atopic asthma
3 Middle age — endobronchial neoplasm
4 Old age — left ventricular failure

  (NB: wheeze does *not* occur in hypersensitivity pneumonitis)

CLINICAL SIGNS OF RESPIRATORY DISEASE

Diagnostic clues from sputum examination
1 Copious, purulent, pungent — bronchiectasis, lung abscess
2 Copious, pink, frothy — acute left ventricular failure
3 Copious, clear, watery — alveolar cell carcinoma

4 Rubbery brown plugs — allergic bronchopulmonary aspergillosis
5 'Anchovy sauce' — amoebic abscess
6 Melanoptysis (jet-black fibrotic particles)— coalworker's pneumoconiosis with progressive massive fibrosis
7 'Blood oyster' (frank blood embedded within mucopurulent sputum) — TB
8 Rusty staining of mucoid sputum — early pneumococcal pneumonia

Clinical components of clubbing
1 Soft tissue swelling
2 Loss of nailfold angle (>150°)
3 Exaggerated curvature of long axis of nail
4 Increased nailbed fluctuation ('boggy') on pressure
5 May be associated with wrist/metacarpal tenderness (HPO)

Differential diagnosis of basal crackles with clubbing
1 Bronchiectasis — coarse crackles (may be unilateral)
2 Asbestosis
3 Idiopathic fibrosing alveolitis } —bibasilar fine end-inspiratory crackles

Clinical significance of basal dullness
1 Stony — pleural effusion
2 'Non-stony'
   a) Loss of aeration (consolidation, abscess)
   b) Loss of lung volume (collapse, fibrosis)

Examination of the patient with bronchiectasis
1 Copious purulent sputum (foul-smelling if anaerobic)
2 Clubbing, coarse crackles
3 Look for
   a) Nasal discharge and or polyps
   b) Dextrocardia
   c) Hepatosplenomegaly
   d) Enlarged kidneys } —due to reactive amyloidosis

Causes of hepatomegaly in respiratory disease
1 Chronic venous congestion in cor pulmonale
2 Metastatic liver disease (in lung cancer)
3 Spurious (ptosed liver) in emphysema

Peripheral oedema: pathogenesis in respiratory disease
1 Right ventricular failure
2 Sequelae of chronic systemic venous congestion
   a) 'Cardiac cirrhosis'
   b) Protein-losing enteropathy
   c) Nephrosis
3 Membranous nephropathy (paraneoplastic)
4 Yellow nail syndrome (lymphoedema)
5 Fluid retention due to corticosteroid administration

OBSTRUCTIVE SLEEP APNOEA

Sleep apnoea: presenting complaints
1 Snoring (in obstructive variety); insomnia
Nocturnal choking and/or panic attacks
Hypnagogic hallucinations; nightmares

2 Disorientation after waking
Excessive daytime somnolence (→ car accidents)
3 Morning headaches (CO_2 retention)
4 Depression, personality change
5 Impotence; nocturnal enuresis; reduced libido
6 Related to aetiology, e.g. myxoedema, acromegaly

Complications of sleep apnoea
1 Systemic hypertension (70%)
2 Pulmonary hypertension
Impaired diurnal pulmonary function (70%)
3 Polycythaemia
4 Nocturnal cardiac arrhythmias (incl. bradycardia)
5 Cor pulmonale (40%)
Respiratory failure
Unexpected death during sleep

Treatment modalities in obstructive sleep apnoea
1 Weight loss
2 Nocturnal nasal C-PAP (continuous positive airways pressure)
3 Medroxyprogesterone acetate
4 Tracheostomy

INVESTIGATING RESPIRATORY DISEASE

Electrophoretographic clues in respiratory diagnosis
1 α-1 pallor — emphysema due to α_1AT deficiency
2 Hypogammaglobulinaemia — may underlie chronic bronchitis
3 Polyclonal gammopathy — sarcoidosis (inter alia)

Diagnosis of α-1-antitrypsin deficiency
1 Family history of emphysema or childhood liver disease
(neonatal hepatitis ± infantile cirrhosis)
2 Development of symptomatic emphysema in a young patient (< 40 years) or in a non-smoker; rarely, may manifest as mesangiocapillary glomerulonephritis
3 Basal hyperlucency on CXR
4 Panacinar (-lobular) emphysema on lung biopsy
5 α-1 pallor on electrophoresis
   ↓ α_1AT levels on quantitative assay
   PiZZ (i.e. homozygous) phenotype

Sputum microscopy in atopic asthma: features
1 Eosinophils
2 Charcot-Leyden crystals (eosinophil derivatives)
3 Creola bodies (clumps of bronchiolar epithelial cells)
4 Curschmann's spirals (bronchiolar casts)

TESTING LUNG FUNCTION

Lung function tests: typical disease patterns
1 Obstructive airways disease
   a) ↑ Residual volume (RV)
   b) ↓ FEV_1/VC (< 70%)
   c) ↑↑ RV/TLC (total lung capacity)
   (NB: VC and TLC may be normal in 'pure' emphysema)

2 Restrictive lung disease
   a) ↓ RV, VC, TLC
   b) N, ↑ FEV_1/VC
   c) N, ↑ RV/TLC

Lung function monitors in large airway disease
1 FEV_1/VC
2 PEFR (peak expiratory flow rate)
3 V_{max} (density-dependence of maximal expiratory flow)
4 Airways resistance

Lung function monitors in small airway disease
(e.g. subclinical lung dysfunction in smokers with normal FEV_1)
1 Maximal mid-expiratory flow rate (MMFR) at 50% and 25% VC
2 Single-breath nitrogen washout studies (slope of phase III)
   Closing volume
3 Flow-volume curves (also useful in extrathoracic obstruction)
4 Frequency-dependence of dynamic compliance — most sensitive test, but invasive (oesophageal balloon required)
5 $V_{max\ 50}$
6 Other — ↑ RV; ↓ $FEV_{3.0}$; ↓ DL_{CO}; postural changes in P_aO_2

Abnormalities of the peak expiratory flow rate (PEFR)
1 Reduced
   a) Obstructive airways disease (e.g. asthma)
   b) Respiratory muscle weakness
   c) Poor technique
2 Normal or increased — restrictive lung disease (e.g. fibrosis)

ARTERIAL BLOOD GAS ANALYSIS

Clues to the interpretation of arterial blood gases
1 ↓ P_aO_2 normalizing on 100% oxygen; ↑ P_aCO_2 — alveolar hypoventilation (e.g. overdose, Pickwickian, Guillain-Barré)
2 ↓ P_aO_2 normalizing on 100% oxygen; normal or low P_aCO_2 — V/Q mismatch (NB: *severe* mismatching may cause elevated P_aCO_2)
3 ↓ P_aO_2 *not* correcting with 100% oxygen; normal P_aCO_2 — shunting (intrapulmonary or intracardiac)
4 Normal or slightly reduced P_aO_2; ↓↓ P_aO_2 on exercise, normalizing with 100% oxygen; normal or low P_aCO_2
   a) Diffusion defect (rare)
   b) Altitude
5 P_aO_2 <60 mmHg, P_aCO_2 >45 mmHg — exclude inadvertent venous (non-arterial) blood sample

Differential diagnosis of increased alveolar-arterial (A-a) oxygen gradient*
(*P_aO_2/R, where $R = 0.8$ normally; normal A-a gradient <15 mmHg)
1 Ventilation/perfusion mismatching, e.g.
   a) Airways obstruction
   b) Pulmonary embolism

2 Shunt
   a) Intrapulmonary (e.g. ARDS, pulmonary oedema)
   b) Intracardiac (e.g. Eisenmenger's syndrome)
3 Diffusion defect (minor contribution to pathophysiology of fibrotic and emphysematous lung disease; V/Q mismatch is more important)

Tissue hypoxia with normal cardiorespiratory capacity
1 Hypoxaemia despite normal A-a gradient
   a) Alveolar hypoventilation
   b) ↓ F_iO_2 (e.g. altitude)
2 Normal P_aO_2 with increased oxyhaemoglobin affinity
   a) Massive transfusion of stored blood (↑ citrate → ↓ 2,3DPG)
   b) Bicarbonate administration in ketoacidosis
   c) Profound hypothermia/acidaemia/hypophosphataemia/myxoedema
   d) High-affinity Hb (e.g. Köln, Chesapeake)
   e) Carbon monoxide poisoning
3 Cyanide intoxication
4 Hyperviscosity
5 Anaemia

Acid-base disturbances in respiratory disease
1 Acute respiratory acidosis (ventilatory failure) — 10 mmHg ↑ P_aCO_2 → 1 mEq/l ↑ HCO_3^- (tissue buffering)
2 Chronic respiratory acidosis (incl. 'acute-on-chronic' exacerbations, e.g. of chronic bronchitis)
   a) 10 mmHg ↑ P_aCO_2 → 3 mEq/l ↑ HCO_3^- (increased renal reabsorption of HCO_3^- and increased acid excretion)
   b) High base excess
3 Acute respiratory alkalosis (e.g. secondary to ketoacidosis) — 10 mmHg ↓ P_aCO_2 → 2 mEq/l ↓ HCO_3^-
4 Chronic respiratory alkalosis (e.g. 'pink puffer') — 10 mmHg ↓ P_aCO_2 → 5 mEq/l ↓ HCO_3^- (rarely <15 mmol/l)

Clinical manifestations of carbon dioxide retention
1 P_aCO_2 > 80 mmHg: progressive impairment of consciousness
   Central cyanosis seen at rest if HbO_2 saturation <85%
2 Neurological
   a) Flapping tremor
   b) Hyporeflexia; muscle twitching
   c) Sweating
   d) Headache
3 Vascular
   a) Hypertension
   b) Bounding pulse
   c) Warm extremities (cf. peripheral cyanosis)
   d) Oedema, tender pulsatile liver *if* cor pulmonale present
4 Ocular
   a) Miosis
   b) Retinal vein distension
   c) Papilloedema
5 P_aCO_2 > 120 mmHg: extensor plantar responses; coma

Clinical significance of central cyanosis

1 Alveolar hypoventilation (type II respiratory failure), e.g. due to sedative overdose
2 Right-to-left shunting ($\uparrow F_iO_2 \rightarrow \uparrow P_aO_2$)
3 Mechanical — superior vena caval obstruction
4 Normal P_aO_2
   a) Polycythaemia vera
   b) Low-affinity Hb (e.g. Kansas, Hammersmith)
5 *Severe V/Q* mismatching (type I respiratory failure), e.g. due to massive pulmonary embolism

RESTRICTIVE LUNG DISEASE

Lung function monitors in restrictive lung disease

1 Post-exercise A-a (alveolar-arterial oxygen) gradient or HbO_2 desaturation
2 DL_{CO}
3 Static compliance
4 VC, TLC (e.g. in myasthenia gravis)

Additional disease monitors in fibrosing alveolitis

1 Cellularity of bronchoalveolar lavage (see below)
2 Gallium-67 scanning (taken up by macrophages; semi-quantitative)
3 Transbronchial biopsy (generally restricted to initial diagnosis)

Conditions affecting measurement of diffusing capacity

1 ↑ DL_{CO}
   a) Alveolar haemorrhage
      — Goodpasture's syndrome (may indicate recent bleed)
      — Idiopathic pulmonary haemosiderosis
      — Mitral stenosis
   b) Acute asthma
   c) Physiological — high-output states (incl. exercise); altitude
   d) Polycythaemia
2 ↓ DL_{CO}
   a) Pulmonary fibrosis
   b) Severe *V/Q* mismatching
      — Emphysema
      — Pulmonary embolism
      — Pneumonectomy
   c) Anaemia (NB: may complicate alveolar haemorrhagic states)

BRONCHOALVEOLAR LAVAGE (BAL)

Indications for bronchoalveolar lavage

1 Therapeutic (heparin/acetylcysteine) lavage
   a) Pulmonary alveolar proteinosis
   b) Cystic fibrosis/bronchiectasis
   c) Asthma with mucus plugging
2 Diagnostic (saline) lavage
   a) Opportunistic infections
   b) Confirmation of asbestos exposure
3 Research: interstitial lung disease (see below)

Normal composition of BAL fluid

1 Macrophages — 90%
2 Lymphocytes — 7–9%
3 Polymorphs — < 3% (usually <1%)

BAL cell counts in disease

1 Smokers
   a) Overall increase in cellularity (up to 5-fold)
   b) Reduced number of activated T-cells
   c) Reduced function of macrophages and lymphocytes
2 Fibrosing alveolitis
   a) Increased polymorphs (5–50%) in active disease
   b) Prognosis worse if >10% polymorphs (esp. if gallium +)
   c) Prognosis may be better *if* lymphocytosis present
3 Sarcoidosis
   a) Lymphocytosis (up to 40%; predominantly T-helper cells)*
   b) May be predictive of steroid-responsiveness
4 Hypersensitivity pneumonitis
   — Lymphocytosis (cf. fibrosing alveolitis)
5 Histiocytosis X
   — Histiocytosis X cells (containing 'X bodies')
   — Cholesterol-laden macrophages ('foam cells')

Indications for bronchography in suspected bronchiectasis

1 Prerequisite — potentially operable (i.e. fit) patient
2 Recurrent localized pneumonia
3 Severe haemoptysis

BRONCHOSCOPY

Indications for bronchoscopy

1 Rigid (under general anaesthesia)
   a) Removal of foreign body
   b) Therapeutic lavage
   c) Large biopsy required
2 Fibreoptic
   a) CXR suggesting primary endobronchial neoplasm
   b) Haemoptysis and/or positive sputum cytology
   c) Assessment of stridor or localized wheeze
   d) Unexplained diffuse lung disease or CXR opacities
   e) Diagnosis of suspected opportunistic (e.g. invasive fungal) infection, esp. in immunosuppressed patient

Contraindications to bronchoscopy

1 Severe hypoxaemia (any cause, esp. respiratory)
2 Severe asthma
3 Severe pulmonary hypertension
4 Severe haemoptysis
5 Cardiovascular instability (e.g. recent infarct)
6 Hepatitis B, HIV infection, or untreated TB
7 Unavailability of experienced bronchoscopist

Contraindications to transbronchial biopsy

1 Coagulopathy
2 Uraemia
3 PEEP

NB: SVC obstruction is *not* generally regarded as a contraindication to bronchoscopic biopsy

---

*Peripheral blood: lymphopenia, relative excess of *suppressor* T-cells

Diagnostic significance of lung granulomata
1 Caseating
 a) Tuberculosis
 b) Some atypical mycobacteria
2 Sarcoidosis
3 Histoplasmosis (and other fungal infections)
4 Hypersensitivity pneumonitis
5 Wegener's granulomatosis
6 Churg-Strauss syndrome (perivascular granulomata)
7 Berylliosis
8 Histiocytosis X
 Lethal midline granuloma
 Lymphomatoid granulomatosis

PLEURAL DISEASE

Diagnostic aspects of pleural effusions
1 Transudate (< 30 g/l protein; often bilateral)
 a) Cardiac failure, constrictive pericarditis
 b) Cirrhosis, nephrosis
 c) Myxoedema
 d) Meigs' syndrome
  (i.e. transudate and/or peripheral oedema
  suggest that local pathology is unlikely)
2 Uniformly bloodstained effusion
 a) Metastatic carcinoma (i.e. to pleura)
 b) Pulmonary infarction
 c) Primary TB (parapneumonic effusion)
3 Chylous effusion (positive Sudan III stain)
 a) Trauma (esp. endoscopy or surgery)
 b) Lymphomas
 c) Other masses compressing the thoracic duct
 d) Nephrosis, cirrhosis (uncommon)
 e) Spurious ('pseudochylous' effusions due to high
  cholesterol in TB/rheumatoid effusions; Sudan III
  negative)
4 Elevated amylase
 a) Oesophageal perforation (salivary isoenzyme)
 b) Pancreatitis
5 Low glucose
 a) Rheumatoid arthritis
 b) Empyema formation in parapneumonic effusion
6 pH
 a) < 6.0 — oesophageal rupture
 b) < 7.2 — implies empyema formation (and
  thereby implies need for thoracostomy drainage)

Predominant lateralization of specific effusions
1 Left-sided
 a) Pancreatitis (if right-sided, suspect pseudocyst)
 b) Pericarditis
 c) Perinephric abscess
 d) Oesophageal perforation
2 Right-sided
 a) Cardiac failure
 b) Tuberculosis
 c) Meigs' syndrome
 d) Catamenial
 e) Ascites; peritoneal dialysis
 f) Hydatid disease, subphrenic abscess

Possible indications for pleural biopsy
1 Suspected tuberculosis (biopsy should be cultured)
2 Suspected malignant pleural effusion; cytology
 negative
3 Suspected granulomatous disorder

RADIOGRAPHIC DIAGNOSIS OF LUNG DISEASE

Upper zone CXR infiltrates: differential diagnosis
1 Tuberculosis, aspergillosis, *Klebsiella* pneumonia
2 Silicosis
3 Histiocytosis X
4 Radiation fibrosis
5 Ankylosing spondylitis
6 Hypersensitivity pneumonitis (long-standing)

Lower zone CXR infiltrates: differential diagnosis
1 Idiopathic pulmonary fibrosis
2 Pulmonary fibrosis due to connective tissue disease
3 Asbestosis
4 Bronchiectasis
5 Cytotoxic-induced lung disease
6 Pulmonary haemosiderosis
7 Aspiration
8 Hypersensitivity pneumonitis (acute)

Radiographic localization of mediastinal masses
1 Any section
 a) Aortic aneurysm
 b) Lymphoma/metastatic carcinoma (i.e. nodes)
2 Superior mediastinum
 a) Thymoma
 b) Retrosternal thyroid
 c) Zenker's diverticulum
3 Anterior/middle
 a) Dermoid cyst/teratoma
 b) Bronchogenic/pericardial cyst
 c) Morgagni diaphragmatic hernia
4 Posterior
 a) Neurogenic tumours (and other paravertebral
  masses)
 b) Bochdalek diaphragmatic hernia (cf. Morgagni)
 c) Achalasia, hiatus hernia

Indications for special CXR projections
1 (Lateral) decubitus — suspected small pleural
 effusion, esp. if subpulmonic
2 Expiratory
 a) Suspected pneumothorax
 b) Suspected segmental bronchial occlusion (esp.
  child inhaling foreign body)
3 Erect — suspected perforation of abdominal hollow
 viscus
4 Penetrated PA
 a) Suspected left atrial enlargement
 b) Suspected left lower lobe collapse
5 Oblique
 a) Visualization of pleural plaques
 b) Suspected rib fracture(s)
6 Apical lordotic — visualization of lesions in lung
 apex

Differential diagnosis of unilateral hemithorax transradiancy
1 Pneumothorax

2 Mastectomy
3 Pulmonary embolism
4 Emphysematous bullae
5 Macleod's syndrome, Swyer-James

Significance of the apparently elevated hemidiaphragm
1 Phrenic nerve palsy
2 Segmental/lobar collapse (→ tracheal deviation) or resection
3 Subpulmonic effusion (decubitus film → diagnosis)
4 Subphrenic collection
5 Massive hepatomegaly
6 Diaphragmatic rupture (e.g. post-traumatic) or dysfunction (e.g. herpes zoster affecting C4 nerve root)

Interstitial vs alveolar infiltrates
1 Interstitial ('honeycombing,' e.g. sarcoidosis)
   a) 'Ground glass' appearance (e.g. asbestosis, berylliosis)
   b) Reticular appearance (e.g. idiopathic pulmonary fibrosis)
   c) Nodular appearance (e.g. histoplasmosis, pneumoconiosis)
2 Alveolar (e.g. pulmonary oedema, pneumonia)
   a) Fluffy opacities
   b) Air bronchograms
   c) Lobar or segmental distribution
   d) Rapid evolution

Clinically important causes of 'honeycomb lung'
1 Idiopathic fibrosing alveolitis
2 Sarcoidosis
3 Scleroderma
   Rheumatoid arthritis (± effusion)
4 Pneumoconiosis; silicosis; berylliosis
   Asbestosis (± 'holly-leaf' pleural plaques)
5 Hypersensitivity pneumonitis (long-standing)
   Histiocytosis X
6 Lymphangitis carcinomatosa
   Alveolar cell carcinoma

Clinically important causes of bilateral hilar adenopathy
1 Sarcoidosis
   — Typically symmetrical lymphadenopathy
   — Patient usually looks well
2 Lymphoma
   — Typically asymmetrical lymphadenopathy
   — Patient often looks ill

Differential diagnosis of hilar calcification
1 TB
2 Silicosis ('egg-shell' appearance)
3 Histoplasmosis

Disseminated interstitial nodules: differential diagnosis
1 Previous varicella pneumonia, esp. if adult-onset
2 Histoplasmosis; hydatid disease
3 Miliary TB
4 Mitral stenosis (microlithiasis pulmonale due to secondary pulmonary haemosiderosis)
5 Malignancy
   a) Metastases, e.g. from germ-cell primary

   b) Lymphangitis carcinomatosas
   c) Bronchoalveolar cell carcinoma
6 Sarcoidosis, pneumoconiosis, Caplan's syndrome

Common causes of pulmonary cavitation
1 Infection
   a) TB
   b) *Klebsiella pneumoniae, Staph. aureus*
   c) Invasive aspergillosis, nocardiosis, actinomycosis
   d) Amoebiasis
   e) Pneumococcal (serotype 3)
   f) Aspiration (anaerobes and mixed flora)
2 Pulmonary infarction
   a) Septic emboli
   b) Bland emboli (with secondary infection)
   c) Vasculitis (e.g. PAN, Wegener's)
3 Malignancy

Radiographic pointers to bacterial diagnosis of pneumonia
1 Lobar consolidation with pleural effusion — pneumococcus
2 'Bulging' fissure
   a) *Klebsiella* (classical)
   b) Pneumococcus (common)
3 Periosteal reaction — *Actinomyces* spp.
4 Superior segment of right lower lobe involved — aspiration
5 Right middle lobe collapse/consolidation — malignancy

Investigation of bronchiectasis
1 CXR
   a) 'Tramline' bronchial thickening
   b) Dextrocardia (Kartagener's)
2 Bronchography, *if*
   a) Severe haemoptysis
   b) Recurrent localized pneumonia
   c) Optimization of postural drainage required
   d) Lobectomy being considered in fit young patient
3 Aetiology
   a) Sweat test, immunoglobulins (in children)
   b) Nasal cilia biopsy for electron microscopy (immotile cilia)
   c) AFBs; *Aspergillus* precipitins/skin test
4 Complications
   a) Sputum culture (for *S. aureus, Ps. aeruginosa*)
   b) Protein electrophoresis; biopsy (for amyloid)

Radiographic features of miscellaneous disorders
1 Asbestosis
   a) Calcified pleural plaques (esp. diaphragmatic)
   b) Bibasilar interstitial fibrosis
   c) 'Shaggy' pericardial silhouette
2 Pulmonary infarction
   a) Usually normal
   b) Area(s) of linear atelectasis
   c) (Small) pleural effusion(s)
   d) Wedgeshaped peripheral lesion(s), apex towards hilum
   e) Elevated hemidiaphragm (if collapse)
   f) Enlarged pulmonary artery, reduced peripheral vascular calibre
3 Emphysema

a) Hyperinflation (DD_x = asthma)
— Hyperlucent lungfields ('black lungs')
— 'Flat' low hemidiaphragms
— Visible 11th rib
— Small, narrow heart shadow
b) Bullae
c) Pulmonary artery diameter >2 cm (pulmonary hypertension)

Main indications for invasive diagnosis of pulmonary infiltrates
1 Percutaneous needle aspiration
a) Cavitating infiltrates
b) Peripheral infiltrates
2 Bronchoscopy
a) Infiltrate of presumed infective aetiology
b) Infiltrate of presumed neoplastic aetiology
3 Bronchoalveolar lavage
a) Presumed opportunistic infection*
b) Cytology of peripheral infiltrates
4 Open lung biopsy — histopathology required, e.g.
a) Drug-induced lung fibrosis
b) Radiation pneumonitis

MANAGING RESPIRATORY DISEASE

ASTHMA

Unexpected death in acute asthma: risk factors
1 Recent discharge from hospital
2 Overdependence on inhaled sympathomimetics and underutilization of systemic steroids
3 Inadequate monitoring of lung function at night
4 Intravenous administration of aminophylline in patients already receiving maintenance oral theophylline

Considerations in assessing asthma severity
1 Patient's assessment of severity
Request for admission by patient or family
2 Previous admission(s) for stabilization
3 History of steroid requirement, esp. if recent reduction or suspected non-compliance
4 Rapid symptomatic development (labile disease)
5 Insufficient lung function to use usual inhalers
6 Iatrogenic factors
a) Inappropriate sedation
b) Precipitation by aspirin or β-blockers

Clinical criteria favouring hospitalization in acute asthma
1 General demeanour
a) Difficulty speaking
b) Sweaty, anxious, irritable
c) Exhausted; confused; sitting forward
2 Central cyanosis
3 Accessory muscle use
Intercostal recession
Tracheal tug (descends on inspiration)

4 Tachycardia >150/min
Tachypnoea >28/min
Forced expiratory time >4 seconds
Blood pressure
a) Paradox* >20 mmHg
b) Pulsus paradoxus (i.e. palpable paradox)
c) Hypotension (ominous)
5 'Quiet' (grossly hyperexpanded) chest
6 PEFR < 200 l/min
FEV_1 < 1 litre or too incapacitated to perform these tests adequately
7 CXR — pneumothorax
ECG — P pulmonale or right ventricular strain
8 $P_a co_2$ >40 mmHg

NB: Presence of one or more of these signs on presentation may justify admission; persistence of any one sign following bronchodilator therapy makes urgent admission mandatory

Therapeutic approach to the young patient with asthma
1 Occasional mild symptoms, no severe acute attacks — intermittent bronchodilator
a) $β_2$-Sympathomimetics (e.g. salbutamol inhaler), or
b) Antimuscarinics (e.g. ipratropium bromide)
2 Occasional mild symptoms with some severe acute attacks — intermittent bronchodilator supplemented with short courses of corticosteroid during acute attacks
3 Frequent troublesome symptoms
a) Continuous prophylaxis with inhaled sodium cromoglycate
b) If no benefit from this, try inhaled beclomethasone
c) Use intermittent bronchodilator when needed
d) Supplement with steroids during acute exacerbations
4 Refractory nocturnal symptoms — bedtime dose of slow-release theophylline may help (also useful in patients unable to use inhalers)

Pharmacokinetic considerations in theophylline therapy
1 *Higher* dose may be required in
a) Cigarette smokers
b) Chronic alcohol ingestion without liver damage
c) Children <12 years
d) Treatment with phenytoin, carbamazepine, barbiturates; rifampicin, isoniazid; sulphinpyrazone
2 *Reduce* dose in
a) Hepatic insufficiency
b) Cardiac failure; fever; pregnancy
c) Elderly patients
d) Treatment with erythromycin; cimetidine; propranolol; oral contraceptives; allopurinol
3 *Overdosage* may precipitate — hypokalaemia ; hyperglycaemia; acidosis; convulsions
If supportive measures fail, haemoperfusion may be useful if plasma theophylline levels exceed 50 mg/l

---

*Defined as systolic drop of >12 mmHg on inspiration
†Parenteral $β_2$-agonists may also cause hypokalaemia

---

*May also require open lung biopsy

Principal indications for inhaler therapy in pulmonary disease

1 Sodium cromoglycate — prophylaxis for children with extrinsic (i.e. allergic or exercise-induced) asthma
2 Anticholinergics (e.g. ipratropium bromide) — COAD > asthma (prophylaxis)
3 β_2-agonists (e.g. salbutamol) — asthma (acute)
4 Corticosteroids (e.g. beclomethasone diproprionate) — asthma > COAD (prophylaxis)

PRINCIPLES OF VENTILATORY SUPPORT

Potential hazards of oxygen therapy

1 Carbon dioxide retention
2 Reduced bronchial ciliary activity; drying of secretions
3 Adult respiratory distress syndrome
4 Potentiation of radiation — or cytotoxic-induced pneumonitis
5 Retrolental fibroplasia in neonates

Indications for assisted ventilation

1 Apnoea
2 Ineffective cough
3 Inadequate ventilation ($P_a\text{co}_2 > 45$ mmHg) due to
   a) Unconsciousness (any cause, incl. postanaesthesia)
   b) Flail segment, asynchronous respiration
   c) Guillain-Barré, myasthenia gravis
   d) Severe asthma

DOMICILIARY OXYGEN

Indications for long-term low-flow oxygen therapy

1 Prerequisites
   a) Age <70 years
   b) No other major illness
   c) Cessation of smoking (carboxyhaemoglobin <3%)
2 Stable chronic airflow obstruction with
   a) $P_a\text{O}_2$ <55 mmHg on room air
   b) $P_a\text{co}_2$ >45 mmHg (esp. if associated with oedema)
   c) FEV_1 < 1.5 litres and FVC < 2 litres
3 Controversial — palliation of severe hypoxaemic lung disease
   a) Stable airflow obstruction without elevated $P_a\text{co}_2$
   b) Advanced restrictive lung disease

Contraindications to long-term low-flow oxygen therapy

1 Obstructive sleep apnoea (this may be treated, however, with C-PAP — continuous positive airway pressure)
2 Respiratory muscle weakness
3 Ventilatory impairment due to kyphoscoliosis

Benefits of long-term oxygen therapy in chronic lung disease

1 Subjective relief from dyspnoea
2 Improved exercise tolerance
3 Reduced pulmonary artery pressure
4 Fewer hospital admissions
5 Prolonged survival

DRUG THERAPY OF RESPIRATORY DISEASE

General principles of steroid therapy in respiratory disease

1 Allergic bronchopulmonary aspergillosis — maintenance prednisolone up to 10 mg/day may be indicated in patients with frequent exacerbations
2 Hypersensitivity pneumonitis — maintenance therapy may be justified only if avoidance of antigen proves impossible
3 Fibrosing alveolitis — some benefit from initial dose of 40 mg/day prednisolone, esp. if
   a) Cellular biopsy with desquamation
   b) > 10% lymphocytosis on lavage (unusual)
4 Adult respiratory distress syndrome — probably no value in established disease
5 Wegener's granulomatosis
   a) Prednisolone useful when combined with cyclophosphamide
   b) This combination probably also of value in Churg-Strauss syndrome and lymphomatoid granulomatosis

Presumptive management of pneumonia in adults

1 Mild community-acquired pneumonia, treatable at home — amoxycillin 500 mg t.d.s. orally
2 Severe community-acquired pneumonia, in hospital
   a) Erythromycin 1 g i.v. q 6 h (covers *Mycoplasma*, pneumococci, *Legionella*, most staphylococci and *C. psittaci*)
   b) ±Ampicillin 1 g i.v. q 6 h (provides additional cover for pneumococci, and for *Haemophilus influenzae*)
3 *Legionella* strongly suspected — erythromycin 1 g q 6 h **plus** rifampicin 600 mg b.d. Staphylococcal pneumonia suspected (e.g. postinfluenza) — flucloxacillin 2 g i.v. q 4–6 h (± aminoglycoside/fusidic acid)
4 Hospital-acquired pneumonia — i.v. β-lactamase (e.g. ampicillin) plus aminoglycoside (e.g. gentamicin) Aspiration pneumonia suspected — add metronidazole to cover anaerobes (or penicillin)
5 Pneumonia in the neutropenic patient — antipseudomonal β-lactamase (e.g. ticarcillin) plus aminoglycoside (e.g. tobramycin)
6 Pneumonia in patients with weight loss, lymphadenopathy and/or oral candidiasis (i.e. ?AIDS) — consider cotrimoxazole/pentamidine to cover *P. carinii*

NB: chest physio is of **no** proven value in lobar pneumonia

Acute mountain sickness (AMS): approach to management

1 Pathogenesis of AMS — altitude-induced hypoxaemia leads to respiratory alkalosis which then limits the ventilatory response to hypoxia (i.e.

until acclimatization occurs, with reduction of extracellular fluid bicarbonate levels)
2 Symptoms of AMS — arise from cerebral oedema
3 Prevention of AMS
  a) Slow ascent
  b) Temporary (immediate) descent if symptoms develop
4 Medical prophylaxis (NB: adjunctive only to above measures) — acetazolamide 250 mg b.d. from 48 hours pre-ascent
5 Treatment of incipient AMS — add 3% CO_2 to inhaled air. This increases $P_{a}CO_2$ levels and abolishes respiratory alkalosis, thus inducing a secondary improvement in ventilation, oxygenation and cerebral perfusion
6 Treatment of established AMS — dexamethasone (for cerebral oedema)

UNDERSTANDING RESPIRATORY DISEASE

ADULT RESPIRATORY DISTRESS SYNDROME

Diagnostic criteria for adult respiratory distress syndrome
1 Previously normal lung function
2 Acute onset of respiratory distress following a precipitating event
3 CXR — widespread infiltrates (sparing apices and costophrenic angles)
4 P_{aO2} <60 mmHg despite F_{iO2} = 60% (due to shunting)
  P_{aCO2} normal or low
5 Reduced pulmonary compliance ('stiff lungs')
  Pulmonary hypertension (> 30/15 mmHg) usual
  Pulmonary capillary wedge pressure normal (<18 mmHg)
6 Clinical improvement with assisted ventilation (volume-cycled, patient-initiated) using positive end-expiratory pressure (PEEP) of 8–15 cm H_2O to increase the functional residual capacity (and hence to increase compliance and thus reduce intrapulmonary shunting)

Common antecedents of adult respiratory distress syndrome
1 Sepsis (incl. pneumonia, Gram-negative septicaemia)
2 Aspiration (incl. drowning)
3 Inhalation (smoke, oxygen, chlorine)
4 Multiple trauma
5 Massive transfusion

NB: ARDS *may* also occur in neutropenic patients even though neutrophils are implicated in the pathogenesis of ARDS

GRANULOMATOUS LUNG DISEASE

Indicators of disease activity in sarcoidosis
1 Symptoms

2 Investigations related to specific organ involvement (e.g. CXR, DL_{CO})
3 Bronchoalveolar lavage
  a) Increased overall cellularity
  b) Up to 40% lymphocytes (predominantly helper T-cells)
  c) ↓ IgG:albumin ratio (cf. allergic alveolitis)
4 Gallium-67 scan
  a) A sensitive index of disease activity in patients with established disease and prior scan uptake
  b) Extrapulmonary uptake (parotid, nodes) supports diagnosis but does not exclude lymphoma
5 Serum angiotensin-converting enzyme (ACE)
  a) Elevated in 70% of patients with active (acute) disease
  b) Useful in monitoring response to steroids in patients with documented elevations
  c) *Not* of routine value in initial diagnosis (also elevated in Gaucher's, silicosis, miliary TB, and miscellaneous granulomatous disorders)
  d) Serum lysozyme and transcobalamin II are similar potential indices of disease activity, albeit similarly insensitive and non-specific
6 Serum and/or urinary calcium (if elevated)
  Hypergammaglobulinaemia (polyclonal)
  Lymphopenia (relative excess of suppressor T-cells; cf. BAL)

Main features distinguishing chronic from acute sarcoidosis
1 Age of presentation — older (>30 years) patients
2 CXR
  a) Pulmonary infiltrates
  b) No hilar adenopathy
3 Skin
  a) Lupus pernio common
  b) Erythema nodosum unusual
4 Mikulicz syndrome (parotidomegaly and facial palsy) common
5 Therapeutic response — steroid-resistant
6 Prognosis — poor

Cardiac manifestations of sarcoidosis
1 Heart block — first-degree/RBBB/complete heart block
2 Arrhythmias — SVT/VT/ventricular ectopic beats
3 Mitral valve disease
4 Pericarditis
5 Congestive cardiac failure
6 Sudden death

Indications for corticosteroids in sarcoidosis
1 Intractable constitutional symptoms
2 Progressive lung disease
3 Hypercalcaemia* and/or persisting hypercalciuria
4 Hypersplenism
5 Vital organ involvement
  a) Heart
  b) CNS
  c) Eye

*May also respond to chloroquine

Hypersensitivity pneumonitis*: making the diagnosis
(*extrinsic allergic alveolitis)
1 Clinical
  a) Recurrent dyspnoea 4–6 hours after antigen exposure
  b) Dry cough; no wheezing
  c) Fevers, progressive weight loss
2 CXR: mid- and lower zone mottling (in acute phase) upper zone mottling (in chronic fibrosis)
3 Lung function tests — restrictive (transient in acute phase)
4 Blood gases — low P_{aO2} and P_{aCO2}
  Diffusion capacity — low DL_{CO}
5 Precipitins
  a) Do *not* indicate pathogenicity (possible exception: budgerigar exposure)
  b) Do *not* correlate with disease activity
  c) Tend to *exclude* diagnosis if negative
6 Total serum IgE levels — typically normal
  Eosinophilia — absent
7 Bronchoalveolar lavage
  a) Lymphocytosis
  b) ↑ IgG:albumin ratio
8 Transbronchial biopsy
  a) Granulomata
  b) Bronchiolitis, mononuclear infiltrate
9 Inhalation provocation (the definitive diagnostic test)
  a) Improvement on cessation of exposure
  b) Relapse on rechallenge

ASPERGILLOSIS

Clinical spectrum of *Aspergillus*-related pulmonary disease
1 Allergic bronchopulmonary aspergillosis — treat with bronchodilators and/or steroids
2 Aspergilloma ('fungus ball') — treat conservatively or surgically
3 Invasive aspergillosis — treat urgently with i.v. amphotericin B + 5-FC

Bronchopulmonary aspergillosis: diagnostic criteria
1 Clinical setting: exacerbation of asthma in an atopic patient
2 Expectoration of rubbery brown sputum plugs which repeatedly yield aspergilli on culture
3 CXR
  a) Upper lobe pulmonary infiltrates
  b) Peripheral linear shadowing
4 Peripheral eosinophilia > 1000/ml
5 Elevated total serum IgE (> 2000 ng/ml)
  Elevated specific IgE to *A. fumigatus* (cf. aspergilloma)
  Elevated specific IgG to *A. fumigatus* (cf. invasive aspergillosis); IgE:IgG >2
6 Immediate skin reactivity to *A. fumigatus* (i.e. positive prick test or intradermal test)
7 Precipitating antibodies to *A. fumigatus* antigen (weakly positive)
8 Bronchoscopy/bronchography — proximal saccular upper lobe bronchiectasis
9 Resolution of symptoms, eosinophilia, sputum

positivity and radiographic appearances with use of long-term systemic steroids (prednisone 0.5 mg/kg daily × 2 weeks, then alternate days × 2 months, then taper) (cf. **invasive** aspergillosis: diagnose by lung biopsy, treat with i.v. amphotericin B and 5FC)

LUNG INFECTIONS

Predispositions to specific pulmonary infections
1 Tuberculosis (incl. reactivation)
  a) Silicosis
  b) Alcoholism
  c) Gastrectomy or jejunoileal bypass
  d) Active measles; uncontrolled diabetes mellitus
  e) Iatrogenic immunosuppression
2 *Mycobacterium kansasii/avium-intracellulare*:
  a) Pre-existing lung disease
3 Anaerobic infections (abscess, aspiration pneumonia)
  a) Obtunded consciousness; general anaesthesia, alcoholism
  b) Poor dental hygiene
  c) Achalasia, scleroderma, Riley-Day syndrome
4 *Klebsiella* spp — alcoholism, derelict lifestyle
5 *Ps. aeruginosa* ⎱ cystic fibrosis
  Staph. aureus ⎰ (bronchial colonization)
6 *Ps. pyocyanea* — humidifier/ventilator therapy
7 *Nocardia asteroides*
  a) Pulmonary alveolar proteinosis
  b) Chronic granulomatous disease of childhood
8 *Staph. aureus*
  Serratia marcescens ⎱ heroin addiction
  Candida spp. ⎰
9 *Pneumocystis carinii* ⎱ transplantation
  Cytomegalovirus   ⎰ (immunosuppression) AIDS
10 Aspergilloma
  a) Old tuberculous cavities
  b) Emphysematous bullae, lung cysts
  c) Apical cavities in ankylosing spondylitis
  d) Cystic fibrosis, atopic asthma

Differential diagnoses in pneumonic presentations
1 Failure to respond to ampicillin (penicillin) in community-acquired pneumonia
  a) 'Atypical' pneumonias (q.v.)
  b) Viral (e.g. adenovirus, varicella, measles)
  c) *Staph. aureus, Klebsiella*
  d) Tuberculosis
2 Pneumonia in recent Asian migrant
  a) Tuberculosis
  b) *Ps. pseudomallei* (melioidosis)
3 Pneumonia in bird-fanciers
  a) Psittacosis (exclude allergic alveolitis)
4 Pneumonia in meatworkers
  a) Q fever
5 Postinfluenza pneumonia — *Staph. aureus*, pneumococci
6 Eosinophilic pneumonia
  a) Tropical diffuse — filariasis (*Wuchereria bancrofti*)

b) Tropical localized — ascariasis (Löffler's syndrome)
c) Non-tropical localized — aspergillosis
d) Toxic (e.g. nitrofurantoin, toluene)

ATYPICAL PNEUMONIA

The atypical pneumonias: which ones are they?
1 Mycoplasma pneumonia (*M. pneumoniae*)
2 Legionnaire's disease (*L. pneumophila*)
3 Q fever (*Coxiella burneti*)
4 Psittacosis (*Chlamydia psittaci*)
5 TWAR (*Chlamydia pneumoniae*: p. 190)

Clinical aspects of *Mycoplasma* pneumonia
1 Occurrence
 a) Slowly spreading epidemics
 b) Long incubation period
 c) Insidious onset
2 Course
 a) Initial URTI slowly transforms to (and terminates as) LRTI
 b) Family members often also affected
 c) Clinical relapse following treatment often occurs
3 Extrapulmonary manifestations
 a) Arthralgias/-itis
 b) Headaches, meningism ± aseptic meningitis
 c) Substernal discomfort (tracheobronchitis)
 d) 'Cold' autoimmune haemolysis ± anaemia
 e) Ear pain (classical but uncommon) due to bullous or haemorrhagic myringitis
 f) Erythema multiforme
 g) Myopericarditis
4 Diagnosis
 a) Routine sputum non-diagnostic
 b) Throat swab may (eventually) yield positive cultures
 c) Definitive diagnosis established by serology (CFT)
 d) Resistant to β-lactams

Distinguishing features of psittacosis
1 Avian exposure
2 Epistaxis
 Photophobia; thrombophlebitis (→ pulmonary infarction)
 Myalgias, confusion, stupor
3 Signs
 a) Splenomegaly (± anicteric hepatomegaly)
 b) Horder's spots (may simulate rose spots of typhoid)
 c) Proteinuria
4 Investigations
 a) Positive serology (CFT); even low-titre generally suffices for diagnosis in acute phase
 b) Transbronchial biopsy → cytoplasmic inclusions (LCL bodies) within macrophages

Distinguishing features of Q ('query') fever
1 Not transmitted from arthropods
 No rash
 Negative Weil-Felix reaction } cf. other rickettsioses

2 Pleuritic chest pain
3 Weight loss (may be dramatic)
4 Granulomatous hepatitis (→ about 20%)
5 Culture-negative endocarditis (usually *de novo*) requiring valve replacement (typically, aortic)

Clinical spectrum of Legionnaires' disease
1 Commoner in
 a) Smokers
 b) Debilitated patients
 c) Males aged about 50–60 years
 d) Moderate (about 30 g/day) alcohol intake
2 No documented person-to-person spread
 Nosocomial transmission not infrequent
 Water-containing receptacles implicated as disease reservoir
3 Distinguishing clinical features
 a) High fever, rigors
 b) Encephalopathy ± headache
 c) Gastrointestinal upset
 d) Transient azotaemia; haemoproteinuria
4 Investigations
 a) Hyponatraemia (SIADH); also seen in other bacterial pneumonias
 b) Hypophosphataemia
 c) Transient liver function test abnormalities
 d) Negative routine cultures
5 Diagnosis
 a) Most rapid — direct fluorescence (DFA) on open lung biopsy (or pleural fluid)
 b) Dieterle silver impregnation stain on sputum
 c) Culture of lung biopsy or pleural fluid in medium containing charcoal yeast-enriched (CYE) agar with alphaketoglutarate or cysteine/iron in 5% CO_2
 d) Serology (indirect fluorescent antibody — IFA)
 — Four-fold rise to > 1:128 (usually takes 2 weeks)
 — Single titre of > 1:256 indicates infection at some stage (past or present)
6 Management
 a) IV fluids if hypovolaemic (diarrhoea, sweats)
 b) Electrolyte homeostasis
 c) Erythromycin 2–4 g/day i.v. ± rifampicin 600 mg/day (continue for 2 weeks, even though defervescence occurs within 48 hours)
 d) PEEP if in respiratory failure (10–20%)

OTHER ASPECTS OF RESPIRATORY DISEASE

Neurological precipitants of respiratory failure
1 Neuromuscular
 a) Myasthenia gravis
 b) Polymyositis, myotonic dystrophy
2 Neuropathy
 a) Guillain-Barré syndrome
 b) Diphtheria, acute intermittent porphyria
3 Anterior horn cell disease
 a) Polio
 b) Motor neurone disease
4 Spinal cord lesion

a) Trauma
   Tumour; demyelination
5 Brainstem
   a) Cerebrovascular accident
   b) Encephalitis; polio; tumour; demyelination

Miscellaneous respiratory diseases
1 Pulmonary alveolar proteinosis
   a) Protean clinical manifestations, highly variable prognosis
   b) Sputum → PAS-positive lipoprotein within epithelial cells
   c) CXR → diffuse infiltrates, perihilar 'rosette'
   d) Not infrequently complicated by opportunistic infection, esp. *Nocardia* (which may in turn metastasize to brain)
   e) Symptomatic patients may benefit from therapeutic lavage (avoid corticosteroids)
2 Idiopathic pulmonary haemosiderosis
   a) Age of onset < 20 years
   b) Sputum → haemosiderin-laden macrophages
   c) Presents with haemoptysis ± iron-deficiency anaemia

d) Diffuse (predominantly basal) infiltrates on CXR
e) No renal disease; negative immunofluorescence and anti-GBM Ab (cf. Goodpasture's)
f) Subclinical disease activity is proportionate to the DL_{CO}
3 Yellow-nail syndrome
   a) Presents in old age usually
   b) Greenish-yellow nail discolouration and dystrophy
   c) Associated with recurrent pleural effusions, peripheral lymphoedema, chronic chest infections and myxoedema
4 Immotile cilia syndrome
   a) Genetic aetiology; includes Kartagener's syndrome (in 50%)
   b) Other manifestations include otitis media, nasal polyposis and infertility (esp. in males: 95%)
   c) Affected females may develop salpingitis, but usually remain fertile (as in cystic fibrosis)
   d) Ultrastructural defect of dynein arms in bronchial/nasal cilia, and in sperm, has been well characterized using electron microscopy

Reviewing the Literature: Respiratory Medicine

13.1 Law C M, Marchant J L, Honour J W et al 1986 Nocturnal adrenal suppression in asthmatic children taking inhaled beclomethasone dipropionate. Lancet i: 942–944

Study of 19 children showing dose-dependent suppression of cortisol diurnal rhythm following inhaler steroid therapy

13.2 Siegel D, Sheppard D, Gelb A, Weinburg P F 1985 Aminophylline increases the toxicity but not the efficacy of an inhaled β_2-adrenergic agonist in the treatment of acute exacerbation of asthma. American Review of Respiratory Disease 132: 283–286

Clinical study which cast further doubts on the routine usefulness of theophylline derivatives

13.3 Fanta C H et al 1986 Treatment of acute asthma: is combination therapy with sympathomimetics and methylxanthines indicated? American Journal of Medicine 80: 5–10

Study of 157 patients concluding that sympathomimetic therapy alone is equally effective in most acutely ill asthmatics, and that routine i.v. aminophylline is therefore not indicated as part of emergency management

13.4 Sears M R et al 1987 75 deaths in asthmatics prescribed home nebulizers. British Medical Journal 294: 477–480

This analysis suggested that delay in using corticosteroids was the main danger in using nebulized β-agonist therapy, rather than β-agonist toxicity

13.5 Stover D E et al 1984 Bronchoalveolar lavage in the diagnosis of diffuse pulmonary infiltrates in the immunosuppressed host. Annals of Internal Medicine 101: 1–7

66% diagnostic yield in series of 97 patients with pulmonary infiltrates of uncertain cause. Particularly impressive accuracy was seen in the diagnosis of opportunistic infections (83% yield) and pulmonary haemorrhage, (78%). Together with other studies these results suggest that lavage may be superior to bronchoscopic biopsy in this setting, and in some centres it has replaced open lung biopsy as the investigation of choice. Moreover, unlike percutaneous biopsy, there is no risk of pneumothorax or haemorrhage

13.6 Hornbein T F 1989 The cost to the central nervous system of climbing to extremely high altitude. New England Journal of Medicine 321: 1714–1719

Major learning deficits were found in mountaineers ascending to 8400 metres during testing 1–30 days following return. Greater deficits occurred in subjects who had a greater ventilatory response, perhaps indicating that cerebral vasoconstriction induced by hypocapnia plays a role in cerebral damage

13.7 Goldstein R S, Ramcharan V, Bowes G, McNicholas W T, Bradley D, Phillipson E A 1984 Effect of supplemental nocturnal oxygen on gas exchange in patients with severe obstructive lung disease. New England Journal of Medicine 310: 425–429

The majority of patients in this study achieved oxyhaemoglobin saturations of > 90% while only minor elevations of P_{aCO2} (generally < 6 mmHg) were noted: frank obstructive sleep apnoea occurred in 20%

13.8 Medical Research Council Working Party 1981 Long term domiciliary oxygen therapy in chronic hypoxic cor pulmonale complicating chronic bronchitis and emphysema. Lancet i: 681–686

A randomized study confirming improved survival in

recipients of continuous low-flow oxygen with chronic hypoxaemia

13.9 Adams J S, Sharma O P, Gacad M A et al 1983 Metabolism of 25-hydroxyvitamin D_3 by cultured pulmonary alveolar macrophages in sarcoidosis. Journal of Clinical Investigation 72: 1856–1860

Study suggesting that the hypercalcaemia of sarcoidosis arises due to inappropriate extrarenal activation of 25-hydroxy-D3 by alveolar macrophages rather than to end-organ hypersensitivity

13.10 Burrows B et al 1989 Association of asthma with serum IgE levels and skin-test reactivity to allergens. New England Journal of Medicine 320: 271–277

Unlike allergic rhinitis, prevalence of asthma was found to be tightly related to the serum IgE level in this study of 2567 'allergic' patients, suggesting that 'intrinsic' (as opposed to 'extrinsic') asthma may be a spurious concept

Rheumatology

Physical examination protocol 14.1   You are asked to examine a patient with rheumatoid arthritis

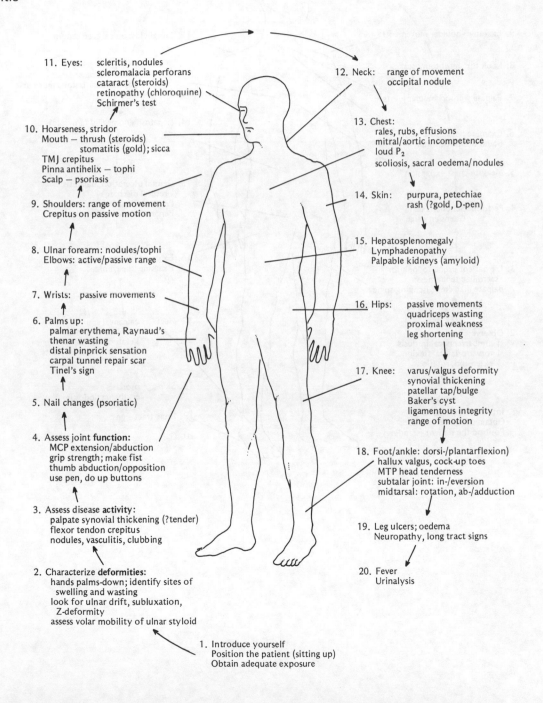

11. Eyes: scleritis, nodules
            scleromalacia perforans
            cataract (steroids)
            retinopathy (chloroquine)
            Schirmer's test

10. Hoarseness, stridor
    Mouth − thrush (steroids)
            stomatitis (gold); sicca
    TMJ crepitus
    Pinna antihelix − tophi
    Scalp − psoriasis

9. Shoulders: range of movement
   Crepitus on passive motion

8. Ulnar forearm: nodules/tophi
   Elbows: active/passive range

7. Wrists: passive movements

6. Palms up:
   palmar erythema, Raynaud's
   thenar wasting
   distal pinprick sensation
   carpal tunnel repair scar
   Tinel's sign

5. Nail changes (psoriatic)

4. Assess joint **function:**
   MCP extension/abduction
   grip strength; make fist
   thumb abduction/opposition
   use pen, do up buttons

3. Assess disease **activity:**
   palpate synovial thickening (?tender)
   flexor tendon crepitus
   nodules, vasculitis, clubbing

2. Characterize **deformities:**
   hands palms-down; identify sites of
     swelling and wasting
   look for ulnar drift, subluxation,
     Z-deformity
   assess volar mobility of ulnar styloid

1. Introduce yourself
   Position the patient (sitting up)
   Obtain adequate exposure

12. Neck: range of movement
            occipital nodule

13. Chest:
    rales, rubs, effusions
    mitral/aortic incompetence
    loud P_2
    scoliosis, sacral oedema/nodules

14. Skin: purpura, petechiae
            rash (?gold, D-pen)

15. Hepatosplenomegaly
    Lymphadenopathy
    Palpable kidneys (amyloid)

16. Hips: passive movements
            quadriceps wasting
            proximal weakness
            leg shortening

17. Knee: varus/valgus deformity
            synovial thickening
            patellar tap/bulge
            Baker's cyst
            ligamentous integrity
            range of motion

18. Foot/ankle: dorsi-/plantarflexion)
    hallux valgus, cock-up toes
    MTP head tenderness
    subtalar joint: in-/eversion
    midtarsal: rotation, ab-/adduction

19. Leg ulcers; oedema
    Neuropathy, long tract signs

20. Fever
    Urinalysis

Physical examination protocol 14.2   You are asked to examine a young man with chronic low back pain

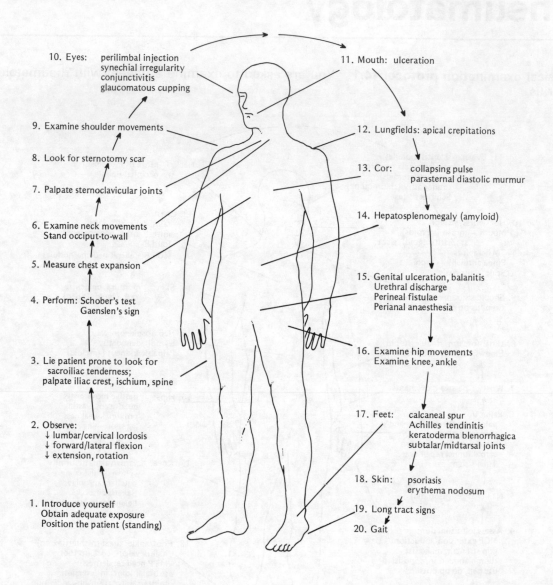

10. Eyes: perilimbal injection
synechial irregularity
conjunctivitis
glaucomatous cupping

9. Examine shoulder movements

8. Look for sternotomy scar

7. Palpate sternoclavicular joints

6. Examine neck movements
Stand occiput-to-wall

5. Measure chest expansion

4. Perform: Schober's test
Gaenslen's sign

3. Lie patient prone to look for
sacroiliac tenderness;
palpate iliac crest, ischium, spine

2. Observe:
↓ lumbar/cervical lordosis
↓ forward/lateral flexion
↓ extension, rotation

1. Introduce yourself
Obtain adequate exposure
Position the patient (standing)

11. Mouth: ulceration

12. Lungfields: apical crepitations

13. Cor: collapsing pulse
parasternal diastolic murmur

14. Hepatosplenomegaly (amyloid)

15. Genital ulceration, balanitis
Urethral discharge
Perineal fistulae
Perianal anaesthesia

16. Examine hip movements
Examine knee, ankle

17. Feet: calcaneal spur
Achilles tendinitis
keratoderma blenorrhagica
subtalar/midtarsal joints

18. Skin: psoriasis
erythema nodosum

19. Long tract signs

20. Gait

Diagnostic pathway 14.1   This patient has unusual hands. What sort of process do you think is responsible?

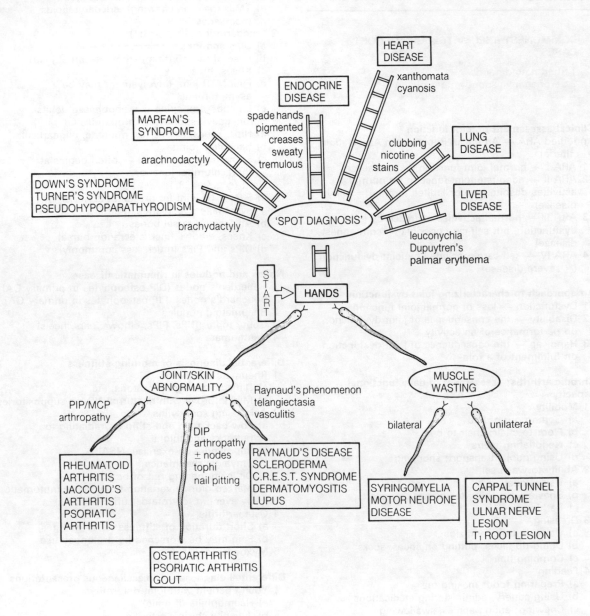

CLINICAL ASPECTS OF RHEUMATIC DISEASES

COMMONEST RHEUMATOLOGICAL SHORT CASES

1 Rheumatoid hands
2 Seronegative spondyloarthropathy

Clinical assessment of joint function
(modified ARA — American Rheumatism Association — criteria)
1 ARA I — normal joint function (= no disease)
2 ARA II — adequate joint function for normal activities despite pain or limited motion (= early disease)
3 ARA III — normal activities restricted by joint dysfunction, but self-care possible (= commonest disease)
4 ARA IV — self-care precluded by joint dysfunction (= severe disease)

An approach to characterizing joint dysfunction
1 Dysfunction — loss of normal joint function
2 Disability — the consequence of joint dysfunction on performance of an activity
3 Handicap — the consequence of joint dysfunction on fulfilment of a role

Chronic arthritis: assessment of daily functional capacity
1 Mobility
   a) Getting out of bed
   b) Floor to chair; chair to bed
   c) Negotiating stairs
   d) Using public transport; shopping
2 Ability to wash self
   a) Using toilet
   b) Shaving, brushing teeth, cutting nails
   c) Bathing
3 Dressing
   a) Using buttons and zips
   b) Doing up laces; putting on shoes, socks
   c) Combing hair
4 Feeding
   a) Preparing food; making tea
   b) Using cutlery; administering medications
   c) Chewing; eating apples, swallowing
5 Housework
   a) Turning taps, keys, dials
   b) Making beds; using telephone
   c) Hanging washing

DIAGNOSTIC PATTERNS IN CLINICAL RHEUMATOLOGY

Patterns of joint involvement in rheumatic disease
1 Rheumatoid arthritis ($\female : \male = 3:1$)
   a) MCPs, PIPs, wrists
   b) Knees, ankles
   c) Lateral MTPs, subtalar/midtarsal joints
   d) Cervical spine, incl. atlanto-axial joint
   e) TMJs (pain on chewing); cricoarytenoids (hoarseness)
2 Osteoarthritis ($\female : \male = 3:1$)
   a) DIPs and PIPs
   b) Base of thumb (first carpometacarpal joint)
   c) Knees, hips
   d) First MTP joint (involvement may be asymptomatic)
   e) Lumbosacral spine (i.e. apophyseal joints)
3 Seronegative spondyloarthropathies ($\male > \female$)
   a) Hips, knees, ankles (asymmetric, oligoarticular)
   b) Sacroiliac joints
   c) Spine (i.e. spondylitis) — often begins at thoracolumbar junction
4 Gout ($\male : \female = 8:1$)
   a) First MTP joint (at presentation in 75%; eventually supervenes in 90%)
   b) Ankles and tarsal bones
   c) Knees, elbows (incl. olecranon bursa)
   d) DIPs and PIPs (much less commonly)

Nodes and nodules in rheumatic disease
1 Heberden's nodes (DIP osteophytes in primary OA)
   Bouchard's nodes (PIP osteophytes in primary OA)
2 Rheumatoid nodules
3 Gouty tophi (DIPs, PIPs, elbows, ears, heels)
4 Xanthomata

Differential diagnosis of morning stiffness
1 Rheumatoid arthritis
   a) Difficulty doing up buttons, etc.
   b) May improve with nocturnal NSAID suppositories
2 Ankylosing spondylitis
   a) Low back pain and stiffness radiating to buttocks and thighs
   b) Improved with exercise, NSAIDs
3 Polymyalgia rheumatica
   a) Difficulty getting out of bed
   b) *Marked* diurnal variation (may be asymptomatic by evening; cf. rotator cuff syndrome)
4 Osteoarthritis
   a) Short duration of stiffness (< 15 minutes)
   b) Pain may be worsened by prolonged use
5 Myxoedema

Differential diagnoses of miscellaneous presentations
1 Young patient with joint deformity
   a) Haemophilia (if male)
   b) Juvenile chronic arthritis
   c) Syringomyelia, Riley-Day (i.e. Charcot joint)
2 Charcot's joints
   a) Tabes dorsalis (→knee)
   b) Syringomyelia (→shoulder, elbow)
   c) Diabetes melilitus (→foot)
   d) Leprosy (lepromatous)
   e) Overzealous administration of intra-articular steroids
3 Acute monarthritis
   a) Septic
   b) Seronegative (incl. 'reactive')
   c) Haemarthrosis (±trauma)

d) Crystal-induced
— (Pseudo) gout
— Triamcinolone (arthritis occurs a few hours after joint injection)
4 Transient polyarthritis
a) SLE
b) Rheumatic fever, SBE, serum sickness
c) Parainfectious — e.g. hepatitis B, gonorrhoea
d) Reiter's syndrome, 'reactive' arthritides
e) Henoch-Schönlein purpura
5 Arthropathy affecting DIPs
a) Primary (familial) osteoarthritis
b) Psoriatic arthritis
c) Juvenile chronic arthritis; RA
d) Gout, sarcoidosis, haemochromatosis
e) Multicentric reticulohistiocytosis

—*if* extensive involvement of other joints

6 Sternoclavicular arthritis
a) Ankylosing spondylitis
b) Narcotic addiction
c) Tietze's syndrome
7 Chondrocalcinosis
a) Old age
b) Joint trauma (e.g. menisceal injury of knee)
c) Familial
d) Gout, OA, RA, Paget's
e) Metabolic predisposition
— Hyperparathyroidism; hypophosphatasia; hypomagnesaemia
— Haemochromatosis; ochronosis
— Acromegaly; myxoedema
— Wilson's disease

Clinical patterns suggesting misdiagnosis
1 'Osteoarthritis' with MCP (esp. 2nd and 3rd) involvement ±chondrocalcinosis on X-ray: suspect
a) Haemochromatosis
b) Wilson's disease
2 'Psoriatic arthritis' with pustular skin lesions and/or prominent eye involvement: suspect
a) Reiter's syndrome
3 'Ankylosing spondylitis' with negative HLA-B27 in a female, suspect
a) Psoriatic arthritis
b) Inflammatory bowel disease
4 Postdiarrhoeal 'reactive arthritis' followed by development of mucocutaneous lesion, suspect
a) Reiter's syndrome
b) Inflammatory bowel disease

EXAMINATION OF SPECIFIC JOINTS

Examination of the hip
1 Check for leg shortening (e. g. collapsed femoral head in OA)
2 Test movements — flexion, abduction, rotation
3 If indicated, test for suspected fixed flexion deformity of the hip (Thomas's test) — with the patient lying supine, flex the contralateral hip to straighten lumbar spine (and thus tilt pelvis to neutral); flexion of ipsilateral hip indicates fixed flexion deformity
4 If indicated, look for Trendelenburg sign (downward tilt of contralateral pelvis when weight-bearing on affected hip) — indicates severe joint or (esp. if bilateral) neuromuscular disease

Differential diagnosis of elbow lesions
1 Rheumatoid nodule
2 Gouty tophus
3 Olecranon bursa (e. g. due to gout, trauma)
4 Synovial cyst (different location to above)
5 Skin lesions
a) Tendon xanthoma
b) Pseudoxanthoma elasticum
c) Psoriasis
d) Subcutaneous calcification in CREST syndrome

Clinical diagnosis of shoulder pain
1 All movements restricted (incl. passive abduction *and* rotation) — *articular/capsular disease*
a) 'Frozen shoulder' (adhesive capsulitis)
b) Rheumatoid arthritis
c) Other synovitis, e.g. septic arthritis
2 Movements restricted in abduction only (passive rotation *normal*) — *rotator cuff injury* (→ 'painful arc')
a) Supraspinatus tendinitis
b) Infraspinatus tendinitis (active external rotation may be painful)
c) Subscapularis tendinitis (active internal rotation may be painful)
d) Bicipital tendinitis (localized tenderness; active supination may be painful)

CHARACTERISTICS OF SPECIFIC SYNDROMES

Adhesive capsulitis ('frozen shoulder'): natural history, therapy, and prognosis
1 *Pain* usually worsens within the first year of onset
2 *Function* usually improves over the first two years
3 >50% of patients are left with some residual dysfunction
4 Best managed with gentle active movements

Repetitive strain injury*: clinical features
1 Usually unilateral
2 Pain most often affects hand, shoulder girdle, and neck
3 Common symptoms
a) Proximal muscular 'tightness'
b) Weakness of handgrip
c) Hand numbness and/or paraesthesiae
4 *Not* associated with muscle wasting
No objective reproducible neurological deficit
5 Best treated by continuing normal limb activity

Carpal tunnel syndrome: physical findings
1 Wasting of thenar eminence

---

*Also called 'chronic regional pain syndrome' or 'localized fibromyalgia syndrome', i.e. **not** tenosynovitis/tendinitis

2 Weakness of thumb opposition and abduction
3 Sensory loss of the first three digits
4 Positive Tinel's sign
   Positive Phalen's test (numbness/pain reproduced by flexing wrists for one minute)
5 Predisposing stigmata, e. g.
   a) Rheumatoid arthritis ⎫—common in clinical
   b) Pregnancy   ⎬ practice
   c) Acromegaly   ⎫
   d) Myxoedema   ⎬—common in exams only

RHEUMATOID ARTHRITIS (RA)

Clinical assessment of disease activity
1 History
   a) Presence of constitutional symptoms
   b) Duration of morning stiffness
   c) Recent involvement of new joints
   d) Recent reduction in range of joint movement
2 Physical examination
   a) Number of *tender* swollen joints
   b) Degree of soft-tissue swelling/tenderness
   c) Ring size at proximal   ⎫— research
      interphalangeal joints   ⎬ measures
   d) Grip strength   ⎬ only
   e) Walking time for given distance ⎭

Differential diagnosis of impaired hand function in RA
1 Active disease — synovitis and/or tendinitis
2 Inactive disease — joint deformity
3 Tendon rupture
4 Carpal tunnel syndrome

Differential diagnosis of impaired walking in RA
1 Active disease (esp. metatarsal head involvement)
2 Inactive disease — joint deformity, muscle contractures
3 Muscle wasting (secondary to synovitis/deformity/steroids)
4 Peripheral neuropathy, mononeuritis multiplex
5 Spastic paraparesis (cervical myelopathy)

Diseases which may mimic rheumatoid arthritis
1 Psoriatic arthritis (*must* be rheumatoid factor negative)
2 Juvenile chronic arthritis (polyarticular RF+ subtype)
3 Rheumatic fever (arthritis typically spares neck and PIP joints)
   Postrheumatic fever (Jaccoud's) arthritis
4 SLE, MCTD, scleroderma
5 Other
   a) Relapsing polychondritis
   b) Multicentric reticulohistiocytosis
   c) Erosive osteoarthritis
   d) Calcium pyrophosphate deposition disease

Rheumatoid arthritis or osteoarthritis? Some comparisons
1 RA — Predominant DIP involvement rare
   OA — Predominant MCP involvement rare

2 RA — Disease manifestations include ulnar deviation at MCPs
   OA — Disease manifestations include first carpometacarpal joint involvement (clinically and radiologically)
3 RA — Tenderness on palpating dorsally subluxed ulnar styloid ('piano key' sign)
   OA — Tenderness on palpating first carpometacarpal joint
4 RA — Elbow disease manifests initially by reduced elbow extension due to predominant ulnar-humeral joint involvement
   OA — Elbow disease manifests initially by reduced supination due to predominant radio-humeral joint involvement
5 RA — First sign of neck involvement is reduced rotation
   OA — First sign of neck involvement is reduced lateral flexion

PATHOGENETIC MECHANISMS IN RHEUMATOID ARTHRITIS

Mechanisms of splenomegaly in rheumatoid arthritis
1 Primary disease manifestation (normal neutrophil count)
2 Felty's syndrome
3 Sjogren's syndrome
4 Amyloidosis

Mechanisms of muscle wasting in rheumatoid arthritis
1 Systemic hypercatabolism (i.e. wasting parallels weight loss)
2 Disuse atrophy
3 Inflammatory (vasculitic) myositis
4 Neuropathic
   a) Vasculitis
   b) Entrapment
   c) Splint-induced nerve compression (shouldn't happen)
5 Iatrogenic
   a) Corticosteroid myopathy
   b) Polymyositis/myasthenia gravis due to penicillamine (rarely causes wasting)

Mechanical basis of rheumatoid deformities
1 *Rupture* of flexor/extensor tendons is the most important mechanical complication; indicated by loss of *active* (but not passive) movements beginning in one finger and progressing (without treatment) to involve all. Therapy — repair of ruptured tendon(s), wrist synovectomy and excision of ulnar head to prevent further rupture
2 Ulnar deviation — subluxation of extensor tendons at MCP joints due to synovitic capsular ligamentous stretching
3 Swan-neck deformity — PIP joint hyperextension and compensatory DIP joint flexion due to interossei contractures and/or shortening of extensor tendon(s)
4 Bouttonière deformity — PIP fixed flexion contracture (with DIP hyperextension) due to division of extensor hood with consequent volar

slipping (or even detachment and rupture) of extensor tendon from middle phalanx
5 Mallet finger deformity — stretching or rupture of the extensor insertion into the dorsum of the terminal phalanx
6 Z-deformity of the thumb — MCP flexion and IP hyperextension due to either prolapse of the metacarpal head between the long and short extensor tendons, or rupture of the thumb flexor
7 'Piano-key' sign (hypermobility of a dorsally subluxated ulnar styloid) — laxity of the radioulnar joint

Pathogenesis of anaemia in rheumatoid arthritis
1 Active inflammatory ('chronic') disease (anaemia reflects disease *activity*, not *chronicity*)
2 Felty's syndrome
3 Iatrogenic
  a) Aspirin/NSAID-induced GI bleeding (NB: parenteral iron may cause arthritic 'flare')
  b) Gold/penicillamine-induced hypoplastic anaemia
  c) Sulphasalazine-induced haemolysis

COMPLICATIONS OF RHEUMATOID ARTHRITIS

Renal disorders in rheumatoid arthritis
1 Amyloidosis (nephrosis)
2 Renal tubular acidosis (in Sjögren's syndrome)
3 Analgesic nephropathy
4 Transient reversible proteinuria due to gold or penicillamine
  Nephrosis due to gold, penicillamine
  Goodpasture's syndrome due to penicillamine
5 NSAID-induced (usually benign) renal disease, e. g.
  a) Interstitial nephritis (→ haematuria, usually without proteinuria; may continue treatment)
  b) Nephrosis (rare)
  c) See also page 264

NB: *glomerular* disease as a primary disease manifestation of RA is uncommon and not characterized by specific pathology

Pulmonary manifestations of rheumatoid arthritis
1 Pleural disease (pleurisy, effusions)
2 Fibrosing alveolitis, interstitial fibrosis
3 Bronchiolitis obliterans (→ acute, often fatal, obstructive lung syndrome; may appear clinically and radiologically normal)
4 Pulmonary arteritis/hypertension
5 Nodules; may lead to
  a) Cavitation
  b) Bronchopleural fistulae
  c) Caplan's syndrome
6 Stridor due to
  a) Cricoarytenoid arthritis
  b) Nodule on vocal cords
7 Recurrent lower respiratory tract infections (Sjögren's)
8 Iatrogenic
  a) Asthma (salicylates)
  b) Allergic/fibrosing alveolitis (gold)
  c) Goodpasture's (D-penicillamine)
  d) Interstitial fibrosis (methotrexate, chlorambucil)

Rheumatoid complications with male predilection
1 'Rheumatoid lung' (fibrosis, effusions, nodules, pleurisy)
2 Accelerated vasculitis (e.g. → mononeuritis multiplex)
3 Mitral valvular regurgitation
  a) Commoner postmortem finding than aortic regurgitation
  b) *Rarely* of clinical significance (cf. AI)

Diagnosis of Felty's syndrome
1 Defining criteria
  a) Seropositive rheumatoid arthritis, *plus*
  b) Splenomegaly, *plus*
  c) Neutropenia
2 Frequent concomitants
  a) Serious infections
  b) Leg ulcers ⎫
  c) Mononeuritis multiplex ⎬ — (vasculitic)
  d) Anaemia, thrombocytopenia
  e) Lymphadenopathy, hepatomegaly
  f) Sjögren's syndrome
  g) Pigmentation, weight loss
3 Investigational clues
  a) Thrombocytopenia despite active disease
  b) Hypocomplementaemia
  c) Positive ANA, high-titre RF (IgM)
4 Response to medical therapy — leucocyte count may (paradoxically) be improved following gold administration
5 Response to splenectomy
  a) Arthritis not affected
  b) Leucopenia usually improves at least temporarily, though lasting benefit often absent
  c) Infections may (theoretically) be increased in frequency or severity

Bad prognostic indicators in rheumatoid arthritis
1 Insidious onset
  Polyarticular presentation
  Marked (>10%) weight loss
2 Fever; nodules; necrotizing scleritis; lung fibrosis; neuropathy
  Lymphadenopathy, splenomegaly (±Felty's/Sjögren's)
  Purpura (any cause)
  Amyloidosis
3 Early onset and/or rapid progression of erosions
4 Marked normochromic anaemia
  Thrombocytosis; eosinophilia (unless gold-induced)
  Hypoalbuminaemia, polyclonal gammopathy
  Markedly elevated ESR/acute phase reactants
5 Markedly elevated rheumatoid factor (IgM)
  Positive neutrophil-specific ANA
  Cryoglobulinaemia
6 HLA–DRw3 or –DRw4

CRYSTAL ARTHROPATHIES

Presentations of calcium pyrophosphate deposition disease
1 Asymptomatic capsular calcinosis or chondrocalcinosis (i. e. radiologic diagnosis) — 30%

2 Pseudogout (→knee, wrist) — 30%
3 Accelerated symmetric osteoarthritis — 30%
4 Pseudorheumatoid arthritis — 5%
5 Pseudoneuropathic arthritis (Charcot-like joint) — rare

Clinical spectrum of abnormal hydroxyapatite deposition

1 Supraspinatus tendinitis
2 Periarthritis in chronic haemodialysis
3 Milwaukee shoulder (destructive atrophic arthritis of the shoulder with activated enzymes and large quantities of hydroxyapatite crystals in synovial fluid)
4 Calcinosis associated with scleroderma, dermatomyositis
5 Myositis ossificans
6 Repeated intra-articular steroid injections into small finger joints

SERONEGATIVE SPONDYLOARTHROPATHIES

Ankylosing spondylitis: manoeuvres on clinical examination

1 Chest expansion (if <5 cm, indicates costovertebral involvement)
2 Schober's test — positive if full lumbar flexion fails to increase by >5 cm the distance between L5 and a point 15 cm above (indicative of lumbar disease)
3 Occiput to wall — failure of approximation suggests loss of cervicothoracic lordosis
4 Straight leg raising — suggests malingering if normal in patient with apparent gross impairment of forward flexion
5 Examination of peripheral joints, esp. hips and sternoclavicular joints.

Potential complications of ankylosing spondylitis

1 HLA-B27 co-variables
  a) Enthesopathy
    — Plantar fasciitis
    — Achilles' tendinitis
  b) Anterior uveitis
  c) Chronic prostatitis
2 Aortic incompetence (due to aortitis; cf. RA, where valve dysfunction arises due to valvulitis or nodules)
  Pericarditis; cardiac conduction defects
  Chest pain due to costovertebral joint disease
3 Restrictive lung function
  a) Impaired chest wall excursion
  b) Apical pulmonary fibrosis
4 Cauda equina syndrome
5 Amyloidosis
6 Leukaemia (esp. CGL) ⎤—if treated with spinal
  Bone sarcomas   ⎦ irradiation

Ankylosing spondylitis in females

1 Neck involvement and peripheral arthritis more common
2 Extra-articular manifestations more common
3 Radiological changes milder
4 True incidence may be underestimated

Clinical patterns of psoriatic arthritis

1 Oligoarticular asymmetric type (70%): 'sausage' digits (dactylitis) represent flexor tendon sheath effusions (also seen in Reiter's)
2 Distal interphalangeal joint type (15%): typically occurs with psoriatic nail disease (pitting, hyperkeratosis, onycholysis)
3 Pseudorheumatoid type
  a) Seronegative
  b) Affects males and females equally
  c) Arthritis severity varies with skin disease
4 Ankylosing spondylitis-type
  a) HLA-B27 positive in 75% only (i. e. less common than in ankylosing spondylitis or Reiter's, though still common)
5 Arthritis mutilans
  a) Often associated with sacroiliitis
  b) 'Telescoping' digits
  c) 'Opera-glass' deformity (may be painless)
  d) X-ray — 'pencil-in-cup' appearance

Rheumatic aspects of inflammatory bowel disease

1 A non-deforming asymmetric arthritis, principally affecting knees, ankles and PIPs, occurs in approximately 15%
2 This peripheral arthritis tends to occur at least 6 months following the onset of bowel disease. Its severity reflects that of the bowel disease; colectomy abolishes it
3 Erythema nodosum, uveitis, mouth ulcers and pyoderma occur in association with peripheral arthritis in IBD
4 Spondylitis/sacroiliitis occurs in approximately 5%, may predate the onset of bowel symptoms, and is associated with HLA-B27. It is independent of bowel disease activity and unaffected by colectomy, and there is no sex predilection
5 Arthritis and spondylitis in Whipple's disease remits with appropriate antibiotic therapy and has no recognized HLA association

Differential diagnosis of genital and oral ulceration

1 Reiter's syndrome
  Behçet's syndrome
2 Crohn's disease
3 Pemphigus
4 Erythema multiforme
5 Syphilis, herpes simplex
6 Strachan's (orogenital) syndrome

Reiter's vs. Behçet's syndrome: the clinical distinction

1 Reiter's
  a) Male:female = 10: 1
  b) Painless ulcers
  c) Predominant ocular manifestation: conjunctivitis
  d) Long-term ocular disability rare
  e) Long-term joint disability frequent (50%) — usually mild, but may on occasion be mutilating
  f) Spondylitis/sacroiliitis frequent
  g) HLA association — B27
  h) Infection seems important in pathogenesis
  i) Rx: NSAIDs
2 Behçet's
  a) Male:female = 2:1
  b) Painful ulcers

c) Predominant ocular manifestation: uveitis
d) Long-term ocular disability almost invariable
e) Long-term joint disability rare
f) Spondylitis/sacroiliitis uncommon
g) HLA associations: B12; B5 (ocular disease, esp. in Japanese; colitis)
h) Racial factors seem important in pathogenesis
i) R_x: immunosuppressives (e.g. cyclosporin)

Clinical spectrum of Behçet's syndrome
1 Eye disease (commoner in males, Japanese, HLA–B5; occurs in 80%)
   a) Uveitis → pain, photophobia, blurred vision
   b) Hypopyon; conjunctivitis, scleritis, phthisis bulbi
   c) Retinal venulitis → 'battlefield' fundus, CRV occlusion
   d) Optic neuritis
2 Genital ulceration, erythema nodosum (commoner in females; occurs in 80%; associated with non-deforming arthritis)
3 Mouth ulceration (98%)
4 Thrombophlebitis (30%)
   a) Sterile pustules at venepuncture sites
   b) CRV occlusion
5 CNS disease (30%)
   a) Aseptic meningitis
   b) TIA-like episodes
   c) Cranial nerve palsies
6 Colitis (30%)
   a) May lead to perforation
   b) Associated with HLA–B5
   c) Clinically overlaps with inflammatory bowel disease
      Spondylitis/sacroiliitis, when present, linked to HLA–B27

OCULAR SEQUELAE OF RHEUMATIC DISEASES

Uveitis: aetiological categorization
1 Seronegative arthritides (including inflammatory bowel disease)
   a) *Severe* in
      — Behçet's
      — Juvenile chronic arthritis (ANA + pauciarticular type)
   b) *Common* in
      — Ankylosing spondylitis
      — Reiter's syndrome (though conjunctivitis commoner)
   c) *Rare* in psoriatic arthropathy
2 Infection
   a) Toxoplasmosis, toxocara
   b) Leptospirosis, syphilis, TB, brucellosis, gonorrhoea
3 Sarcoidosis
4 Vogt-Koyanagi syndrome (chronic uveitis, recurrent aseptic meningitis, vitiligo, alopecia)
5 Idiopathic (60%) ± HLA–B27

Anterior vs posterior uveitis
1 Anterior uveitis (iritis)
   a) Uniocular (acute) presentation usual
   b) Painful red eye:

— Circumcorneal ('ciliary') hyperaemia
— Photophobia
— Discharge
c) Visual acuity unaffected, unless complicated by:
   — Anterior vitreous inflammation (iridocyclitis, hypopyon)
   — Corneal opacification (band keratopathy)
   — Cataracts, glaucoma (esp. if topical steroids used)
d) Slit-lamp examination may reveal posterior synechiae
e) Signs of chronicity — miosis/keratopathy/cataracts/glaucoma
f) Treated with mydriatics, topical and/or systemic steroids
2 Posterior uveitis (choroidoretinitis)
   a) Binocular (chronic) presentation usual
   b) Painless white eye
   c) Reduced visual acuity
      — Vitreous debris ('floaters')
      — Macular oedema
      — Retinopathy
   d) Fluorescein angiography reveals retinal venous leakage
   e) Treated with steroids, cytotoxics, surgery

Ocular manifestations of rheumatoid arthritis
1 Keratoconjunctivitis sicca (in 20–30%)
2 Scleral disease
   a) Episcleritis (hyperaemia) — good prognosis: sclera heals
   b) Scleritis — intermediate prognosis: sclera scars
   c) Scleromalacia perforans — poor prognosis: sclera sloughs
3 Scleral nodules and/or vasculitis
4 Iatrogenic
   a) Corneal opacities
      Pigmentary retinopathy } — chloroquine
   b) Cataracts — steroids

Differential diagnosis of band keratopathy
1 Juvenile chronic arthritis (ANA+, RF–, pauciarticular type)
2 Long-standing hyperparathyroidism
3 Long-standing renal failure
4 Long-standing sarcoidosis
5 Long-term chloroquine treatment (NB: corneal microdeposits also occur with amiodarone or chlorpromazine therapy)

Ocular complications of corticosteroid therapy
1 Herpes simplex keratitis (esp. with topical steroids)
2 Papilloedema (benign intracranial hypertension)
3 Cataract
4 Glaucoma

INVESTIGATING RHEUMATIC DISEASES

SEROLOGICAL ASSESSMENT OF RHEUMATIC DISEASE

The acute phase reactants
1 Grossly elevated in inflammatory conditions:

a) C-reactive protein
b) Serum amyloid-A (SAA) component } — ↑ In RA/JCA; normal in SLE
2 Moderately elevated in inflammatory conditions
   a) $α_1AT$, orosomucoid, $α_1$ acid glycoprotein
   b) Haptoglobin, caeruloplasmin, AT III
   c) $C_3(C_4, C_9)$
   d) Fibrinogen, plasminogen; factors V, VIII
   e) Ferritin
3 Decreased in inflammatory conditions
   a) Albumin, prealbumin
   b) Transferrin, iron, TIBC
   c) Fibronectin

Potential clinical value of C–reactive protein estimations
1 Reportedly correlates more closely than ESR with
   a) Radiographic progression of joint damage
   b) Disease response to gold/penicillamine — in rheumatoid arthritis
2 Reportedly useful in monitoring activity of
   a) Ankylosing spondylitis
   b) Juvenile chronic arthritis
3 Reportedly helpful in distinguishing infective episodes in
   a) SLE
   b Sicca syndrome } ↑ ↑ CRP in infection; normal in active disease
4 Grossly elevated values may reportedly aid in distinguishing
   a) Rheumatoid arthritis (from SLE)
   b) Crohn's disease (from ulcerative colitis)
   c) Bacterial meningitis (from viral)
   d) Pyelonephritis (from cystitis)

Rheumatoid factors: clinical correlations
1 RA latex (human IgG) — most sensitive test
2 Rose-Waaler (rabbit IgG) — most specific test
3 Marked elevation in RA
   a) Rheumatoid lung disease
   b) Felty's, Sjögren's
4 Marked elevation in non-rheumatic conditions
   a) SBE
   b) Myeloma
   c) Cryoglobulinaemia

Grossly elevated ESR in rheumatoid arthritis
1 Highly active synovitis
2 Extra-articular vasculitis
3 Development of amyloidosis
4 Sjögren's syndrome
5 Septic arthritis

RADIOLOGICAL ASSESSMENT OF RHEUMATIC DISEASE

Classical X–ray signs of common rheumatic disorders
1 Rheumatoid arthritis
   a) Most diagnostic — cortical erosions in MCP joints, ulnar styloid, carpal bones, and feet
   b) Early signs
      — Soft-tissue swelling
      — Juxta-articular osteoporosis (non-specific)

c) Late signs — joint subluxation, narrowing, deformity, atlantoaxial subluxation
2 Primary (familial) osteoarthritis
   a) Osteophyte formation
   b) Subchondral sclerosis (*no* periarticular osteoporosis)
   c) Joint space narrowing
   d) Loose bodies
   e) Sparing of metacarpophalangeal joints
3 Chondrocalcinosis — calcification of cartilage in
   a) Knee
   b) Wrist
   c) Symphysis pubis
   d) Intervertebral discs
4 Reiter's syndrome
   a) Periostitis contiguous with affected joints
   b) Calcaneal spurs
   c) Asymmetric joint erosions sparing hands
   d) Asymmetric sacroiliitis
5 Charcot (neuropathic) joint
   a) Both sides of joint exhibit destructive changes and sclerosis
   b) Loose bodies present within joint; soft tissue swelling
   c) No osteoporosis

Differential diagnosis of radiographic erosions in hands
1 Rheumatoid arthritis
2 Gout
3 Psoriatic arthritis
4 Sarcoidosis
5 Miscellaneous
   a) Gaucher's
   b) Albright's (polyostotic fibrous dysplasia)
   c) Osteitis fibrosa cystica ('brown tumours')
   d) Aneurysmal bone cyst, non-ossifying fibroma

The abnormal spinal radiograph: features and diagnosis
1 Ankylosing spondylitis
   a) Vertebral 'squaring'
   b) Syndesmophyte formation (→ 'bamboo spine')
   c) Romanus lesion (erosion of anterosuperior vertebral body)
   d) Apophyseal joint fusion
   e) Sacroiliac joint erosion, sclerosis or fusion
   f) Hip joint erosions
2 DISH (diffuse idiopathic skeletal hyperostosis; Forestier's disease)
   a) Heavy ossification of paraspinal ligaments
   b) Olecranon and/or calcaneal spurs
   c) Preservation of disc height
   d) Normal sacroiliac joints
3 Pott's disease (spinal TB)
   a) Gibbus (acute anterior angulation)
   b) Paraspinal mass
   c) Narrowing of disc space
   d) Vertebral body collapse (often affecting vertebrae in contiguity)
4 Metastatic carcinoma
   a) Obliteration of pedicle in P–A view
   b) Discrete lytic (and/or sclerotic) lesions throughout spine
   c) Multiple levels of vertebral collapse

5 (Old) Scheuermann's disease (benign adolescent osteochondritis) — residual stigmata of vertebral epiphyseal osteochondritis
6 Straight back syndrome (often associated with marfanoid habitus and/or mitral valve prolapse) — marked reduction of A–P chest diameter on lateral CXR

Differential diagnosis of sacroiliitis
1 Ankylosing spondylitis
2 Other seronegative arthritides — psoriatic, Reiter's, juvenile chronic arthritis
3 Inflammatory bowel disease; 'reactive' spondyloarthritis
4 Infection
   a) Septic arthritis
   b) TB
   c) Brucellosis
5 Recurrent polyserositis (familial Mediterranean fever)
6 Ochronosis

Atlanto-axial subluxation: diagnosis and management
1 Pathogenesis
   a) Odontoid erosion
   b) Ligamentous destruction
2 Occurrence
   a) Rheumatoid arthritis
   b) Juvenile chronic arthritis
   c) Ankylosing spondylitis
3 Diagnosis — >2.5 mm displacement of odontoid peg on atlas seen on flexion cervical spine radiograph
4 Management if symptomatic
   a) MRI scan — may show mass of inflammatory tissue
   b) If positive MRI scan, proceed to surgery
      — Transoral anterior approach for resection of inflammatory tissue ± odontoid peg, *plus*
      — Posterior cervical fusion
5 Management if asymptomatic
   a) Cervical collar when driving
   b) Check for A–a subluxation (with lateral flexion/extension cervical spine films) prior to general anaesthesia
   c) Spinal rather than general anaesthesia for elective surgery if possible

INVASIVE ASSESSMENT OF JOINT DISEASE

Indications for joint aspiration
1 Diagnosis
   a) Septic arthritis
   b) Crystal synovitis
2 Therapy — massive effusion interfering with joint function
3 Diagnosis and therapy — haemarthrosis

Indications for joint injection
1 Diagnosis

   a) Arthrogram for suspected menisceal (knee) tears
   b) Arthrogram for suspected (ruptured) Baker's cyst
2 Therapeutic
   a) Intra-articular corticosteroids
   b) 'Medical synovectomy' (yttrium[90])

Indications for diagnostic arthroscopy
1 Unexplained monarthritis
2 Suspected mechanical derangement (e. g. menisceal tear, cruciate ligament rupture)
3 Histologic diagnosis sought (e. g. suspected villonodular synovitis)

Important diagnoses on synovial biopsy
1 Tuberculous arthritis
2 (Pigmented) villonodular synovitis
3 Amyloidosis
4 Ochronosis (alkaptonuria)
5 Synovial tumours (e. g. haemangioma)

ANALYSIS OF SYNOVIAL FLUID

Non-inflammatory effusions: characteristics and causes
1 Characteristics
   a) Synovial fluid white cell count $<2 \times 10^9$/l
   b) High viscosity
   c) Negative fibrin clot
2 Causes
   a) Osteoarthritis
   b) Post-traumatic
   c) Sympathetic (e. g. adjacent to osteomyelitis)
   d) Myxoedema
   e) Amyloidosis
   f) Sickle-cell disease
   g) Hypertrophic pulmonary osteoarthropathy

Synovial fluid leucocyte counts in health and disease
1 Normal — $<0.2 \times 10^9$/l
2 'Non-inflammatory' synovitis (see below) — $<2.0 \times 10^9$/l — e. g. osteoarthritis
   a) $0.2-5 \times 10^9$/l (av. 0.5×10^9/l)
   b) 10–30% polymorphs
3 Inflammatory synovitis
   a) Septic arthritis
      — $5-500 \times 10^9$/l (av. 50×10^9/l)
      — 80–100% polymorphs
   b) Gout
      — $2-300 \times 10^9$/l (av. 15×10^9/l)
      — 60–95% polymorphs
   c) Reiter's syndrome
      — $2-50 \times 10^9$/l (av. 20×10^9/l)
      — 50–90% polymorphs
   d) Rheumatoid arthritis
      — $2-100 \times 10^9$/l (av. 10×10^9/l)
      — 50–75% polymorphs

Other joint fluid abnormalities
1 Low glucose level
   a) Septic arthritis
   b) Reiter's syndrome
   c) Rheumatoid arthritis (also low in rheumatoid effusions)

2 Complement levels
  a) Elevated in Reiter's syndrome
  b) Low in rheumatoid arthritis, SLE, gout, sepsis
  (Note that *plasma* complement levels may be
  similarly low in active SLE, but elevated in active
  rheumatoid arthritis. Hence, synovial:serum
  complement ratio is typically <10% in RA without
  systemic vasculitis. When RA is complicated by
  systemic vasculitis, however, plasma complement
  levels are usually also low
3 Cytology
  a) Phagocytosed leucocytes — Reiter's syndrome
  b) 'Ragocytes' — rheumatoid arthritis
  c) Haemosiderin-laden *macrophages* — recurrent
     haemarthroses
  d) Haemosiderin-laden *synovial cells* —
     haemochromatosis

Differential diagnosis of haemarthrosis

1 Haemophilia
2 Major trauma (e. g. fracture communicating with
  joint)
  Minor trauma in anticoagulated patient
3 Joint tumours, incl. pigmented villonodular
  synovitis
4 Charcot joint; arthritis mutilans
5 Calcium pyrophosphate deposition disease
6 'Traumatic tap' — distinguish from true
  haemarthrosis by centrifuging aspirate and
  demonstrating absent xanthochromia

Crystal arthropathies: findings on joint aspiration

1 Gout
  a) Needleshaped urate crystals
  b) Strongly negative birefringence on polarized
     microscopy
  c) Angle of extinction — parallel
  d) Crystals may be found in non-inflamed joints in
     gouty patients
2 Pseudogout
  a) Rhomboid-shaped pyrophosphate crystals
  b) Weakly positive birefringence
  c) Angle of extinction — oblique
3 Rheumatoid arthritis may mimic crystal synovitis
  due to presence of cholesterol crystals in chronic
  effusions
4 Hydroxyapatite crystals may be visualised on
  electron microscopy in osteoarthritis or other
  arthritides, especially when bone destruction
  present
5 Post-steroid injection flare (4–12 hours afterwards)
  is probably due to steroid crystals

HLA IN RHEUMATIC DISEASE

Relative indications for tissue typing in rheumatic disease

1 Older male child (11–16 years) with oligoarthritis, *if*
  probability of ankylosing spondylitis seems around
  50% using combined clinical and radiological
  criteria (i. e. if diagnosis of inflammatory back
  disease seems neither very likely nor unlikely):
  B27-positive indicates 90% probability of

ankylosing spondylitis (and hence reduced risk of
chronic anterior uveitis)
  B27–negative indicates 15% probability of
  ankylosing spondylitis (and hence increased risk of
  chronic anterior uveitis; see p. 306)
2 Controversial — DR3 screening to predict patients
  at increased risk of renal toxicity from
  gold/penicillamine

NB: *No* absolute — or routine— indications currently
exist

HLA associations in rheumatoid arthritis

1 DR4
  a) Increased incidence of (seropositive) disease
2 DR3
  a) Increased incidence of strongly seropositive
     (aggressive) variant
  b) Increased incidence of major side-effects (esp.
     heavy proteinuria, cytopaenia) from gold,
     penicillamine
  c) Increased incidence of Sjögren's syndrome,
     which may in turn be associated with either of
     the above two trends
3 DR2
  a) Decreased incidence of disease
  b) Increased incidence of stomatitis due to gold
     therapy

MANAGING RHEUMATIC DISEASE

Therapeutic emergencies in rheumatic disease

1 Atlanto-axial subluxation
  a) Tends to affect RA patients on long-term steroids
  b) Rx — surgical decompression and fusion for
     progressive symptomatic disease
2 Temporal arteritis
  a) Draw blood for ESR as soon as diagnosis
     suspected
  b) Rx — prednisone 20–60 mg/day (high doses
     used if ocular involvement)
  c) Treatment may be commenced as soon as ESR
     sample drawn — biopsy appearances unaffected
     by up to 48 hours of steroids
3 Septic arthritis
  a) Drain joint, Gram-stain, culture, sensitivity
  b) Rx — intravenous antibiotics
4 Vasculitic complications
  a) Mononeuritis multiplex; digital gangrene, bowel
     infarction
  b) Rx — high-dose steroids, cytotoxic drugs
5 Iridocyclitis
  a) May complicate seronegative
     spondyloarthropathy (*not* RA)
  b) Rx — mydriatics, topical/systemic steroids
  Episcleritis
  a) May complicate RA (*not* seronegative
     spondyloarthropathies)
  b) Rx — topical steroids, NSAIDs, or systemic
     steroids
6 Iatrogenic — GI bleed, blood dyscrasia, adrenal
  dysfunction

a) Identify and cease offending medication
b) Rx — supportive

GENERAL MEASURES IN RHEUMATIC DISORDERS

Rationâle of exercise in joint disease
1 To maintain or restore muscle strength around joint
2 To maintain or restore range of joint movement
3 To prevent or minimize periarticular osteoporosis

Principles of occupational therapy in rheumatic disease
1 Provision of appliances to reduce joint strain
   a) Work splints (for wrists)
   b) Removable splints (for unstable knees)
   c) Cervical collars (hard or soft)
2 Provision of appliances to improve function
   a) Special shoes and insoles, non-slip mats
   b) Walking sticks, wheelchairs, walking frames
   c) Shopping cart
3 Home visits to assist in household adaptation for activities of daily living
   a) Toilet aids, handrails, electric toothbrush
   b) Tap turners, electric can opener, large-handled cutlery
   c) Bookrest, page-turner, push-button phone, electric typewriter

Principles of physiotherapy in rheumatoid arthritis
1 *Night splinting* to rest joints in a position of function (esp. knees, wrists)
   Serial splinting to reverse early deformities such as knee flexion, (NB: bedrest usually exacerbates wasting and deformity in patients with active disease)
2 *Passive exercises* to maintain range of joint movement
   Isometric exercises to maintain muscle power
   Active exercises to maintain muscle power as well as range of joint movement
3 Facilitation of exercise using
   a) Ultrasound
   b) Heat
   c) Hydrotherapy

Management of nerve or tendon compression in rheumatoid arthritis
1 **S**plinting (esp. wrist or knee)
2 **S**ystemic treatment (e.g. gold)
3 **S**teroid injection (use soluble preparation to reduce risk of neurolysis)
4 **S**urgical decompression
5 **S**ynovectomy (esp. wrist or knee)

Effects of good posture/physiotherapy on ankylosing spondylitis
1 *No* effect on rate of ankylosis
2 *Mild* reduction in pain
3 *Major* reduction in disability (e. g. eventual ankylosis occurs in erect, rather than kyphotic, posture)

NON-STEROIDAL ANTI-INFLAMMATORY DRUGS (NSAIDs)

Points to consider in NSAID prescribing
1 NSAIDs may improve joint *function* by reducing pain and inflammation; they do not, however, appear to reverse the course of the arthropathy
2 The maximal tolerated dose of any given NSAID should be prescribed before being discarded as ineffective
3 Several NSAIDs may need to be tried before finding an acceptable drug
4 In general, different NSAIDs should *not* be combined

Non-steroidal anti-inflammatory drugs: toxicity
1 Gastrointestinal — dyspepsia, gastritis, ulceration* (esp. with high-dose aspirin, indomethacin)
2 CNS — headache, confusion, dizziness (esp. indomethacin)
3 Blood dyscrasias (esp. with phenylbutazone — aplastic anaemia, agranulocytosis, haemolytic anaemia, thrombocytopenia[†])
4 Nephrotoxicity
   a) Precipitation of acute renal failure
   b) Oedema (sodium retention); nephrosis (rare) ⎬ — see also page 264
   c) Papillary necrosis
   d) Interstitial nephritis
5 Unusual — bullous dermatoses, hepatitis, aseptic meningitis, hypersensitivity reactions

ASPIRIN

Aspirin as first-line therapy
1 Juvenile chronic arthritis
2 Rheumatic fever
3 Rheumatoid arthritis
4 Seronegative
5 Spondyloarthropathies (except AS) ⎬ — In USA only
   Soft tissue rheumatism

* NB: The reported association of aspirin with Reye's syndrome makes close monitoring mandatory in children younger than 12 requiring aspirin therapy

Predispositions to aspirin hepatotoxicity
1 Juvenile chronic arthritis
2 Reiter's syndrome
3 Chronic active hepatitis
4 Rheumatic fever
5 SLE

Presentations of aspirin sensitivity
1 Urticaria, bronchospasm, anaphylaxis
2 Pyrexia of unknown origin

---

*Sulindac and ibuprofen are probably the least ulcerogenic of these drugs. In general, however, patient tolerance of any one drug is quite unpredictable.
†Phenylbutazone now only indicated for control of refractory ankylosing spondylitis under hospital supervision

3 Pneumonitis
4 Pancreatitis
5 Proctocolitis
6 Ulceration of the oesophagus

Aspirin toxicity: the clinical spectrum

1 Anti-inflammatory action requires daily dosage of 2–4 g/day
2 Gastrointestinal intolerance is the commonest cause of noncompliance at these dosage levels
3 Tinnitus and vertigo are dose-related toxicities which may be clinically useful in regulating drug dosage. Hearing loss may necessitate treatment cessation; salicylate levels and/or audiograms may be useful in monitoring
4 Iron-deficiency anaemia may be precipitated in the absence of gastrointestinal symptoms; hypoprothrombinaemia occurs rarely
5 High-dose regimens are uricosuric, whereas low-dose administration may lead to hyperuricaemia and gout
6 Hepatotoxicity typically manifests as asymptomatic transaminase elevation which often normalizes even if the drug is continued at the same dosage. It occurs more commonly in young patients

REMITTIVE DRUG THERAPY

Diseases treatable with remittive drug therapy

1 Gold
   a) Rheumatoid arthritis
   b) Sjögren's syndrome (reportedly higher incidence of drug reactions; sicca syndrome alone may not respond)
   c) Psoriatic arthritis
   d) Juvenile chronic arthritis
   e) Pemphigus (steroid-sparing)
2 D-Penicillamine
   a) Rheumatoid arthritis ⎫
   b) Cystinuria   ⎬ → proteinuria in 25%
   c) Wilson's disease (→ proteinuria in 5%)
   d) Psoriatic arthritis
   e) Heavy metal poisoning
3 Chloroquine
   a) SLE (esp. joint and skin involvement)
   b) Juvenile chronic arthritis
   c) Rheumatoid arthritis
   d) *Contraindicated* in psoriatic arthritis
4 Sulphasalazine
   a) Rheumatoid arthritis
   b) Seronegative spondyloarthropathies

Gold: toxicity

1 Pruritic rash
   a) Occurs in 30% of treated patients
   b) May mimic lichen planus, pityriasis rosea
   c) Frequently preceded by development of peripheral eosinophilia
   d) More common with aurothiomalate than with aurothioglucose or (oral) auranofin
2 Stomatitis, mouth ulcers; auranofin → diarrhoea
3 Leucopenia, thrombocytopenia — constitute an absolute indication for treatment cessation; in acute management heavy metal chelators may be indicated
4 Proteinuria
   a) Occurs in 5% of treated patients
   b) If <1 g/day, drug may be cautiously reintroduced following normalization of protein excretion
   c) If >1 g/day, cease gold therapy indefinitely
5 Nephrosis
   a) Occurs in 1% of treated patients
   b) Recovery may take 18 months
6 Rare — fibrosing alveolitis, enterocolitis, cholestasis, peripheral neuropathy

D-Penicillamine: toxicity

1 Loss of taste, anorexia, nausea
   a) Occurs in 25%
   b) Improves with continued treatment
2 Proteinuria (25%), nephrosis (5%)
3 Thrombocytopenia (10%)
4 Early rash (10%) within first month — treatment may be reintroduced
   Wrinkly skin (elastosis serpiginosa perforans)
   Late (pemphigus-like) rash: occurs in 5%; if severe, cease treatment
5 Rare — SLE, myasthenia gravis, polymyositis, Goodpasture-like syndrome
6 Lack of efficacy (25%) — similar incidence to gold, and more likely if previously unresponsive thereto

TREATING RHEUMATOID ARTHRITIS

Rheumatoid arthritis: indications for remittive therapy

1 Symptomatic young patients (esp. females) with polyarticular disease and high levels of rheumatoid factor
2 Development of radiological erosions within the first year of symptomatic disease
3 Symptomatic disease activity despite optimal anti-inflammatory medication for 6 months
4 Development of extra-articular disease affecting vital organ function

Prescribing strategy in rheumatoid arthritis

1 First-line therapy — symptomatic treatment only
   a) NSAIDs
   b) Aspirin 3–4 g/day (popular in USA only)
2 Second-line therapy — remittive drugs (may reverse X–ray erosions)
   a) Gold (intramuscular or oral)
   b) D-Penicillamine
   c) Sulphasalazine
   d) (Hydroxy) chloroquine
3 Third-line therapy — failure of conventional remittive drugs
   a) Cytotoxics (azathioprine, cyclophosphamide)
   b) Systemic corticosteroids
4 Experimental therapy — total nodal irradiation

NB: nocturnally administered slow-release NSAIDs (oral or suppositories, e. g. indomethacin) may help minimize morning stiffness in RA

Indications for systemic steroids in rheumatoid arthritis

1 Development of stridor
2 Necrotizing scleritis
3 Pleuropericarditis
4 Other manifestations of extra-articular vasculitis which threaten to impair vital organ function, e.g. mononeuritis multiplex
5 Persistent arthritic activity despite adequate trial of remittive treatment

SYSTEMIC STEROIDS IN RHEUMATIC DISEASE

Prescribing steroids in rheumatoid arthritis

1 Uncommonly indicated
2 If considered necessary, treatment should be aimed towards a specific goal (i. e. considered a temporizing measure only)
3 Treatment should be low-dose: 5–7.5 mg prednisone/day max.
4 To minimize adrenal suppression, aim to use a single morning dose only
5 Alternate-day steroids don't work in RA; if symptoms appear well-controlled on alternate-day steroids, then the patient probably doesn't need steroids at all

Potency and toxicity of various corticosteroids

1 30 mg cortisone acetate
   = 25 mg hydrocortisone
   = 5 mg (methyl)prednis(ol)one, triamcinolone
   = 1 mg dexamethasone, betamethasone
2 Hydrocortisone causes major sodium retention; hence useful in adrenal replacement therapy, but not otherwise
3 Triamcinolone, given systemically, is the most myopathic of the corticosteroids; therefore only used topically
4 Prednisone is a pro-drug; hence in *severe* liver disease, better to use prednisolone (the active metabolite)

ACTH or prednisone? Pros and cons of ACTH therapy

1 Disadvantages of ACTH
   a) Expensive
   b) Painful (daily intramuscular injections)
   c) Difficult to adjust or taper dosage
   d) Greater salt/fluid retention than prednisone (reflecting greater mineralocorticoid effect)
   e) Pigmentation; bruising; occasional severe allergic reactions
2 Advantages of ACTH
   a) For juvenile chronic arthritis patients: less stunting of growth
   b) For hospitalized patients with early severe inflammatory arthritis — no adrenal suppression, hence easier to discontinue than oral steroids
   c) For polymyositis/dermatomyositis/multiple sclerosis patients — less muscle wasting than oral steroids (androgen effect)
   d) For postmenopausal female patients in

particular — less osteoporosis (↑ androstenedione → ↑ oestrone by peripheral conversion)

INTRA-ARTICULAR STEROIDS

Potential indications for intra-articular steroids

1 Systemic treatment contraindicated (e. g. blood dyscrasia induced)
2 Systemic treatment inadequate to control inflammation at one or more joints
3 Troublesome oligoarticular inflammation not warranting systemic therapy (e. g. peripheral joint disease in seronegative spondyloarthropathy)
4 To assist mobilization (and deformity reduction) in rehabilitation
5 Rapid analgesia required

Intra-articular steroids: which joints?

1 Common — knee, shoulder
2 Less often — ankle, elbow, fingers
3 Rare — hip

Intra-articular steroid therapy: potential morbidity

1 Crystal-induced synovitis (manifests as a 'flare' of pain and swelling a few hours after injection; commoner with triamcinolone)
2 Charcot-like arthropathy (i. e. severe joint destruction, though probably **not** due to loss of pain sensation)
3 Cushing's syndrome
4 Septic arthritis, *or*
5 Suppression of inflammatory signs, e.g. in septic arthritis complicating RA

ANTIMALARIALS IN RHEUMATIC DISEASE

Potential hazards of antimalarial chemotherapy

1 Chloroquine is traditionally avoided in psoriatic arthritis due to the risk of precipitating a pustular exacerbation of the skin disease (which may in turn be indistinguishable from the keratoderma blenorrhagica of Reiter's syndrome)
2 Chloroquine should not be administered in full antirheumatic dosage to SLE patients with known coexisting porphyria cutanea tarda; there is a recognized association between the two disorders. When the drug is administered in this context, the patient should be phlebotomized on at least two prior occasions and the drug given in low-dose twice-weekly schedule
3 Oculotoxicity may include cycloplegia (→ transient visual blurring) and corneal microdeposits (rarely culminating in band keratopathy) in addition to the well-known retinopathy

Features of chloroquine retinopathy

1 Occurrence is commoner with
   a) Renal impairment
   b) SLE
   c) Concomitant probenecid therapy
   d) Daily dosage >150 mg *base* per day (i.e.

>250 mg chloroquine phosphate/sulphate or 400 mg hydroxychloroquine)
2 Occurrence cannot be predicted by onset of visual symptoms (these are more commonly due to presbyopia or cycloplegia in any case)
3 Slit-lamp examination every 4–6 months is regarded as mandatory, though the benefit remains unproven. The best screening tests are
 a) Observation of the foveal reflex
 b) Charting the pericentral visual fields to a red object
4 The classic 'bull's eye' macula may supervene despite early cessation of therapy

THE HYPERURICAEMIC PATIENT

Aetiology of hyperuricaemia in childhood
1 Associated with gout in childhood
 a) HGPRTase deficiency (Lesch-Nyhan syndrome)
 b) PRPP synthetase overactivity
2 Not associated with gout in childhood
 a) Acute leukaemia (esp. lymphoblastic; esp. post-chemotherapy)
 b) Chronic haemolysis (e. g. sickle-cell disease)
 c) Lead poisoning
 d) Von Gierke's; Gaucher's
 e) Severe diabetes mellitus, hypertriglyceridaemia

Management aspects of gout and hyperuricaemia
1 Modalities available for treating acute gouty arthritis
 a) Colchicine (traditional remedy; major GI toxicity)
 b) NSAIDs (now more popular than colchicine)
 c) Joint aspiration
 d) Intra-articular corticosteroids
2 Drugs inhibiting uricosuric (probenecid, sulphinpyrazone) efficacy — i.e., avoid these:
 a) Thiazides
 b) Ethambutol
 c) Low-dose salicylate
 d) Cyclosporine

Exclusive indications for allopurinol administration
1 Tophaceous gout, *or* gouty bony erosions
2 Recurrent troublesome acute gouty attacks
3 Recurrent urate calculi, *or* recurrent oxalate calculi associated with hyperuricosuria
4 Prevention of uric acid nephropathy in patients at risk for tumour lysis syndrome (p. 142) about to commence chemotherapy
5 *Massive* urate overproduction (>7.2 mmol/24 hour urinary excretion) despite low-purine alcohol-restricted diet, esp. if family history of renal disease

NB: Asymptomatic hyperuricaemia or uncomplicated gout are **not** indications for maintenance allopurinol

Allopurinol: toxicity
1 Major hypersensitivity reactions (toxic epidermal necrolysis, vasculitis, eosinophilia) may be heralded by apparently trivial episodes of rash or fever
2 Major reactions are more common in the presence of renal impairment and/or diuretic therapy, and may lead to renal failure
3 Hepatotoxicity is an uncommon but serious sequela
4 Ampicillin rashes are more frequent in allopurinol-treated patients
5 Allopurinol potentiates
 a) 6MP, azathioprine (four-fold)
 b) Warfarin (weak effect)

OPERATIVE OPTIONS IN JOINT DISEASE

Rheumatoid arthritis: the place of surgery
1 Resection of metatarsal heads (for forefoot pain due to MTP subluxation)
2 Total articular arthroplasty (ideal for hip)
3 Excision arthroplasty
 a) Excision of radial head in severe erosive elbow arthritis
 b) Resection of distal ulna as part of wrist synovectomy
4 Synovectomy (tends to improve symptoms for about 2 years)
 a) Knee — for symptomatic Baker's cyst unresponsive to intra-articular steroids
 b) Wrist — for nodular tenosynovitis refractory to remittive therapy
5 Miscellaneous
 a) Silastic MCP joint replacement (deformity recurs)
 b) Immediate tendon reanastomosis for rupture
 c) Posterior cervical fusion for atlanto-axial subluxation
 d) Decompression of entrapment neuropathies
 e) Splenectomy in Felty's syndrome

Total hip replacement: indications and complications
1 Indications
 a) Patient older than 50 with unrelieved hip pain of arthritic aetiology
 b) Any patient with permanent loss of hip mobility (<45° flexion, <10° abduction) leading to reduced activity (unable to climb stairs, etc.)
2 Complications
 a) Implant loosening
 b) Infection of bone–cement interface
 c) Metal sensitivity (→loosening)
 d) Mechanical failure
 e) Postoperative thromboembolism despite prophylaxis

Arthrodesis or osteotomy? Clinical considerations
1 Arthrodesis
 a) Favoured joints — wrist; ankle (subtalar joint only)
 b) Less popular — knee, hip, tarsal, 1st MCP
 c) Best for young (20–30) patients
 d) Optimally indicated in monarthritis since reduced joint mobility is less significant
 e) Indicated in preference to osteotomy if X-ray reveals destruction of joint architecture
2 Osteotomy
 a) Favoured joints — hip, knee
 b) Best for patients younger than 50

c) Optimally indicated in painful joints of adequate stability in which improved mobility is not a priority
d) Indicated in preference to arthrodesis if X-ray confirms asymmetrical disruption of joint architecture

Anaesthetic considerations in patients with rheumatic disease
1 Rheumatoid arthritis
  a) If cervical spine X-ray shows atlanto-axial subluxation and/or odontoid erosion in an asymptomatic patient, protect with soft collar and opt for spinal anaesthesia if possible
  b) If atlanto-axial subluxation or odontoid erosion is radiologically apparent in a patient with progressive symptoms due to cord compression, assess further with MRI and consider cervical spine surgery (p. 299) prior to elective operation
  c) If temporomandibular joint disease evident, anticipate difficult endotracheal intubation (though rarely a major problem in RA; cf. in JCA)
2 Ankylosing spondylitis
  a) Lower cervical spondylosis and/or TMJ disease may make intubation difficult
  b) Costovertebral joint involvement may restrict lung ventilation
3 Juvenile chronic arthritis — intubation may be a **major** problem if micrognathia present

Patient selection for 'medical synovectomy'
(i.e. intra-articular instillation of, say ^{90}yttrium)
1 Most effective for recurrent knee effusions of inflammatory origin
2 Pregnancy, or any risk thereof, constitutes an absolute contraindication
3 Youth is a relative contraindication in view of the theoretical risk of leukaemogenesis
4 Ideally the joint to be injected should be devoid of gross synovial thickening or severe destructive changes
5 An adequate trial of rest, physiotherapy, systemic drug therapy and intra-articular steroids should precede medical synovectomy

PAGET'S DISEASE

Treatable causes of pain in Paget's disease
1 Osteoarthritis (hip, knee) due to limb deformity
2 Pseudogout
3 Nerve entrapment
4 Microfractures due to cortical expansion
5 Pathological fracture
  a) Disease-related
  b) Supervening osteosarcoma
  c) Diphosphonate use

Indications for commencement of specific chemotherapy
1 Serum alkaline phosphatase >1000 U/l

2 Severe bone pain unresponsive to conservative measures
3 Intractable angina or heart failure (if due to Paget's)
4 Progressive deformity of weight-bearing long bones or skull base, esp. in relatively young patients
  Osteolytic lesions with cortical thinning of long bones, esp. if painful
5 Hypercalcaemia (precipitated by immobilization or trauma) and/or radio-opaque renal calculi
6 Neurological sequelae
  a) Spinal cord compression
  b) Peripheral nerve entrapment
  c) Visual failure due to macular degeneration
  d) Progressive deafness accompanied by tinnitus

Drug treatment: relative indications and contraindications
1 Calcitonin
  a) Indications
    — Severe bone pain requiring rapid relief
    — Painful osteolytic lesions
    — Hypercalcaemia/symptomatic hypercalciuria
    — Failure or toxicity of alternative therapy
  b) Contraindications
    — Resistance due to neutralizing antibodies
    — Unsuitability of parenteral administration and ongoing expense
2 Biphosphonates
  a) Indications
    — Predominant skull involvement
    — Mild to moderate bone pain
    — Incomplete clinical or biochemical response to calcitonin
  b) Contraindications
    — Severe bone pain (may be worsened)
    — Development of otherwise unexplained fractures (may complicate treatment courses of >6 months)
    — Known (pre-existing) osteolytic lesions
    — Development of diarrhoea while on treatment
3 Mithramycin
  a) Indications
    — Failure or toxicity of first-line agents
    — Severe or life-threatening hypercalcaemia
  b) Contraindications
    — Thrombocytopenia
    — Severe renal or hepatic dysfunction

UNDERSTANDING RHEUMATIC DISEASE

POLYMYALGIA RHEUMATICA

Diagnostic criteria for polymyalgia rheumatica (PMR)
1 Age >50
2 ESR >50 mm/h
3 Bilateral shoulder/pelvic girdle morning stiffness
  a) Symptomatic episodes >1 hour duration, *and*
  b) Clinical history >1 month duration
4 Response to low-dose (≤15 mg/day prednisone equivalent) steroids

5 Minor criteria
 a) Weight loss, night sweats, fever
 b) Symmetrical proximal muscle tenderness
 c) Elevated alkaline phosphatase/GGT
 d) Normocytic anaemia
 e) Positive joint scintigraphy (i. e. synovitis — but *no* myositis or vasculitis/giant-cell arteritis in pure PMR)
 f) Normal CPK, EMG, muscle biopsy

Exclusion of coexisting temporal arteritis
1 50% of temporal arteritis patients have symptoms of PMR
2 50% of *all* PMR patients (i. e. with or without symptoms of temporal arteritis) will be found to have giant-cell arteritis on temporal artery biopsy
3 10–20% of patients with *clinically pure* PMR will be found to have temporal arteritis on biopsy
4 False-negative biopsies may occur due to presence of 'skip lesions' (term refers to distribution of *abnormal* arterial segments) leading to sampling error; if a 2 cm biopsy is taken, however, the false-negative rate is <5%
5 Height of initial ESR *cannot* be used to predict disease severity or likelihood of complications
6 With proper management, the diagnosis of giant-cell arteritis is *not* associated with reduced life expectancy

INFECTION AND JOINT DISEASE

Infections commonly associated with arthritis
1 *S. aureus*, esp. in intravenous drug abusers
2 *S. albus*, esp. in prosthetic joints
3 *Salmonella* spp., esp. in hyposplenic patients (typically in association with osteomyelitis or spondylitis)
4 *H. influenzae*, esp. in children
5 *N. gonorrhoeae*, esp. in young women
6 Lyme disease (spirochaetal aetiology)

Infections commonly associated with arthralgias
1 Associated with arthralgias alone
 a) Influenza A
 b) Coxsackie B, EBV, mumps
 c) Mycoplasmas
 d) Brucellosis
2 Associated with arthralgias ± arthritis
 a) Hepatitis B
 b) Rubella (incl. rubella vaccine)
 c) Parvovirus
 d) Arboviruses — Ross River, Sinbis, Chikungunya
 e) Disseminated gonococcal infection

Reactive arthritis: occurrence and manifestations
1 Aetiology
 a) Postdysenteric
  — *Shigella flexneri*
  — *Salmonella* spp.
  — *Yersinia enterocolitica*
  — *Campylobacter jejuni*
 b) Venereal — *Chlamydia trachomatis*

2 Symptoms
 a) Knee and ankle pain 1–3 weeks following infection
 b) Enthesopathy (tenosynovitis, plantar fasciitis)
 c) Low back pain
3 Urethritis may occur as a manifestation of the postdysenteric variety (e. g. in prepubertal children)
4 Joint fluid is sterile
5 The initial episode generally settles over about 3 months
6 Long-term prognosis is good, although about 50% will have symptom recurrence

OTHER ARTHROPATHIES

Juvenile chronic arthritis: a working classification
1 Systemic onset ('Still's disease')
 Age of onset <16 years
 Quotidian fever usual ± leucocytosis
 Transient non-pruritic rash exhibiting Koebner phenomenon
 ± Polyserositis, hepatosplenomegaly, lymphadenopathy
 50% progress to polyarticular disease, while 50% remit
 The acute phase is associated with small but significant mortality
 Commonest cause of death is amyloidosis
 RF–, ANA–
2 Polyarticular non-systemic (true 'juvenile rheumatoid arthritis')
 90% female; late childhood onset
 Majority progress to severe adult disease
 RF+ (100%) ANA+ (75%)
3 Pauciarticular disease with chronic uveitis (50%) and knee disease
 90% female, early childhood onset
 Significant joint disability uncommon; severe eye disease common
 RF–, ANA+ (50%)
4 Pauciarticular disease with sacroiliitis, hip disease and acute uveitis (10%)
 90% male
 May progress to typical ankylosing spondylitis
 RF–, ANA–
 HLA-B27+ (75%)

Clinical aspects of miscellaneous arthropathies
1 Jaccoud's (post-rheumatic fever) arthropathy
 a) Moderately severe rheumatic heart disease
 b) History of severe, prolonged or recurrent rheumatic fever
 c) Minimally symptomatic, albeit grossly deforming, arthropathy
 d) Voluntarily reducible ulnar deviation and PIP hyperextension
 e) Good hand function despite degree of deformity
 f) No erosive or destructive changes on X-ray
 g) Rheumatoid factor negative
2 Palindromic rheumatism

a) Equal incidence in males and females
b) Asymptomatic between exacerbations
c) Typically affects hand, wrists, carpal tunnel
d) May evolve to typical RA or SLE
e) 90% rheumatoid factor negative at diagnosis
3 Relapsing polychondritis
  a) Associated with autoimmune disease in 30%
  b) Leads to fever, arthralgias, episcleritis, swollen floppy ears
  c) Nasal septum involvement → nasal collapse ('saddle nose')
  d) Laryngeal disease → hoarseness, respiratory obstruction
  e) Tracheobronchial degeneration → recurrent infections, sudden death
  f) Approx. 10% →
    — Aortic valvular incompetence/aneurysm
    — Mitral valve prolapse
  g) Responds to corticosteroid administration

Rheumatological manifestations of sickle-cell disease
1 Gout
2 Sickle crisis →
  a) Lower limb arthralgias, myalgias
  b) Acute synovitis with non-inflammatory effusion
3 'Hand-foot' syndrome (dactylitis due to periostitis, marrow expansion and/or infarction)
4 Secondary haemochromatotic arthropathy (transfusional iron overload)
5 Septic arthritis (or osteomyelitis), esp. due to *Salmonella* spp. if hyposplenic
6 Aseptic (avascular) necrosis

AVASCULAR NECROSIS OF BONE

Avascular necrosis of the femoral head: predispositions
1 Primary (Perthes' disease: epiphyseal osteochondritis)
2 Local trauma
  a) Slipped epiphysis (often bilateral in overweight children)
  b) Femoral neck fractures
  c) Traumatic dislocation
3 Sickle-cell disease (including sickle trait)
4 Hypercoagulable states, e.g.
  a) Hb C disease
  b) Paroxysmal nocturnal haemoglobinuria
  c) Nephrotic syndrome; pregnancy
5 SLE, rheumatoid arthritis
  Corticosteroid administration
  Renal transplantation
6 Alcoholism, cirrhosis, pancreatitis
7 Myxoedema
8 Gaucher's disease
9 Caisson (decompression) disease; hyperbaric oxygen
10 Therapeutic irradiation

Diagnosing avascular necrosis of the femoral head
1 X-ray of abducted hip — irregularity of femoral head, translucent band, sclerosis
2 $^{99}Tc^m$ diphosphonate scan — low isotope uptake (only useful in post-traumatic cases)
3 CT scan — subchondral rarefaction
4 MRI — clear definition of area of ischaemic necrosis

Reviewing the Literature: Rheumatology

14.1 Keat A et al 1987 *Chlamydia trachomatis* and reactive arthritis: the missing link. Lancet i: 72–74

A small study documenting 100% correlation of chlamydial antigen (detected by monoclonal antibodies) in joint material of patients with sexually acquired reactive arthritis; conventional cultures of joints and genital tract yielded some false negatives

14.2 Granfors K et al 1989 *Yersinia* antigens in synovial-fluid cells from patients with reactive arthritis. New England Journal of Medicine 320: 216–221

Study documenting that in patients experiencing arthritis following systemic *Yersinia* infection microbial antigen can be identified in the synovial fluid cells of affected joints

14.3 Res P C M et al 1988 Synovial fluid T cell reactivity against 65 KD heat shock protein of *Mycobacteria* in early chronic arthritis. Lancet ii: 478–481

Another lead to the holy grail of rheumatological aetiopathogenesis?

14.4 Hochberg M C 1986 Auranofin or D-penicillamine in the treatment of rheumatoid arthritis. Annals of Internal Medicine 105: 528–33

Auranofin (oral gold) was only slightly less effective than D-penicillamine in treating RA, but was associated with significantly fewer side-effects

Van der Heijde D M et al 1989 Effects of hydroxychloroquine and sulphasalazine on progression of joint damage in rheumatoid arthritis. Lancet i: 1036–1038

Dutch double-blind randomised study of 60 patients, showing significantly greater efficacy of sulphasalazine in preventing erosions than the antimalarial, and thus establishing the status of sulphasalazine as a major (and relatively non-toxic) remittive drug in RA

14.5 Ehsanullah R S B et al 1988 Prevention of gastroduodenal damage induced by non-steroidal anti-inflammatory drugs: controlled trial of ranitidine. British Medical Journal 297: 1017–1021

In this multicentre European study, duodenal ulcer was found to be as common as gastric ulcer in NSAID-treated patients; ranitidine effectively prevented duodenal, but not gastric, ulcers

14.6 Graham D Y et al 1988 Prevention of NSAID-induced gastric ulcer with misoprostol: multicentre double-blind, placebo-controlled trial. Lancet ii: 1277–1279

The PGE$_1$ analogue misoprostol proved effective in preventing gastric ulceration in this study of 420 patients receiving NSAIDs

Rashad S et al 1989 Effect of non-steroidal anti-inflammatory drugs on the course of osteoarthritis. Lancet ii: 460–462

Randomised study of 105 arthritic patients showing that aggressive NSAID therapy was in fact associated with more rapid joint destruction than was milder treatment, raising doubts as to the 'benign' nature of NSAID therapy.

14.7 Singer J Z, Wallace S Z 1986 The allopurinol hypersensitivity syndrome: unnecessary morbidity and mortality. Arthritis and Rheumatism 29: 82–87

Report emphasizing that inappropriate prescription of allopurinol for asymptomatic mild-to-moderate

hyperuricaemia risks occurrence of severe idiosyncratic reactions in up to 5% of patients, esp. those receiving concurrent diuretic therapy

14.8 Mathews J A et al 1987 Back pain and sciatica: controlled trials of manipulation, traction, sclerosant and epidural injections. British Journal of Rheumatology 26: 416–423

Randomized British trial of 513 patients which concluded that manipulation may be effective therapy in back pain patients with impaired straight leg raising but without neurological deficit.

14.9 Deyo R A et al 1986 How many days of rest for acute low back pain? A randomized clinical trial. New England Journal of Medicine 315: 1064–1070

In this trial, two days of bedrest was equally as good as one week in treating acute back pain

CHAPTER 15

Skin disease

Physical examination protocol 15.1 You are asked to examine a patient who has recently developed a rash

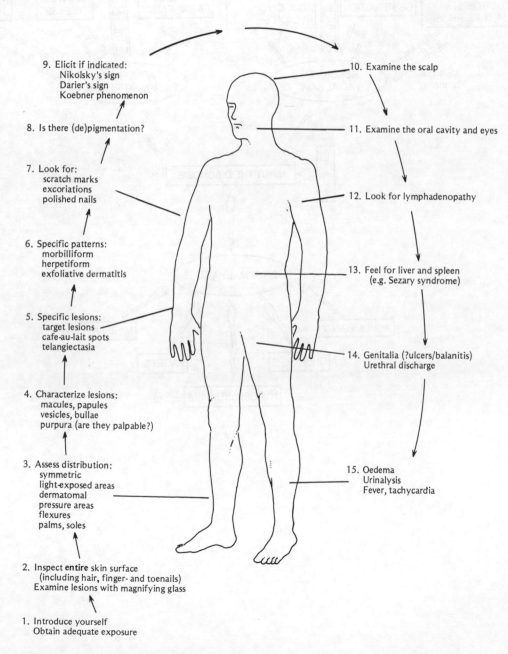

9. Elicit if indicated:
   Nikolsky's sign
   Darier's sign
   Koebner phenomenon

8. Is there (de)pigmentation?

7. Look for:
   scratch marks
   excoriations
   polished nails

6. Specific patterns:
   morbilliform
   herpetiform
   exfoliative dermatitis

5. Specific lesions:
   target lesions
   cafe-au-lait spots
   telangiectasia

4. Characterize lesions:
   macules, papules
   vesicles, bullae
   purpura (are they palpable?)

3. Assess distribution:
   symmetric
   light-exposed areas
   dermatomal
   pressure areas
   flexures
   palms, soles

2. Inspect **entire** skin surface
   (including hair, finger- and toenails)
   Examine lesions with magnifying glass

1. Introduce yourself
   Obtain adequate exposure

10. Examine the scalp

11. Examine the oral cavity and eyes

12. Look for lymphadenopathy

13. Feel for liver and spleen
    (e.g. Sezary syndrome)

14. Genitalia (?ulcers/balanitis)
    Urethral discharge

15. Oedema
    Urinalysis
    Fever, tachycardia

Diagnostic pathway 15.1   This patient has a spot diagnosis — what is it?

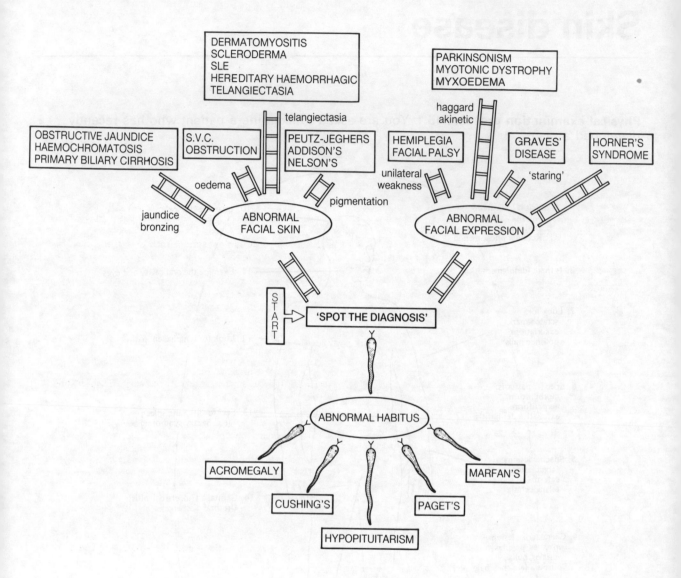

CLINICAL ASPECTS OF SKIN DISEASE

COMMONEST DERMATOLOGICAL SHORT CASES
1 Purpura
2 Psoriasis (± arthropathy)

Eponymous signs of skin disease
1 Nikolsky's sign — seen in
  a) Pemphigus (esp. foliaceous)
  b) Porphyria (PCT, EP, VP)
  c) Staph scalded skin syndrome
  Refers to palpable separation of stratum corneum from underlying epidermis (leading to blister formation) as a result of mild shearing stress
2 Darier's sign — seen in urticaria pigmentosa
  Refers to whealing of macule on rubbing
3 Koebner phenomenon — seen in
  a) Psoriasis
  b) Still's disease
  c) Lichen planus
  d) Viral warts
  Denotes development of skin lesions on areas of local trauma (e.g. along scratch marks) due to papillary layer disruption

Skin rashes: diagnostic checklist for examinations
1 Purpuric
  a) Vasculitis (is it palpable?)
  b) Haematological (dependent distribution?)
2 Bullous or blistering
  a) Pemphigus, bullous pemphigoid
  b) Dermatitis herpetiformis (though more typically vesicular)
  c) Porphyria cutanea tarda
  d) Drug-induced
3 Exfoliative or plaque-like (?lymphoma)
4 Drug eruption (always mention)
5 Secondary syphilis (never hurts to mention)
6 Suggesting systemic disease, e.g.
  a) Herpes zoster
  b) Eruptive xanthomata
  c) Pretibial myxoedema
  d) Erythema nodosum
  e) Acanthosis nigricans

Clinical patterns in skin disease
1 Asymmetric
  a) Fungal
  b) Contact dermatitis
  c) Zoster (dermatomal)
2 Widespread symmetrical maculopapular
  a) Drug eruption
  b) Exanthem
3 Palms and soles
  a) Erythema multiforme, Stevens-Johnson syndrome
  b) Reiter's; pustular psoriasis
  c) Secondary syphilis
  d) Toxic shock; atopic eczema; 'pink disease'
4 Flexures
  a) Psoriasis
  b) Seborrheic dermatitis
  c) Fungal, eczema, intertrigo
5 Limbs
  a) Flexor aspects
    — Eczema
    — Lichen planus
    — Bullous pemphigoid
  b) Extensor aspects
    — Psoriasis
    — Erythema multiforme
    — Dermatitis herpetiformis
6 Pruritic
  a) Lichen planus
  b) Dermatitis herpetiformis
  c) Drug eruptions
  d) Eczema, contact dermatitis, scabies

SKIN LESIONS OF GENERAL MEDICAL SIGNIFICANCE

Medical conditions associated with pruritus
1 Obstructive jaundice (e.g. PBC)
2 Chronic renal failure
3 Polycythaemia rubra vera ('aquagenic') — exclude iron deficiency
4 Hodgkin's disease; also CLL, lung cancer
5 Thyrotoxicosis; hypothyroidism
6 Oestrogens — pregnancy, oral contraceptives
7 Parasitic infestations, esp. trichinosis
8 Drugs, esp. narcotic abuse

Erythema nodosum: associated underlying conditions
1 **S**arcoidosis
2 **S**ulphonamides (and other drugs)
3 **S**treptococci (and TB, leprosy, toxoplasmosis)
4 Inflammatory bowel disease

Miscellaneous erythemas: diagnostic significance
1 Erythema induratum — tuberculosis
2 Erythema ab igne — myxoedema, peripheral neuropathy
3 Erythema marginatum — transient truncal rash in rheumatic fever
4 Erythema gyratum repens — internal malignancy
5 Necrolytic migratory erythema — glucagonoma

FACIAL RASHES

The central facial rash: diagnostic possibilities
1 SLE
2 Acne rosacea
3 Lupus pernio
4 Dermatomyositis
5 Porphyria cutanea tarda
6 Secondary syphilis

Differential diagnosis of facial telangiectases
1 Scleroderma
2 Hereditary haemorrhagic telangiectasia
3 Chronic liver disease (spider naevi)
4 Carcinoid syndrome
5 Ataxia telangiectasia (involve conjunctiva also)

Photosensitive skin rashes: predispositions
1 SLE
2 Porphyrias — cutanea tarda, erythropoietic
3 Drugs
   a) Chlortetracycline
   b) Chlorpropamide
   c) Chlorpromazine

DISORDERS OF PIGMENTATION

Likely causes of diffuse hyperpigmentation in short cases
1 ACTH
   a) Addison's disease
   b) ACTH-secreting tumour
   c) Nelson's syndrome
2 Chronic renal failure
3 Haemochromatosis
4 Primary biliary cirrhosis
5 Porphyria cutanea tarda
6 Drug-induced (e.g. busulphan)

Differential diagnosis of discrete hypopigmented areas
1 Vitiligo
2 Tinea versicolor
3 Tuberculoid leprosy
4 'Ash-leaf macules' of tuberose sclerosis
5 Morphoea (localized patches of scleroderma)

SKIN APPENDAGES

Diagnostic features of the fingernails in systemic disease
1 Clubbing, nicotine stains — cigarette-induced lung cancer
2 Pitting — psoriasis
3 Subungual splinters — infective endocarditis
4 Telangiectasia, nailfold infarcts — collagen-vascular diseases
5 'Half-and-half' (Lindsay's) nails — renal failure
6 Leuconychia — hypoalbuminaemia, esp. in chronic liver disease
7 Koilonychia (spoon nails) — chronic iron deficiency
8 Onycholysis — thyrotoxicosis
9 Yellow nails — lymphatic hypoplasia (with chylous effusions)
10 Blue lunules — Wilson's disease
11 Periungual fibromata — tuberous sclerosis
12 Candida — autoimmune hypoparathyroidism

Aetiological significance of splinter haemorrhages
1 Trauma
2 Infective endocarditis
3 Trichinosis (transverse splinters)

INVESTIGATING SKIN DISEASE

Immunological aids to clinical dermatology
1 Pemphigus vulgaris
   a) Circulating antibodies to intercellular cement (70%)

   b) Direct fluorescence → epidermal staining of intercellular cement with IgG, C_3
2 Bullous pemphigoid ⎫ Circulating antibodies to basement membrane (60%)

Cicatricial pemphigoid
Herpes gestationis ⎬ Direct fluorescence → linear IgG and/or C_3 at dermoepidermal junction (i.e. subepidermal)
3 Dermatitis herpetiformis
   a) ± Circulating reticulin antibodies (25%)
   b) Direct fluorescence → IgA in dermal papillae (incl. normal skin)
4 SLE — direct fluorescence → linear IgM, IgG or C_3 at dermoepidermal junction in normal and affected skin ('lupus band')
   Discoid LE — negative fluorescence in normal skin
5 Erythema multiforme — negative direct and indirect immunofluorescence

The bullous dermatoses: how to tell them apart
1 Pemphigus vulgaris
   a) Mucosal involvement typical:
      Recurrent oral ulceration is often the major manifestation
      May also cause conjunctivitis, genital ulceration; nasal, scalp or umbilical involvement
   b) Age of onset 40–60; runs 'malignant' course
   c) Bullae are small, flaccid, fragile (rarely intact); present as erosions and heal without scarring
   d) Histology reveals 'acantholytic' cells
   e) Autoimmune association; frequently only responds to *massive* steroid doses (120–240 mg prednisone/day)
   f) Rarely remits spontaneously
2 Bullous pemphigoid
   a) Mucosal involvement rare — primarily affects flexor aspects of extremities
   b) 80% patients > 70 years old
   c) Bullae are large, tense, non-fragile
   d) No acantholytic cells
   e) May respond to relatively low initial doses of steroid (e.g. 40 mg prednisone/day)
   f) May remit spontaneously; self-limiting (albeit recurrent) course
3 Cicatricial (benign mucous membrane) pemphigoid
   a) Primarily affects conjunctivae, mouth, pharynx
   b) Classically afflicts middle-aged women
   c) Tense blisters, often leading to prominent atrophic scars
   d) Complicated by entropion, symblepharon, dysphagia
   e) Requires long-term corticosteroid therapy
4 Dermatitis herpetiformis
   a) Most typically manifests with (herpetiform) vesicles
   b) May affect scapulae, sacrum, scalp, and extensor aspects of knees, elbows; buttocks
   c) Associated with pruritus, eosinophilia, intestinal villous atrophy, and HLA B8/DRw3
   d) May respond to dapsone (short-term), gluten-free diet (long-term); may be aggravated by iodine ingestion

5 Other
 a) Porphyria cutanea tarda
  — Atrophic scars on light-exposed regions
  — Facial hypertrichosis; pigmentation
 b) Acquired epidermolysis bullosa — atrophic
  scarring associated with amyloidosis, internal
  malignancy
 c) Pellagra
  — Affects light-exposed regions
  — → 'Casal's necklace'

MANAGING SKIN DISEASE

DRUG ERUPTIONS

Immunological mechanisms of drug-induced skin reactions
1 Type I reaction (immediate hypersensitivity):
 urticaria — commonly caused by
 a) Penicillin, sulphonamides
 b) Aspirin
 c) Sera, contrast media
2 Type II reaction (cytotoxic): e.g. thrombocytopenic
 purpura — commonly caused by
 a) Quinine
 b) Methyldopa
 c) Gold
3 Type III reaction (vasculitis): e.g. drug-induced
 lupus — commonly caused by
 a) Hydralazine, procainamide
 b) Sulphonamides
 c) Penicillin
4 Type IV reaction (delayed hypersensitivity): contact
 dermatitis — commonly caused by
 a) Topical antihistamines
 b) Topical neomycin

Clinical patterns of drug-induced skin reactions
1 Toxic erythema (β-lactams, gold, allopurinol,
 carbamazepine)
2 Fixed drug eruption (barbiturates, phenolphthalein)
3 Morbilliform (penicillin)
4 Erythroderma (gold)
5 Erythema multiforme (sulphonamides,
 phenylbutazone)

Clinical spectrum of drug-induced bullous disease
1 Erythema multiforme, e.g.
 trimethoprim/sulphamethoxazole
2 Photosensitization, e.g.
 a) Psoralens
 b) Demeclocycline
 c) Nalidixic acid
3 Porphyria cutanea tarda, e.g.
 a) Oral contraceptives
 b) Stilboestrol (in prostate cancer)
4 Fixed drug eruption (→ hands, feet, penis), e.g.
 a) Quinine — in tonic water
 b) Phenolphthalein — in laxatives
5 Following coma → skin necrosis, e.g. barbiturates
6 Pemphigus-like rash — penicillamine

7 Pemphigoid-like rash, e.g. frusemide
8 Pellagra-like rash — isoniazid
9 Vasculitis → haemorrhagic bullae, e.g. allopurinol
 (esp. in renal failure and/or concomitant diuretic
 therapy)

Distinguishing features of the Stevens-Johnson syndrome (erythema multiforme affecting mucous membranes)
1 Systemic illness (fever, arthralgias)
2 Purulent and/or pseudomembranous conjunctivitis
 often associated with corneal ulceration/perforation
 or symblepharon
3 Buccal ulceration and bullous stomatitis ±
 genital/anal ulcers
. Acute (or recurrent) bloodstained crusting of
 swollen lips

Drug eruptions: miscellaneous characteristics
1 Rashes due to drug hypersensitivity are classically
 symmetrical, truncal, pruritic and associated with
 eosinophilia
2 *Sensitization* to drug occurs most frequently with
 topical use and least frequently with oral use
3 Drug rashes are distinctly *unlikely* with
 a) Digoxin
 b) Erythromycin
 c) Benzodiazepines
 d) Hormones, vitamins

Conditions predisposing to ampicillin rashes
1 Infectious mononucleosis (EBV)
2 CMV infection
3 Chronic lymphocytic leukaemia
4 Concurrent allopurinol treatment

Antineoplastic efficacy of synthetic retinoids
1 Regression of preneoplastic lesions
 a) Oral leukoplakia
 b) Senile actinic keratoses (incl.
  transplant-associated lesions)
2 Reduction of new tumours in xeroderma
 pigmentosum patients
3 Responses sometimes seen in established mycosis
 fungoides

UNDERSTANDING SKIN DISEASE

Medical consequences of ultraviolet radiation
1 UV-A (320–400 nm, long-wavelength u.v., 'black
 light')
 a) Low energy, high skin penetration
 b) Present in solar radiation all day
 c) Implicated in pathogenesis of skin ageing,
  photosensitive drug eruptions and porphyria
  rashes
 d) *High-dose* (therapeutic) UV-A irradiation with
  psoralen photosensitization (PUVA) may cause
  skin SCCs
2 UV-B (290–320 nm, medium-wavelength u.v.)

a) High energy, high skin penetration
b) Attenuated by ozone layer
c) Present in solar radiation mainly 10 a.m.–3 p.m.
d) Responsible for sunburn
e) Implicated in pathogenesis of skin SCCs, BCCs and melanomas
f) Also implicated in pathogenesis of cataract
g) Absorbed by PABA-containing sunscreens
3 UV-C (200–290 nm, short-wavelength u.v.)
a) High energy, low skin penetration
b) Used in sterilizing lamps
c) May cause sunburn in mountain climbers (less ozone)

Classical cutaneous complications of cancer
1 Skin infiltration or metastases — esp. breast cancer, melanoma
2 Erythroderma — Sézary syndrome, mycosis fungoides
3 Excoriations (pruritus) — Hodgkin's disease, polycythaemia vera
4 Herpes zoster — esp. myeloma, lymphoma, chronic lymphocytic leukaemia
5 Dermatomyositis (esp. steroid-resistant variant in adults) — many causes, e.g. ovarian/gastric/lung cancer
6 Radiotherapy effects
a) Early — erythema, desquamation
b) Late — discolouration, atrophy, fibrosis, telangiectasia
7 Rare
a) Acanthosis nigricans (widespread, mucosal, pruritic)
b) Gastrointestinal adenocarcinomas, esp. gastric
c) Thrombophlebitis migrans — mucin-secreting adenocarcinomas, esp. pancreatic
d) Necrolytic migratory erythema — glucagonoma
e) Systemic nodular panniculitis (Weber-Christian disease) — pancreatic acinar-cell carcinoma
f) Xanthomatosis — multiple myeloma
g) Post-proctoscopic periorbital 'pinch' purpura — myeloma with supervening amyloidosis
8 Not associated with any *specific* tumour type
a) Erythema gyratum repens
b) Acquired hypertrichosis lanuginosa ('malignant down')
c) Bullous pyoderma gangrenosum
9 Unproven associations
a) Pemphigoid
b) Psoriatic exacerbations
c) Erythema multiforme
d) Bowen's disease

URTICARIA

Urticarial problems in clinical practice
1 Ordinary urticaria
a) May be immunologically (IgE-) mediated, e.g. reactions to insect stings or drugs
b) May also be non-immunologically mediated: histamine-containing foodstuffs (e.g. frozen tuna), arachidonic acid pathway inhibitors (e.g. aspirin), mast-cell degranulation induction (e.g. opiates)
c) Topical therapy generally ineffective; oral antihistamines and/or exclusion diets may be useful
2 Chronic urticaria
a) Defined as recurrent lesions for 3 months ± arthralgias, adenopathy, abdominal pain
b) Mediated by histamine, *not* IgE; prick tests negative
c) Precipitating dietary factor identifiable in 25%
d) H2-receptor antagonists sometimes useful; steroids contraindicated
3 Cholinergic urticaria
a) Affects head and upper trunk, esp. in young patients
b) Transient painful pruritic lesions with 'blush'
c) Rapid skin cooling may abort an attack
4 Cold urticaria — *familial*
a) Autosomal dominant; usually presents in infancy
b) Rash may appear only several hours after cold exposure
c) Associated with fever, arthralgias, and leucocytosis
5 Cold urticaria — *acquired*
a) Rash occurs within minutes of skin contact with cold water or ice (diagnostic test); syncope may ensue
b) May cause sudden death in young people (esp. drowning)
6 Solar urticaria
a) Weal occurs within 30 seconds to 3 minutes of sun exposure
b) Localized to sun-exposed areas; tolerance may develop
c) Differential diagnosis includes SLE and drug reactions
7 Pressure urticaria
a) Affects pressure areas, e.g. feet, buttocks, back
b) Tender swelling occurs 2–12 hours after pressure injury
8 Scratch urticaria (delayed dermographism)
a) Redness, weal and itch occur hours after scratching
b) Distinct from *simple dermographism*, which affects 5% of the population and is *not* pruritic
9 Vasculitic urticaria
a) Serious condition which may be life-threatening
b) Painful non-pruritic skin lesions; usually last >24 hours
c) ± fever, abdominal pain, arthritis, glomerulonephritis
d) Hypocomplementaemia (C_3, C_4, THC), high ESR usual
10 Angioneurotic oedema
a) Affects mucocutaneous junctions: lips, eyes, penis
b) Large tender swellings, often pruritic
c) Glottal oedema may be a complication, esp. when angioedema occurs in the context of anaphylaxis

NB: urticaria does **not** occur in association with hereditary angio-oedema (C1-INH deficiency)

SKIN SYNDROMES

Sweet's syndrome: acute febrile neutrophilic dermatosis

1 Manifests with tender erythematous skin plaques
→ head and neck, upper limbs esp.) associated
with fever and neutrophilia
2 May be accompanied by arthritis, conjunctivitis,
mouth ulcers, or proteinuria
3 20% of patients will be found to have an
associated malignancy (e.g. acute leukaemia); such
patients tend to have more severe skin lesions
and/or associated cytopenias
4 Symptoms are generally steroid-responsive, and
may resolve within 2–3 months in patients without
underlying malignancy

The dysplastic naevus ('B-K mole') syndrome: features

1 Naevi typically 5–15 mm in diameter
2 Characterized by irregular borders and variegated
colour
3 Distributed predominantly over trunk, but also
sun-deprived areas
4 Often more than 100 in number
5 Continue to appear after age 35
6 Histology
a) Melanocytic hyperplasia
b) Cytologic atypia
c) Spindle-shaped melanocyte 'nests'
d) Lymphocytic superficial dermal infiltrates
7 Autosomal dominant transmission
8 Risk of developing melanoma approaches 100% in
DNS patients with positive family history of
melanoma

Reviewing the Literature: Skin Disease

15.1 Garden J M, Freinkel R K 1986 Systemic absorption of topical steroids: metabolic effects as an index of mild hypercortisolism. Archives of Dermatology 122: 1007–1010

Five psoriasis patients treated with topical steroid sustained rapid and long-lasting reduction of cortisol with increases in insulin and peripheral white cell count. Reports of actual Cushing's syndrome induced by topical therapy, however, have been confined to patients with (i) large skin areas treated, (ii) liver disease, or (iii) high skin:mass ratio (e.g. babies)

15.2 Henseler T, Wollff K, Honigsmann H, Christophers E 1981 Oral 8-methoxypsoralen photochemotherapy of psoriasis: the European PUVA study. Lancet i: 853–837

The use of PUVA leads to 90% response rates but cannot be recommended for maintenance (prophylactic) therapy of severe psoriasis

15.3 Stern R S, Laird N, Melski J et al 1984 Cutaneous squamous cell carcinoma in patients treated with PUVA. New England Journal of Medicine 310: 1156–1161

Study showing an increased incidence of skin SCCs (but not BCCs) following therapy for psoriasis using PUVA

15.4 Kraemer K H et al 1988 Prevention of skin cancer in xeroderma pigmentosum with the use of oral isotretinoin. New England Journal of Medicine 318: 1633–1637

63% reduction of tumour incidence during 2 years of treatment with 13-cis-retinoic acid, followed by a 9-fold increase on cessation

15.5 Peck G L, Olsen T G, Yoder F W et al 1979 Prolonged remission of cystic and conglobate acne with 13-cis-retinoic acid. New England Journal of Medicine 300: 329–333

The first report of this dramatic breakthrough in the management of intractable acne vulgaris. Side effects of the retinoid derivative include skin desquamation and dry eyes

15.6 Lammer E J et al 1985 Retinoic acid embryopathy. New England Journal of Medicine 313: 837–841

59 pregnancies exposed to uninterrupted isotretinoin therapy yielded 12 abortions and 21 malformed infants (esp. ear malformations, other craniofacial abnormalities, and thymic defects), making this drug one of the most potent teratogens known

15.6 Olsen E A et al 1986 Dose-response study of topical minoxidil in male pattern baldness. Journal of the American Academy of Dermatology

Double-blind placebo-controlled trial of minoxidil (a vasodilator with hirsutism as a side-effect) in 89 patients, showing that the 2% cream had a significant effect on hair restoration. Overall, however, the efficacy is unpredictable and expensive, and only a minority of patients benefit cosmetically

15.7 Brice S M et al 1989 Detection of herpes simplex virus DNA in cutaneous lesions of erythema multiforme. Journal of Investigative Dermatology 93: 183–187

Demonstration of HSV nucleic acid sequences in EM target lesions using polymerase chain reaction-derived DNA and in-situ hybridisation, suggesting a possible pathogenetic (i.e. as well as epidemiologic) role for the virus

15.8 Raynaud F et al 1989 A cAMP binding abnormality in psoriasis. Lancet i: 1135–1137

Discovery of a biochemical defect within psoriatic patients' erythrocytes. The defect was expressed in milder form in unaffected family members, and was reversed by retinoid therapy

Recommended reading

1. BEST INVESTMENT: Your own notes

These are always the most useful revision material since they are (or at least should be) custom-designed to cover your own weaknesses. Don't underestimate their value

2. BEST CLINICALLY-ORIENTED TEXTBOOK: Your patients' notes

When it comes to learning clinical medicine, there's no substitute for getting out on the wards. Cajole, bribe or blackmail your seniors into demonstrating physical signs and the techniques for eliciting them; armed with this knowledge, find out where 'the cases' are, team up with a similarly-motivated colleague, and proceed to grill each other on your respective performances. Watch one, do one, teach one: that's how medicine's been for time immemorial, and it's not about to change in your lifetime

3. BEST GENERAL TEXTBOOK: *Oxford Textbook of Medicine*

Like expensive and weighty stethoscopes, expensive and weighty textbooks are not a prerequisite for passing medical exams. Owning one decent reference book can make life easier, however, and is probably worthwhile in the long run. Despite its arm-breaking weight, poor indexing, paucity of clinical detail, and at times eccentric commentary, the *Oxford* is probably the safest choice for a reference text; although many prefer the time-tested American alternatives (Harrison's, Cecil) or their clones (Stein, Kelley). So take your pick!

4. BEST MCQs: MKSAP (Medical knowledge self-assessment program)

For candidates who need a 'quiz-show' format to sustain their interest in the lead-up to an exam, this American Medical Association publication is clearly the best (it includes excellent state-of-the-art summaries of each subspecialty in addition to the self-assessment questions) provided that either you or your library can afford it. If not, look for other publications which feature detailed and authoritative answers: Lawrence & Hunter's *MCQs in General Medicine* and the *Pre-Test* series fall into this category

5. BEST ARMCHAIR AIDS FOR THE TEXTBOOK-WEARY

a) *Wolfe Medical Atlas* series, and
b) Merck, Sharpe and Dohme *Heart Sounds* cassettes (great for pre-exam insomnia)

Both should be available from your local medical library

6. BEST EDITORIALS: *British Medical Journal*

Up-to-date summaries of important (and fashionable) topics can be found here; an afternoon scanning the last 6–12 months' issues prior to your exam could be well spent

7. BEST ORIGINAL ARTICLES: *Lancet, New England Journal of Medicine*

These are the only two journals containing original articles worth perusing on a regular basis. So how do you get the most out of such articles when your time is limited? Try this: (i) skim through the Abstract — if the conclusions are earth-shattering, read the Introduction and Discussion; (ii) if (much more commonly) the Abstract sounds less than earth-shattering, just read the Introduction — in most cases it will provide a concise summary of a topical clinical problem as well as pointing out uncertainties in current knowledge. The latter is an important goal which traditional medical textbooks rarely achieve

317

8. BEST REVIEW ARTICLES: *Medicine International, Hospital Update, British Journal of Hospital Medicine*

Review articles in any journal are worth a look since they often provide more thoughtful information than that found in textbooks; they occur in greatest profusion in these journals

9. BEST SUBSPECIALTY TEXTS

The limitations of having to rely on library stock for your reading are obvious. The book you want may be unavailable, stolen, out-of-date, or chained to the library shelf; or it may be so badly defaced that reading it becomes an archaeological exercise. Nonetheless, borrowing library books has two definite advantages: first, it's cheap, and second, it provides some incentive to read the thing within a given time interval.

The following recommendations are for those exam candidates who feel they need more in-depth or background information on a specific subject than is provided in *Medicine for Examinations* and/or their general reference textbook

Cancer medicine
Short and readable:
UICC Manual of Clinical Oncology Springer-Verlag, Berlin
Reference:
De Vita VT et al (eds.) *Cancer: Principles and Practice of Oncology* Lippincott, Philadelphia

Cardiology
Short and readable:
Schlamt R C, Hurst J W *Handbook of the Heart*. McGraw-Hill, New York
Reference:
Braunwald E (ed.) *Heart Disease*. Saunders, Philadelphia

Endocrinology
Short and readable:
Watts N B, Keffer J H *Practical Endocrinology* Lea and Febiger, Philadelphia
Reference:
Wilson J D, Foster D W (eds) *Williams' Textbook of Endocrinology* Saunders, Philadelphia

Gastroenterology
Short and readable:
Christensen J *Bedside Logic in Diagnostic Gastroenterology* Churchill Livingstone, Edinburgh
Reference:
Sleisenger M H et al (eds) *Gastrointestinal Disease* Saunders, Philadelphia

Haematology
Short and readable:
Isbister J P, Pittiglio D H *Clinical Haematology: a Problem-oriented Approach* Williams & Wilkins, Baltimore

Reference:
Jandl J H *Blood*. Little, Brown & Co, Boston

Immunology
Short and readable:
Male D *Immunology: an Illustrated Outline*. Gower, London
Reference:
Samter M (ed) *Immunologic Diseases*. Little, Brown & Co, Boston

Infectious disease
Short and readable:
Emond R T D, Rowland H A K *Diagnostic Picture Tests in Infectious Disease* Wolfe Medical, London
Reference:
Mandell G L et al (eds) *Principles and Practice of Infectious Disease* Wiley, New York

Metabolism, nutrition and genetics
Reference:
Stanbury J B et al (eds) *The Metabolic Basis of Inherited Disease* McGraw-Hill, New York

Neurology
Short and readable:
Weiner W J, Goetz C G *Neurology for the Non-neurologist* Lippincott, Philadelphia
Reference:
Walton J *Brain's Diseases of the Nervous System* Oxford University Press, Oxford

Pharmacology & toxicology
Short and readable:
Greenblatt D J, Shader R I *Pharmacokinetics in Clinical Practice* W B Saunders, Philadelphia
Reference:
Goodman L S, Gilman A G et al *The Pharmacological Basis of Therapeutics* MacMillan, New York

Psychiatry
Short and readable:
Burns A S et al *MCQs and Short Notes in Psychiatry* Wright, Bristol
Reference:
Kaplan H I, Sadock B S *Comprehensive Textbook of Psychiatry* Williams and Wilkins, Baltimore

Renal medicine
Short and readable:
Whitworth J A, Lawrence J R *Textbook of Renal Disease* Churchill Livingstone, Edinburgh

Respiratory medicine
Short and readable:
West J B *Pulmonary Pathophysiology* Williams and Wilkins, Baltimore
Reference:
Murray J F et al (eds) *Textbook of Respiratory Medicine* Saunders Philadelphia

Rheumatology
Short and readable:
Moll J M H *Manual of Rheumatology* Churchill

Livingstone, Edinburgh
Reference:
Katz W Z *Diagnosis and Management of Rheumatic Diseases* Lippincott, Philadelphia

Skin disease
Short and readable:
Fitzpatrick T B et al *Color Atlas and Synopsis of Clinical Dermatology* McGraw-Hill, New York

Reference:
Rook A et al (eds) *Textbook of Dermatology* Blackwell, Oxford

10. BEST BOOK FOR PASSING MEDICAL EXAMS:

. . . .? I'm afraid I'll have to leave this one up to you.

Afterword

Medical training has always been a long process, and it's getting longer all the time — it's not unusual any more to train for 20 years and still be searching for a 'proper job' at the end of it. Is it any wonder, then, that the popularity of medical careers is declining as we approach the 21st century?

During the early years of training, issues such as these seem somewhat unreal: things are too busy on the wards to encourage introspection, and besides, there always seems to be another *exam* lurking over the horizon. In a way this makes life simpler: there is always more study to do, even when the clinical action has ended for the day.

Laudable sentiments. There is a danger here, however: the danger of turning into an 'exam bore'. Not that there is anything wrong with working hard, of course, but it doesn't have to become an obsession. If it does, you risk career 'burn-out', disillusion, even despair.

So what's the alternative?

We all know that the pursuit of a medical career is a competitive business. My aim in this book has been to show that it *is* possible to learn (and hence compete) efficiently, and that it *isn't* necessary to waste half your life poring over mammoth textbooks — in other words, it *is* possible to make time for other pursuits. If *Medicine for Examinations* succeeds in helping you even a little way towards this goal, it will have been a worthwhile exercise.

And once you have made time, have the courage to recognize what you are good at—what you enjoy, whether it be within medicine or without it—and do it.

Abbreviations

α_1AT	alpha-1-antitrypsin	A-V	atrioventricular, arteriovenous
αFP/AFP	alpha fetoprotein	AVM	arteriovenous malformation
αHBD	hydroxy butyrate dehydrogenase	βHCG	beta-subunit of human chorionic gonadotrophin
A_2	aortic component of second heart sound	BAL	dimercaprol
A-a	alveolar-arterial (oxygen)	BCC	basal cell carcinoma
Ab	antibody	BCG	bacillus Calmette-Guérin
ACE	angiotensin-converting enzyme	b.d.	twice-daily (dosage)
AChRAb	acetylcholine receptor antibody	BJP	Bence-Jones protein
ACTH	adrenocorticotrophic hormone	BP	blood pressure
AD	autosomal dominant	BSP	bromsulphthalein
ADH	antidiuretic hormone (vasopressin)	BUN	blood urea nitrogen
ADP	adenosine diphosphate	C1-7(8)	cervical vertebra (nerve root)
AF	atrial fibrillation	$C_{3,4}$(etc.)	complement components
AFB	acid-fast bacilli	Ca	cancer
Ag	antigen	Ca^{2+}	calcium
AI	aortic incompetence	CABG	coronary artery bypass graft
AIDS	acquired immunodeficiency syndrome	c-abl	cellular oncogene abl
AIHA	autoimmune haemolytic anaemia	CAH	chronic active hepatitis
ALA	aminolaevulinic acid	cALLA	common ALL-antigen
ALL	acute lymphoblastic leukaemia	cAMP	cyclic adenosine monophosphate
ALT	alanine aminotransferase (SGPT)	CAPD	chronic ambulatory peritoneal dialysis
AMOL	acute myelomonocytic leukaemia	CCF	congestive cardiac failure
ANA	antinuclear antibody	CCK	cholecystokinin
ANF	atrial natriuretic factor	CCl_4	carbon tetrachloride
Ang	angiotensin	CDCA	chenodeoxycholic acid
ANLL	acute non-lymphocytic (usually myeloblastic) leukaemia	CEA	carcinoembryonic antigen
A-P	antero-posterior	cf.	confer (compare, contrast)
APML	acute promyelocytic leukaemia	CFT	complement fixation test
APTT	activated partial thromboplastin time	CGDC	chronic granulomatous disease of childhood
APUD	amine precursor uptake and decarboxylation	CGL	chronic granulocytic leukaemia
AR	autosomal recessive	CHAD	cold haemagglutinin disease
ara-C	cytosine arabinoside	CHOP	cyclophosphamide, hydroxydaunorubicin (doxorubicin, Adriamycin), Oncovin (vincristine), prednisone
ARDS	adult respiratory distress syndrome		
ASD	atrial septal defect	C_1-INH	C_1-esterase inhibitor
ASO	antistreptolysin O	Cl^-	chloride
AST	aspartate aminotransferase (SGOT)	CLL	chronic lymphocytic leukaemia
AT-III	antithrombin III	CMC	chronic mucocutaneous candidiasis
ATG	antithymocyte globulin	CMT	Charcot-Marie-Tooth disease
atm	atmospheres (pressure)	CMV	cytomegalovirus
ATN	acute tubular necrosis	c-myc	cellular oncogene myc
ATP	adenosine triphosphate	CN	cranial nerve(s)

CNS	central nervous system	ESR	erythrocyte sedimentation rate
COAD	chronic obstructive airways disease	EUA	examination under anaesthesia
Con-A	Concanavalin A	F VIII$_c$	coagulant moiety of factor eight
c-onc	cellular oncogene	Fab	antibody fragments
C-PAP	continuous positive airways pressure	FAB	French-American-British (classification)
CPK	creatine phosphokinase	5-FC	flucytosine
c.p.s.	cycles per second	FDPs	fibrin degradation products
CRA	central retinal artery	Fe	iron
CREST	calcinosis, Raynaud's, oesophageal	FEV$_1$	forced expiratory volume in one second
	dysfunction, sclerodactyly, and	FFP	fresh frozen plasma
	telangiectasia (syndrome)	F_iO_2	concentration of inspired oxygen
CRF	chronic renal failure	FMF	familial Mediterranean fever
	corticotrophin-releasing factor	FSH	follicle-stimulating hormone
CRP	C-reactive protein	FTA-ABS	fluorescent treponemal antibody
CRV	central retinal vein		absorption test
CSF	cerebrospinal fluid	FTI	free thyroxine index
CT	computed tomography	5FU	5-fluorouracil
CTS	carpal tunnel syndrome	GABA	γ-aminobutyric acid
CVA	cerebrovascular accident	GBM	glomerular basement membrane
CVP	chlorambucil, vincristine, prednisone	GBS	Guillain-Barre syndrome
CXR	chest X-ray	GFR	glomerular filtration rate
2-D	two-dimensional (real-time)	GGT	gamma-glutamyl transpeptidase
DAT	direct antiglobulin (Coombs') test	GH(RF)	growth hormone (releasing factor)
dDAVP	de-amino D-arginine vasopressin	GHPS	gated heart pool scan
	('desmopressin')	GIP	glucose-dependent insulinotrophic
DCA	dichloroacetate		polypeptide ('gastric inhibitory peptide')
DD$_x$	differential diagnosis	GI(T)	gastrointestinal (tract)
DES	diethylstilboestrol	GN	glomerulonephritis
DFA	diffuse fibrosing alveolitis	GnRH	gonadotrophin-releasing hormone
DFO	desferrioxamine	G6PD	glucose-6-phosphate dehydrogenase
DHCC	dihydroxycholecalciferol	GTT	glucose tolerance test
DHEA	dehydroepiandrosterone	GVHD	graft-versus-host disease
DHFR	dihydrofolate reductase	Gy	Gray (100 rad)
DIC	disseminated intravascular coagulation	HbA$_{1c}$	glycosylated haemoglobin
DIP	distal interphalangeal joint	HBcAg	hepatitis B core antigen
DISIDA	(see HIDA)	HBeAg	hepatitis B 'e' antigen
DL$_{co}$	diffusing capacity to carbon monoxide	HbO$_2$	oxyhaemoglobin
	(transfer factor)	HBsAG	hepatitis B surface antigen
DNS	dysplastic naevus syndrome	HbSC	sickle-C haemoglobin
2,3-DPG	2,3-diphosphoglycerate	HbSS	(homozygous) sickle-cell haemoglobin
dsDNA	double-stranded deoxyribonucleic acid	HBV	hepatitis B virus
DTs	delirium tremens	HCC	(25) hydroxycholecalciferol
DTH	delayed-type hypersensitivity	HCG	human chorionic gonadotrophin
DVT	deep venous thrombosis	HCL	hairy cell leukaemia
D$_x$	diagnosis	HCO$_3^-$	bicarbonate
EACA	epsilonaminocaproic acid	HDL	high-density lipoprotein
EB(V)	Epstein-Barr (virus)	HHV	human herpesvirus
ECG	electrocardiogram	(5)-HIAA	hydroxyindoleacetic acid
ECHO	enteric cytopathic human orphan (virus)	HIDA	technetium-labelled iminodiacetic acid
ECOG	Eastern Co-operative Oncology Group		derivative
	(criteria)	HIV	human immunodeficiency virus
EDTA	ethylenediamminetetraammonium	HLA	human leucocyte antigen
EEG	electroencephalogram	HPO	hypertrophic pulmonary
ELISA	enzyme-linked immunosorbent assay		osteoarthropathy
EM	electron microscopy	HPT	hyperparathyroidism
EMG	electromyography	HS	hereditary spherocytosis
EN	erythema nodosum	HSP	Henoch-Schönlein purpura
ENT	ear, nose and throat	HSV	herpes simplex virus
EP	erythropoietic protoporphyria	5HT	5-hydroxytryptamine (serotonin)
EPG	electrophoretogram	HTLV	human T-cell leukaemia virus
ER	oestrogen receptor	H-V	His-ventricle
ERCP	endoscopic retrograde	H-X	histiocytosis X
	cholangiopancreatogram	HZ	herpes zoster
esp.	especially	^{131}1	radioiodine

IAT — indirect antiglobulin (Coombs') test
IBD — inflammatory bowel disease
IBS — irritable bowel syndrome
ICU — intensive care unit
IDL — intermediate density lipoproteins
IEPG — immunoelectrophoretogram
IF — immunofluorescence
IFA — indirect fluorescent antibody
IFN — interferon
Ig — immunoglobulin
IGF-1 — insulin-like growth factor I (somatomedin C)
IHC — idiopathic haemochromatosis
i.m.(i) — intramuscular (injection)
INH — isoniazid
IP — interphalangeal (joint)
iPTH — immunoreactive parathyroid hormone
IQ — intelligence quotient
ITP — idiopathic thrombocytopenic purpura
IUD — intrauterine device
i.v.(i) — intravenous (injection)
I-V — interventricular
IVC — inferior vena cava
IVP — intravenous pyelogram
JCA — juvenile chronic arthritis
JVP — jugular venous pressure
K^+ — potassium
LAHB — left anterior hemiblock
LBBB — left bundle branch block
LCAT — lecithin-choline acetyltransferase
LDL — low-density lipoprotein
L-DOPA — *levo-d*ihydr*oxy*phenyla*l*anine
LE — lupus erythematosus
Leu-1, 3a — monoclonal antibodies to T-cell subpopulations
LFTs — liver function tests
LGV — lymphogranuloma venereum
LH — luteinizing hormone
LMN — lower motor neurone
LOS — lower oesophageal sphincter
LP — lumbar puncture
LPHB — left posterior hemiblock
LRTI — lower respiratory tract infection
LV(H) — left ventricle (hypertrophy)
MAO(I) — monoamine oxidase (inhibitor)
MBC — minimal bactericidal concentration
MCHC — mean corpuscular haemoglobin concentration
MCP — metacarpophalangeal (joint)
MCQ — multiple choice question
MCT — medullary carcinoma of the thyroid
MCTD — mixed connective tissue disease
MCV — mean corpuscular volume
M:E — myeloid:erythroid (ratio)
MEA — multiple endocrine adenomatosis
MESNA — sodium-2-mercaptoethanesulphonite
MF — myelofibrosis
MIBG — metaiodobenzylguanidine
MIC — minimal inhibitory concentration
MIF — migration inhibitory factor
MLC — mixed lymphocyte culture
MND — motor neurone disease
MOPP — mustine (nitrogen mustard), Oncovin (vincristine), procarbazine, prednisone

6-MP — 6-mercaptopurine
MRC — Medical Research Council (UK)
MRI — magnetic resonance imaging
mRNA — messenger RNA
MS — mitral stenosis
MSU — midstream urine (specimen)
MTP — metatarsophalangeal (joint)
MVP — mitral valve prolapse
N — normal
NADH — nicotinamide
Na^+ — sodium
NAP — neutrophil alkaline phosphatase (score)
NB — note well
NBT — nitroblue tetrazolium
NMR — nuclear magnetic resonance
NSAIDs — non-steroidal anti-inflammatory drugs
NSU — non-specific (-gonococcal) urethritis
OA — osteoarthritis
OCs — oral contraceptives
OX (2, 19, K) — Weil-Felix reactions
P_2 — pulmonary component of second heart sound
PA — pernicious anaemia
P-A — postero-anterior
PABA — *para*-aminobenzoic acid
P_aCO_2 — arterial partial pressure of carbon dioxide
PAN — polyarteritis nodosa
P_aO_2 — arterial partial pressure of oxygen
P_AO_2 — alveolar partial pressure of oxygen
PAS — periodic acid-Schiff *or* ρ-aminosalicylic acid
PBC — primary biliary cirrhosis
PBG — porphobilinogen
PCK — polycystic kidneys
PCP — phenycyclidine ('angel dust')
PCR — polymerase chain reaction
PCT — porphyria cutanea tarda
PCV — packed cell volume (haematocrit)
PCWP — pulmonary capillary wedge pressure
PDA — patent ductus arteriosus
PDGF — platelet-derived growth factor
PEEP — positive end-expiratory pressure (ventilation)
PEFR — peak expiratory flow rate
PERLA — pupils equal, react to light and accommodation
PGI_2 — prostacyclin
Ph^1 — Philadelphia (chromosome)
PHA — phytohaemagglutinin
PI — prothrombin index
PICA — posterior inferior cerebellar artery (lateral medullary) syndrome
PIP — proximal interphalangeal joint
PiZZ — phenotype for homozygous α1AT deficiency
PMR — polymyalgia rheumatica
PNH — paroxysmal nocturnal haemoglobinuria
p.o. — orally
PR — per rectal
p.r.n. — as necessary
PRV — polycythaemia rubra vera
PS — pulmonary stenosis
PT — prothrombin time

PTC	percutaneous transhepatic cholangiogram
PTH	parathyroid hormone
PTTK	partial thromboplastin time (with kaolin)
PTU	propylthiouracil
PUO	pyrexia of unknown origin
PUVA	psoralens/ultraviolet light (UV-A wavelength)
PVB	cis-platinum, vinblastine, bleomycin
q 4 h	every (four hours)
q.i.d.	four times daily
Q-T$_c$	corrected Q-T interval
q.v.	which sees (i.e. discussed elsewhere)
RA	rheumatoid arthritis
RBBB	right bundle branch block
RBC	red blood cell
RDW	red-cell distribution width (anisocytosis)
REM	rapid eye movement
RF	rheumatoid factor
RIA	radioimmunoassay
RNP	ribonucleoprotein
RPGN	rapidly progressive glomerulonephritis
RPR	rapid plasma reagin
RSV	respiratory syncytial virus
RTA	renal tubular acidosis
RV	right ventricle
R$_x$	treatment
SAP	serum alkaline phosphatase
SBE	subacute bacterial endocarditis
SCA	sickle-cell anaemia
SCC	squamous cell carcinoma
SCID	severe combined immunodeficiency
SCLC	small-cell lung cancer
SHBG	sex hormone binding globulin
SIADH	syndrome of inappropriate ADH secretion
SLE	systemic lupus erythematosus
Sm	Smith (antibody)
Spp.	species
SRS-A	slow-reacting substance of anaphylaxis
ssDNA	single-stranded DNA
SSPE	subacute sclerosing panencephalitis
SVC	superior vena cava
SVT	supraventricular tachycardia
SXR	skull X-ray
t$^{\frac{1}{2}}$	half-life
T2-12	thoracic vertebrae nos 2–12
TB	tuberculosis
TBG	thyroid-binding globulin
Tc	technetium
TC	transcobalamin
TCC	transitional cell carcinoma
t.d.s.	three times daily
TdT	terminal deoxytransferase
TF	transferrin
6-TG	6-thioguanine
TGB	thyroglobulin
T$_H$	helper T-cell
THC	total haemolytic complement
TI	tricuspid incompetence
TIA	transient ischaemic attack
TIBC	total iron-binding capacity
TLC	total lung capacity
TMJ	temporomandibular joint
TNM	tumour/nodes/metastases
tPA	tissue plasminogen activator
TPHA	treponema pallidum haemagglutination
TPI	treponema pallidum immobilization
TPN	total parenteral nutrition
TRH	thyrotropin-releasing hormone
T$_s$	suppressor T-cell
TSH	thyroid-stimulating hormone (thyrotropin)
TSI	thyroid-stimulating immunoglobulin
TT	thrombin time
TTP	thrombotic thrombocytopenic purpura
TXA$_2$	thromboxane A$_2$
UDP	uridine diphosphate
UMN	upper motor neurone
URTI	upper respiratory tract infection
UTI	urinary tract infection
UV	ultraviolet
VC	vital capacity
VDRL	Venereal Disease Research Laboratory (reaginic test)
VEB	ventricular ectopic (premature) beat
VER	visual evoked response
VF	ventricular fibrillation
VIP	vasoactive intestinal peptide
VLDL	very low density lipoprotein
VP	variegate porphyria
V/Q	ventilation perfusion
VSD	ventricular septal defect
VT	ventricular tachycardia
VWF	von Willebrand factor
WAS	Wiskott Aldrich syndrome
WBC	white blood cell
WCC	white cell count
WDLL	well-differentiated lymphocytic lymphoma
WPW	Wolff-Parkinson-White (syndrome)
WR	Wassermann reagent (test)
XD	X-linked dominant
XR	X-linked recessive
ZES	Zollinger-Ellison syndrome

Index

Palpation
  apex beat, failure, 45
  Palpitations, 59
Pancoast's syndrome, 22
Pancreatic cancer, 20–1
Pancreatic polypeptide, 119 *see
    also* PPoma
Pancreatitis, 108
Panhypogammaylobulinaemia, 123
Panhypopituitarism, 91
Papillary necrosis, 262
Papillary thyroid carcinoma, 34
Papillitis, 218
Papilloedema, 218
Papillomavirus, 35, 178, 187
Pappenheimer bodies, 133
Paracetamol, 241
Paralysis, periodic
  hyperkalaemic, 236
  hypokalaemic, 83, 236
Paraparesis, 224–5
Paraprotein, 23
Paraproteinaemia, 158
Parasitic infections, 157, 177 186
    *see also specific
      infections/organisms*
Parathyroid hormone,
    immunoreactive, 199
Paratrigeminal neuralgia, 221
Parenteral nutrition, 203
Paresis of the insane, general, 233
Parietal lobe lesions, 217
Parkinson's disease and
    parkinsonism, 211, 232, 233
Parvoviruses, 124, 178
Peak expiratory flow rate, 277
Pellagra, 195, 313
Pellagra-like rash, 195
Pelvic irradiation, 27–8
Pelviureteric junction translucency,
    262
Pemphigoid
  bullous, 312
  cicatricial, 312
Pemphigus vulgaris, 312
D-Penicillamine, 302
Penicillins, 135, 169, 185
Pentopril, 57
Peptic ulceration, 112–13, 113,
    270
Peptide hormones, 97, 118
Perianal lesions, 191
Pericarditis, constrictive, 64
Peritoneal dialysis, 265, 266
Peritoneovenous shunting, 114
Pes cavus, 235
pH disturbances, 277
Phaeochromocytoma, 85, 90
Pharmacology, 239–47
  clinical aspects, 240–1
  literature review, 246, 318
  management, 241–3
  understanding, 243–6
    see also Drugs
Pharyngitis, 184, 191
Phenobarbitone, 230, 231
Phenothiazines, 28

Phenytoin, 230, 231
Philadelphia chromosome, 136, 137
Phlebotomy, 140, 240
Phospholipase A$_2$ inhibitors, 245
Phospholipids, autoantibodies,
    160–1
Photocoagulation, 94
Photosensitivity, 140, 312, 313
Physiotherapy, 301
Pick's disease, 233
Pigmentation disorders, 312
Pinealoma, 99
'Pink puffer', 275
Pituitary disorders, 82, 85, 86–8, 89
Pituitary tumours, 82, 91
Plasma exchange, 162, 236
Plasma proteins
  abnormalities, 158
  drug binding, 243
Plasmapheresis, 162
Plasmodium spp., 177, 184
Platelet function tests, 139–40
Plethysmography, impedance, 71
Pleural disease, 279
Pleuritic pain, 275
Pneumococcal infections, 185, 187
Pneumocystis carinii, 168, 182 184
Pneumonia, 280, 294–5, 285
  epidemic, (TWAR), 190
  refractory, 275
Pneumonitis, 143, 278, 282, 284
Poisoning, 240, 241–2
Polya gastrectomy, 113
Polyarteritis nodosa, 155, 159
Polyarthritis, 292
Polycythemia, 132
Polycythemia vera, 137, 138
Polychondritis, 307
Polycystic kidney disease, 259,
    269, 270
Polycystic ovaries, 85
Polydipsia, 82, 261, 262
Polymyalgia rheumatica, 292,
    305–6
Polymyositis, 156, 228
Polypeptide hormones, 97, 118
Polyserositis, recurrent, 201
Pontine haemorrhage, basal, 216
Popliteal nerve palsy, lateral, 225
Porphobilinogen, urinary, 140
Porphyria(s), 140, 241
Porphyria cutanea tarda, 313
Portal-systemic shunting, 114
Portal venous hypertension, 104
Postphlebitic syndrome, 71
Postural hypotension, 68
Posture
  abnormal, 225
  good, in ankylosing spondylitis,
    301
Potassium-sparing diuretics, 264
Potassium therapy, 93
Pott's disease, 298
PPoma, 120
Praecordium, 45–6
Prednisone, 302
Pregnancy, 96

anticoagulants in, 54
breast cancer in, 33
cardiac conditions exacerbated
    in, 70
drugs in, 245–6
epilepsy in, 231
Graves' disease in, 93
liver disease in, 121, 122
Preload reducers, 58
  predominant, 57
Premalignant diseases/syndromes,
    31, 35
Presenile dementia, 250
Probenecid, 263
Probucol, 67
Procainamide, 241
Procarbazine, 27
Proctitis, 184, 190
Proctocolitis, 190
Prohormones, 97
Prolactinomas, 82
Prolymphocytic leukaemia, 138
Promyelocytic leukaemia, acute,
    137
Propylthiouracil, 92
Prostacyclin, 245
Prostaglandins, 245
Prostate-specific antigen, 22–3
Prostatic carcinoma, 34
Prosthetic joints, 186
Prosthetic valves, 54, 186, 202
Proteinosis, alveolar, 286
Proteinuria, 258–9, 261, 302
Protozoan parasitic infections, 188
    *see also specific
      infections/organisms*
Pruritus, 302, 311
Pruritus ani, 190
Pseudocholinesterase deficiency,
    240
Pseudo-Cushing's syndrome, 90
Pseudogout, 300
Pseudohermaphroditism, 86
  female, 86
  male (testicular feminization
    syndrome), 86, 98
Pseudohyperaldosteronism, 90
Pseudohyponatraemia, 203
Pseudohypoparathyroidism, 98,
    200, 261
Pseudomonal endocarditis, 62
Pseudomonas spp., 186, 284
  aeruginosa, 185, 284
Pseudopapilloedema, 218
Pseudo-parkinsonism, 251
Pseudoxanthoma elasticum, 197
Psittacosis, 190, 285
Psoriatic arthritis, 293, 296
Psychiatric disorders, 247–53, 268
  clinical aspects, 248–50
  investigation, 252
  literature review, 253–4, 318
  management, 250–2
  physical examination, 247
  understanding, 250, 268
Psychosis, 248
Ptosis, 213, 220